A. Moritz

Oral Laser Application

A. Moritz

Oral Laser Application

F. Beer, K. Goharkhay, U. Schoop, M. Strassl,
P. Verheyen, L. J. Walsh, J. Wernisch, E. Wintner

with contribution from

R. Blum, C. Maiorana, A. Peschek, G. Romanos, F. Schwarz

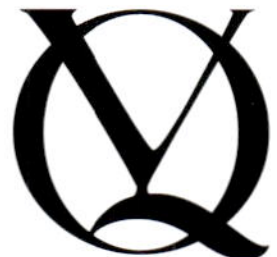

Quintessenz Verlags-GmbH
Berlin, Chicago, Tokio, Barcelona, Istanbul, London, Mailand, Moskau,
Mumbai, Paris, Peking, Prag, São Paulo, Seoul und Warschau

Brithish Library Cataloguing in Publication Data
Moritz, A.
Oral laser application
1. Lasers in Dentistry
I. Title II. Beer, F.
617.6'05
ISBN–10: 1850971501

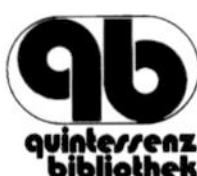

editing: Compuscript, Ireland
image handling: Quintessenz Verlags-GmbH, Berlin
production: Ina Steinbrück, Quintessenz Verlags-GmbH, Berlin
print: freiburger graphische betriebe, freiburg

ISBN: 1-85097-150-1
Printed in Germany

Foreword

For many years now – actually already decades – research in laser supported therapies in dental, oral and craniomandibular sciences is progressing steadily. In the beginning it was only in some branches of this scientific field where significant therapeutic advantages compared to conventional forms of treatment could be reached, but by now this development already includes all branches of dentistry and integrates them into the spectrum of laser supported dental treatment. A great variety of different wavelengths always presents new possibilities of use with constantly new – partly almost unbelievable – accomplishments.

The experiences that could be collected during many years in the Research Center for Clinical Laser Technology in the Department of Conservative Dentistry at the Vienna University Clinic of Dental, Oral and Craniomandibular Sciences have been summarized in this book. In the beginning there were many sceptics, but today no one can deny the results of meticulous studies, that clearly and conclusively document the achievements reached by supportive laser therapy. Everyone who wants to conduct conscientious dentistry in the future inevitably has to integrate the advantages of laser substitution into his or her therapeutic strategy.

This book contains not only a comprehensive introduction to the basics of laser technology, but covers also the specific and accurate use of lasers in all branches of dentistry. Clear guidelines also point out the limits of the possibilities of application, which is of particular importance considering that incorrect, uncritical adjustment of the equipment can lead to serious tissue damage and compromise the success of the therapies.

We should always bear in mind that it has to be the duty of every responsible physician, for the good of the patients entrusted to his or her care, to make use of all the possibilities provided by modern medical science and apply them in accordance with the oath of the University of Vienna
...doctrinam, qua nunc polletis, cum industria vestra culturos tum omnibus incrementis, quae progrediente tempore haec ars ceperit, aucturos, usum et facultatem vestram ad salutem et prosperitatem hominum studiose conversuros,...

This book is an important milestone on the way to a successful future of dental, oral and craniomandibular science, which is no longer thinkable without laser therapy.

Prof. Wolfgang Sperr MD, DMD
Honorary President ESOLA

Preface

There is almost no field of dentistry where development took place at such a tearing pace in recent years as in the field of laser dentistry. Therapy concepts, that seemed merely fiction some years ago, are long since reality and form a valuable part in the spectrum of possible therapies. By now it is comparatively easily accomplished to conserve teeth by means of laser-supported endodonty, which would have been a safe bet for extraction until recently. Today lasers allow for a low-pain preparation, they help us to solve partly severe aesthetic problems by means of laser-supported dental bleaching and dramatically improve the chances for success in periodontal treatment.

In the field of oral surgery the use of lasers has become an established method a long time ago, which enables the surgeon to work safely and efficiently. These are only a few examples of the enormous spectrum of applications for lasers in dentistry, but this fact already conveys one problem:

The great amount of therapy concepts and wavelengths that is available today makes it difficult even for experienced users to keep track of all the applications that seem possible and useful. On this account it seems appropriate to collect the knowledge of numerous authors gathered in many years of laser dentistry in this atlas. This book is addressed to beginners and students in the field of laser dentistry, who are provided with a valuable guide book to the integration of lasers in their practice concept, as well as to experienced physicians, who can use this book to keep their knowledge up to date.

Apart from being a guide to clinical practice, this book offers a detailed examination of the literature in the field of laser dentistry published up to the present and motivates the reader to delve into the latest scientific findings. You can also find a detailed description of the physical basics of laser application, the understanding of which is very important for an efficient use of the different wavelengths.

I would like to thank all the people who contributed to this book for their patience and dedication, they all have played a vital role in the realisation of this piece of work. At this point I would like to commend Mr Boris Spieler, whose sophisticated illustrations substantially added value to this book. I would also like to express my sincere thanks to Professor Sperr, who made it possible for me from the start to engage scientifically and clinically in the subject of laser dentistry. I hope that this book meets with great interest from all readers and I wish you all an exciting reading time with this piece of (Laser-)literature.

Prof. Andreas Moritz MD, DMD
President der ESOLA

Authors

DDr. Beer, Franziska
Secretary General ESOLA
Medizinische Universität Wien
Bernhard-Gottlieb-Universitäts-kliniken
Währingerstraße 25a
1090 Vienna, Austria

Dr. Blum, Romain
Coordinator for Practitioners ESOLA
25, Rue Rabatt
6475 Echternach, Luxemburg

Ass. Prof. DDr. Goharkhay, Kawe
Medizinische Universität Wien
Bernhard-Gottlieb-Universitäts-kliniken
Währingerstraße 25a
1090 Vienna, Austria

Prof. Dr. Maiorana, Carlo
Vice-President ESOLA
University of Milan
Dept. Oral Surgery
Via della Commenda 10,
20122 Milan, Italy

Prof. DDr. Moritz, Andreas
President ESOLA
Medizinische Universität Wien
Bernhard-Gottlieb-Universitäts-kliniken
Währingerstraße 25a
1090 Vienna, Austria

Dr. Peschek, Antonia
Medizinische Universität Wien
Bernhard-Gottlieb-Universitäts-kliniken
Währingerstraße 25a
1090 Vienna, Austria

Prof. Dr. Romanos, Georg
Clinical Professor of Implant Dentistry
New York University
120 West 15th Street, App. 4K
10011 New York, NY
United States of America

Ass. Prof. DDr. Schoop, Ulrich
Medizinische Universität Wien
Bernhard-Gottlieb-Universitätskliniken
Währingerstraße 25a
1090 Vienna, Austria

Priv. Doz. Dr. Schwarz, Frank
Heinrich-Heine-Universität
Poliklinik für Zahnärztliche Chirurgie und Aufnahme
Moorenstr. 5
40225 Düsseldorf, Germany

DI Strassl, Martin
Technische Universität Wien
Institut für Photonik
Gusshausstraße 27
1040 Vienna, Austria

Prof. Dr. Walsh, Laurence J.
University of Queensland
School of Dentistry
200 Turbot Street
4000 Brisbane, Australia

Prof. Dr. Wernisch, Johann
Technische Universität Wien
Institut für Festkörperphysik
Wiedner Hauptstraße 8-10
1040 Vienna, Austria

Prof. Dr. Wintner, Ernst
Technische Universität Wien
Institut für Photonik
Gusshausstraße 27
1040 Vienna, Austria

DDS Verheyen, Peter
Treasurer ESOLA
Breekiezel 36
3670 Gruitrode, Belgium

Contents

chapter 1 Basic Information on Lasers

1.1 Introduction **1**

1.2 The Nature, Properties and Sources of Light **3**
1.2.1 What is light? 3
1.2.2 Properties of Light 4
1.2.3 Sources of Light 8

1.3 Optical Concepts for the Function of a Laser **11**
1.3.1 Stimulated Emission and Amplification in a Laser Medium 11
1.3.2 Basic Scheme of a Laser 13
1.3.3 Level Schemes of Real Lasers 15
1.3.4 The Laser Resonator and its Output Radiation 18
1.3.5 Specific Frequency and Temporal Operation Regimes of Lasers 23

1.4 Laser Media, Power Input and Optical Output **29**
1.4.1 Laser Media 29
1.4.2 Pumping Methods and Schemes 33
1.4.3 Geometrical and Frequency Conversion of the Laser Output 34

1.5 Specific Lasers Relevant for Oral Applications **38**
1.5.1 Excimer Lasers 38
1.5.2 Argon ion Laser 39
1.5.3 Helium-Neon Laser 40
1.5.4 Semiconductor Diode Lasers 41

1.5.5 Ruby and Alexandrite Lasers 45
1.5.6 Titanium-Sapphire Laser 47
1.5.7 Neodymium and Ytterbium Lasers 49
1.5.8 Holmium and Holmium-Thulium Lasers 51
1.5.9 Erbium and Erbium-Chromium Lasers 52
1.5.10 Carbon Dioxide Laser 53

1.6 Textbooks and References 55
1.6.1 Textbooks 55
1.6.2 References 55

chapter 2 Laser Safety

2.1 Introduction 57

2.2 Maximum Permissible Exposure 59

2.3 Laser Classes 60
2.3.1 Class 1 60
2.3.2 Class 2 60
2.3.3 Remarks on Laser Classes 1M and 2M 61
2.3.4 Class 3A (old Class) 61
2.3.5 Class 3B 61
2.3.6 Special Class 3B (old classification) 61
2.3.7 New Class 3R 62
2.3.8 Class 4 63

2.4 Secondary Hazards 64
2.4.1 Common Hazards 64
2.4.2 Vapours and Dusts 66

2.5 Protective Measures 67
2.5.1 Laser Protective Eyewear 67
2.5.2 Organizational Protective Arrangements 69
2.5.3 Technical Protective Arrangements 69

2.6 Standards and Legal Rules 71
2.6.1 Laser Safety Officer 71
2.6.2 Legal Scope 72
2.6.3 Behavior in the Case of Incidents and Accidents 72

chapter 3 Cavity Preparation

3.1 **Overview. 75**
3.1.1 Development of the Laser – Assisted Cavity Preparation 75

3.2 **Technologies for Cavity Preparation. 77**
3.2.1 Indication-specific Problems 77
3.2.2 Conventional Methods – Rotating Instruments 78
3.2.3 Kinetic Cavity Preparation – KCP 80
3.2.4 Preparation Lasers 80

3.3 **Laser-supported Cavity Preparation. 86**
3.3.1 Er:YAG and Er,Cr:YSGG Lasers 86
3.3.2 Surface Characteristics of Laser-prepared Cavities 90
3.3.3 Adhesion and Margin Tightness of Laser-prepared and Adhesive Techniques-treated Cavities 93
3.3.4 Caries-preventing Properties of Laser-prepared Cavities. 99

3.4 **Mechanisms of Ablation 100**
3.4.1 Overview. 100
3.4.2 Physical Factors Influencing on Ablation Efficiency and Quality 101
3.4.3 Physical Limitations for Present-day Laser Systems 111
3.4.4 Conclusion for the Specifications of Laser Systems Optimized for Minimal Collateral Effects on Dental Hard Tissues. 112
3.4.5 Future Perspectives 113

3.5 **Other Laser Types. 122**
3.5.1 The CO_2 Laser 122
3.5.2 The Nd:YAG Laser. 122
3.5.3 The Ho:YAG Laser. 123

3.6 **Practical Procedure in Laser-assisted Cavity Preparation – Clinical Work 124**
3.6.1 Application of the Rubber Dam 124
3.6.2 Display of the Cavity 124
3.6.3 Caries Removal. 125
3.6.4 Completion of the Cavity 125
3.6.5 Choice of Parameters 126

3.7 **Clinical Cases. 127**
3.7.1 Cavity Preparation Class I, II and III 127
3.7.2 Fissure Sealing 127
3.7.3 Veneer 128
3.7.4 Gold Inlay 129
3.7.5 Ceramic Inlay 130
3.7.6 Maryland Bridge. 132

3.7.7 Esthetic Front Restoration 134
3.7.8 Esthetic Reconstructions. 134

3.8 References 136

chapter 4 Photopolymerization

4.1 Introduction 139

4.2 In General 141

4.3 Photopolymerization Reaction 150

4.4 Laser Photopolymerization versus Traditional Methods 153

4.5 Improved Clinical Performance of Laser Cured Materials 161

4.6 Caries Prevention by Laser and with Laser Activated Fluoride 162
4.6.1 Laser Preventive and Laser-Fluoride Effects on Enamel with the Argon Laser 162
4.6.2 Mechanisms of Action: Enamel 164
4.6.3 Mechanisms of Action: Root Surfaces 166

4.7 General Considerations 167

4.8 Clinical Procedue of Photopolymerization by an Argon Laser 169

4.9. Clinical Cases. 172
4.9.1 Introduction. 172
4.9.2 Esthetic Dentistry 173
4.9.3 High Caries Sensitivity 178
4.9.4 Functional Problems 181
4.9.5 Orthodontic Problems 182
4.9.6 Periodontal Problems 183
4.9.7 Pediatric Dentistry 184
4.9.8 Geriatric Dentistry 185
4.9.9 Prosthetic Dentistry 187

4.10 References 189

chapter 5 Caries Prevention

5.1 Introduction 193

5.2 Conventional Treatment Methods 195

5.3 Laser Application in Preventive Dentistry 196
5.3.1 Historical Aspects 196
5.3.2 Light Interactions with Dental Hard Tissues 196
5.3.3 Scattering and Absorption Parameters 197
5.3.4 Mechanism of Laser Irradiation and Improved Caries Resistance 200

5.4 The Caries Preventing Effect of CO_2 Lasers 204
5.4.1 The Influence of Wavelength and Pulse Duration 205
5.4.2 The Influence of the Pulse Number 207
5.4.3 The Influence of Wavelength and Fluence 208
5.4.4 Oral Safety Parameters 210
5.4.5 Surface Morphology 211
5.4.6 The Problem of Cracking 212
5.4.7 Polished Enamel 213
5.4.8 Unpolished Tooth Crowns 214
5.4.9 Pulse-Width Effects on Unpolished Human Enamel 214
5.4.10 Combined Effect of CO_2 Laser Irradiation and Fluoride Treatment 216
5.4.11 Clinical Aspects 217

5.5 The Caries Preventing Effect of Argon Lasers 219
5.5.1 Oral Safety Parameters 219
5.5.2 Surface Morphology 221
5.5.3 Combined Effect of Argon Laser Irridiation and Fluoride Treatment 222
5.5.4 Clinical Aspects 224

5.6 The Caries Preventing Effect of Nd:YAG Lasers 225
5.6.1 Oral Safety Parameters 227
5.6.2 Surface Morphology 228
5.6.3 Combined Effect of Nd:YAG Laser and Fluoride Treatment 229
5.6.4 Clinical Aspects 231

5.7 The Caries Preventing Effect of Er:YAG, Er,Cr:YSGG, Ho:YAG and UV Lasers 232

5.8 Conclusion 234

5.9 References 235

chapter 6 Lasers in Endodontics

6.1 Introduction **241**
6.1.1 The Importance of Endodontics in Dentistry 241
6.1.2 Identifying Endodontic Problems 241

6.2 Conventional Working Methods **253**
6.2.1 Chemo-mechanical Disinfections 253
6.2.2 Laser-supported Root Canal Sterilization 254

6.3 Description of the Different Wavelengths **268**
6.3.1 The Nd:YAG Laser 268
6.3.2 The Diode Laser 274
6.3.3 The Er:YAG and Er,Cr:YSGG Lasers 275

6.4 Root Canal Shaping **278**

6.5 Apex Sealing **281**

6.6 Safety in Laser Treatment **284**

6.7 Indications **288**

6.8 Practical Procedure **290**
6.8.1 Preparation of the Entrance Cavity 290
6.8.2 Root Canal Preparation 290
6.8.3 Laser Treatment 296
6.8.4 Root Canal Filling 298

6.9 Clinical Cases **300**

6.10 Future Perspectives **306**

6.11 References **309**

chapter 7 Pulp Capping and Pulpotomy in Permanent and Primary Teeth

7.1 Direct Pulp Capping . . . 315
7.1.1 Introduction . . . 315
7.1.2 Conventional Pulp Capping . . . 316
7.1.3 Laser-Assisted Pulp Capping . . . 318
7.1.4 Laser Doppler Flowmetry . . . 312

7.2 Pulpotomy . . . 323
7.2.1 Introduction . . . 323
7.2.2 Success Rates . . . 323
7.2.3 Procedure . . . 324

7.3 References . . . 329

chapter 8 Laser-Assisted Periodontal Therapy

8.1 Introduction . . . 333
8.1.1 General . . . 333
8.1.2 Specific Problems of the Indication . . . 333

8.2 Laser Versus Conventional Therapy . . . 343
8.2.1 Conventional Therapy . . . 343
8.2.2 Laser . . . 344
8.2.3 Impact of the Different Lasers on Tissues . . . 346
8.2.4 Pro and Contra the Respective Lasers – Literature Discussion . . . 347

8.3 Practical Procedure . . . 365
8.3.1 Anamnesis . . . 365
8.3.2 Clinical Preparation . . . 367
8.3.3 Modus Operandi . . . 367

8.4 Case Reports . . . 371
8.4.1 Clinical Case Report . . . 371

8.5 References . . . 374

chapter 9 Dentin Hypersensitivity

9.1 Introduction 377
9.1.1 Theories of Dentin Sensitivity 378
9.1.2 Natural Pulpal Defense Mechanisms 380

9.2 Conventional Treatment Methods 382
9.2.1 Therapy Requirements 382
9.2.2 Historic Treatment Methods 382
9.2.3 Common Agents 382

9.3 Laser Application for Dentin Hypersensitivity Treatment 386
9.3.1 Low Output Power (Low-level) Lasers 386
9.3.2 Middle Output Power Lasers 387
9.3.3 Direct Method 390
9.3.2 Indirect Method 390

9.4 Clinical Procedure in Treatment of Hypersensitive Dentin 397

9.5 Case 398

9.6 References 399

chapter 10 Laser-Assisted Bleaching

10.1 Introduction 407

10.2 In General 408
10.2.1 Causes of Tooth Discoloration 408
10.2.2 Extrinsic Discolorations 408
10.2.3 Intrinsic Discolorations 409
10.2.4 Treatment Options 413

10.3 Bleaching 416
10.3.1 Chemistry of Hydrogen Peroxide 416
10.3.2 Bleaching Mechanism of Teeth 417
10.3.3 Safety of Bleaching 418

10.4 Laser versus Conventional Means 420

10.5 Clinical Procedure 429
10.5.1 Diagnosis and Treatment Planning 429
10.5.2 Clinical Procedure 429

10.6 **Clinical Cases** **433**
10.6.1 Introduction 433
10.6.2 Yellow Discolorations 435
10.6.3 Lightening of a Single Tooth and Internal Bleaching of a Single Dead Tooth 437
10.6.4 Brown Discolorations 439
10.6.5 Grey Discolorations and Tetracycline Staining 440
10.6.6 Trouble Shooting 443

10.7 **References** **446**

chapter 11 Laser-Atlas Surgery

11.1 **Introduction** **449**

11.2 **Specific Problems in the Context of Surgical Indications** **450**

11.3 **Conventional Therapy** **452**

11.4 **Laser Therapy** **454**

11.5 **Lasers Used in Dental Surgery** **463**
11.5.1 Surgical Lasers Used at Present 463
11.5.2 Summary 466

11.6 **Indications** **467**

11.7 **Frequently Asked Questions When Using a Laser** **468**

11.8 **Practical Proceedings** **470**

11.9 **Indications and Cases** **472**
11.9.1 Benign Tumors 472
11.9.2 Leukoplakias and Precancerous Lesions 484
11.9.3 Oral Lichen Planus 488
11.9.4 Mucocele/Ranula 488
11.9.5 Preprosthetic Surgery 491
11.9.6 Frenotomy 492
11.9.7 Implantology/Peri-implantitis 493
11.9.8 Periodontal Surgery 494

11.10 **References** **496**

chapter 12 Photoactivated Disinfection (PAD)

12.1 Introduction 503

12.2 Photodynamic Therapy – the Origins of PAD 505

12.3 Principles of PAD 506

12.4 Photosensitizers 507

12.5 Clinical Aspects of the PAD Technique 509

12.6 Laser Used in PAD 510

12.7 Laboratory and Clinical Studies of PAD 511

12.8 Safety Issues with PAD 514

12.9 Summary and Conclusions. 515

12.10 References 516

chapter 13 Low Level Laser Therapy (LLLT)

13.1 Introduction 521

13.2 Mechanism of Action. 523

13.3 Cellular Effects of LLLT During Wound Healing 525

13.4 LLLT and Neural Tissues. 528

13.5 Clinical Applications of LLLT 530

13.6 Frontiers of Clinical Practice for LLLT 533

13.7 LLLT Technology 534

13.8 LLLT Equipment 535

13.9 Conclusions 537

13.10 References 538

Index 541

1

Basic Information on Lasers

E. Wintner and M. Straßl

1.1 Introduction

The laser[*1] was demonstrated for the first time in 1960 by Maiman[1] after the pioneering theoretical work of Basov, Prokhorov and Townes[2]. The name laser, representing an elegant acronym formed out of the initials of "light amplification by stimulated emission of radiation", was not used in the early days, rather the more conservative expression "visible maser"[*2] which was developed on the basis of the same idea more than 10 years earlier. This fact represents the doubts that existed at the time as to whether laser function in the visible light regime might be possible at all; a similar scientific question has arisen in recent years with respect to the feasibility of an X-ray laser. In both cases the fundamental problem was the likelihood of stimulated emission[*3] in the respective wavelength regime which is essential for laser function and was described for the first time by Einstein in 1917[3]. Now, the realization of some version of the X-ray laser really does seem possible, potentially contributing a great deal to medical applications of lasers which are already extremely numerous and indispensable, with oral laser applications being an interesting branch of them.

Typical lasers, which emit in the visible and the adjacent areas of the UV and IR wavelengths (from 158 nm down[*4] to the 10 µm of the CO_2 laser), comprise a large number of individual laser materials (e.g., excimer lasers, ion lasers, semiconductor diode lasers, rare-earth[*5] or transition metal[*6] ion-doped solid-state lasers and, providing the longest wavelength in this list, the above-mentioned CO_2 laser, all of which are applied in oral medicine) and laser oscillator setups working in the continuous wave (cw) or

*1 I.e. the ruby laser, a typical metal ion (Cr^{3+})-doped and flashlamp pumped solid-state laser (see later sections for such details).
*2 Similar acronym, where the letter m stands for microwave.
*3 Stimulated emission can happen only if incoming radiation causes the emission of radiation with the same properties such as wavelength, direction, polarization and phase. This is the opposite of spontaneous emission as explained later!
*4 In fact, ultraviolet and infrared refer to the frequency of light, whereas otherwise thinking in terms of wavelength is predominant.
*5 E.g. Nd^{3+}, Yb^{3+}, Ho^{3+}, Er^{3+} being relevant in this context.
*6 E.g. Ti^{3+}, Cr^{3+} being relevant in this context.

pulsed regime. Pulses of laser emission might last characteristically for microseconds, nanoseconds, picoseconds or even femtoseconds[*7], each of the temporal regimes standing for a typical laser operation mode. All of these mentioned pulse durations are typically generated by a rather limited number of specific types of lasers and they play a useful role even in the narrow field of oral laser applications.

The development and application of lasers emitting rather collimated[*8] and more or less intensive beams of generally narrow bandwidth coherent light[*9], in association with increasingly sophisticated optical and electro-optical components, has been recognized as a new field of optical science called photonics, comprising aspects of quantum optics, electro-optics, and linear and nonlinear optics[*10]. The combination of photonic approaches with medical applications nowadays is a very prospective and innovative field showing aspects of maturity on the one hand, but being the object of continuous innovation with respect to new lasers employed, or new treatment technologies applied, on the other hand.

This chapter on "Basic information on lasers" is organized in such a way that even a reader inexperienced in laser physics can follow the explanations and descriptions. In particular, the drawings, specifically prepared for this publication, and with a consistent use of colour, are an innovative means of presentation. A few introductory concepts on light as an electromagnetic wave are offered, followed by laser concepts, an overview of laser media and pumping schemes as well as the options for changes of output beam characteristics. A selected number of specific lasers relevant in dental medical applications are described in such detail that at least their basic functioning is understandable.

Expressions and aspects, usually unfamiliar to the expected readers, are explained or, in order not to interrupt the flow of information in the main text, illustrated by footnotes. Special physical details are elucidated in separated blocks of text called "Detail 1-X" which are printed in a smaller font. These are to provide detailed information on fundamentals in a more mathematical form, or specific data on the lasers chosen to be covered in this book on dental laser applications.

*7 The latter two together are called "ultra-short" light pulses, being 10^{-12} or 10^{-15} s long, respectively.

*8 Beam with low divergence, i.e., angular width.

*9 Property of a wave having systematic phase relations between different sections along or orthogonal to its propagation axis.

*10 If optical properties of matter characteristically represented by the index of refraction n and the absorption coefficient α depend only on the wavelength λ, optics are considered linear; if properties are intensity-dependent in addition, we talk about nonlinear optics.

1.2 The Nature, Properties and Sources of Light

1.2.1 What is Light?

According to modern physics, light has a dual nature, with properties of waves or particles[*11]. It depends on the wavelength (or equivalently, the frequency) and on certain circumstances to determine which character will dominate. Nowadays, the concept of light reaches far beyond the visible spectrum (VIS), which extends from ~ 400 to 800 nm. Ultraviolet light (UV) extends to shorter wavelengths and down to X-rays (starting, according to general agreement, at around 50 nm, as so-called soft X-rays): this wide range of invisible radiation of higher energy may be divided into near, middle and far ultraviolet (UV-A, -B, -C, respectively), vacuum ultraviolet[*12] (VUV, from about 200 nm downwards) and extreme ultraviolet (EUV) beyond ~ 100 nm. On the other side of VIS, there is infrared light[*13] (IR), distinguished as near infrared (NIR, up to 3.0 µm), middle infrared (MIR, up to ~ 50 µm) and far infrared (FIR, up to some tenths of mm wavelength), also called THz radiation[*14]. This double naming is, i.e. wavelength or particles, typical for the transition stage between to different concepts of generation as well as measurement: the wave being generated by transitions between energetic atomic or molecular levels and measured according to optical principals such as by spectrometer, the particle being yielded by electric devices and counted by electronic measurement tools.

If we assign a wavelength to radiation, we implicitly anticipate the wave nature: light is an electromagnetic wave of transversal type as depicted in Fig. 1-1. According to Maxwell's equations[*15], a temporal change of the electric field $\vec{E}$ induces a curl of the magnetic field $\vec{B}$ and vice versa. The three directions involved, i.e., the vectors $\vec{E}$ and $\vec{B}$ and the direction of propagation (usually labeled z), are mutually orthogonal. By convention, $\vec{E}$ is defined as the polarization direction of a light wave. Usually, transversal waves, like sound waves in some solid material, need a medium for propagation. After many years of uncertainty in this respect, the famous 1881 experiment by Michelson[*16] proved decisively that

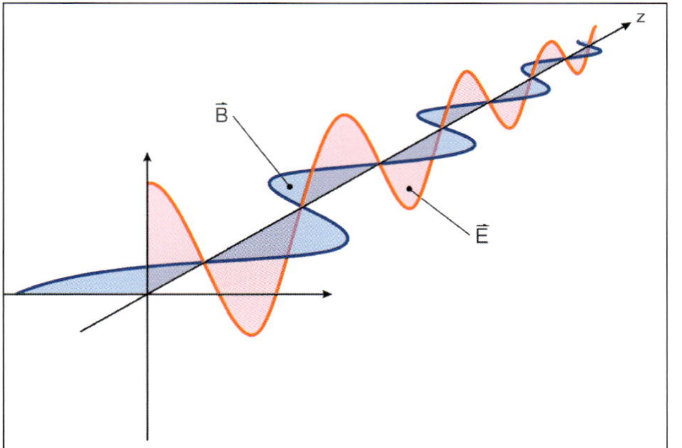

Fig 1-1 Electromagnetic wave in free space: transversal nature expressed by the polarization parallel to the electric field $\vec{E}$; the magnetic field $\vec{B}$ is orthogonal to it as well as to the direction of propagation.

*11 Both concepts, however, are rather old: Descartes († 1650) founded the "emission or corpuscular theory", later supported by Newton († 1727). Huygens († 1695) was the first to propound the "wave or undulation theory", which was strongly backed by the experiments of Young († 1829) and Fresnel († 1827).

*12 Vacuum ultraviolet is absorbed in air and hence cannot propagate in a normal environment without substantial attenuation.

*13 First described in 1800 by Herschel as part of the spectrum of the sun.

*14 I.e. radiation of a few THz (10^{12} Hz) compared to VIS in the range of about 500 THz.

*15 By J.C. Maxwell in 1862, published as "Treatise on Electricity and Magnetism (1873)".

*16 Michelson thereby ended speculation about the existence of a so-called "ether", a fictive propagation medium for light giving rise to the crusial question as to which inertial system the ether would reside in.

light needs no medium, but that free that space allows it to propagate at the well-known speed of light $c = 3 \times 10^8$ ms^{-1}. It should be mentioned also that light only in a vacuum strictly observes the conditions of transversality. In some anisotropic media, as well as in waveguides or resonators, this may be different; hence we stress names like *TEM* (transverse electromagnetic) modes (see Fig. 1-8).

If we talk about light in a more general manner, we nevertheless anticipate the applicability of optical concepts such as diffraction, reflection, and refraction, which are the physical principles underlying diffraction gratings, reflective coatings for mirrors, and refraction in lenses, respectively. In this context, refraction is the limiting factor, as it requires media that are reasonably transparent to allow a refractive beam to be formed and to propagate over reasonable distances. Based on transparency of optical materials in this wider sense, a more general range of optics can be defined between ~ 200 nm and ~ 22 μm[*17]. Within this range it is possible to design optical instruments based on more or less conventional glassy or crystalline materials[*18], even incorporating reflective and anti-reflective coatings. A much simpler version of optics (in terms of the phenomena to be used) is employed in the case of EUV and FIR, which are based only on reflection and diffraction.

Since radio waves came into use, their exploitation has steadily extended from kilometre to metre and finally millimetre waves[*19]; in this their wave-like nature always was predominant and evident despite the fact that measurement emphasized the high frequency character. On the other hand, on the shortest wavelength end of the electromagnetic spectrum, for X-rays and γ-rays[*20], indications of (photon) energy always supported the underlying particulate character[*21]. The visible optical electromagnetic radiation, i.e., light as we usually call it, lies right in the middle of the applicability the two concepts. Depending on the situation, the wave or the particle nature may predominate, and physics, i.e., in this case optics, takes the liberty of employing the respective model.

If we, for instance, discuss the absorption of light, the concept of the photo effect[4] is really useful and seemed to be a strict law until "two-photon absorption"[*22] was discovered[5], starting the field of nonlinear optics. This turned out to be a rather wide and comprehensive new discipline in optics nearly exclusively based on the laser.

1.2.2 Properties of Light

Corresponding to its wave nature, light can be described either by a wavelength λ, a frequency f or ν, or a wavenumber $\bar{\nu}$ (see Detail 1-1). If the particle aspect is in the foreground, the photon energy E_{ph} may be specified. It is evident that one of these quantities is sufficient to cover the wavelength-related aspect. As for a transversal wave, the polarization $\vec{E}$ has to be indicated. The phase φ is also important if the wave is to be accurately characterized[*23].

So far, we have assumed monochromatic light, which represents a rather idealistic situation. All

*17 According to the lower and upper wavelength absorption edges of materials as different as BaF_2 or ZnSe, respectively.

*18 As an example, silicon may represent an excellent material for lenses for wavelengths above 1.1 μm (i.e., below the absorption edge of this semiconductor) although it is generally known as a black and opaque crystal far from useful in conventional optics.

*19 Corresponding to "Long or Short Wave" (> hundreds of kHz), "Ultra-Short Wave or FM" (~ 90-110 MHz; as written on radio sets), and finally frequencies of satellite receivers or mobile phones in the > GHz regime, respectively.

*20 Typically ~ 25 eV – 25 keV and > 25 keV, respectively; 1 eV = 1.602×10^{-19} J.

*21 Planck founded quantum theory in 1900, Einstein discovered the photo effect in 1905 assuming light quanta.

*22 Simultaneous absorption of two photons, obviously contradicting Einstein's Nobel prize-honoured discovery of 1905.

*23 It is important to note that only now, after the successful advent of ultra-short laser pulses, access to the determination of the absolute phase of light is possible.

the above-mentioned quantifiers are subject to a certain width of variation, termed bandwidth of wavelength $\Delta\lambda$, or of frequency Δf or $\Delta\nu$, or also of wave number $\Delta\bar{\nu}$. All these quantities are interrelated, although in a somewhat more complicated way than the corresponding absolute ones mentioned above (also explained in Detail 1-1). Polarization can also vary: unpolarized light, however, has to be distinguished from random polarization[*24].

A new aspect is to be considered if the phase is not varying systematically with time at a certain location or between different positions within the laser beam: temporal or spatial coherence. Only if the sources (see Section 1.2.3) generate light in a consistent way and emit it in phase-correlated oscillations can coherent light be produced. The average time between breaks of phase correlation is called coherence time t_c, the distance light can travel within that time coherence length ℓ_c. An ideal light wave has infinite dimension and infinite duration. At every position within it, and at any time, there is an amplitude and a consistent phase relation according to the laws of wave propagation expressed by the general wave equation (see Detail 1-1). One special solution to it is a planar wave where all the phase fronts (locations of the same phase) are planes and the amplitude stays constant at all times. In this case, the wave has also one absolutely precise direction expressed by the wave vector $\vec{k}$. Another special solution to the wave equation, met frequently in nature, is spherical waves. In this case, the wave spreads from one origin to all directions; hence, its amplitude decreases with the square of the distance of propagation. In these cases, the waves can be monochromatic having one precise value of ν or ω[*25].

Real light waves are circumscribed and hence subject to diffraction, i.e., the distribution of amplitude over the cross section varies during propagation. In simple terms, the wave becomes, according to the diffraction laws, broader after having been forced to pass through an aperture[*26]. There is only one type of lateral distribution of light that never changes its mathematical characteristics throughout the temporal course of propagation: the Gaussian beam (see Fig. 1-7) which has a bell-shaped[*27] distribution of amplitude as well as intensity over its cross section. In the case of a confined light distribution, called a beam, the direction of propagation is not sharply defined but is distributed over a certain range $\Delta\vec{k}$ of $\vec{k}$-vectors. For a realistic light wave, the frequency is not infinitely exact but lies within a certain bandwidth expressed by $\Delta\lambda$, Δf or $\Delta\nu$, or $\Delta\bar{\nu}$. The light beam may also have started or may end at a certain time; this fact is closely related to the imprecision of the frequency[*28].

It is important to know that for all wave phenomena the so-called Fourier limitations hold: a wave cannot be simultaneously infinitely "precise" in cross section (Δx) and direction ($\Delta\vec{k}$), nor simultaneously in time (Δt) and frequency ($\Delta\nu$):

$$\Delta x \times \Delta\vec{k} \geq C_1$$
$$\Delta t \times \Delta\nu \geq C_2$$

where both C_1 and C_2 are constants for a certain pulse depending on its shape in space and time, respectively. This is the same wave-related back-

*24 The former may stand for a wide range of polarizations being present simultaneously in most kinds of conventional light, the latter for a random walk of the polarization vector with time – the usual property of most types of lasers.

*25 It should be emphasized that the frequency remains the same as in a vacuum if the wave enters into a medium, but the wavelength is shortened according to the index n.

*26 The most simple situation is caused by a slit: the light intensity distribution behind is proportional to $(\sin x/x)^2$. It can be most easily remembered as the narrower the slit the wider the diffraction angle behind.

*27 The square of a Gaussian function is also such a function, however having different curvature.

*28 A very useful tool to analyze temporarily varying waves is Fourier analysis: a periodic wave can be expressed by a Fourier series of up to infinite elements of harmonic frequencies. A single temporal wave packet is usually analyzed by Fourier integrals giving a clear interrelation between time- and frequency-related aspects. Details lie beyond the scope of this book.

Detail 1-1.

Formal characterizations of light properties and their interrelations.

Wave-related properties

$\lambda . \nu = c$	λ wavelength in vacuum ν or f frequency, $\nu \equiv f$, c speed of light in vacuum (phase velocity)
$\lambda_n \nu = c/n$	λ_n wavelength in a medium with refractive index n
$n = c/c_n$	c_n speed of light in a medium with index n
$\omega = 2\pi\nu$	ω angular frequency
$\bar{\nu} \equiv 1/\lambda$	$\bar{\nu}$ wave number
$\vec{k} = (2\pi/\lambda)\ (\vec{k}/\lvert k \rvert)$	$\vec{k}$ wave vector (direction of propagation) $(\vec{k}/\lvert k \rvert)$ unit vector in direction of propagation
$I = \sqrt{\varepsilon\varepsilon_0/\mu\mu_0}E^2$	I light intensity or power density or irradiance $[W/At]$ W energy A area t time E magnitude of vector $\vec{E}$
$Z = \sqrt{\mu\mu_0/\varepsilon\varepsilon_0}$	$\varepsilon_0 = 8.858 \cdot 10^{12}\ As/Vm$ permittivity of vacuum $\mu_0 = 4\pi \cdot 10^{-7}\ Vs/A$ permeability of vacuum
$n = \sqrt{\varepsilon\mu}$	ε relative permittivity, μ relative magnetic permeability $Z = 377\ \Omega$ *for* $n = 1$ *vacuum resistivity*
$\rho = I/c$	ρ energy density $[W/V]$, V volume

Quantum-related properties

$E_{ph} = h\nu = \hbar\ \omega$	E_{ph} photon energy
$\vec{p} = \hbar\ \vec{k}$	$\vec{p}$ momentum of a photon
$\hbar \equiv h/2\pi$	$h = 6.626 \cdot 10^{-34}\ Js$ Planck's quantum
$F = I/E_{ph}$	photon flux (number of photons/At)
$\Phi = \rho/E_{ph}$	photon density (number of photons/V)

Bandwidth and coherence

$\Delta\nu = -(c/\lambda^2)\cdot\Delta\lambda$	$\Delta\nu$ frequency bandwidth
$\Delta\bar{\nu} = \Delta\nu/c = -(1/\lambda^2).\Delta\lambda$	$\Delta\bar{\nu}$ width of wave numbers
$\Delta\nu/\nu = -\Delta\lambda/\lambda$	$\Delta\lambda$ width of wavelength
$\ell_c = c.t_c$	ℓ_c coherence length t_c coherence time

Wave equations, refraction and absorption

$\left(\frac{\partial^2}{\partial x^2}+\frac{\partial^2}{\partial y^2}+\frac{\partial^2}{\partial z^2}-\frac{1}{c^2}\frac{\partial^2}{\partial t^2}\right)\vec{E}\,(x, y, z, t) = 0$	generalized wave equation
$E(z,t) = E_0\cos(\omega t - kz) = (E_0/2)\exp\text{-}i(kz\text{-}\omega t) + c.c.$	magnitude of the electric field of a planar wave
$E(r,t) = \frac{E_0}{r}\cos(\omega t - kr) = \frac{E_0}{r}\exp{-i(kr\text{-}\omega t)} + c.c.$	magnitude of the electric field of a spherical wave
$r = \sqrt{x^2 + y^2 + z^2}$	radius from the origin of wave
$n_1 \sin\alpha_1 = n_2 \sin\alpha_2$	**Snell's law of refraction** (between medium 1 and 2)
$dI/dx = -\alpha I(x)$ or equivalently (atomistic view) $dI/dx = -\sigma_{12}N_1I(x)$	differential versions of **Beer's law of absorption,** the latter expressed for a two-level system (see Fig 1-4). Hence, $\alpha = \sigma_{12}N_1$ in this case. (σ_{12} absorption cross section [A], A area, N_1 occupation number of energy level 1).

ground which underlies Heisenberg's uncertainty relation expressed for space and momentum as well as time and energy[*29]. Going from an ideal unlimited wave to an ideal pulse confined in space and time, we consider a Gaussian pulse of characteristic temporal shape (see Section 1.3.5) as is commonly produced by mode-locked lasers. Such a pulse is called Fourier limited and, mathematically, can be treated exactly. Hence, it is the basis of model calculations describing the interaction of short pulses with matter, i.e., tissue in the context of this book.

*29 Observe the relations between $\vec{k}$ and $\vec{p}$ as given in Detail 1-1 which correspond to a multiplication by $\hbar$. To avoid any misunderstanding: waves of matter as considered in wave mechanics are probability waves (the amplitude having no physical meaning, but the square of it corresponds to probability).

1.2.3 Sources of Light

Light is to be encountered everywhere in our daily life but we do not spend too much time thinking about where it comes from, apart from the sun. Thinking in terms of physics, sunlight or the light from stars is emitted from a hot body. If this is a "black" body it may be described by Planck's law of radiation (see Detail 1-3) which shows an infinite bandwidth with a clear temperature-dependent maximum, e.g., lying in the green in the case of the sun. If the light is modified by matter as it travels, characteristic parts may be missing, known as an absorption spectrum[*30]. If certain hot atoms or molecules emit light, as is the case in flames, for instance, it may be called an emission spectrum showing details corresponding to the atomic nature[*31]. Thermally generated light, as mentioned before, has no specific direction, and neither precise frequency nor distinct phase. According to the previous statements it is non-coherent[*32].

In this context, it is useful to spend a short time on the inner structure of an atom as depicted in Fig. 1-2. Several electrons according to the positive charge of the nucleus (N^+) normally[*33] "circle" around it. Niels Bohr was the first to describe electronic orbits as simply being elliptic trajectories[*34]. According to quantum theory we think about electron "clouds", meaning the sum of locations around the nucleus where there is a finite probability for the electrons to reside. These are called orbitals. Their shapes and energies as well as angular momenta[*35] can be very systematically derived and calculated involving unique quantum numbers as typical parameters for their categorization. Electrons can only hop between such orbitals thereby gaining or losing energy, which often is exchanged radiatively by photons, the quanta of light. For such changes of orbital, electrons and the respective photon (angular momentum 1 $\hbar$!) must observe conservation rules for energy, momentum and angular momentum[*36].

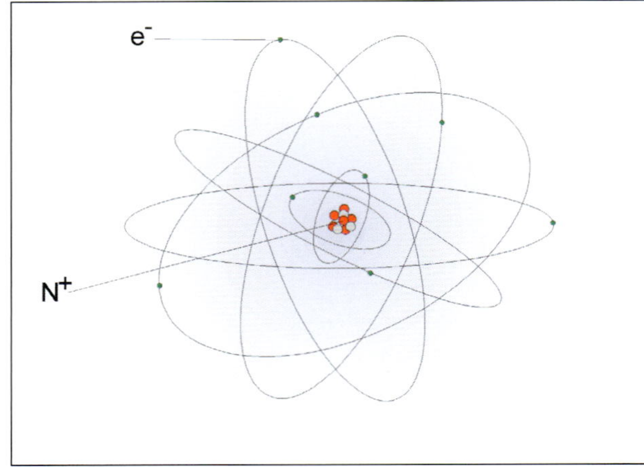

Fig 1-2 Simple model of an atom: it consists of the nucleus (N^+) and electrons (e^-) moving around it. Orbitals as drawn in the figure represent in reality no precise trajectories but rather diffuse zones of non-vanishing probability of occupation.

Atoms with their electrons in certain orbitals are said to be in a quantum state. Additionally, it must be considered that atoms are normally always in motion. Atoms may be bound together into molecules[*37] having similar but more complicated orbitals. Molecules having a non-symmetric

*30 In the case of the sun and stars, their atmosphere absorbs certain parts of the frequency spectrum which are characteristic for the elements or molecules therein. Hence, this gives us information about composition.

*31 The analysis of emission and absorption spectra is called spectroscopy. By this method, researchers have gained most of the information about the structure of atoms.

*32 To be correct: a certain amount of, even very little, coherence is present in any light. The coherence length may be in the worst case just of atomic dimensions (Å). Hence, a more correct expression is partial coherence.

*33 Of course, only if the atom is uncharged. If there are more electrons, we talk about a negative or anion, in the opposite case a positive or cation.

*34 Only by the assumption that certain ones are stable, could the atom be explained. Out of this, quantum theory eventually evolved. Previous understanding would have claimed continuous radiation of moving electrons finally causing catastrophic collision with the nucleus.

*35 Most interestingly, angular momentum has the same physical dimension as Planck's quantum h. Therefore, this property is essential in atomic theory as well as elementary particle description (Bose or Fermi particle nature, $m\hbar$ or $\hbar/2$, respectively; m being an integer).

*36 These are called the selection rules, in some cases not allowing any transition, at least via normal photons consisting of "electric dipole" radiation. If a transition is forbidden in this sense, the state may be called quasi-stable. There are other kinds of electromagnetic radiation called "magnetic dipole", "electric quadrupole" and "magnetic quadrupole" radiation following other selection rules, however lying beyond the scope of this text.

*37 If orbitals overlap and electrons are common to both or several atoms they are in a lower energetic state due to the exchange energy set free. This fact characterizes covalent bonds.

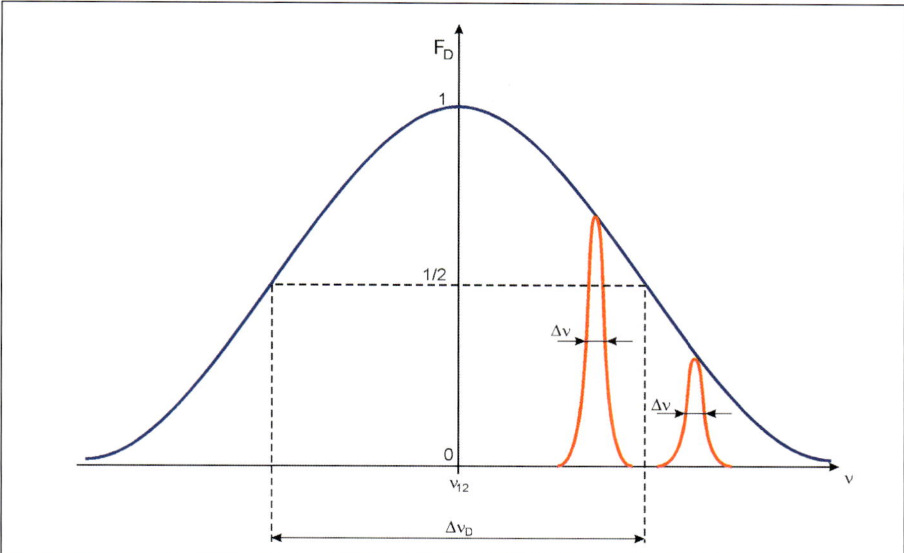

Fig 1-3 Doppler broadening in a gas: at finite temperature average width $\Delta\nu_D$, consisting of frequency-shifted atomic emissions originally having the natural linewidth $\Delta\nu$. (ν_{12}, frequency of resting atom; F_D, Gaussian curve function for Doppler broadening in a gas indicating the relative number of atoms with frequency shifted by ν).

shape may rotate and thereby assume different rotation states with discrete energies. Furthermore, molecules may vibrate in various modes also corresponding to discrete vibration states with associated discrete energies. Therefore, the most common quantum state of a molecule may be a rotational vibrational electronic state[*38]. All transitions between such states may go ahead with the emission of photons[*39].

Even if the emitters of light create certain light frequencies characteristic to them, a detector may see different ones. The reason is the Doppler shift in the case where either the source or the detector of light is moving. More frequently, a wide mixture of frequencies originates within a gas at some finite temperature which when measured at a detector gives rise to a markedly broadened spectrum as is depicted in Fig. 1-3. According to Maxwell's distribution of velocities of gas molecules at a certain temperature, different Doppler shifts occur even for equal atomic emissions, which overlap to a much wider bandwidth. This is a typical example for inhomogeneous broadening characterized by different quantitative effects on different subgroups (in this example applying to groups of atoms having different velocities) which at least in principle could be selected. Homogeneous broadening is just the contrary. There are various other broadening mechanisms that apply under other circumstances, e.g., the strong crystalline binding forces in solid-state matter.

All artificial light sources, such as light bulbs, electron discharge tubes etc., or even fluorescent media[*40], can be attributed to the kind of emitters as described above. The laser represents a very special light source: it is very directed, has a fairly narrow band (compare Detail 1-2), is fairly well polarized and coherent to a high degree. Most important of all, it can be made to be very intensive, which is described best by the quantity "brightness" (see Detail 1-11). As will be shown later, the essential difference responsible for all this is based on the origin of this kind of light via stimulated emission as opposed to all other light sources, which are based on spontaneous emission. With all these properties, the availability of

*38 There are new artificial words such as ro-vibr-onic or vibr-onic which are self-explanatory if written in such a way!

*39 Generally, transitions can also happen upon collisions with a partner molecule, e.g., within condensed matter or with a container wall. In this case also, non-radiative transitions occur frequently.

*40 Excited media, such as products of chemical reactions, can produce luminescent light. If it is emitted in fractions of seconds one calls it fluorescence, if it is delayed even for many hours it is named phosphorescence.

Detail 1-2.
Examples for linewidths of emissions from various media employed for lasing under the conditions indicated.

Medium	wavelength	frequency	Broadening mechanism
He-Ne (300 K)	0.633 μm	1.5 GHz	Doppler, inhomogeneous
Ar ion (2000 K)	0.488 μm	4.0 GHz	Doppler, inhomogeneous
CO_2:10 mbar, 300 K	10.6 μm	60 MHz	Doppler, inhomogeneous
CO_2: 1 bar, 300 K	10.6 μm	4 GHz	collisions, homogeneous
CO_2: 10 bar, 300 K	10.6 μm	150 GHz	overlapping rotational levels
KrF excimer	0.248 μm	10 THz	overlapping vibration levels
Rh6G dye	0.6 μm	80 THz	overlapping vibration levels
Ruby laser	0.694 μm	330 GHz	lattice vibrations, homogeneous
Nd:YAG	1.06 μm	120 GHz	lattice vibrations, homogeneous
Nd:glass	1.06 μm	7.5 THz	strong effect by static E-fields, inhomogeneous
GaAs diode	0.89 μm	10 THz	energy bands in periodic lattice

laser radiation initially revolutionized physics with respect to spectroscopy, and later many fields of application including metrology, optical data storage and transmission, laser chemical and biological interactions and, last but not least, materials processing, with dental laser applications being a small fraction of them.

1.3 Optical Concepts for the Function of a Laser

1.3.1 Stimulated Emission and Amplification in a Laser Medium

The first important feature to be discussed in this section is the threefold interaction between light and matter: absorption, spontaneous emission and stimulated emission, shown in Fig. 1-4. All three of them are indispensable for laser function. In many cases, energy is deployed within the laser medium by the absorption of an optical pump source, which might be a flash lamp or arc lamp or, following a much more modern concept, a highly efficient diode laser. This absorption process is indicated by the transfer of an electron from energy level E_1 to E_2[*41]. Spontaneous emission, which is one possible mechanism for the reciprocal electronic transition E_2 to E_1, is the result of typical radiative decay of excited electronic states[*42] (corresponding to higher energy levels than the lowest possible) of atoms or molecules. This follows quantum mechanical rules of probability without recognizable classical causality, and is in many respects comparable to radioactive decay of excited or unstable nuclear states. Stimulated emission representing the complementary decay mechanism, on the contrary, can only occur if a photon interacts with an atom in the excited state causing[*43] the emission of a second, identical photon (with respect to direction, frequency, phase and polarization). In the case of the laser in general, a few spontaneous photons will always have the desired direction of laser operation, determined by the resonator axis, so that they can be repetitively duplicated in the laser medium, eventually establishing a beam (super-radiation, see section 1.3.4) which, if storage within the oscillator occurs, represents a transversal mode (see section 1.3.4). As the already existing photons stimulate the emission of exactly matching ones, net amplification[*44] of the initial radiation takes place given that absorption

*41 We consider only two energy levels in this exemplary analysis. In general, all atoms or molecules have an infinite number of energy levels, but only the ones interacting have to be taken into account. Throughout this laser chapter, we keep the same colour code for energy levels; i.e., the ground level is represented by a blue colour, and the upper level, being the starting point of stimulated emission, is depicted by yellow. The end level of stimulated emission is shown in green if different from the ground level (see Fig. 1-6a and b).

*42 An electronic state describes the configuration of the electrons with respect to the nucleus (nuclei) of an atom (molecule) characterized by quantum numbers defining energy, angular momentum etc. The ground state is always stable, the excited states decay with typical decay times τ according to $N_i(t) = N_i(t=0)e^{-t/\tau}$, where N_i is the occupation number of a state (the number of atoms or molecules per unit volume being in a certain state) at time t.

*43 Stimulated emission as well as "stimulated" absorption have a classical analogue within the context of harmonic oscillators driven by external forces; causality is observed! The most simple example is a children's swing: it can be pushed or slowed down depending on the phase of the periodic driving force.

*44 As absorption and stimulated emission are equally probable, the higher energy level has to have a higher occupation called inversion (which is a non-thermal non-equilibrium situation).

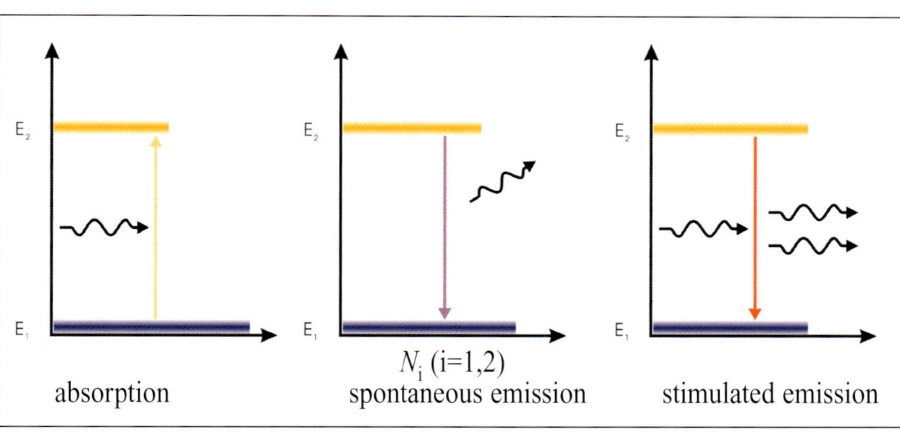

Fig 1-4 Interaction of light and matter illustrated for the example of a two-level system: N_i, population density (i.e., number of atoms per volume occupying energy state E_1 or E_2). The waved arrows left of the vertical transition arrow symbolize incoming photons, the ones on the right side emitted photons (in case of spontaneous emission with random phase and direction indicated).

Detail 1-3.
The probability of stimulated versus spontaneous emission (Fig. 1-4 following Einstein's calculation) amplification

Transition probability of absorption ($1 \rightarrow 2$): $P_{12}^{abs} = B_{12}\rho(v) = \sigma_{12}F$
Transition probability of spontaneous emission ($2 \rightarrow 1$): $P_{21}^{sp} = A_{21} = 1/\tau_{21}$
Transition probability of stimulated emission ($2 \rightarrow 1$): $P_{21}^{sp} = B_{21}\rho(v) = \sigma_{21}F$
$\rho(v)$ spectral energy density of radiation field $[W/Vv]$, τ_{21} spontaneous lifetime,
σ_{12} and σ_{21} $[A]$ cross sections for absorption and emission, respectively.
A_{21}, B_{12}, B_{21} traditional symbols dating back to Einstein (in reality just A und B used)

Stationary equilibrium: equal rates for transitions $1 \rightarrow 2$ and $2 \rightarrow 1$!

$$\frac{d}{dt}N_1 = \left(\frac{d}{dt}N_2\right)^{sp} + \left(\frac{d}{dt}N_2\right)^{st} \quad \frac{d}{dt}N_i = N_iP_{ij} = N_i\sigma_{ij}F \qquad (i=1,2;\ j \neq i)$$

$$N_1B_{12}\rho(v) = N_2(A_{21}+B_{21}\rho(v))$$

$$\rho(v) = \frac{N_2A_{21}}{N_1B_{12}-N_2B_{21}} = \frac{A_{21}/B_{21}}{(N_1/N_2)\ (B_{12}/B_{21})-1}$$

$$\rho(v) = \frac{A_{21}}{B_{21}} \frac{1}{\frac{B_{12}}{B_{21}}\exp\ (E_2-E_1)/\ kT-1}$$

We use Boltzmann's statistics (as an approximation for high energies compared to kT;
$k = 1.381 \cdot 10^{-23}\ J/K$,
$kT = 25.9$ meV at 300 K):
$N_1/N_2 = \exp(E_2-E_1)/kT$

being equivalent to Planck's formula for black body radiation which is valid at (thermal) equilibrium:

$$\rho(v) = \frac{8\pi hv^3}{c^3} \frac{1}{\exp(hv/kT)-1}$$

In **case of identity**: **comparison** of **numerator** and **denominator**:

$A_{21}/B_{12} \equiv 8\pi hv^3/c^3$ ratio of stimulated to spontaneous emission drops by the 3rd power of the frequency.
$B_{12} \equiv B_{21}$ absorption und stimulated emission are equally probable at all temperatures.
$E_2 - E_1 = hv$ corresponds to the assumption of Bohr's atomic model.

Generalized Beer's law of absorption, and amplification:

$$dI = dI|_a + dI|_{st} \Rightarrow \frac{dI}{dx} = -\sigma N_1I + \sigma N_2I$$ absorption and stimulated emission counteract.

Integration over medium thickness d yields:
$I/I_0 = \exp\ (\sigma(N_2-N_1)d) = G = \exp(gd)$
G amplification, g gain coefficient; $g = \sigma(N_2-N_1)$ is only positive yielding amplification for $N_2 > N_1$ being called inversion. For small values gd, $G \approx 1 + gd$ is a good approximation.

is weaker or negligible. Eventually, an equilibrium between losses and gain is reached allowing the laser to emit a continuous wave (cw), i.e., at nearly constant power, in cases where no additional operational conditions are implied (e.g., any kind of switching or modulation process).

1.3.2 Basic Scheme of a Laser

Fig. 1-5 shows the basic scheme of each laser comprising the laser medium (green box), which is energetically excited by an external source (yellow arrow). Furthermore, light can travel to and fro many times along a defined axis by being repeatedly reflected by mirrors of different reflectivity R forming an optical oscillator or resonator (traditionally also called a cavity[*45]). As depicted in (a) and (c), the laser oscillator stores light via the multiple reflections of its mirrors, but also emits light through the partially transmitting outcoupling mirror (it couples the interior of the cavity, where generally the intensity of light or photon flux[*46] is much higher[*47], with the "outside world", allowing us to make use of the radiation). It will be shown later that the properties of the cavity (generally the specifications of its mirrors) determine the optical properties of the beam. If we could "fill" the cavity with radiation at one instant of time, it would emit a beam which, however, would lose its intensity exponentially because every oscillator is subject to loss (by intention via outcoupling or unavoidably via mirror losses, diffraction, scattering or absorption). In order to compensate for those losses, yielding a balance and thereby allowing continuous emission, amplification of exactly the size of losses has to take place (compare (b) where one can observe a frequency-dependent gain line and idealized constant unavoidable losses). Thus, a "loss-

*45 Referring rather to the microwave situation where radiation has to be enclosed from all sides within a hollow cavity of comparable dimensions to the wavelength. In case of a laser the cavity is typically 10^6 times larger than λ and hence needs only two mirrors to enclose the directed radiation.

*46 Photon flux F means the number of photons per time and area, corresponding to intensity I (power per area, W/cm^2) divided by the photon energy (dimension of F [cm^{-2}]). The alternating use of wave-related expressions and expressions referring to (quasi) particles (e.g., quanta, such as photons) is characteristic to physics dealing with quantum phenomena.

*47 The transmittivity (relates transmitted intensity to incoming intensivity) of the outcoupling mirror M_2, $T_2 = 1-R_2$ (reflectivity defined correspondingly), determines the ratio between emitted radiation and intra-cavity radiation; e.g., if $T_2 = 0.05$ (5 %), then inside the cavity the intensity is 20 times higher! Depending on the gain in the laser medium, one can always find an optimum for R_2 or T_2.

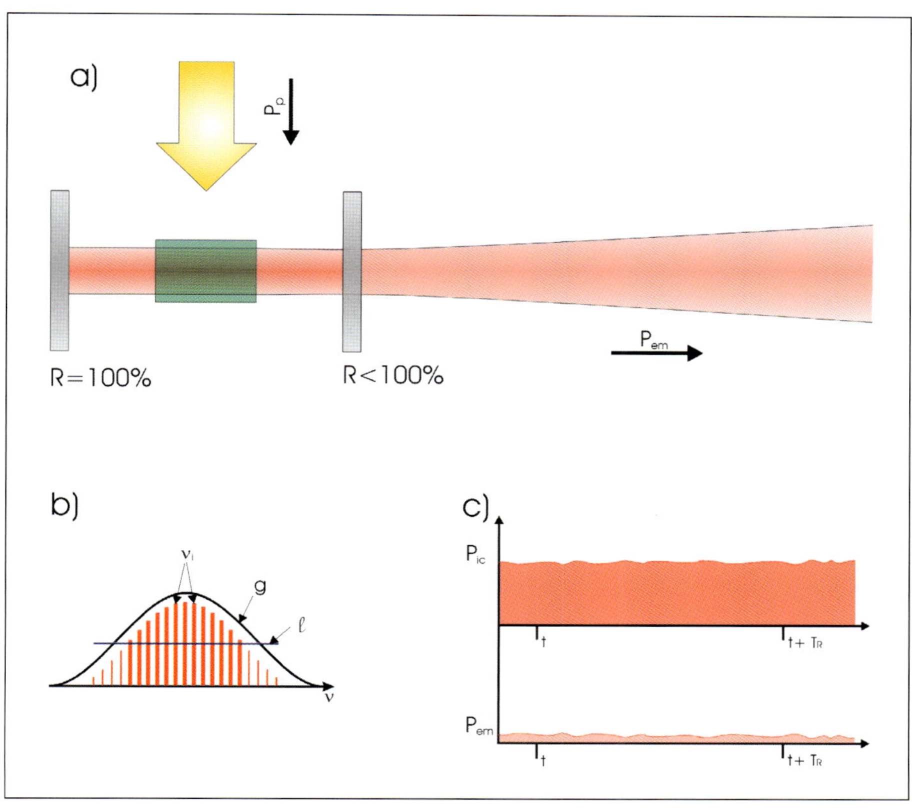

Fig 1-5 Free running laser.
(a) Basic scheme of a laser consisting of a resonator and an amplifying medium.
(b) Description in the frequency regime (several modes having frequency ν_i with random relative phase).
(c) Description in the temporal regime, (top) intracavity, (bottom) outcoupled (power fluctuations due to mode interference);
T_R, resonator round-trip time;
P_p, pump power;
P_{ic}, intracavity power;
P_{em}, emitted power;
g, gain;
l, loss.

Detail 1-4.
Threshold condition of lasers.

Rate equations based on a four-level system as depicted in Fig.1-6b: Assumptions:
Between levels 3 and 2 as well as 1 and 0 very fast transitions take place, hence lifetimes τ_3 and $\tau_1 << \tau_2$ (spontaneous emission 2→1)! Therefore the total population density (of lasing atoms) $N = N_2 + N_0$; N_1 und $N_3 \cong 0$,

$$\frac{d}{dt}N_2 = W_p N_0 - BE_{\mathrm{ph}}\Phi N_2 - \frac{N_2}{\tau_2} \qquad (1)$$

W_p normalized pump rate, level $0 \rightarrow 3$ $[t^{-1}]$, $B = \sigma_{21}c/E_{\mathrm{ph}}$
Interpretation of (1): N_2 is increased via the pump level E_3 by the pump rate W_p while it is reduced by stimulated and spontaneous emissions

$$\frac{d}{dt}\Phi = BE_{\mathrm{ph}}\,\Phi N_2 - \frac{\Phi}{\tau_c} \qquad (2)$$

Φ photon density $[V^{-1}]$, $\tau_c = d/c(1\text{-}RT)$ lifetime of photons in the cavity,with d length of cavity and medium, R reflectivity of outcoupling mirror, T transmission of cavity
Interpretation of (2): Φ is increased by stimulated emission and decreased by cavity losses; contributions by spontaneous emission are neglected!

These are coupled nonlinear differential equations: general solution rather complicated; however under special conditions very useful results (relaxation oscillations).

Stationary solutions:
If in Equ. (2) $\frac{d\Phi}{dt} \cong 0$, this marks the **threshold**, as any minimum increase beyond zero will cause amplification of Φ:

$$N_{2,\mathrm{th}} = \frac{1}{\tau_c BE_{\mathrm{ph}}} = \frac{1-RT}{\sigma_{21}d} \qquad (3)$$

At the same time this is a **stationary condition**!
The stationary photon density follows from Equ. (1) by $\frac{dN_2}{dt} = 0$

yielding
$$\Phi_s = \frac{W_p N_{0,\mathrm{th}} - N_{2,\mathrm{th}}/\tau_2}{BE_{\mathrm{ph}}N_{2,\mathrm{th}}}.$$

Using (3) the result becomes
$\Phi_s = \tau_c N_{0,\mathrm{th}}\,(W_p - W_{p,\mathrm{th}}) \approx \tau_c N\,(W_p - W_{p,\mathrm{th}})$,

where
$$W_{p,\mathrm{th}} = \frac{N_{2,\mathrm{th}}}{N_{0,\mathrm{th}}}\;\frac{1}{\tau_2}. \qquad (4)$$

For most 4-level lasers $N_{0,th} \approx N$; $W_{p,th}$ is called the threshold pump rate. According to (4) the **output power** of a laser through a cross sectional area A is $P = A(1\text{-}R)E_{ph}c\Phi_s$ (being linear with respect to pumping beyond the threshold). For most solid-state lasers, including the semiconductor laser, this is clearly the case (comp. Fig. 1-34).

free" oscillator[*48] is approximated which would potentially have zero frequency bandwidth for every mode (if there were no perturbations, as is well known from harmonic oscillator theory[*49]). This view represents an alternative understanding of the laser compared to the concept of starting it from a few photons to be amplified until cw equilibrium is reached. Nevertheless, it is from the latter view that the threshold concept of a laser is derived.

1.3.3 Level Schemes of Real Lasers

If light passes through matter, it is slowed down by a factor *n*, called the index of refraction ($n = c/c_n$, *c* being the phase velocity of light in vacuum and c_n the velocity in matter), and exponentially attenuated following Beer's law $I_d = I_0 . e^{-(\alpha+\beta)d}$, with I_0 being the incoming intensity and I_d the transmitted intensity through a layer of thickness *d*. In this context we will neglect scattering (coefficient β) and consider only on the absorption coefficient α. Under normal linear optical circumstances, $\alpha = \alpha(\lambda)$ and is always positive. However, it is possible under nonlinear optical conditions that the occupation of a higher energy level is greater than the occupation of a certain lower level (contrary to the probability of thermodynamics) so that net amplification takes place. Such a situation is called population inversion, and it may be characterized formally by a negative temperature, to be seen easily in the example of Boltzmann statistics (see the detailed explanation of the probability of stimulated emission in Detail 1-3). This inversion cannot be achieved by strong pumping of a two-level system, like the one depicted in Fig. 1-4, because the probabilities of absorption and stimulated emission are the same. Hence, once the occupations N_2 and N_1 are the same, no net change will take place because the rates of absorption and of stimulated emission in this case are the same (spontaneous emission becomes unimportant under strong pumping conditions because it is independent of the radiation field). We need three-level and four-level systems (as schematically shown in Fig. 1-6) in order to practically realize inversion and hence amplification. The width of these levels can vary over a wide range from the narrow natural linewidth to the very broad width of energetic bands[*50] amounting to some tens of percent.

In a three-level system (Fig. 1-6a), the atoms or molecules[*51] are raised from ground level *0* to level *2* by a pumping mechanism. If the material is such that, after level *2* has been reached, it decays rapidly[*52] in a radiative or non-radiative manner to the longer lifetime[*53] level *1*, then in this way a population inversion can be obtained between levels *2* and *1*. In a four-level laser, atoms are raised from the ground level to level *3*. If the atom or molecule then decays rapidly to level *2*, where it should remain as long as possible, a population inversion can be obtained accordingly between levels *2* and *1*. Once oscillation starts in such a four-level laser, however, the atoms will be transferred to level *1* via stimulated emission (and negligible spontaneous emission). For continuous wave operation of a four-level laser it is necessary, therefore, that the transition $1 \rightarrow 0$ should also be ultra-fast to keep level *1* at a lower population than level *2*.

*48 Very often characterized by a high quality factor (Q) that is theoretically ∞.
*49 Harmonic oscillators can be realized in mechanical (weight with spring), electrical (L-C circuits), atomic (electron in an atom) or nuclear systems; in reality they are always damped and sometimes excited by periodic forces.
*50 In quantum mechanics, the natural width of an energy level is defined by its lifetime. Additional influences such as crystal fields or the Doppler effect of moving particles act by broadening. In some cases, e.g., the diode laser, the overlap of many levels results in a broad band (compare also Detail 1-2 and Fig. 1-3).
*51 From now on, if we say just atoms we also mean molecules etc. as laser media.
*52 In atomic systems, "rapidly" typically means femtoseconds (fs) or picoseconds (ps), i.e., ultra-fast transitions.
*53 Very useful excitation storage lifetimes of solid-state lasers are typically between µs and ms, and are called quasi-stable. Excimer and diode lasers unfortunately have only ns lifetimes, allowing no substantial excitation storage.

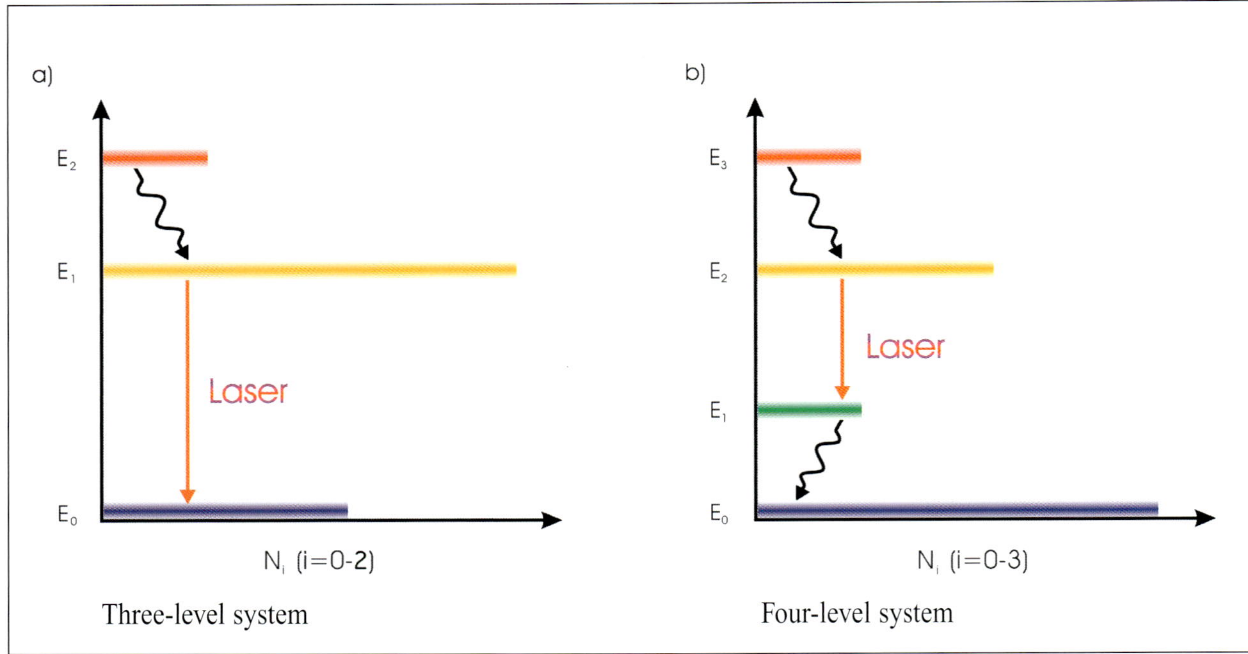

Fig 1-6 Level systems of lasers: E, energy; N_i, $(i=0–3)$ occupation density. To achieve inversion, separate pump levels (E_2 or E_3, red) must be available. From there, fast, mostly non-radiative transitions ($\tau \approx 10^{12}$ s) lead down to the upper laser level (E_1 or E_2, yellow). In case of the three-level system the laser transition directly connects to the ground level (E_0, blue), which has to be less populated than the upper (only achievable by hard pumping). In the four-level system a separate lower laser level (E_1, green) is available, which is effectively emptied by a fast transition to the ground state and allows easy realization of inversion.

Detail 1-5.
Schawlow-Townes formula for theoretical laser bandwidth to be compared with realistic bandwidths indicated in Detail 1-2.

At any time, spontaneous emission with its random phase adds to the instantaneous intra-cavity radiation thereby changing its phase with time and this causes frequency broadening:

$$\Delta\nu = \pi E_{ph}(\Delta\nu_c)^2 \mu P$$
$$\Delta\nu_c = (1-R)c/2\pi L$$
$$\mu = N_2/(N_2-N_1)_{th}$$

$\Delta\nu$	frequency bandwidth of monomode laser
$\Delta\nu_c$	bandwidth of the passive cavity,
P	laser (intra-cavity) power
L	length
R	reflectivity of mirror
$(N_2-N_1)_{th}$	threshold inversion

Quantitative examples:

HeNe laser: $\lambda = 632$ nm, $\nu = 5\cdot10^{14}$ Hz, $E_{ph} = 3.3\cdot10^{-19}$ J, $P = 1$ mW, $L = 10$ cm, $R = 99\%$, $\mu = 1 \Rightarrow \Delta\nu = 5\cdot10^{-2}$ Hz.
In practice, it is nearly impossible to realize such a narrow line width, because off variations in L.

Diode laser: $\lambda = 850$ nm, $\nu = 3.5\cdot10^{14}$ Hz, $E_{ph} = 2.3\cdot10^{-19}$ J, $P = 3$ mW, $L = nl = 3.5\cdot300$ µm, $R = 30\%$, $\mu = 3 \Longrightarrow \Delta\nu = 1.5\cdot10^{6}$ Hz. In reality, the bandwidth is 10 to 100 times larger, as a result of modulations of n according to fluctuations of electron density.

So far, we have seen how one can use a three- or four-level system of a given material to produce a population inversion. Whether a system will work in one of these schemes (or whether it will work at all!) depends on whether the various conditions stated above are fulfilled. We could, of course, ask why one should bother with a more complicated four-level scheme if a three-level scheme already seems to offer a suitable way of establishing population inversion. The answer is simple because in the four-level system the so-called lower laser level *1* is nearly unpopulated because of the fast transition into the ground level, so that inversion can be easily achieved. In a three-level system the so-called upper laser level *1* has to be heavily pumped via level *2* to become more populated than the ground state.

Detail 1-6.
Lifetime in laser levels and cross sections for stimulated emission.

lasertype	λ	τ_2	τ_1	σ_{21}
HeNe	633 nm	10–20 ns	12 ns	$3 \cdot 10^{-13}$ cm^2
Ar^+	488 nm	9 ns	0.4 ns	
excimer (KrF)	248 nm	1–10 ms	< 1 ps	10^{-16} cm^2
GaAs diode	800 nm	4 ns		10^{-16} cm^2
CO_2 low pressure high pressure	10600 nm	1–10 ns	100 ns 1 ns	10^{-16} cm^2
Rh6G dye	600 nm	5 ns	≤10 ps	$2 \cdot 10^{-18}$ cm^2
Ti:S $\parallel$ to c-axis $\nparallel$ to c-axis peak	670–1100nm	3.2 μs	ns	$4.1 \cdot 10^{-19}$ cm^2 $2.0 \cdot 10^{-19}$ cm^2
Nd:YAG	1060 nm	230 μs	30 ns	$8 \cdot 10^{-19}$ cm^2
Ruby	694 nm	3 ms	∞	$2 \cdot 10^{-20}$ cm^2
Yb:YAG 220 K 300 K	1030 nm	950 μs	dept. on T	$7 \cdot 10^{-21}$ cm^2 $2 \cdot 10^{-20}$ cm^2
Nd:glass	1060 nm	300 μs	50–100 ns	$4 \cdot 10^{-20}$ cm^2
alexandrite 300 K 475 K	701–818 nm	260 μs	ns	$7 \cdot 10^{-21}$ cm^2 $2 \cdot 10^{-20}$ cm^2

1.3.4 The Laser Resonator and its Output Radiation

One could easily imagine building a laser – contrary to traditional concepts – by first considering the characteristics of the radiation field required, and later specifying resonator and medium properties. In practice, there are never any plane-parallel waves, as every light source is spatially confined. Diffraction does not allow production and maintenance of a "beam" with sharp edges. As a matter of fact, a Gaussian beam, as shown in Fig. 1-7, and mathematically characterized according to the equations in Detail 1-7, represents the shape of a laterally confined wave which is, as was already mentioned above, easily treated theoretically as well as practically: its amplitude (E[*54]) as well as its intensity (I) distribution follow a Gaussian bell curve[*55], which, in principle extends to infinity, although, with a very rapid loss of height (Fig. 1-7a). A "radius" r has to be voluntarily defined, at a position where the maximum intensity I_{max} is reduced by $1/e^2 = 0.135$, called the Gaussian parameter w. Such a beam has a waist with radius w_0 and extends symmetrically to infinity along the z-axis asymptotically approaching a cone originating in the center of the waist with an angular aperture of 2θ (θ is the divergence angle; compare Fig. 1-7b). The phase fronts, i.e. areas of constant phase φ, are spherical with a radius of curvature $R(z)$ varying with z. There are two z-positions with flat wavefront, i.e., $R = \infty$, at $z = 0$ and $z = \infty$. In this context, it is interesting to recognize that a Gaussian beam represents a partial spherical wave within a cone with, of course,

*54 Light, being an electromagnetic wave, can be characterized by its electric field E as well as by its magnetic field B (both are vectors orthogonal to the propagation axis for a transversal wave). In this context, only the amplitudes are relevant.

*55 $I/I_{max} = \exp(-2r^2/w(z))$ for the intensity at a position z along the propagation axis (beam waist at $z = 0$).

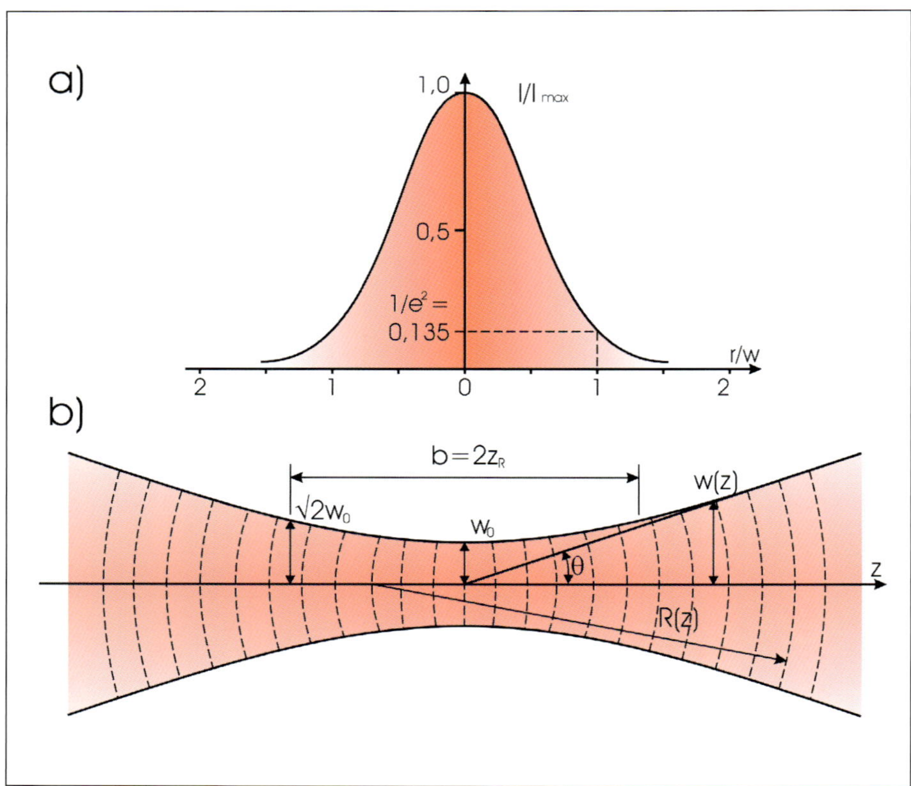

Fig 1-7 Gaussian beam.
(a) Bell-shaped intensity distribution at any cross section at distance z from waist; I, intensity at radial position r; I_{max}, maximum intensity at the z-axis;
(b) longitudinal cut through the rotational symmetric Gaussian beam indicating the beam width as defined in (a) (full lines) and the wave fronts (dashed lines);
w_0, radius of beam waist;
$w(z)$, radius at distance z from the waist;
z_R, Rayleigh length;
$2z_R$, confocal parameter b;
θ, divergence angle; $R(z)$, radius of curvature at distance z.

Detail 1-7.
Mathematical treatment of Gaussian beams.

A Gaussian beam can be represented as a spherical wave with imaginary center (being hard to imagine but mathematically elegant, comp. Detail 1):
Wave center or origin $O\ (x,y,q)$ with $x = 0,\ y = 0,\ q = z+iz_R$ where z_R Rayleigh length

$$E\ (r,z,t) = \frac{E_0}{\sqrt{q^2 + r^2}}\ exp{-i}\ (k\sqrt{q^2 + r^2} - \omega t) \qquad \text{where } r = \sqrt{x^2 + y^2}.$$

The so-called paraxial approximation considering only the area close to the z-axis where $r << |q|$ is

$$E\ (r,z,t) = \frac{B}{q} exp\ (-i\ \frac{kr^2}{2q})\ exp\ i\ (\omega t - kz) \qquad \text{where } B = E_0 exp(kz_R).$$

B represents a generalized amplitude, and $1/q$ is a complex generalized wave parameter which can be split in real and imaginary parts having the following meaning:

$$\frac{1}{q(z)} = \frac{z-iz_R}{z^2 + z^2_R} = \frac{1}{R(z)} - i\frac{2}{kw^2\ (z)} \qquad \text{where } w(z) \text{ beam radius, } R(z) \text{ radius of curvature}$$

$$E\ (r,z,t) \approx \frac{B}{q} exp\left(-\frac{r^2}{w^2\ (z)}\right) exp\left(-i\frac{kr^2}{2R\ (z)}\right) exp\ i\ (\omega t - kz)$$ characterizes the

Gaussian beam representing an approximate solution of the wave equation. In radial direction, its amplitude is expressed by a Gaussian function $exp(-r^2/w^2)$. $I/I_{max} = exp(-2r^2/w^2(z))$ is also a Gaussian ($I \propto E^2$).

The **beam radius** is $w(z) = w_0 \sqrt{1+z^2/z^2_R}$, where $w_0 = \sqrt{z_R\ \lambda/\pi}$.

For $z=z_R w(z_R) = \sqrt{2}\ w(0) = \sqrt{2}\ w_0$. Therefore the cross sectional area of the beam $z = \pm z_R$ is doubled compared to the waist cross section, and hence $b = 2z_R$ is called the focal length or **confocal parameter**.

Divergence: Far away from the waist ($z >> z_R$) the beam radius grows nearly linearly with z: $w(z) = w_0 \cdot z/z_R$. Hence the divergence angle

$$\theta = \lim_{z<<z_R} \frac{w(z)}{z} = \frac{w_0}{z_R} = \frac{\lambda}{\pi w_0}.$$

A comparison with a planar wave propagating through a spherical aperture of diameter $2w_0$ shows that the zero-order diffraction spot (within the first dark ring of the diffraction pattern) is confined within the angle $\theta_1 = 1.22\ \lambda/2w_0 = 0.66\ \lambda/w_0 < \theta$. Therefore the Gaussian beam is called diffraction limited as it diverges weaker than other laterally confined light waves.

Radius of curvature: $R(z) = z + \frac{z_R^2}{z}$
represents the radius of curvature of the parabolic phase fronts of Gaussian beams. There are two special cases: for $z \to 0$ and $z \to \infty$ $R(z) \to \infty$ yielding planar wavefronts. For all $z >> z_R$, $R(z) \approx z$, i.e spheric waves with center at the waist at $z = 0$. As a matter of fact, the Gaussian beam represents a mixture of planar and spheric wave as is depicted in Fig. 1-7.

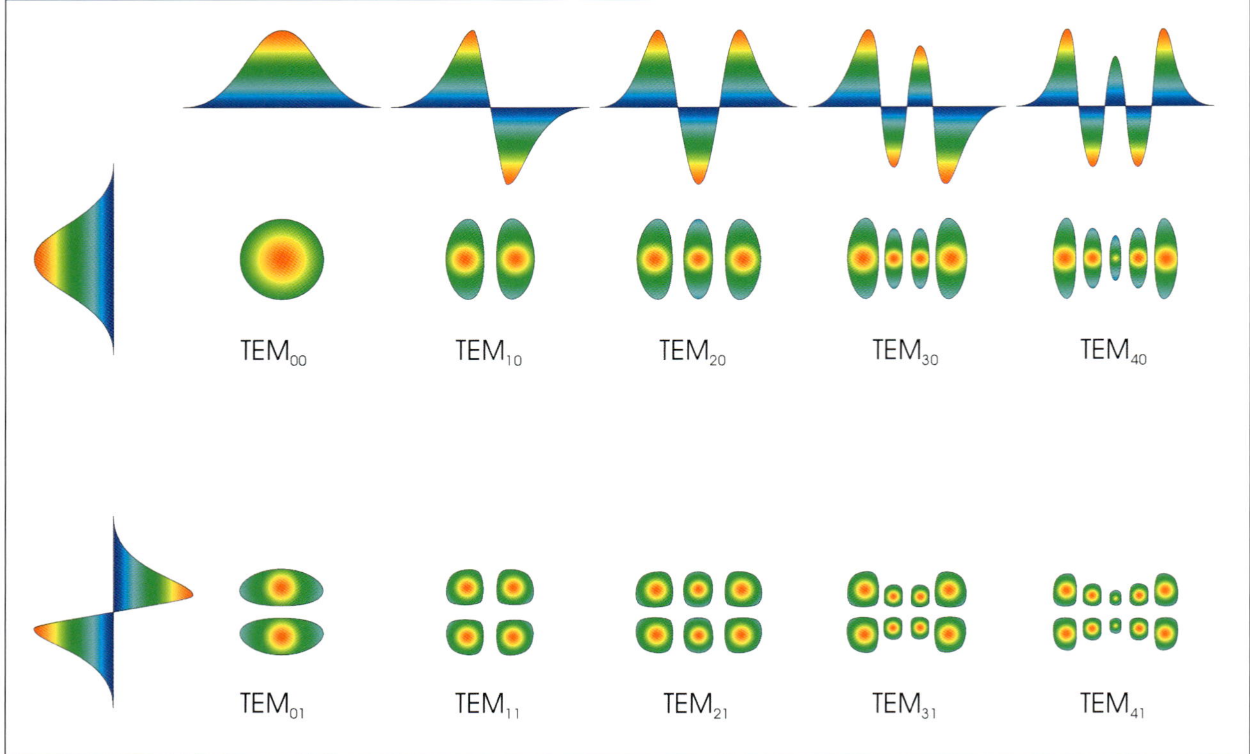

Fig 1-8 TEM laser modes[*59]: two-dimensionally represented by electric field amplitude versus radius and projected intensity shape. Artificial colors relate corresponding amplitude and intensity levels. The uppermost row also illustrates the one-dimensions series of Hermite–Gaussian functions. The symmetry of the lowermost row of intensity patterns refers to rectangular-shaped resonator mirrors.

variable amplitude or intensity distribution over its cross section. If focusing of a Gaussian beam is of specific interest, a pragmatic definition of the depth of focus is quite relevant: in the present context, it is called the confocal parameter[*56] $b \equiv 2z_R$, with z_R being the position on the z-axis where the cross-sectional area is two times the size of the smallest (at the beam waist)[*57].

If a Gaussian beam is focused it stays a Gaussian beam, however, with a different parameter characterizing the width of its bell shape. In mathematical terms, this corresponds to a Fourier transformation, against which a Gaussian function is an invariant. Every distribution of amplitude across the propagation direction z, e.g., along the x-axis, can be represented by a sum of Hermite-Gaussians[*58] as illustrated in Fig. 1-8 (upper row of graphics), the first order Hermite-Gaussian being represented by the Gaussian explained before.

As mentioned above, stimulated emission as the laser amplification mechanism requires the interaction of light with an inverted laser medium. This may already happen without a resonator being based on the feedback of light via mirrors. Already the avalanche-like growth of the number of photons, starting with some spontaneously generated ones, upon only one transition through the long axis of the inverted medium, can yield some kind of "beam" usually called amplified spontaneous emission (ASE) as illustrated in Fig. 1-9. Generally, in such a case the beam quality

*56 Or focal depth.
*57 Hence $w(z = z_R) = \sqrt{2}\, w_0$.
*58 They represent, mathematically speaking, an infinite system of orthogonal functions, also called complete, having the specific property that for every z-position the field distributions are similar, and only $w(z)$ varies.
*59 The abbreviations stand for transversely electromagnetic, with as many zero-transitions along the x- and y-axis as the corresponding integer number indicates.

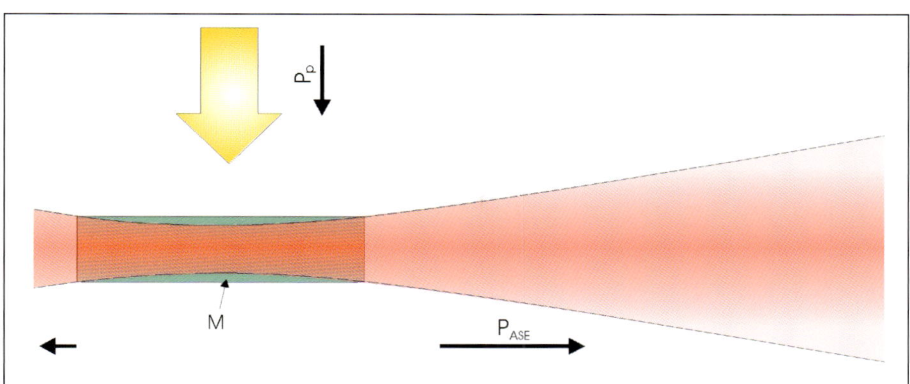

Fig 1-9 Super-radiator. A laser medium M inverted by sufficient pump radiation P_p without resonator mirrors can emit directed radiation P_{ASE} of low coherence and high divergence called amplified spontaneous emission (ASE).

with respect to divergence, smooth intensity distribution[*60] and coherence is rather low. In the case of heavily pumped laser media, e.g., as in the thin disk laser (see Fig. 1-23), care has to be taken to avoid parasitic super-radiation orthogonal to the resonator axis.

For a beam of laser quality to be generated, adequate resonator mirrors have to be put in place: as the phase fronts are spherical, mirrors of the same curvature and with reflectivity observing the above-mentioned considerations have to be inserted at the respective z-position. As a matter of fact, innumerable combinations are possible, and some of them are depicted in Fig. 1-10. The most systematic for mathematical description is the confocal resonator where both concave mirrors have a common focus in the center. It is obvious that a half-size resonator with a plane mirror on one side corresponding to the plane phase front at the beam waist will yield the same output beam characteristics. All the resonator configurations shown are symmetric or half-symmetric and stable[*61], the coplanar one, however, lying at the edge of stability.

All stable resonators generate transversal mode patterns like the ones depicted in Fig. 1-8. Their symmetry depends on the mirrors used, which may be round or rectangular causing corresponding mode patterns, the illustrated ones referring to the latter. It is a general feature that the beam waist of higher order modes is wider than for the lower ones. This represents an easy way to discriminate between modes allowing the laser to oscillate in TEM_{00} mode if an appropriate aperture is integrated in the resonator, although at the price of some additional loss.

There is another kind of characteristic field distribution resulting from the fact that light propagates to and fro within the resonator[*62] yielding standing waves as shown in Fig. 1-11. This is just a drawing of the basic idea, far from realistic geometrical relations where the number of half waves[*63] might be around one million! Standing waves are known to possess nodes and peaks of amplitude or intensity leading to the consequence that around the nodes no stimulated emission can take place, leaving inversion to stay unused. This fact may give rise to the tendency to generate higher-order modes, which have to be filtered out – resulting in further losses as mentioned.

*60 No characteristic field distribution, i.e., transversal mode (like the ones shown in Fig. 1-8), is formed! The excimer laser described in Section 1.5.1 is an example in the context of this book.

*61 "Stable" means that radiation is kept within the resonator for, in principle, an unlimited time, taking just geometrical losses into account. There are also unstable resonators laid out for a few cycles of high amplification, which will not be treated here.

*62 There are also so-called ring resonators (they must be non-planar) where the light path encircles some area in a topological sense. In this case no standing waves are formed!

*63 At λ = 1 µm, a half wave in vacuum is 0.5 µm long; for $m = 10^6$ and an average index of refraction n = 1.5 the resonator length L = 33 cm!

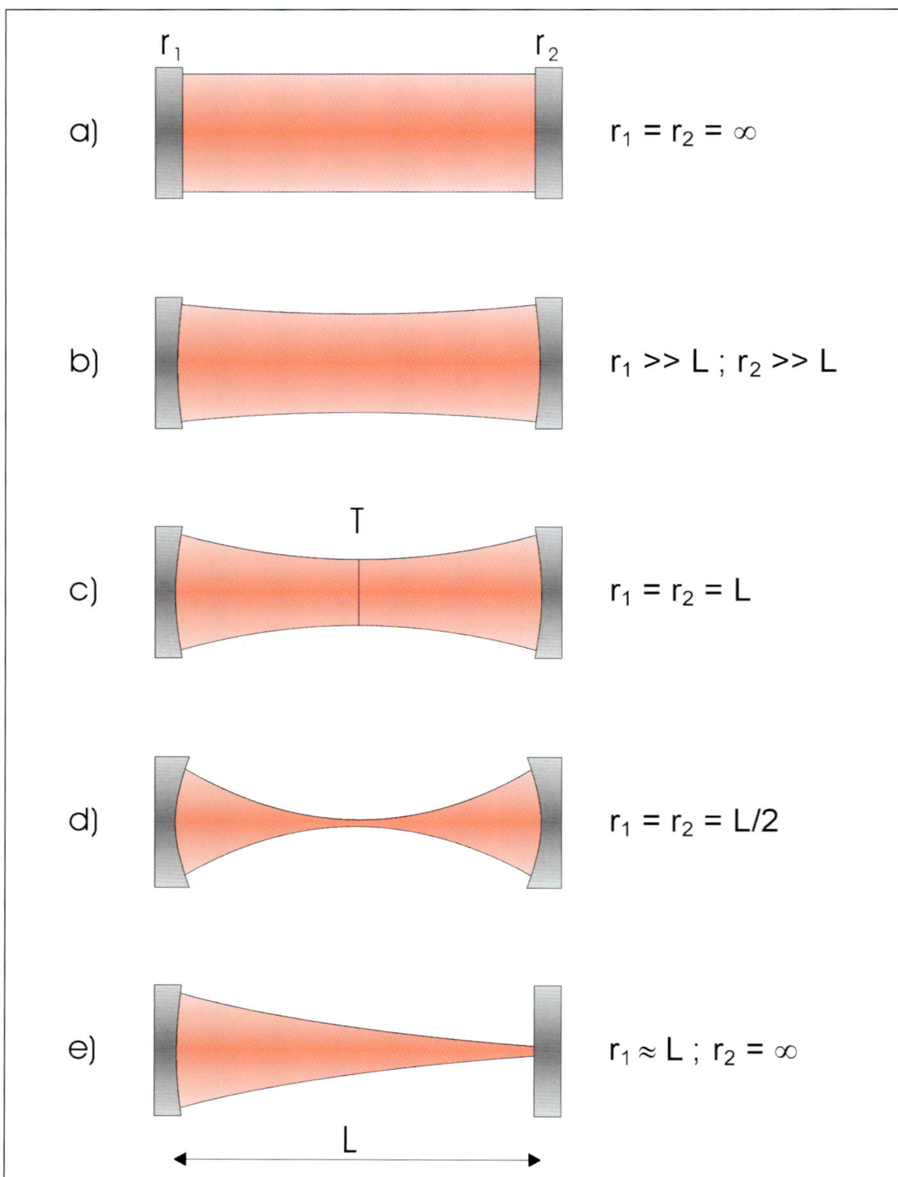

Fig 1-10 The most common stable resonator configurations:
(a) co-planar (plane mirrors),
(b) over-confocal (large radii of curvature),
(c) confocal,
(d) spheric (concentric),
(e) hemi-spheric (half-concentric).

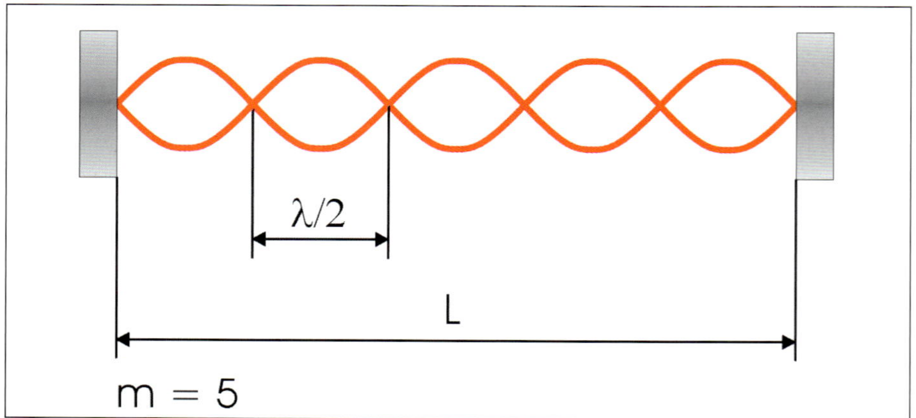

Fig 1-11 Schematic depiction of longitudinal laser modes in the form of standing waves with half wavelength λ periodicity. The mode order *m* in reality is of the order of 10^6.
L, resonator length.

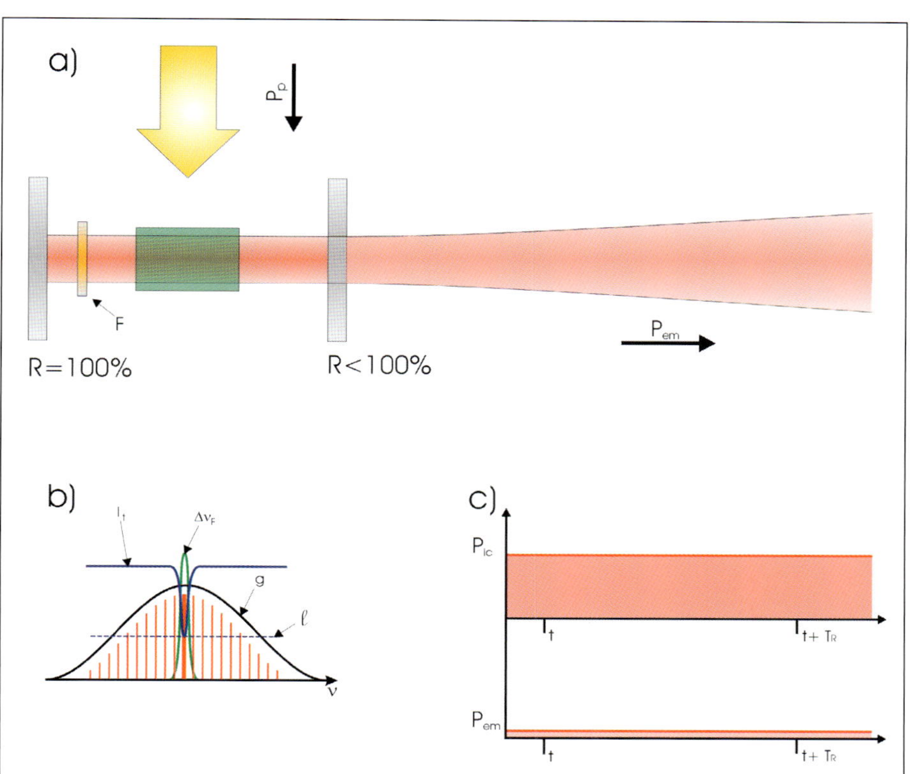

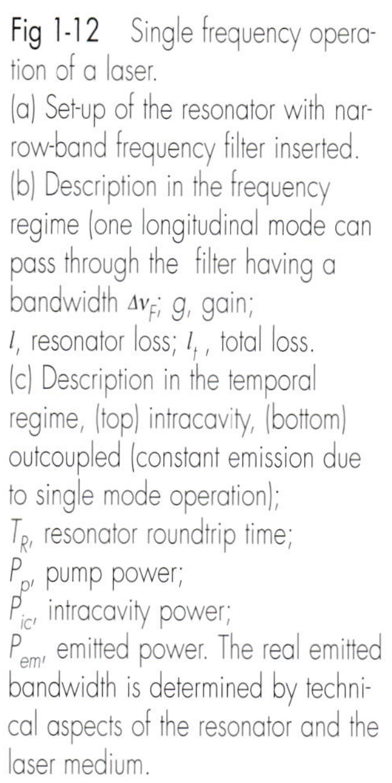
Fig 1-12 Single frequency operation of a laser.
(a) Set-up of the resonator with narrow-band frequency filter inserted.
(b) Description in the frequency regime (one longitudinal mode can pass through the filter having a bandwidth $\Delta\nu_F$; g, gain; l, resonator loss; l_t, total loss.
(c) Description in the temporal regime, (top) intracavity, (bottom) outcoupled (constant emission due to single mode operation);
T_R, resonator roundtrip time;
P_p, pump power;
P_{ic}, intracavity power;
P_{em}, emitted power. The real emitted bandwidth is determined by technical aspects of the resonator and the laser medium.

1.3.5 Specific Frequency and Temporal Operation Regimes of Lasers

As the gain curve already shown in Fig. 1-5 indicates, a laser can support radiation in a more or less wide frequency regime. It may be desirable in certain cases to select and to confine the spectral width of laser emission. This situation is depicted in Fig. 1-12. In (a) the previously depicted resonator is equipped with a spectral filter which might even be tunable. If the laser medium supports several transitions lying tens of nanometres apart, narrowband resonator mirrors might do the selection. In order to select longitudinal modes lying close together, a narrow-band filter of, e.g., a dielectric type can be employed. If, as indicated in Fig. 1-12b, filtering is sufficiently narrow for only one mode to be amplified, this results in single frequency operation. This is a very clearly defined state of laser operation associated with constant coherent[*64] output free of modal interference fluctuations (depicted in Fig. 1-5c).

For many applications pulsed laser operation is very desirable. In some cases, it is sufficient simply to apply the pumping action in a pulsed fashion. In this way microsecond pulses, e.g., of diode laser radiation, can be produced (called quasi-cw to indicate how "long" such pulses are in comparison to much shorter ones, such as ultra-short pulses which will be explained below). If a fast switch[*65] is incorporated within the cavity, Q-switched operation can be achieved (depicted in Fig. 1-13): in this case, the laser medium is pumped typically for the

*64 In real lasers there is always a limited coherence length l_c (the statistical laser beam length between perturbations of phase) between, in general, µm and 10^3 km (see also Section 1.5 describing specific lasers).

*65 Fast switches are acousto-optic or electro-optic: the acousto-optic switch is based on the rapid switching on – and – off of an ultrasonic wave that diffracts light; the electro-optic switch is based on rapide phase changes by the electro-optic effect in conjunction with a polarizer.

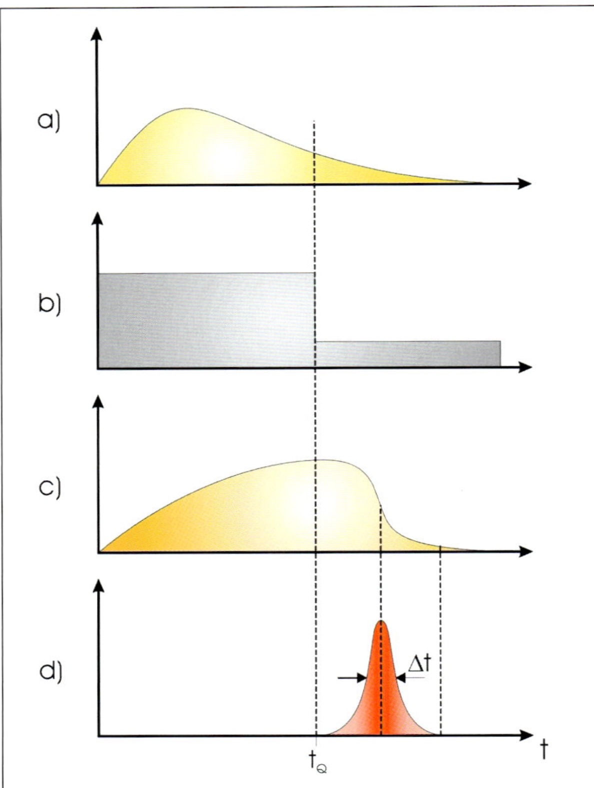

Fig 1-13 Quality switching of a laser resonator.
(a) Pump power, (b) resonator losses, (c) inversion, (d) laser power, all of them versus time *t*. Inversion can be accumulated effectively by inhibiting resonator action during most of the pumping period via switching of artificial resonator losses. Soon after rapid reduction of these losses at the inversion peak a giant pulse of typically ns-duration Δt occurs. t_Q, time of Q-switching.

duration of its spontaneous lifetime*66. This enables the build up of a large inversion, while the switch prevents laser oscillation by blocking the beam path, i.e., making losses very high. At the time of switching, the resonator action is re-established, giving rise to strong stimulated emission. This generates a strong laser pulse of typically nanosecond duration, terminated by gain depletion. The basic idea in this case is to store the energy in the form of electronic inversion to be finally set free via a strong nanosecond pulse.

A sophisticated method of producing much shorter pulses in the pico- and femtosecond range is called mode-locking (Fig. 1-14). The background of this idea is based on beating*67 which, of course, is more complicated in the case of several equally spaced frequencies as represented by longitudinal modes. To yield stable and useful temporal interference, the phase relations of all *N* modes*68 involved (depicted in Fig. 1-14b) have to be fixed*69, resulting in intensity peaks of *N* times the original height (compare Fig. 1-14c, not drawn to scale) and 1/*N* temporal width*70. Hence, laser media of wide bandwidth, nowadays amounting up to 30%, will be the materials of choice for shortest pulses.

There are several ways to force the modes to stay in phase, all of them involving some modulation*71 of loss or gain within the cavity. In Fig. 1-15a, as an example, the most successful modulation method, which is called Kerr lens modulation (KLM), is depicted. It is beyond the scope of this textbook to review mode-locking techniques in more detail. Only the basic idea of the most modern pulse formation theory for femtosecond solid-state lasers such as Ti:sapphire (see section 1.5.6) will be briefly explained here: the high intensity of such a short pulse oscillating within the resonator undergoes non-linear interactions in the laser medium, such as self-phase modulation, i.e., an increase of the index *n**72 depending on intensity. Furthermore, positive dispersion usually is present within the laser medium, a typical linear property as mentioned above. A pulse consisting of many frequencies would be soon

*66 Of the order of hundreds of microseconds for solid-state media.
*67 Beating is well-known as a cosine-like amplitude modulation occurring in the case of interference of two waves that are close to each other in frequency (most popular example: the acoustic beating of two wine glasses).
*68 They can be hundreds of thousands if the medium and the resonator support them.
*69 The term "mode-locking" refers to this fact, standing for a much stronger interaction than mode coupling. "Mode coupling" usually means that energy gradually is shifted from one to another mode, e.g., in optical fibers.
*70 When describing the width of pulses that have no clearly defined edges, the measure FWHM (full width at half maximum) has proven to be most fruitful.
*71 This can be caused by an external influence that must be extremely precise in its timing ("resonant") or by non-linear interaction of the beam with some media (saturation of loss or gain); the former is called active, the latter passive mode-locking.
*72 $n = n_0 + n_2 I$, with n_2 being the so-called non-linear index of refraction which usually is positive.

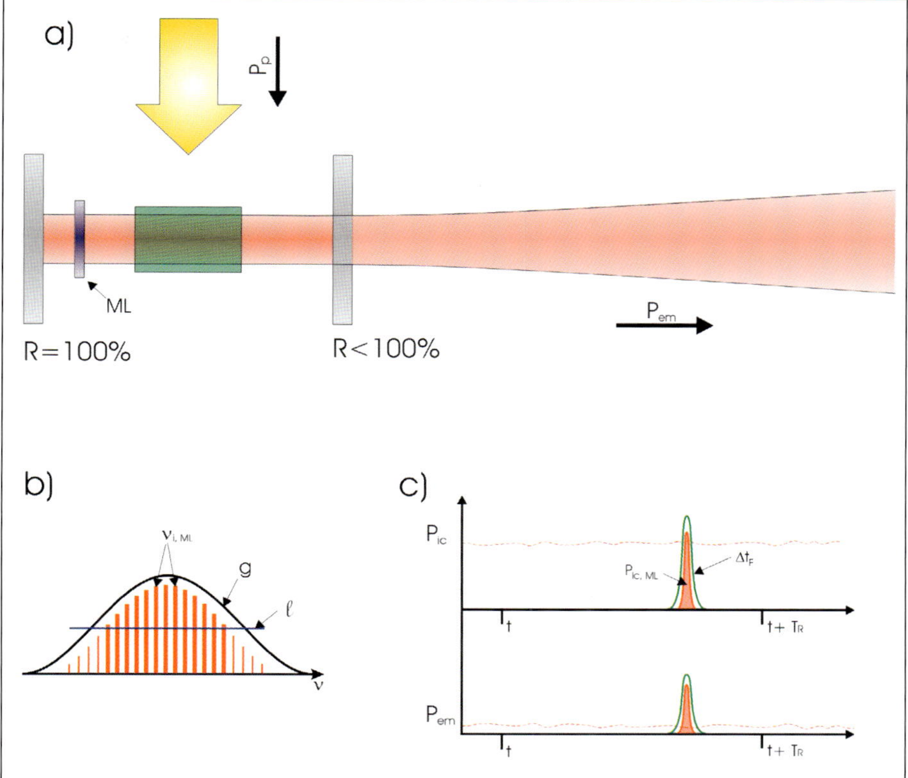

Fig 1-14 Mode-locked laser operation.
(a) Resonator set-up including a modulator for modelocking.
(b) Portrayal of the frequency regime (*N*, number of longitudinal laser modes to be phase locked; *g*, gain; *l*, resonator loss).
(c) Portrayal of the temporal regime: the *N*-locked modes allow constructive interference to form an ultra-short pulse in the resonator having *N*-fold intracavity power $P_{ic,ml}$ compared to the free-running laser power P_{ic} (indicated by the dotted line). By repetitive outcoupling of the pulse from the resonator a train of pulses is formed with intervals between them corresponding to the round-trip time T_R (the peak powers of the pulses are not drawn to scale!). The green line represents an effective temporal filter. P_p, pump power; P_{em}, emitted power.

torn apart if the net dispersion during one round-trip were not close to zero. Hence, negative dispersion is introduced into the cavity, in order to cancel out the originally positive one; the smaller the positive one is, the easier this will be. This sets a requirement for short-pulse laser media which, in the most modern designs of ultra-short pulse lasers, can be (slightly over-) balanced by dielectric cavity mirrors with integrated negative dispersion based on a careful design of the multilayer sequence[*73]. In this case one talks about solitary or soliton-like pulse formation, referring to the stand-alone pulses associated with nonlinear waves called solitons[*74].

Fig. 1-15b contains an easy to understand explanation of a soliton: assuming the three runners depicted represent the different frequencies contained within an ultra-short laser pulse, the group formed by them would disintegrate soon due to their different running speeds[*75]. Under their special conditions, they run on a deformable mattress, which slows down the red leader and accelerates the blue runner thereby keeping them together. The compression of the mattress represents the intensity-dependent change of phase velocity in the propagation (laser) medium. An optical soliton is comparable in this respect, because its intensity, which varyies over its duration, modifies the propagation constant (i.e., the speed of light) in such a way that all frequency components stay together.

*73 Such ultra-broadband mirrors (useful bandwidth up to 300 nm) reflect higher frequencies closer to the surface and lower ones deeper inside the structure, causing less phase delay for the former and more for the latter — constituting negative dispersion.
*74 There are solitons in shallow-water surface waves, in crystals, in optical fibers etc. The latter became interesting for optical communications because pulses representing bits of information can propagate over thousands of kilometres without substantial change of shape, provided there is repetitive amplification.
*75 Blue stands for higher frequency facing larger *n*, i.e., slower phase velocity; vice versa for red.

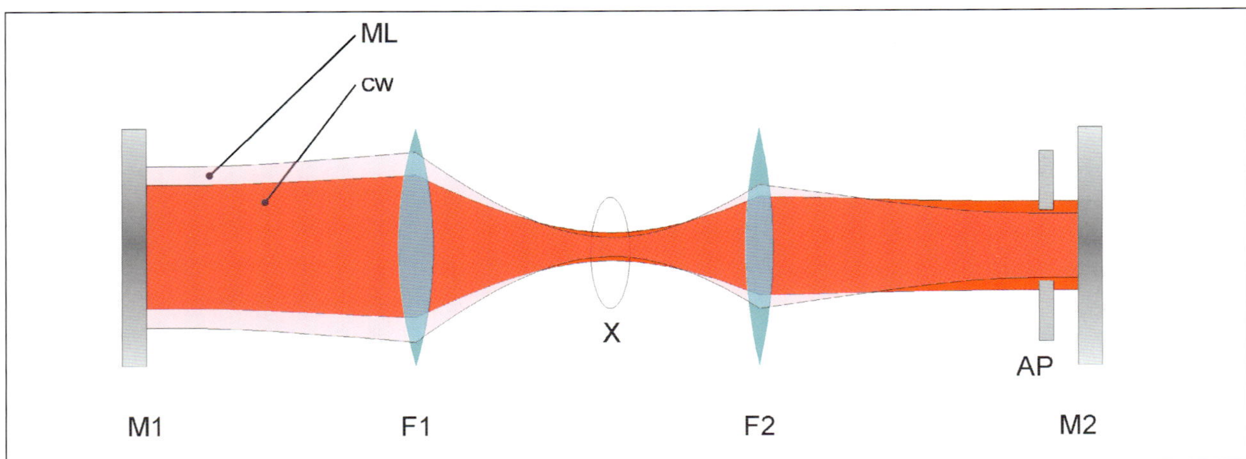

Fig 1-15a Generation of ultra-short pulses in a solid-state laser. Kerr lens mode-locking: according to the (Gaussian) intensity profile across the beam and the nonlinear Kerr effect (see Detail 1-8) an index distribution over the medium cross section X is induced acting as a graded index (GRIN) lens. It is only effective at of high intensities that cause the Kerr effect, and it allows different beam shapes and losses for the two limiting cases of intensity. M_1, M_2 mirrors; F_1, F_2 lenses; *AP*, aperture; *cw*, continuous wave and *ML* mode-locked operation.

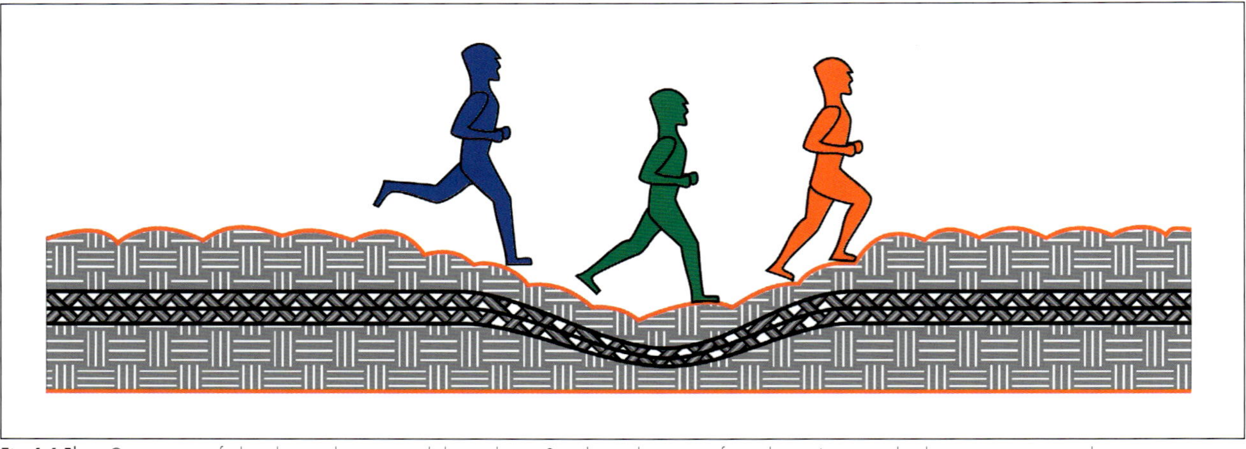

Fig 1-15b Generation of ultra-short pulses in a solid-state laser. Simple explanation of a soliton. An optical soliton represents a solitary intensity peak, which can propagate with unchanged shape over large distances. This is made possible by a constructive interplay between linear and nonlinear properties of the optical medium. In this comparison, three runners of different speed represent the frequency components of a light pulse. They influence their running conditions by their collective interaction (i.e., they compress the mattress by their weight like an intensive light pulse changes the speed of light in the medium where it propagates). They will stay together because the first, normally being the fastest, always has to run uphill, and vice versa.

Progress in ultra-short pulse generation (Fig. 1-16) has been one of the most outstanding in optics: the first operation of the ruby laser was already pulsed in the microsecond range. However, achieving cw emission was the challenging goal in 1960 and the years following. Dye lasers (especially Rhodamine 6G) provided sufficient bandwidth to allow extensive work in the 1970s and 1980s on ultra-fast laser technology and on investigation of ultra-fast phenomena. The corresponding records for shortest dye laser pulses out of the resonator and after external compression were 27 fs and 6 fs, respectively. From the 1990s on, ultra-fast laser technology based on solid-state lasers (mainly Ti:sapphire) was started, yielding most impressive results on "few-cycle

Detail 1-8.
Self-phase modulation along and orthogonal to progagation direction; linear and nonlinear dispersion.

As already indicated in footnote*72, intensity can change the index of refraction, according to $n = n_0 + n_2 I$. In Fig. 1-15 a) the result of this effect named electro-optic or **optical Kerr effect** on the cross section of a beam (i.e. **orthogonal** to z) is depicted leading to focusing in an appropriate medium (Kerr lens).

Most generally expressed, a light wave can be written as

$$\vec{E}\ (x,y,z,t) = \frac{1}{2}\vec{E}_0\,(x,y,z)\ \exp i(\omega t + \varphi\ (x,y,z,t)) + c.c.,$$

where φ represents the phase depending on location and time (the most general implementation of the optical Kerr effect). In the case of ultra-short pulses propagating in a medium, the temporal properties can be expressed by (we only consider $E = |\vec{E}|$ any further)

$$E(t) = A(t)e^{-i[\omega_0 t + \varphi(t)]}$$

where $A(t)$ represents the envelope of the pulse, ω_0 the carrier (i.e. mean) angular frequency and $\varphi(t)$ a time-dependent frequency shift called chirp (the word being derived from the sound sparrows generate).

A general Gaussian pulse as it commonly occurs, has a complex envelope of Gaussian shape

$$E(t) = E_0 \exp(-\gamma t^2)\exp(-i\omega_0 t)$$

with $\gamma = \alpha + i\beta$ (according to intensity dependence of phase) leading to

$$E(t) = E_0 \exp(-\alpha t^2)\exp(-i(\omega_0 t + \beta t^2))$$

where $A(t) = E_0 e^{-\alpha t^2}$ represents the classical Gaussian envelope and $\varphi(t) = \beta t^2$ the chirp.

The instantaneous frequency $\omega_i = \frac{\partial}{\partial t}(\omega_0 t + \beta t) = \omega_0 + 2\beta t$ follows a linear frequency shift as a result of the **optical Kerr effekt**, acting **along propagation**! $\beta > 0$ means linear growing while $\beta < 0$ linear decreasing carrier frequency (positive und negative chirp, respectively).

Due to **dispersion**, the propagation time T of a pulse for a distance L is a function of the angular frequency ω and can be formally expanded in a Taylor series:

$$T(\omega) = T(\omega_0) + D_2(\omega-\omega_0) + (1/2)\,D_3(\omega-\omega_0)^2 + (1/6)\,D_4(\omega-\omega_0)^3 + \ldots$$

where $D_i = (\partial^{i-1}/\partial t^{i-1})T(\omega_0)$ for $i = 2, 3, 4, \ldots$; D_2 is called group delay (linear dispersion); D_3 and D_4 are higher orders of dispersion negatively affecting ultra-short pulses.

Both self-phase modulation leading to chirp and linear dispersion are the two basic ingredients of the **concept of a soliton**.

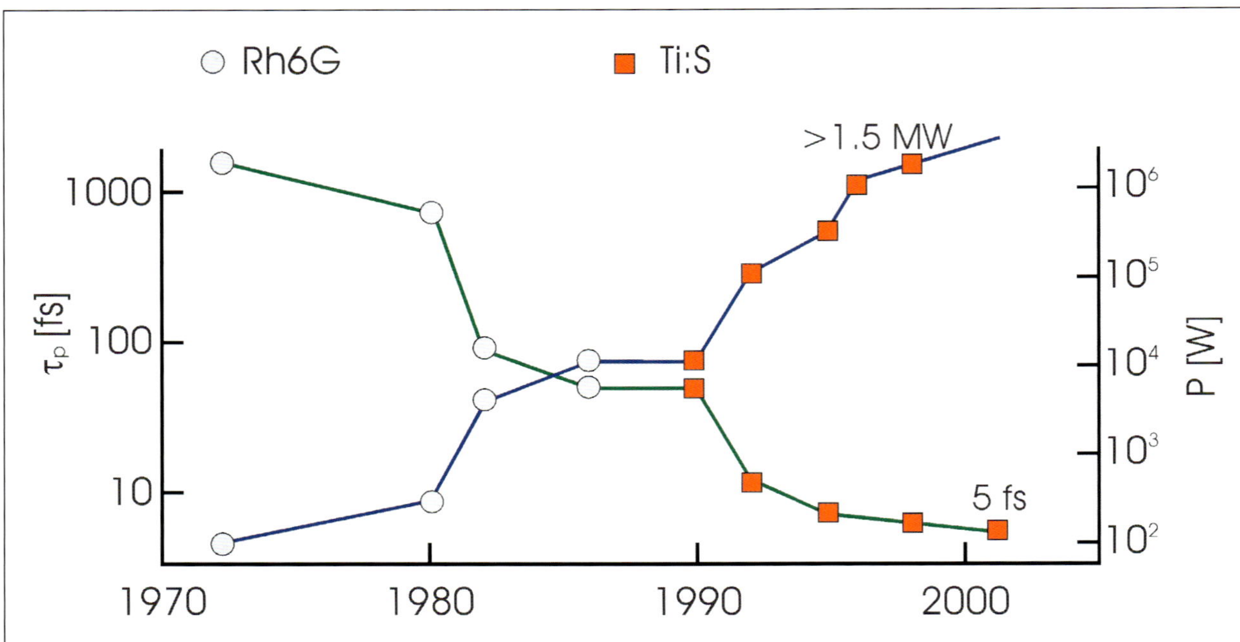

Fig 1-16 Progress in ultra-short pulse generation. Two types of laser, the Rhodamine 6G dye laser and the titanium-sapphire solid-state laser, were mainly responsible for the development of ever-shorter pulses directly emitted from laser resonators. The high peak powers represent a major advantage of ultra-short pulses enabling novel applications, e.g., dental hard tissue ablation with no collateral damage and without pain; τ_p, pulse duration, P, peak power of a pulse.

pulses" around 5 fs duration of substantial power (~ 10 nJ at ~ 100 MHz repetition rate corresponding to ~ 1 W average power) or sub-4 fs pulses of ~mJ energy and kHz repetition rate. The former specifications are going to revolutionize materials processing including that of organic tissue[7]. The latter have opened a new era of nonlinear and time-resolved optics based on attosecond pulses[8] in the soft X-ray range[*76], and are heading towards the realisation of an xraser (X-ray laser).

*76 The "water window" where especially organic, water-containing tissue is rather transparent at ~ 4 nm can be accessed for the first time by coherent radiation from a laboratory source.

1.4 Laser Media, Power Input and Optical Output

1.4.1 Laser Media

Most elements in the periodic system have been involved in some laser action so far, allowing the development of thousands of lasers. However, only some dozens of them have gained practical importance. Generally seen, laser media can be divided into atomic (such as HeNe) or molecular ones (gaseous, e.g. CO_2), further large organic molecules (of type Rh6G in liquid solution), ions (e.g. gaseous Ar^+, solid-state Nd^{3+}), excimers (e.g. KrF^*), semiconductor diodes (e.g. GaAs/GaAlAs), F-centers (e.g. F_2^+), chemical (HF^*)[*77] or even free-electron-based ones[*78].

Gases can be contained within appropriate tubes, which have to be sealed either by special, usually Brewster-type windows (present approach for heavy duty tubes as in the case of Ar laser or CO_2 laser, compare Fig. 1-42 in section 1.5.10 and Detail 1-9) or by dielectric mirrors (current solution for HeNe lasers). The orientations of the incident, reflected and refracted beams in the special case of Brewster's angle are drawn in Fig. 1-17a, the reflectivity[*79] for *S* and *P*[*80] polarizations over the 90° span of incidence angles in Fig. 1-17b. From this it becomes clear that in the *P* case at a certain angle no reflection takes place, i.e., there are no reflective losses at the tube win-

77 "Burning" H_2 and F_2 to form HF (* indicates an excited state) within a resonator can yield powerful laser emission; due to the large scale this is only relevant to the military so far.

*78 Periodically transversally accelerated electrons emitting bremsstrahlung generate coherent radiation under specific conditions; this is large-scale technology not relevant in this context.

*79 Referring to intensity; the reflection coefficient governs amplitude.

*80 *S* and *P* mean "senkrecht" (German, i.e., perpendicular) and parallel, respectively, referring to the orientation of the polarization of the incident light with respect to the plane of incidence (formed by the incident and reflected beams, also containing the vertical onto the reflecting surface).

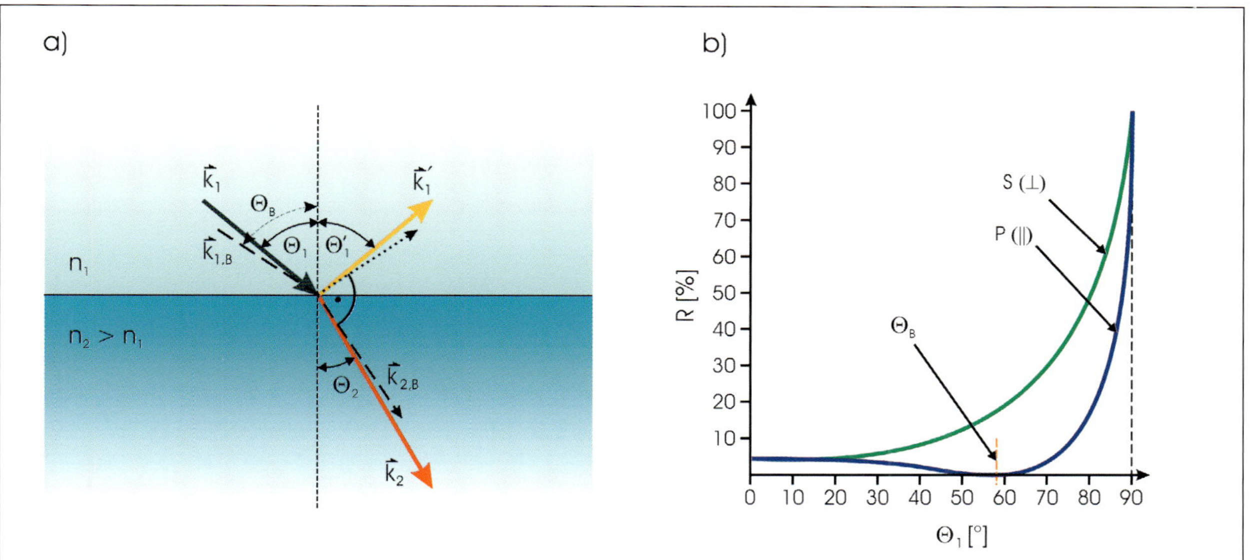

Fig 1-17 Brewster's angle: (a) ray representation and (b) reflectivity R at the interface air/glass (n_1 and n_2, respectively) depending on angle of incidence. $\vec{k}_1$, incident; $\vec{k}_1'$, reflected and $\vec{k}_2$, refracted beams; θ_1, θ_1', θ_2, angles of incidence, reflection and refraction, respectively; θ_B Brewster's angle only existing for *P* (in this case the reflected beam is vertical to the refracted one!); *S*, *P* polarizations (perpendicular) and parallel to plane of incidence between incident and reflected beam).

dows within a resonator. Simultaneously, this means that the output beam is always polarized[*81] accordingly. Normally, gas lasers contain the lasing species only up to a concentration of a few percent. A larger concentration is taken by some gases that are very effective in heat transportation, preferably He. In many cases, there is also a third component mixed in, which effects the removal of unwanted products of the favorable gas discharge excitation. This is done either by such buffer gases or by interactions with the wall (e.g., in the case of the HeNe laser). This latter process imposes a limitation to the maximum power to be generated. Usually, this demands larger cross sections. In the special case mentioned, however, this is excluded as the surface/volume relation becomes prohibitive.

Liquid laser media are primarily dyes dissolved in alcoholic solutions. The most prominent and most efficient of them is Rhodamine 6G[*82], a large aniline-based molecule as shown in Fig. 1-18. Due to their complex nature, dyes allow many vibrational modes, each of them having its characteristic quantized energy. As these energy levels are so densely arranged they overlap, thereby forming wide energy bands as shown in Fig. 1-19.

The levels are drawn in the figure in such a way that the left column contains the *S* levels[*83] defined by the orbit angular momentum zero, and the right column the *T* levels having angular momentum one[*84]. The *S* column represents a wide variety of four-level systems allowing broad-band laser emission. If an appropriate filter is put into the laser, tunable light may be emitted (compare Fig. 1-12); if a temporal modulation is carried out, mode-locking may take place giving rise to the generation of shortest pulses (compare Fig. 1-14 and Fig. 1-16).

Solid-state laser media mostly consist of a host medium with laser ions or molecules embedded in it. The spectroscopic characteristics of the emission reflect to a vast extent the properties of the lasing species; however, they are affected by the internal fields of the solid medium (see also for a comparison Detail 1-2). Preferably, the

Detail 1-9.
Explanation of the origin of Brewster's angle.

If radiation interacts with matter it becomes polarized according to

$$\vec{P}(t) = \chi \otimes \vec{E}(t)$$

where χ is the susceptibility, depending on material and frequency. Both, $\vec{P}$ and $\vec{E}$ are functions of time t. $\vec{P}(t)$ radiates and hence emits an electromagnetic wave again. This process is somewhat delayed by material properties and results in a slower propagation velocity, the origin of the refractive index n. Light emission of this kind obeys the same rules a the emission of radio radiation from an antenna following a $(sin^2\alpha)$ law (α being the angle between direction of propagation and antenna orientation – in our case corresponding to polarization, i.e. to the direction of the electric field $\vec{E}$). As is well known in electrical engineering, an antenna does not radiate parallel to its orientation. In the case of Brewster orientation, the refracted beam is orthogonal to the reflected beam (see Fig. 1-17) and, hence, in the case of *P* polarization there is a corresponding situation that does not allow a reflected beam.

*81 Every laser emitting coherent light is polarized. The direction of polarization will diffuse randomly if no structural element forces it to stay in some orientation.

*82 The Rhodamine and Coumarine dyes were introduced before 1900 as so-called aniline dyes for the coloring of cloth by Badische Anilin- und Sodafabrik (BASF), Germany.

*83 In atoms the orbit quantum number l is always $l \leq n - 1$ with n being the principal quantum number. $l = 0$ is symbolized by s, $l = 1$ by p, $l = 2$ by d, $l = 4$ by f (for historic reasons those letters stand for sharp, principal, diffuse and fundamental spectroscopic line series); for molecules this was taken over, but writing the symbols for states as capitals. *S* and *T* in Fig. 1-19 stand for singlet and triplet according to the multiplicity of lines within an external field (according to the magnetic quantum number).

*84 Due to the selection rules optical transitions between *S* and *T* states are forbidden; only under special circumstances can such intersystem crossing happen.

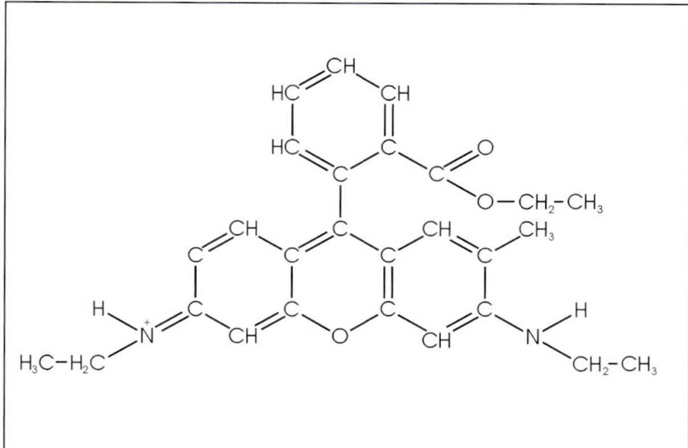

Fig 1-18 Structure of the molecule Rhodamine 6G, which is one of the most important dye laser media.

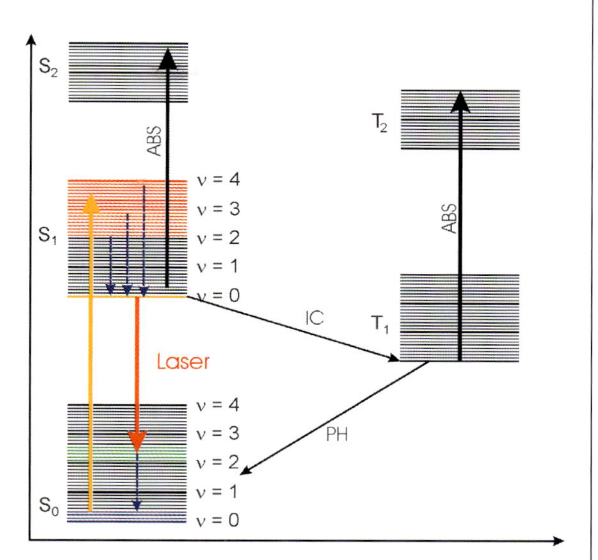

Fig 1-19 Energy level scheme of Rhodamine 6G, revealing broad bands being composed of many overlapping vibrational levels. The vertical bold yellow arrows represents the intended pump absorption, the black arrows indicate excited state absorption (ABS), the red one he tunable laser transition (Laser), all of them only allowed between states of the same type. The blue arrows stand for non-radiative transitions within the bands. Black faint arows between the two coloumn: non-radiative transition (*IC*) between different types of states (S_i singlet, T_i triplet); *PH*, radiative phosphorescence.

medium chosen is a crystal because it may offer optimum heat transportation properties (one of the best being YAG, i.e., yttrium aluminum garnet). If high power has to be generated, along with a demand for larger crystals this may cause technological problems in single crystal preparation. Recently, the concept of polycrystalline ceramic laser media has become extremely successful. Starting from a nanometre-structured material, an optically homogeneous solid is "sintered" together which allows any shape and large sizes. Before, only doped glasses could be manufactured to larger dimensions, although at the cost of smaller heat conductivity, limiting power to typically 0.5 W. In some cases, the larger variation of binding forces in a glass, with respect to a crystal, yielded spectrally broader emissions useful for ultra-short pulse generation.

The doping ions for solid-state lasers are usually taken out of two groups in the periodic system: either rare earths (such as Nd^{3+}, Yb^{3+}, Ho^{3+}, Er^{3+}) or transition metals (such as Cr^{2+}, Cr^{3+}, Cr^{4+}, Ti^{3+}). The former are rather efficient but rather narrow-band, the latter offering the widest spectral widths. The semiconductor laser is different to all of them: it is based on solid semiconductor crystals uniting laser and host properties, thereby containing the highest density of states to be potentially inverted (allowing highest amplification).

Also, solid-state lasers may contain a laser medium confined by Brewster angle cuts, or by facets carrying reflective or anti-reflective coatings depending on the position with respect to the resonator. An actual example is represented by the slab laser as depicted in Fig. 1-20: the laser radiation with $\vec{E}$ polarization (orthogonal to the paper) leaves the medium on both sides without reflective losses and is confined by the resonator mirrors. Another important method of radiation confinement is employed in the slab laser and is to be seen in the figure, i.e., total internal reflection as illustrated in Fig. 1-21. It allows a long propagation path within the laser medium thereby overlapping with even non-focused pump light (e.g., of a diode array; compare Section 1.5.4). Waveguides (employed, e.g., in diode lasers) are based on the same principle of total internal reflection on two

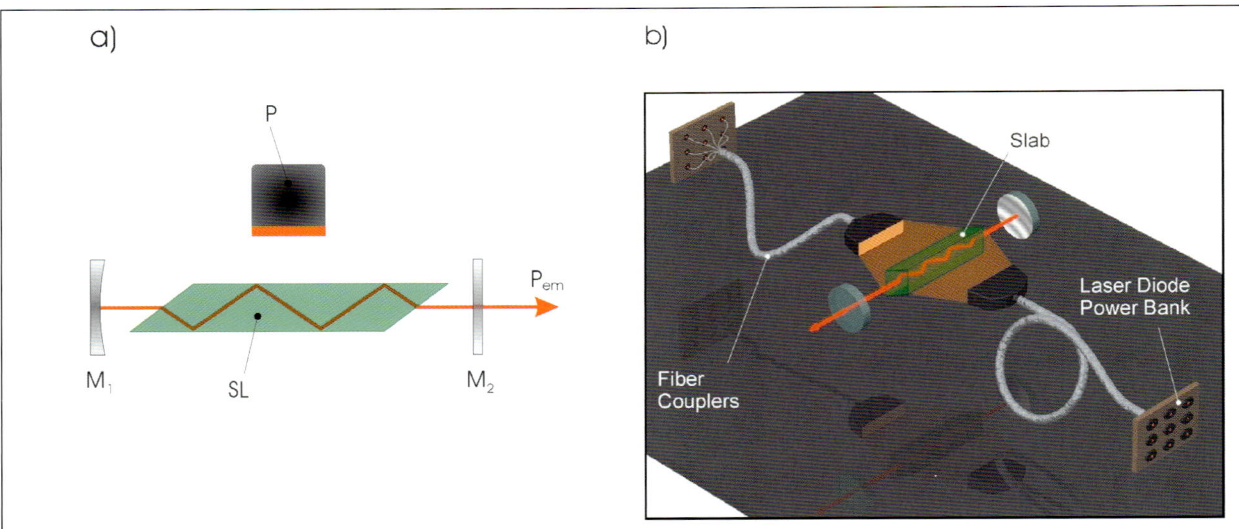

Fig 1-20 Slab laser: (a) resonator scheme including pump source *P*, (b) three-dimensional view[10] above an optical table also depicting stacked array laser diodes being fiber coupled; M_1, M_2, resonator mirrors; P_{em}, emitted radiation.

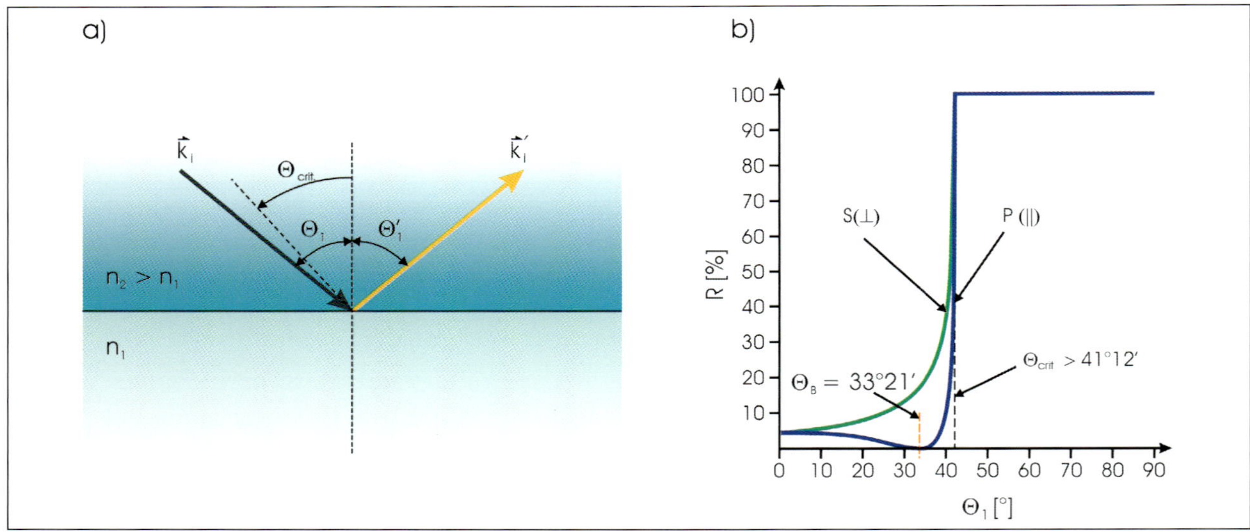

Fig 1-21 Total internal reflection: (a) ray representation and (b) reflectivity *R* at interface glass/air (n_2 and n_1, respectively) depending on the angle of incidence. $\vec{k}_1$, incident and $\vec{k}_1{}'$ reflected beams; θ and θ' are equal angles of incidence and reflection, respectively; θ_B is the internal Brewster's angle (33°21′) only existing for *P*-polarization; θ_{crit} is the critical angle for total internal reflection (41°12′); *S*, *P* are polarizations ("senkrecht" (vertical) and parallel).

interfaces between an optically denser medium in the middle (n_2) and thinner media to the sides (n_1 and n_3)[*85] , exactly as in the slab laser geometry. There are many variations of solid-state laser designs, a representative number of solutions being discussed in Section 1.5.

*85 The condition $n_1 < n_2 > n_3$ has to be fulfilled!

1.4.2 Pumping Methods and Schemes

There is a wide range of options for pumping, in order to transfer energy into the laser medium. Only if pumped hard enough (compare Detail 1-3), is inversion reached so that amplification can take place. The following processes may be employed:

- optical pumping by strong lamps or lasers
- electric pumping by gas discharges
- chemical pumping by reactions yielding excited molecules
- impact pumping by inelastic collisions between partners (impacts of second order)
- electronic pumping by diffusion of carriers in semiconductors
- pumping by acceleration of electrons (free electron laser)

For the lasers covered in this book, only optical, electric, impact and electronic pumping are relevant. Electronic pumping is described in Section 1.5.4 dealing with the semiconductor laser. This is the best laser to date with respect to effectivity (>50%), cost and maintenance. It is the cheapest source of monochromatic light of substantial power and is excellent when used for optical pumping. Fig. 1-22 shows a comparison between a xenon arc lamp, a common traditional optical pump light source, and an AlGaAs diode laser. Obviously, the emission of the latter is much narrower and can be selected by composition in such a way that the emitted wavelength coincides exactly with an absorption band of the laser medium (depicted for Nd:glass in the figure 1-22; compare also Section 1.5.7). Only in the case of much narrower absorption bands or lines, the emission of the diode has to be stabilized because its wavelength is influenced by changes in temperature and current. During diode pumping, heat production which is always detrimental in a laser is reduced; effectivity is thereby simultaneously improved.

Diode laser pump light can be transported through optical fibers as shown in Fig. 1-20b or collimated by a certain amount to hit the active volume of the laser material. In the case of a slab laser this volume is rather elongated, and in the case of the extremely successful thin disk laser (see Fig. 1-23) the pump spot is narrower (*D* is a few mm). Because cooling through the heat sink is so successful, out of ~1 mm^3 of laser crystal, kW power can be extracted. There are also certain versions of other longitudinally pumped solid-state or dye lasers where strong collimation of the pump light is indispensable. In such cases, optical pumping by a conventional laser may still be the method of choice (e.g., a cw dye laser is usually pumped by an Ar laser employing a pump focus of $D = 20$ µm!).

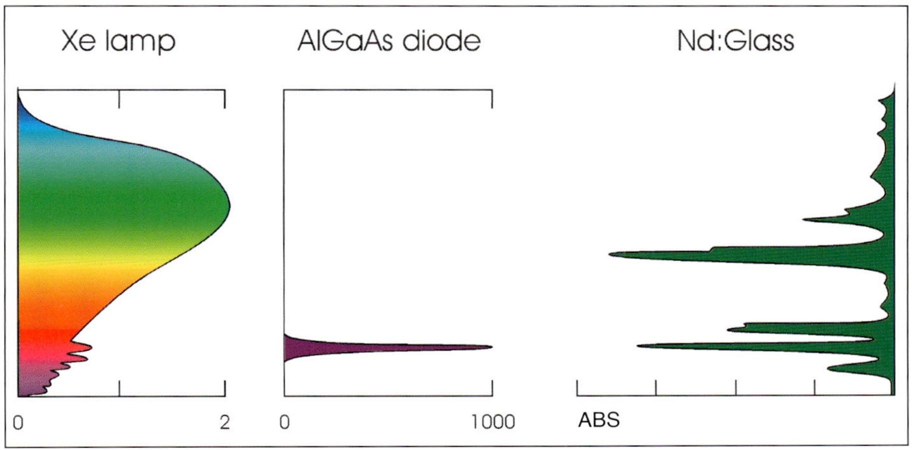

Fig 1-22 Comparison of two optical pump sources: Xe arc lamp and AlGaAs diode laser (spectral intensity given in W/cm^2 nm). To estimate effectivity, the absorption spectrum ABS (in relative units versus wavelength or frequency) of Nd:glass, which is a very common solid-state laser medium, is depicted.[10]

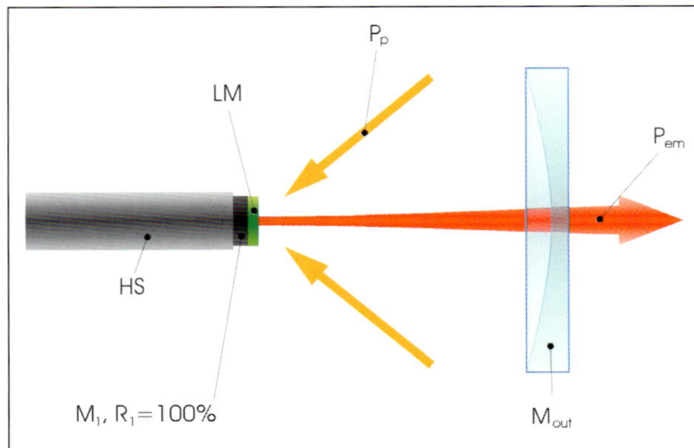

Fig 1-23 Thin disk laser: the pump radiation P_p from – preferably – a set of laser diodes passing through a thin platelet of laser medium *LM* (green, most successfully Yb:YAG) up to 16 times before being completely absorbed. Mounting on a heat sink *HS* exerts very effective cooling. M_1 (with R_1 reflectivity) and M_{out} are resonator mirrors; P_{em}, emitted power.

1.4.3 Geometrical and Frequency Conversion of the Laser Output

In the ideal case, a laser emits a Gaussian beam. By focusing it, another Gaussian is yielded with a narrower waist and more divergence (compare Fig. 1-7)[*86]. The quality of a beam can be expressed by the M^2 factor as defined and explained in Detail 1-10. If $M^2 = 1$ the beam is ideal and is called Fourier limited. Especially in the case of a diode laser as shown in Fig. 1-24, the output deviates strongly from ideal: the beam is even astigmatic with more divergence*[87] in the direction of the narrower dimension of the emitting aperture and thereby creating an elliptic cross section in the far field. In this case, the *M* parameters are different in the two directions that are orthogonal with respect to propagation direction. Nevertheless M^2 can be defined and stays constant in the best case during transformation by special aspheric optics in order to yield a round beam. If the optical system is imperfect, M^2 can only become larger.

Detail 1-10.
Propagation of real laser beams,
beam parameter product.

In the **ideal case,** laser beams are TEM_{00} **Gaussian rays.** These are fully characterized by the wavelength λ and the beam waist w_0. Because w_0 can be adjusted freely, e.g. via lenses, generally the **beam parameter product,** defined as

$$\theta w_0 = \frac{\lambda}{\pi}$$

(units mm·mrad) is observed.
As can be seen easily, for Gaussian beams it is dependent only on λ.

Real beams may be a combination of several transversal modes, overlapping in such a way that the real beam radius $W(z)$ at any position z is larger than $w(z)$ by a constant factor M: $W(z) = Mw(z)$,
and accordingly $\Theta = M\theta$,
with Θ being the divergence of the real beam. If in comparison the same beam waist for ideal and real beams is assumed, the relation

$$\theta = M^2\frac{\lambda}{\pi w_0} \cdot M^2 \geq 1 \text{ holds.}$$

$M^2 \geq 1$ is always valid.
M^2 defines how much the beam deviates from diffraction limitation.

*86 Focusing is one type of Fourier transformation under which a Gaussian beam is invariant.
*87 In the case of astigmatic beams we talk about fast (vertical in Fig. 1-24) and slow axis (horizontal).

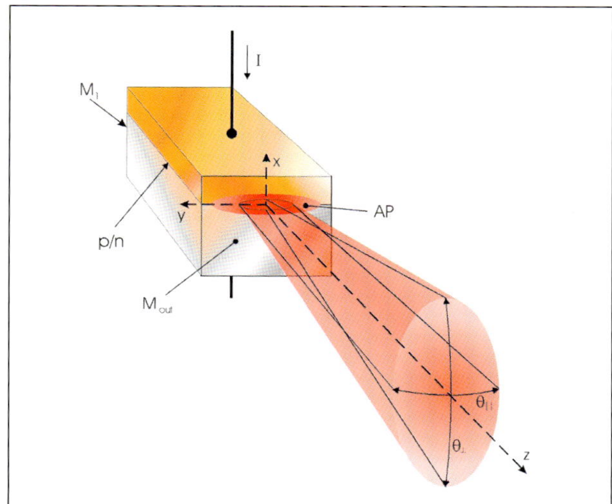

Fig 1-24 Beam characteristic of a laser diode: the astigmatic beam having divergence angles $\theta_{\perp}$ (fast axis) and $\theta_{//}$ (slow axis) emitted from an elliptic active optical aperture *AP* reveals an elliptic cross section in the far field (orthogonal with respect to aperture). M_1 and M_{out} are resonator mirrors (mostly cleaved facets); *I* is the current through the *pn* junction.

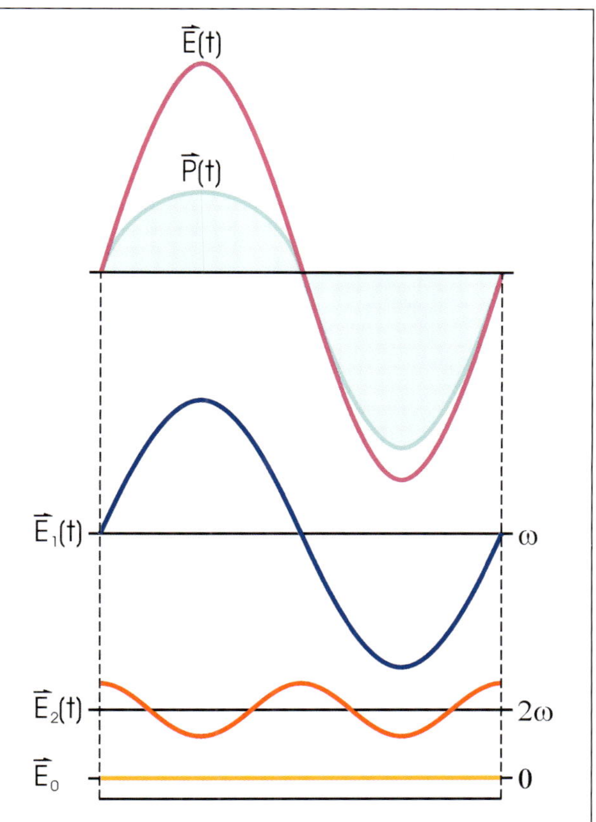

Fig 1-25 Frequency conversion: the oscillating electric field $\vec{E}(t)$ of a light wave incident onto matter creates a non-linear polarization $\vec{P}(t)$ which again emits electromagnetic waves containing components $\vec{E}_1(t)$ with the fundamental frequency ω (first harmonic) as well as $\vec{E}_2(t)$ with the doubled frequency 2ω (second harmonic) and even higher harmonics. Additionally, there is also a constant field component $\vec{E}_0$ (all of them are depicted).

Detail 1-11.
Brightness being a most relevant characterization of light.

The average power of a beam and its collimation (i.e. divergent nature) can be expressed simultaneously by an additional quantity called brightness L, describing the power P per area A and steric angle Ω:

$$L = \frac{P}{A\Omega}.$$

For a given area of beam waist, Ω is determined by M^2 and λ so that

$$L = \frac{P}{\lambda^2 M^4}.$$

This quadratic dependence of brightness on M^2 explains why commercial multimode lasers ($M^2 > 30$) even at average power of several kW have rather poor brightness, this being lower than that of diffraction-limited light sources of only ~100 W.

In many cases, the user is not satisfied with the wavelength or wavelength range a laser can emit. A special phenomenon at high intensity, the non linear frequency conversion, allows frequencies to be changed. Specifically, under such conditions, sum frequencies and difference frequencies can be generated, with frequency doubling being a special case among them. Fig. 1-25 illustrates the aspect of

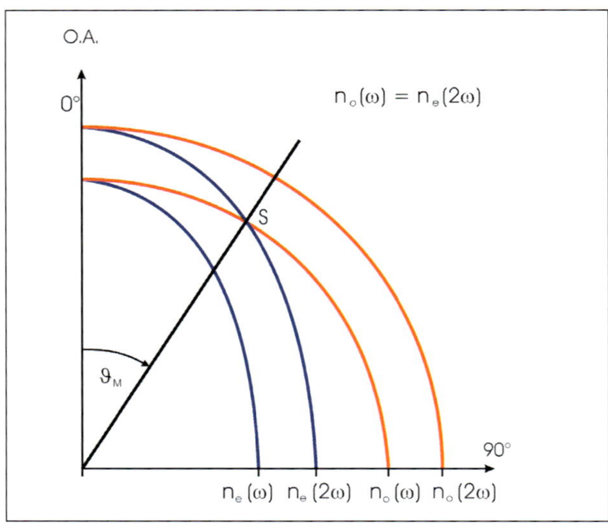

Fig 1-26 Angular phase matching: in crystals with birefringence under special geometric conditions, the same phase velocity for ω and 2ω light can be achieved. n_o and n_e are refractive indices of the othogonally polarized ordinary or extra-ordinary beams at ω or 2ω, respectively. S marks the phase-matching axis inclined at an angle ϑ_m to the optical axis (O.A.).

non linear polarization giving rise to the emission of harmonic waves (second harmonic in this example) representing multiples (the doubled one in this case) of the fundamental angular frequency.

Mathematical aspects of this conversion may be found in Detail 1-12. Generally speaking, such non-linear effects are weak but happen at every point of the trajectory of the beam through appropriate matter[*88]. It looks obvious that one may expect to sum up all small contributions yielding eventually a strong conversion. Unfortunately, in almost every material there is dispersion, and hence the two harmonics do not propagate at the same phase velocity[*89]. As a matter of fact, after a certain propagation distance called coherence length ℓ_c,[*90] the contributions to the second harmonic from along the path of the beam get into antiphase and hence reduce the already existing amplitude, which finally reaches zero before increasing again thereafter. Only by a sophisticated trick can equal propagation velocity for the first and second harmonics be achieved: employing birefringence. Nonlinear frequency generation can also yield orthogonal polarizations for the harmonics[*91] which then may correspond to the ordinary and extra-ordinary beams in a birefringent crystal. At a certain angle from the crystal axis, depicted in Fig. 1-26, $n_e(2\omega)$ and $n_o(\omega)$ may become equal, which allows phase-matched propagation of the fundamental and the second harmonic, eventually turning a substantial[*92] fraction of the fundamental power into second harmonic power. There are also other methods for frequency conversion that, however, are not effectively used in our context.

The higher the harmonic, the lower the yield! This is certainly valid for the third harmonic. For the fourth harmonic one may also proceed via iterated frequency doubling. To increase power and intensity in the area of interaction, sharp focusing may be attempted. This is associated with a small depth of focus and hence a short interaction zone at high intensity. If possible, one may specifically use frequency doubling of pulsed radiation in order to achieve a higher yield[*93]. Finally, considering that within a resonator the power and intensity are much higher, the frequency doubler crystal may be implemented in the cavity so that this represents the only outlet of radiation energy (there is no outcoupling mirror for the fundamental, but a dichroic mirror lets only the second harmonic pass through)[*94].

Detail 1-12.
The nonlinear polarization leading to harmonic waves.

The electric field $\vec{E}$ (or written as components E_i) of a light wave forces electrons in a medium to oscillate and induces dipoles thereby. The density of dipole moments is called $\vec{P}$ (also written as P_i) and should not be confused with polarization of a light wave. The oscillating polarization is again the source of radiation. Generally, the relation

$$P_i = \varepsilon_0(\chi_{ij}^{(1)}E_j + \chi_{ijk}^{(2)}E_jE_k + \chi_{ijkl}^{(3)}E_jE_kE_l + \ldots)$$

is valid it is preferably written in tensor style with $\chi^{(n)}$ being a tensor of stage $n+1$ representing the different orders of susceptibility. In this way it is expressed that, in the general case, $\vec{E}$ and $\vec{P}$ (as well as the emitted light polarization) may be non-parallel.

The magnitude of $\chi^{(n)}$ decreases rapidly with order n:

$\chi^{(1)} \approx 1,\ \chi^{(2)} \approx 10^{-12}\ m/V$

$\chi^{(3)} \approx 10^{-21}\ m^2/V^2$

Therefore the realization of nonlinear frequency mixing based on this background is very often extremely inefficient.

Sum and difference frequency generation, for example, can be easily understood according to the following considerations (assuming two planar incident waves with $\vec{k}_1$ and $\vec{k}_2$ as their wave vectors and ω_1 and ω_2 as their angular frequencies):

$$E_i \propto \exp i\,(\vec{k}_i\vec{x} - \omega_i t)$$

$$P_i^{(2)} = (\omega, \vec{k}) \propto \chi_{ijk}^{(2)}E_j \exp i\,(\vec{k}_1\vec{x} - \omega_1 t)\ E_k \exp i\,(\vec{k}_2\vec{x} - \omega_2 t)$$

Multiplication shows that $\omega = \omega_1 \pm \omega_2$ and $\vec{k} = \vec{k}_1 \pm \vec{k}_2$ and $\vec{P}$ may be non-parallel to either $\vec{E}_1$ and $\vec{E}_2$. A very special case, employed in **phase-matched second harmonic generation** is $\omega = 2\omega_1$
because in this case $\omega_1 = \omega_2$
Thereby the incoming and outgoing waves may be orthogonally polarized (comp. Fig. 1-26).

---

*88 In case of intended frequency doubling no inversion symmetry of the material is allowed.

*89 It is essential in this context that at every point the harmonics are in phase.

*90 Typically being around 10 µm for many non-linear optic materials.

*91 In this case it would be more correct to call it sum frequency generation, even if we deal with 2ω light.

*92 The percentage can be up to > 50%, although limited even at highest intensities by back-conversion into the fundamental via difference frequency generation.

*93 This can often be observed with green beams of Nd lasers: when moved they show a line of points on a screen.

*94 In this way, little green laser pointers based on frequency-doubled Nd vanadate achieve rather high conversion efficencies.

1.5 Specific Lasers Relevant for Oral Applications

In this section the most important lasers for oral use are described, but only in enough detail for their operation to become evident. Knowledge of general aspects, as mentioned in the previous sections, is assumed. The following sequence of subsections is ordered by rising wavelength rather than importance.

1.5.1 Excimer Lasers

The excimer laser is a special gas laser based on unstable molecules called excimers[*95]. They exist only in the excited state for nanoseconds, just long enough for pulsed laser action. The noble gas constituents are confined in a laser tube containing high voltage electrodes as shown in Fig. 1-27. Via discharges, the atoms are excited and form excimers for a short time, whereby an inversion arises. The tube is implemented in a simple unstable resonator that has only a small effect. More typically, the light is generated as amplified spontaneous emission (ASE), and the "laser" is more like a super-radiator (see Fig. 1-9). As the lifetime of the excimers is rather short, ns pulses are emitted and hence there is no time to form a clear mode pattern. The emitted beam has basically the shape of the window, which is indicated in the figure. Detail 1-13 contains the most important performance data. According to the numerous UV lines, this type of laser represents the most important source of such short-wavelength radiation.

95 This is an artificial word combining excited dimer, meaning molecules of two (equal) components. (Compare also the word polymer). This applies only to such molecules as $Ar_2{}^*$, $Kr_2{}^*$, and N_2 and F_2, which are also employed in such a laser set-up but which, of course, represent stable species. Noble gas halides (like ArF), the characteristic excimers, should be properly named exciplex (from excited complex).

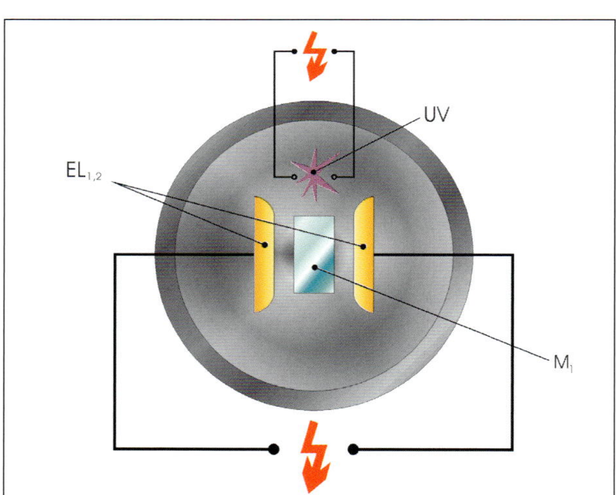

Fig 1-27 Cross section through an excimer laser tube: it contains the high voltage electrodes EL_1 and EL_2 for creating pulsed discharges (in the center the rear laser mirror M_1 is indicated). Via some ionization provided by a UV source, reliable ignition of the discharge can be achieved.

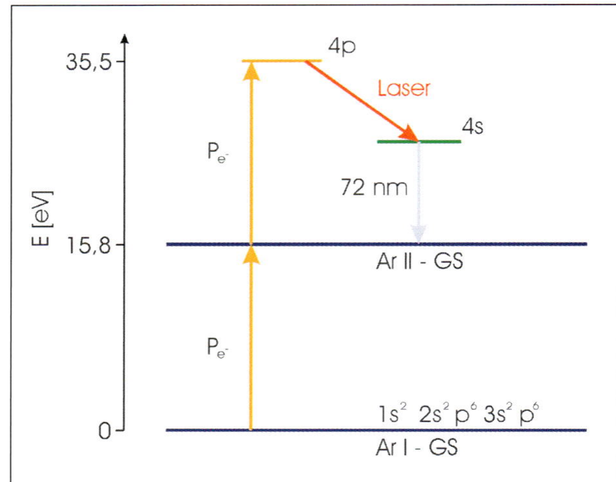

Fig 1-28 Energy levels and excitation process of the argon laser: for the ground state the complete electronic configuration is indicated (the upper index telling the number of electrons in the state). Vertical coordinate: energy *E*, *GS* ground state of neutral Ar I and single-ionized argon Ar II (Ar^+); P_{e}, excitation by electron impact; *Laser*, laser transition.

Detail 1-13.
Typical data of excimer lasers.

Transversal discharge of 30 kV and 10–30 ns duration with electric power density ~100 MW/ℓ needed; repetition rate ~1 kHz, flow of gases ~10 m/s for beam width of 5 mm; gas pressure 1–4 bars; composition: 5–10% active noble gas, 0.1–0.5% halogen, remainder buffer gas (He or Ne). Efficiency: a few percent; 10^5 to 10^7 modes created; $\ell_c \approx 0.1$ mm; $\Delta\lambda \approx$ 1–2 nm; beam profile 10 x 20 mm^2.				
laser gas	λ (nm)	E (mJ)	τ_p (ns)	P_{ave} (W)
F_2*	158	60	10–30	10
ArF*	193	650	10–30	10
KrF*	248	1200	10–30	5
XeCl*	308	600	10–30	10
XeF*	351	400	10–30	10

Excimer laser UV light can ablate tissue very effectively via photochemical interaction[*96] without depositing heat therein. In general, this sounds attractive for dental laser applications. However, the beam has bad characteristics and cannot be transported effectively via optical fibers[*97]. The laser itself is very expensive, and has no potential for reduction of size or cost . The gases have limited lifetime[*98], and some of them are expensive (e.g., Xe) or poisonous and aggressive (e.g., F_2). Short UV wavelengths, especially $\lambda = 248$ nm, are potentially carcerogenic because as they can sever the chromosomes of the cell nuclus.

1.5.2 Argon Ion Laser

From the ionized noble gases (Ne, Ar, Kr, Xe), more than 250 lines within the spectroscopic range from 175 to 1100 nm can be emitted in gas discharges. The higher the ionization state, the shorter are the wavelengths. In this context only the Ar laser is of importance as it can emit cw up to 100 W in the blue-green and up to 60 W in the UV. As is shown in Fig. 1-28, Ar is first ionized-by the impact of electrons, and, upon a second collision, is transferred into the excited state representing the upper laser level. As only highly energetic electrons can contribute to energies in the range of 35 eV, a low quantum efficiency results. Because the $4p$ and $4s$ states are split into many sub-levels, radiation of several transitions will be emitted (see Detail 1-14) if the resonator supports it.

Due to the high discharge currents and the high temperature of the ionized gas, reaching up to 5×10^3 K, very resistive tube materials have to be chosen, such as BeO (most common type) or graphite. A high heat conductivity is especially important. Within the tube, rings of tungsten are positioned to remove the heat to the outer tube surround, and to center the emission. Owing to the high density of electrons (~ 10^{14} cm^{-3}) these are moved to the outer radius of the tube thereby reducing the current density. This can be compen-

*96 In this case, energy-rich photons can break the bonds of complex molecules and turn them into volatile radicals.

*97 Free motion of the output beam is achieved only by employing an articulate arm with mirrors at the joints, which can be rotated. Such a device is bulky, expensive and heavy.

*98 Typically 10^8 shots.

Detail 1-14.
Emission lines of an Argon ion laser.

Gas pressure 1–100 Pa, pure Ar			
385.1–351.1 nm	3 W	528.7 nm	2 W
363.8–333.6 nm	5 W	514.5 nm	10 W
335.8–300.3 nm	2 W	501.7 nm	2 W
305.5–275.4 nm	0.6 W	496.5 nm	3 W
		488.0 nm	10 W
		476.5 nm	3 W
		472.7 nm	1 W
		465.8 nm	1 W
		457.9 nm	1 W
		454.5 nm	1 W
		all lines together	20 W

The UV and visible emissions need different optics. Wavelength selection is mostly achieved by a combination of prism dispersion and mirror adjustment (in this case, for different colors different resonator alignments have to be found!), to some extent also by specified dielectric mirrors.

sated by an external longitudinal magnetic field induced by a coil around the tube. By means of the Lorentz force (oriented vertical to the field and to the radial component of motion) a helical trajectory is achieved, together with a concentration of the discharge along the axis. This reduces wear of the tube wall material and increases the efficiency of the laser. Nevertheless, this type of laser is extremely inefficient[*99], with $\eta < 10^{-3}$.

Owing to the low amplification within the laser (g = 2.7/m) the tube has to be rather long, typically around 1.5 m, and hence only allows small outcoupling (a few percent). This laser is expensive to purchase and to maintain (the tube life is only around 1000 h), and it is space-consuming and demands strong electric and cooling supplies, which is especially inconvenient when mobile use is intended. Within dentistry, the applications are very limited. Nevertheless, this laser is a traditional representative of a well-collimated visible laser that is useful for exciting fluorescence due to the rather short blue and green wavelengths. For the same reason, it was and still is used as a pump source for most cw dye lasers.

1.5.3 Helium–Neon Laser

This type is one of the forerunners of all lasers, which was at first theoretically proposed[*100], and then demonstrated in 1961[*101]. Since then, it has developed into the most investigated laser and the best understood of all. Generally, only the red 632 nm emission was widely applied as a pointing beam, however becoming replaced in recent years by diode lasers of similar wavelength. On the other hand, also other wavelengths became

*99 The typical electric supply specifications are 63 A at 380 V yielding a few Watts of output; nearly all the power has to be cooled away.
*100 By the laser inventors N.G. Basov and A.M. Prokhorov, and Ch.T. Townes in 1958.
*101 By A. Javan at M.I.T, Cambridge, MA.

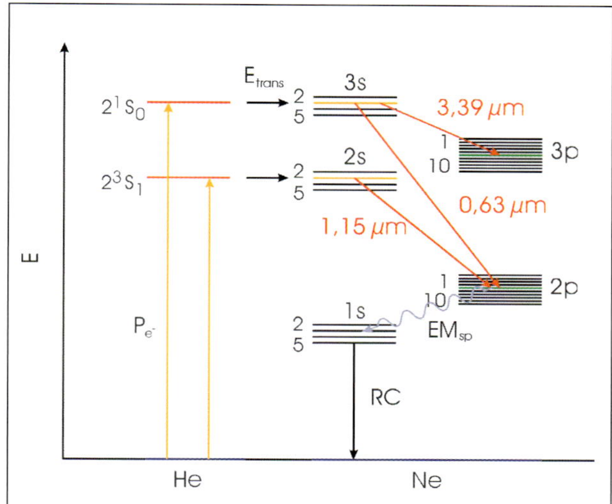

Fig 1-29 Four-level diagram of the HeNe laser: excitation by electron impact P_{e^-} (yellow vertical arrows) mainly affects He which transfers its energy to Ne; red arrows: laser transitions with indicated wavelength; blue waved arrow: spontaneous emission EM_{sp}. Vertical axis: E, energy; E_{trans}, energy transfer (impacts of 2nd kind), RC, recombination at the discharge tube wall.

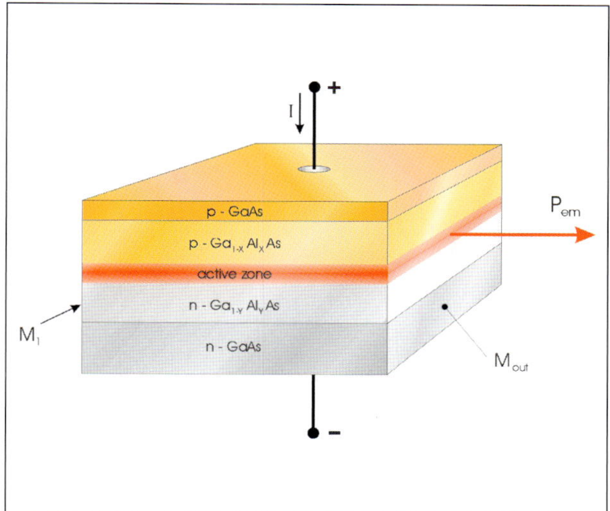

Fig 1-30 Block diagram of a double heterostructure diode laser (example GaAlAs/GaAs): the active zone is the source of radiation which is laterally rather broad in this basic version (no stripe confinement). The cleaved facets represent a simple resonator ("mirror" M_{out}). Light is guided within the active zone by a planar waveguide effect. I, current through the diode, P_{em}, laser radiation.

commercially available within the last decade. The lay-out of levels in Fig. 1-29 depicts all of the important lines (see more in Detail 1-15). It is the classical gas laser of low power (typically a few mW), and, in terms of the emission, is a Ne laser rather than a combination. The performance can barely be increased because collisions with the wall are essential as depicted in the figure. At large diameters, the ratio between volume and surface area becomes more and more unfavorable.

The beams of such lasers are usually of very good quality. The degree of polarization is about 1000:1. The coherence length ℓ_c of commercial products is around 200–300 mm, which even allows holography of small objects. In laser dentistry, only beam-pointing applications are known.

1.5.4 Semiconductor Diode Lasers

Semiconductor lasers need not be diode lasers in all cases. Especially in the early years, it was not possible to produce the newly developed semiconductors with pn-junctions incorporated. Therefore, at least for a while, either optical or electron-beam pumping was employed. Nowadays, the outstanding success of the semiconductor laser is closely linked to the availability of pn-junctions. Even more, double hetero-junctions[*102] are the basic requirement for good performance, as depicted in Fig. 1-30. This concept allowed the first cw room-temperature operation.

*102 A pn-junction represents an electrically conductive connection between two semiconductor regions of the same type but different doping (more precisely called a homojunction). It is named hetero-junction if the two semiconductor layers are similar (e.g., by lattice parameters, otherwise there could be no good electrical contact) but having, e.g., different electronic properties, such as bandgap, and optical properties, such as index of refraction.

Detail 1-15.
Specifications of the HeNe laser.

Gas composition: for red HeNe = 5:1, for infrared at 1.15 µm HeNe = 10:1. Electric supply: 2 kV und 5–10 mA, length of discharge typically ≥ 100 mm. Diameter of capillary D = 1 mm; pressure has to observe $p\ D$ = 500 Pa mm; lifetime 20,000 h.

wavelength λ	power P	bandwidth $\Delta\nu$	gain g
3391 nm	>10 mW	280 MHz	100.000/m
1523 nm	1 mW	625 MHz	
1153 nm	1 mW	825 MHz	
640 nm (red)			
635 nm (red)			
633 nm (red)	>10 mW	1500 MHz	0.100/m
629 nm (red)			
612 nm (orange)	1 mW	1550 MHz	0.017/m
604 nm (orange)			
594 nm (yellow)	1 mW	1600 MHz	0.005/m
543 nm (green)	1 mW	1750 MHz	0.005/m

Generally, if a free flow of carriers is possible via a pn-junction, this will take place as a result of different concentrations and following diffusion laws. The Fermi levels[*103] F_1 and F_2 of the two semiconductor regions with p and n doping, respectively, arrange themselves at the same energy F as shown in Fig. 1-31a). The diffusion voltage U_D stops further diffusion via the build-up of space charges inside the contact zone, also called the carrier depletion zone (being mostly depleted of mobile carriers).

By poling a laser diode in the forward direction[*104], a flow of charge carriers diffuses across the pn-junction. Adjacent to the depletion zone, so-called diffusion zones build up; these contain a non-equilibrium concentration of carriers[*105] (being too high) yielding inversion, as shown in Fig. 1-31b and c. In this way, stimulated emission can occur, yielding gain and making laser action possible. As broad bands (energy range between band edges and Quasi-Fermi levels) are involved, many four-level systems operate simultaneously and hence the emitted radiation is rather broadband[*106]. In the simplest, most often used case, the resonator that is to provide stimulated emission is

*103 The Fermi level indicates the density of electrons in a semiconductor by representing the highest energy occupied by them within the band structure (precisely at 0 K and in thermal equilibrium). Therefore it may lie inside the conduction band of an *n*-semiconductor (see left side in Fig. 1-31a) and inside the valence band of a *p*-semiconductor (see right side in Fig. 1-31a).

*104 In this case the positive electrode is connected to the p-side and vice versa allowing nearly free diffusion of carriers.

*105 In case of non-equilibrium of the semiconductor, local equilibria in the corresponding bands can be observed and characterized by so-called Quasi-Fermi levels.

*106 In this respect the semiconductor laser is comparable to the dye laser.

*107 Cleaving yields surfaces of perfect smoothness. According to the high index of, e.g., GaAs n=3.6, R=0.32, i.e. 32%. Normally, such mirrors are totally inadequate, but the high amplification of diode lasers can easily compensate for that allow easy laser action.

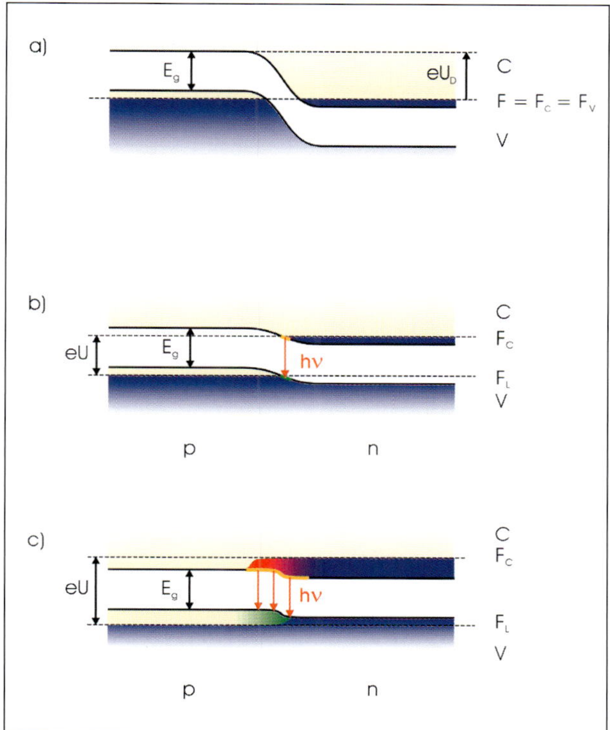

Fig 1-31 Band diagram of a diode laser in three different conditions of applied voltage:
(a) no applied voltage; *p* and *n* layers arrange themselves energetically in such a way that the Fermi level is common to both;
(b) a small forward bias U ($U < U_D$) is applied, causing the bands to reduce their potential steps and thereby allowing the diffusion of carriers;
(c) application of a larger bias U than the bandgap voltage E_g/e allows nearly undisturbed flow of carriers across the junction these accumulate in the diffusion zone on the opposite side and result in an inversion. This band diagram corresponds to a four-level system depicted by the colors selected in this book; U_D, diffusion voltage; U, applied forward bias voltage; C, conduction band; V, valence band; F_c and F_v are corresponding Quasi-Fermi levels.

simply formed between the two end facets, which are produced by simple cleaving[*107] (see Fig. 1-24).

As depicted in Fig. 1-24, the region of inversion or active zone is not geometrically well defined. Only the statistical[*108] fading away of inversion, to mainly the *n*-sidewards, defines the gain region. In order to clearly define the laser volume in current flow direction and to easily invert it, the double hetero-junction was introduced; this consists of a sequence of a high-bandgap *p*-layer, a small active low-bandgap layer which could even be undoped, and a high-bandgap *n*-layer (compare again Fig. 1-30). Charge carriers have to stay within the active layer until they recombine by stimulated or spontaneous emission; however, no diffusion out to the hetero-layers is possible because of potential steps of >100 meV. In this way, thresholds[*109] can be achieved at rather low current densities[*110] of ~1 kA/cm^2.

In most cases, the semiconductors to be employed for diode lasers are III–V compounds[*111], which are normally of a binary nature, like GaAs. In order to be able to generate any desired wavelength and to lattice match the laser layers to simple substrates like GaAs or InP, ternary or quaternary semiconductors are also fabricated (such as InGaAs or InGaAsP, respectively). Si is not suitable for a diode laser as its carrier recombination requires, in addition to e^+ and e^-, the interaction of phonons[*112], and this is incompatible with laser action.

If a hetero-structure is formed as described above, in most cases it also represents a planar waveguide, which confines light by total internal reflection within the active layer with the higher refraction index *n*. Given this design, there is still no lateral confinement of current, amplification and laser light. Hence, the same concept of a het-

*107 Cleaving yields surfaces of perfect smoothness. According to the high index of, e.g., GaAs, $n = 3.6$, $R = 0.32$, i.e. 32%. Normally, such mirrors are totally inadequate, but the high amplification of diode lasers can easily compensate for that and allow easy laser action.

*108 Usual diode lasers are doped in an asymmetrical fashion: the *n*-doping is high (>10^{18} cm^{-3}, labeled n$^+$) while *p*-doping is low (10^{15} cm^{-3}). Hence, current is dominated by electrons (having better mobility, i.e., facing lower resistance) that flow to the p-side and generate inversion only there.

*109 For threshold inversion, densities of 2 x 10^{18} cm^{-3} are required.

*110 For homo-junction diode lasers (i.e., same semiconductor, p and n-doped, compare Fig. 1-24) the threshold current density is ~ 100 kA/cm^2.

*111 Meaning the combination of elements of columns III and V in the periodic system. These are isoelectronic to Si, which is the best semiconductor. Other options are, e.g., II–VI compounds.

*112 This is called indirect recombination; the statistical phases introduced by phonons are in contradiction to stimulated emission of coherent photons.

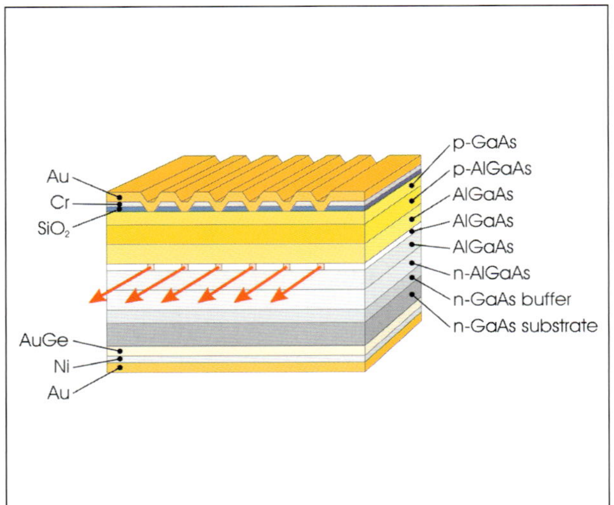

Fig 1-32 GaAlAs/GaAs stripe contact array laser: where the SiO_2 layer is interrupted, optimum stripe contacts for gain guiding are provided. Electrical contacts are not shown.

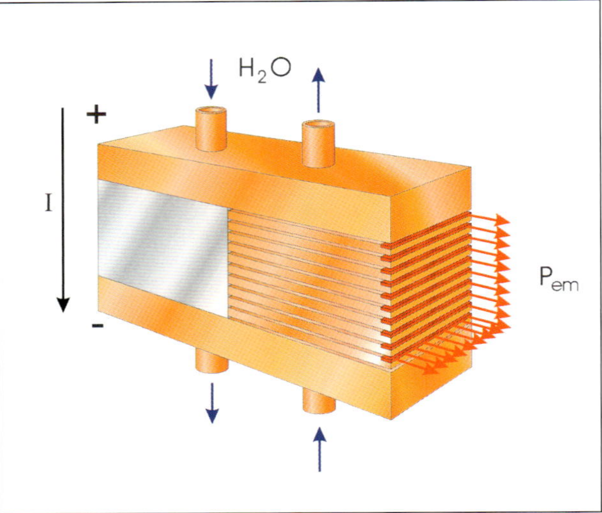

Fig 1-33 Two-dimensionally stacked array with water cooling between the array layers; *I*, current through the array; P_{em}, emitted laser radiation.

ero-structure might be employed in the lateral direction, giving rise to a stripe laser. This type emits light from a rectangular active zone at the facets as depicted in Fig. 1-24, yielding an astigmatic beam. If the emphasis is on highest power, maximum stripe widths of up to 200 µm are possible, but sacrificing transversal monomode operation.

In cases where much higher power is necessary, one has to apply the concept of arrays, i.e., linear monolithic arrangements of several lasing stripes as is illustrated in Fig. 1-32. The individual stripes in this version are defined by the stripe contacts in the top layer, since they allow the current only to flow in stripes, which represents gain guiding[*113]. Operation of these several "individual lasers" on a single substrate (called monolithic) certainly represents an advantage in production. If they are closely spaced and certain coupling schemes are in effect, even more or less coherent output of more than 100 W is achievable.

In cases where a more power is desired, as is the case for certain applications such as pumping of solid-state lasers, stacked arrays can be formed like the one shown in Fig. 1-33. Despite the high efficiency of diode lasers, which can reach up to 50%, the removal of waste heat is one of the most important issues in such types of high-power diode lasers. Sometimes this is achieved by sophisticated water channels between the individual arrays.

Fig. 1-34 uses representative light-current plots to describe the performance of modern diode lasers. The left part shows qualitatively the transition between spontaneous emission-dominated LED operation below threshold and stimulated emission-dominated laser operation above threshold. The right part of the figure indicates the optical output power (left scale) or the voltage to be applied for a certain current (right scale) in a high-power stacked array. The voltage only marginally rises along the wide range of output powers, in good correspondence with aspects mentioned in association with Fig. 1-31.

There are numerous versions of diode lasers far beyond the scope of this book. In this context, diode lasers are, on the one hand, directly used as "soft lasers" for low-intensity interactions such as

*113 Guiding means the confinement of light which can be achieved by gain or by loss, i.e., by a restricted amplification (gain) zone or by a lossless propagation (index waveguiding) zone.

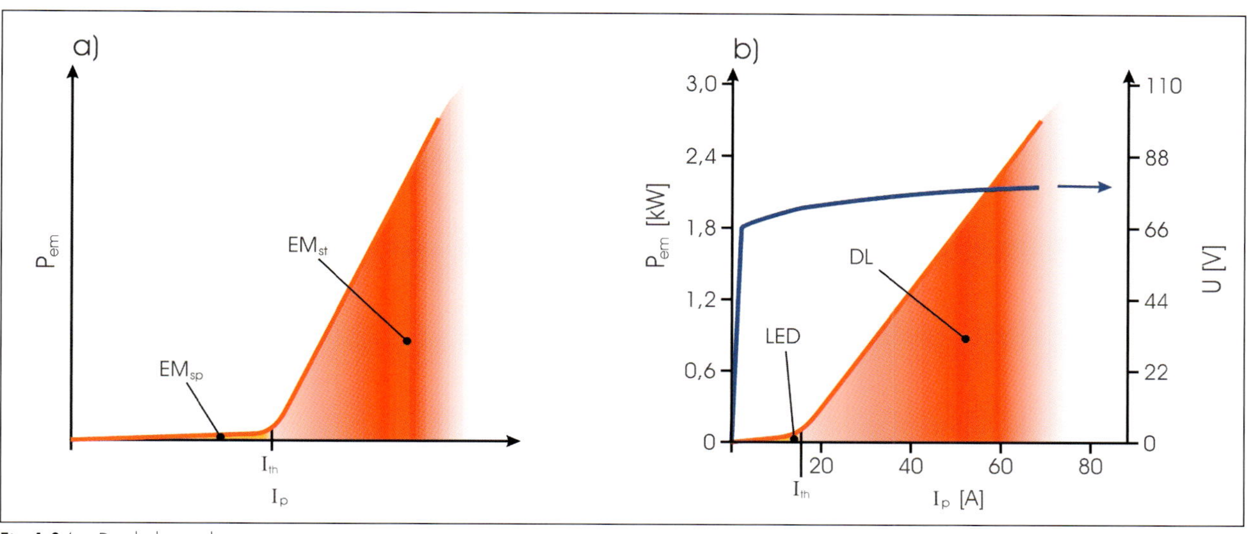

Fig 1-34 Diode laser characteristic:
(a) optical output power P_{em} versus pumping current I_p featuring areas of spontaneous EM_{sp} and of stimulated emission EM_{st} divided at the threshold current position I_{th};
(b) output power P_{em} and applied voltage U versus stimulating current I_p. clearly distinguished from LED regime and laser regime DL .

biostimulation (e.g., increased speed of healing of wounds, removal of pain, even laser acupuncture) or soft-tissue interactions such as sterilization or cutting of gums. On the other hand, they represent the most efficient source of optical energy for pumping other lasers, especially solid-state. Generally, diode laser output can be easily transported via optical fibers, although sometimes coupling in requires high performance (aspheric) optics. Simple diode lasers can be purchased as pigtail options, meaning that fiber coupling is already provided. As a conclusion of this special laser section with the greatest relevance, in Detail 1-16 several practical data on diode lasers are given.

1.5.5 Ruby and Alexandrite Lasers

The following lasers described in this and the next section are called transition metal ion[*114] lasers, the most prominent of them being Cr^{3+} and Ti^{3+} lasers in suitable host crystals. Cr^{3+} doping ions are common to both ruby and alexandrite laser, but details of the energy level structure are different, yielding rather narrow emission for ruby and broad tunability for alexandrite, as indicated in Fig. 1-35 for comparison.

Figure 1-35 (left side) depicts the energy level diagram of ruby. Absorption can take place very efficiently for the upper ($^4T_1$) and the lower ($^4T_2$) pump bands[*115], from where energy transits in less than 1 ns into the upper laser level ^2E which is metastable with a lifetime τ_2 = 3 ms. The ruby laser represents a three-level system requiring an excitation from the ground state of more than 50% of the laser ions. The long lifetime τ_2 favors allowing reasonable pump powers, which are traditionally provided by flash lamps in a typical solid-state laser set-up like the one illustrated in Fig. 1-38.

*114 The name refers to the periodic system; Cr and Ti have 18 electrons in filled orbitals, and the following outer configurations: $3d^5 4s$ for Cr, $3d^2 4s^2$ for Ti. The 3^+-ions have $3d^3$ and $3d$ configuration for the two elements, respectively. These electrons determine the optical properties of the ions and are strongly affected by the electric fields of the host crystal, as they are unshielded by outer shells of other electrons (in contrast to rare earths).

*115 The names of energy levels or bands in this case originate from crystal field theory.

Detail 1-16.
Performance data of cw single-stripe diode lasers with potential relevance for laser dentistry.

Type	wavelengths	output power	threshold current
GaN	>365 nm	50 mW	~ 20 mA
GaAlAs	640–880 nm	100 mW	10 mA
InGaAsP	650–700 nm	10 mW	100 mA
InGaAsP	900–1600 nm	50 mW	10 mA

The example of the ruby laser illustrates very clearly the drawbacks of three-level systems:

- compared to a four-level laser, three-level lasers require high pump intensities because a certain amount of pump power is required just to achieve transparency in the material.
- such lasers absorb the laser emission wavelength unless pumped to inversion. Any portion of the laser crystal that is shielded from the pump light will present a high absorption loss.

Despite these obvious drawbacks, such lasers have other, redeeming features such as desirable wavelengths, or they allow a particular efficient pump method that makes them attractive. Ruby lases in the visible region, it has broad absorption bands particularly well suited for flashlamp pumping, and it has a long fluorescent lifetime and a reasonably large stimulated emission cross section.

Ruby, historically seen, was the first laser, and works on the basis of synthetic ruby crystal rods[*116]. Its Al_2O_3 host crystal[*117] is usually doped by ~$1.5 \cdot 10^{19}$ Cr^{3+} ions per cm^3, giving rise to the reddish color of the crystal. Rod sizes of length $L \leq 30$ cm and diameter $D \leq 2.5$ cm are typically fabricated. To reach the threshold, a pump energy density $\rho_{p,th} \cong 3.2$ J/cm^3 is required; $\rho_p = 800$ J/cm^3 will yield $\rho_{em} \approx 4$ J/cm^3 output energy density (efficiency $\eta \approx 0.5$ %). Operation generally is pulsed: $\tau_p \approx 0.5$ ms for normal (flashlamp pulsed) pumping, $\tau_p \approx 10$ ns for Q-switched, and $\tau_p \approx 20$ ps for mode-locked operation.

Nowadays, the ruby laser is still in much use. Holography can be carried out after achieving a coherence length $\ell_c \geq 1$ m by longitudinal mode number reduction. In medicine, cosmetic work, such as hair removal represents a very large business. Even in dentistry, the red wavelength allows several applications.

In Fig. 1-35 (right side), the alexandrite energy level scheme is shown for comparison with ruby. The crystal field of $BeAl_2O_4$ interacts in a stronger way with the Cr^{3+}-doping, broadening, e.g., the ground state $^4A_2$ greatly by many vibrational levels. For these reasons, this laser represents a three-level and a four-level laser, simultaneously. The narrow emission wavelength range, which exactly corresponds with that of ruby, is of little interest. The broad tunability range of the four-level operation output, λ = 701–818 nm, however, is of much greater relevance. This tunability occurs because the emission of a photon is always coupled to a phonon, the energy being shared in a variable way. Most operational aspects, apart from tunability, are similar to the ruby laser.

*116 Their availability goes back to ruby masers and is another reason for the first laser demonstration, together with the efficient helical flashlamp as pump source. Artificial rubies have been employed in watch bearings for a long time.

*117 In English usually called sapphire; more correct would be, however, corundum: it has the best thermomechanical properties of all solid-state laser materials.

1.5.6 Titanium-Sapphire Laser

Since its laser action was first reported around 20 years ago, the $Ti^{3+}:Al_2O_3$ laser has been the subject of extensive investigations, and today is the most widely used tunable solid-state laser. The Ti:sapphire laser combines a broad tuning range of ~ 400 nm with a relatively large gain cross section that is half of Nd:YAG at the peak of its tuning range (compare Detail 1-6). The energy level structure of the Ti^{3+} ion is unique among transition-metal laser ions in that there are no *d* state energy levels above the upper laser level[*118].

In this material, a Ti^{3+} ion is substituted for an Al^{3+} ion in Al_2O_3. Laser crystals are usually doped by 0.1% Ti^{3+} and exhibit a broad absorption band located in the blue-green region, as can be seen in Fig. 1-36. The great interest in and the importance of the lasers arise from the broad vibronic fluorescence band that allows tunable laser output between 670 and 1100 nm, with the peak of the gain curve around 800 nm. The host crystal sapphire possesses, besides the already mentioned high thermal conductivity, also exceptional chemical inertness and mechanical rigidity. Ti:sapphire lasers have been pumped by a number of optical sources, most commonly Ar^+ lasers and frequency-doubled Nd:YAG or Nd:YLF lasers, the latter nowadays representing the most modern commercial versions. Flashlamp pumping is very difficult to achieve because a very high pump flux is required; nevertheless, it has been done.

This type of laser is most often used on account of its tunability, which can even be increased by generating the second and third harmonics. Furthermore, and most importantly, the Ti:sapphire laser represents the most successful laser for ultra-short pulse generation of picosecond and femtosecond duration. Resonator set-ups for the shortest pulses are very simple because they consist only of the laser medium, a modulating device[*119] and dispersion-compensating mirrors (Fig. 1-14 and Fig. 1-15 illustrate this aspect according to the scope of this book). Repetition

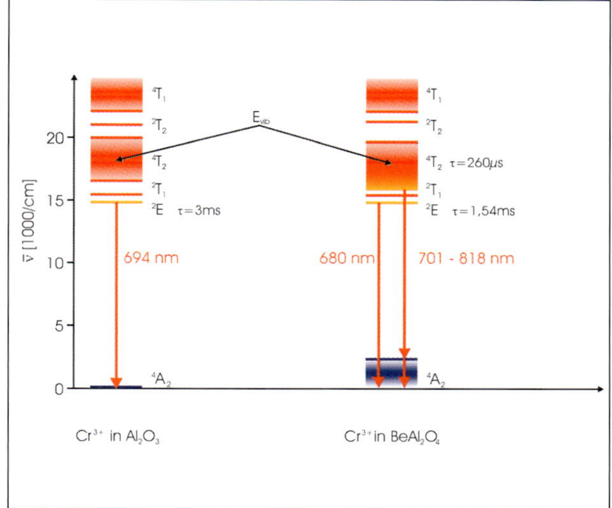

Fig 1-35 Energy bands and levels of the ruby and alexandrite lasers: based on the same lasing ion they are very similar, incorporating three-level systems (see the color code for levels); however, in alexandrite the tunable emission merits special attention. E_{vib}, vibronically broadened energy bands, ν, wave number (1000 cm^{-1}).

rates of resonators are of the order of 100 MHz; in the case of amplification they nowadays lie around 1 kHz with pulse energies ≤ 1 mJ[*120].

Applications of femtosecond pulses with low average power (typically ~100 mW) include, e.g., optical coherence tomography (OCT), a destruction-free optical method[*121] to generate cross-sectional images with a resolution down to sub-cellular levels (~2 μm in three dimensions); this already been successfully tested on dental tissue[9].

*118 This simple energy level structure ($3d^1$ configuration) eliminates the possibility of excited state absorption of the laser radiation, an effect that has limited the tuning range and reduced the efficiency of other transition-metal-doped lasers.

*119 For shortest pulses Kerr-lens modulation (KLM) and semiconductor saturable mirror modulation (SESAM) are employed, yielding $\tau_p \geq 5$ fs in such a simple resonator.

*120 Such "high" values are only achievable by multi-stage amplification which is not yet commercially available and represents only a tool for scientific research ($E_p \approx 1$ mJ, $\tau_p \approx 10$ fs → $P \approx 10^{11}$ W, when focused to D ≈ 50 μm → $I \approx 10^{16}$ W/cm^2!).

*121 OCT is based on longitudinal resolution being determined by the optical coherence length, as it plays a crucial role in Michelson interferometers determining the range of arm difference (characterized by fringe visibility). For ultra-short pulses $\tau_c \leq \tau_p$ (the equality holds in the case of Fourier limited pulses).

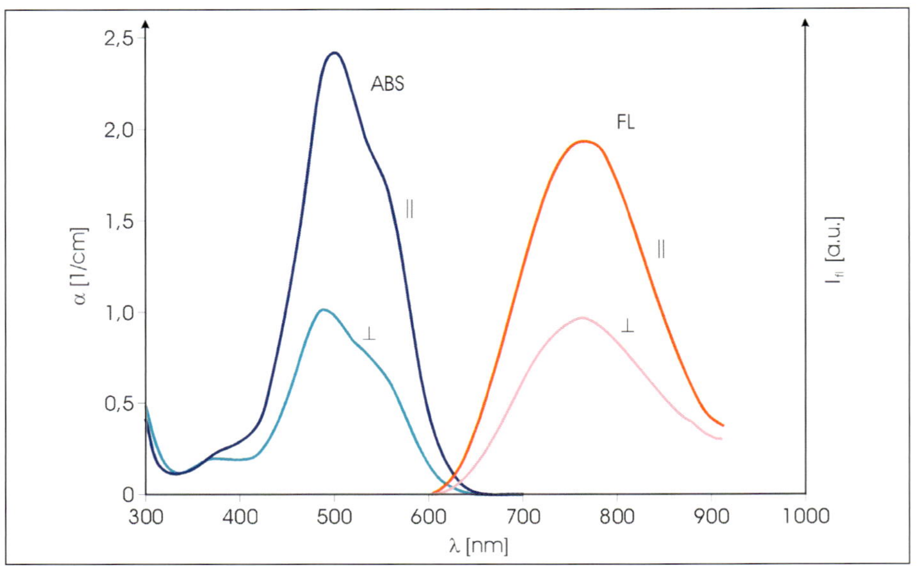

Fig 1-36 Absorption (ABS) and emission (FL) of Ti:sapphire over wide spectral bands revealing anisotropic differences; α, absorption coefficient; I_{fl}, fluorescence intensity.

Amplified ultra-short pulses, which, however, are much longer[*122], represent a new avenue for dental hard-tissue treatment as described in detail in other sections. For these novel applications, other solid-state lasers, such as Nd:YAG or especially Nd:YLF, have proven to be superior, e.g., in efficiency and cost.

*122 There has been a long development of the suggested "best pulse duration" for dental hard tissue treatment over around 5 years: starting at ~100 fs, the present state of the art culminates between 1 and 10 ps.

Detail 1-17.
Laser parameters of Ti:sapphire.

Index of refraction $n = 1.76$, fluorescent lifetime $\tau_2 = 3.2\ \mu s$, peak emission wavelength $\lambda = 795$ nm, stimulated emission cross section at 795 nm (II c-axis) $\sigma_{||} = 2.8 \times 10^{-19}\ cm^2$, quantum efficiency for 0.53 µm pump photons $\eta \approx 1$, saturation fluence $E_s = 0.9\ J/cm^2$. Shortest pulse duration in an oscillator: $\tau_p \approx 5$ fs, average power with sub-10fs pulses: $P_{ave} \leq 1$ W, average power after amplification typically several W

1.5.7 Neodymium and Ytterbium Lasers

The most important solid-state laser is the neodymium laser based on the rare earth ion Nd^{3+}*123. This ion can be incorporated into different host materials, the most important ones being YAG (yttrium aluminum garnet – $Y_3Al_5O_{12}$) and several glasses. YAG offers favorable mechanical and thermo-optical properties allowing its use for cw and pulsed lasers, even of high power.

Fig. 1-37 shows the simplified energy level scheme of the Nd:YAG laser. Most commercial lasers emit the wavelength 1064 nm corresponding to a transition between the $^4F_{3/2}$ and $^4I_{11/2}$ levels. Other laser lines can be seen in Detail 1-18. Excitation is achieved via optical pumping into broad energy bands followed by radiation-less transitions into the upper laser level $^4F_{3/2}$ of this four-level scheme. Heat set free during these transitions is transferred into the crystal lattice, making it evident why good heat conduction is important for a good host. The lower laser level lies around 240 meV above the ground level and hence is essentially unpopulated at room temperature, a crucial requirement for the four-level system.

Commercial YAG rods typically are up to 150 mm in length and up to 10 mm in diameter. The doping concentration is ~ 0.7% (weight) of Nd corresponding to $N = 1.4 \cdot 10^{20}$ cm^{-3}. Typically, a rod 75 mm long and 6 mm in diameter can yield around 300 W with 4.5% efficiency. The laser threshold is reached at ~ 2 kW electrical power of a Kr arc lamp in an arrangement as shown in Fig. 1-38. The drawing shows a hollow cavity with gold-coated internal surfaces revealing an elliptical cross section. The arc lamp is in the other while the laser rod is in one focal line. According to the properties of ellipses, all rays from one focus are reflected (the tangent to the curve represents the "reflecting plane") to the other and vice versa. This hollow cavity is filled with very pure water for cooling of both the lamp and the rod.

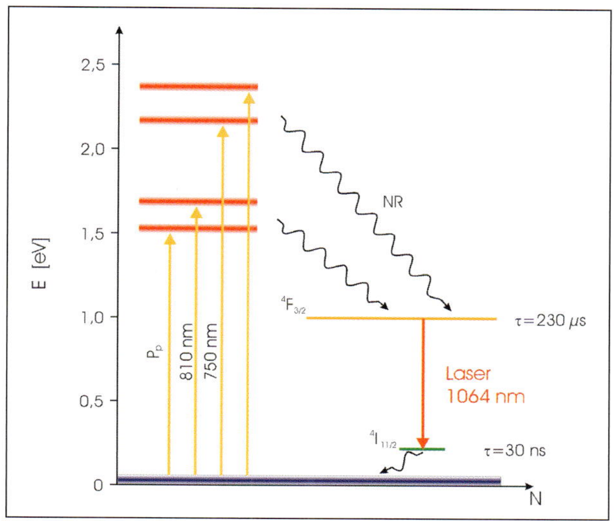

Abb. 1-37 Nd:YAG laser scheme: based on a characteristic four-level system (observe the color code for the levels!) drawn versus population density *N*; *E*, energy, P_p, optical pumping, *NR*, non-radiative transitions.

Thereby, very high pumping efficiencies can be achieved. Most modern designs, however, rely on diode-pumped operation and use GaAlAs/ GaAs laser diode arrangements that pump extremely efficiently around 810 nm. Pulsed operation is achieved in a similar fashion comprising Q-switching and mode-locking (achievable pulse durations 100 ns or 100 ps, respectively). As the infrared wavelength is unfavorable for many applications, generations of second, third and even fourth harmonic is very common. Pulsed operation yields much higher efficiencies in this case as a result of the strong dependence on intensity.

In medicine, this laser has been used for a long time, taking advantage of its greater depth of penetration into tissue and dispersion in tissue as a

*123 The electronic configuration of Nd^{3+} {Kr}$4d^{10}4f^3 5s^2 5p^6$ reveals that the 4*f*-sub shell is only partially filled. Therefore, the influence of the crystal field is weak because of the shielding by the 5*s* and 5*p* electrons. {Kr} stands for full krypton shell.

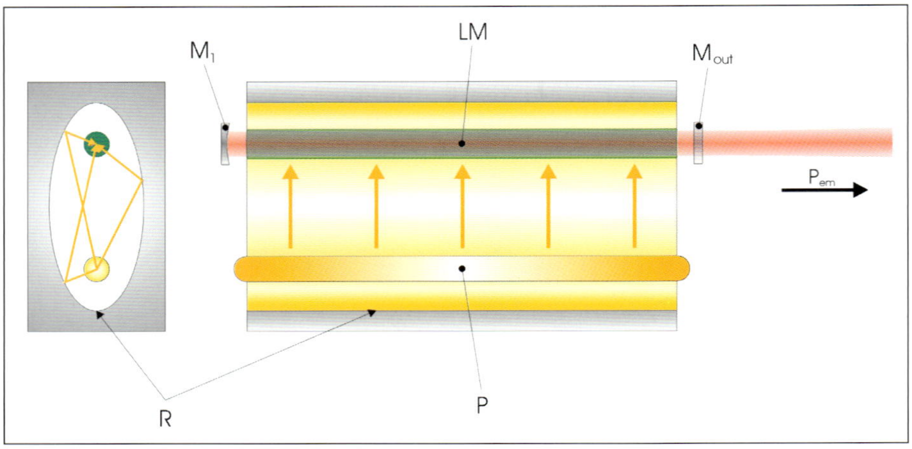

Fig 1-38 Flashlamp pumped cavity of a solid-state laser, e.g., like Nd:YAG, with elliptical cross section: the lamp in one cross-sectional focal point reflects nearly evenly all light onto the laser rod in the second one; *LM*, laser medium; M_1, M_{out}, laser mirrors; *P*, pump intensity of flashlamp; *R*, reflector; P_{em}, emitted laser radiation.

result of scattering. Coagulation stops bleeding effectively and immediately after the cut. This is, e.g., employed in soft tissue treatment in dentistry. Another advantage, especially in comparison with the CO_2 laser, is the propagation through silica fibers allowing for endoscopic use or for fibers to be inserted in root canals, etc.

Yb:YAG has been known for a long time as a laser crystal emitting a wavelength rather similar to that of Nd:YAG (λ = 1030 nm). At first, there was no interest in its application as it lacks any pump bands in the visible. This laser material has only one single absorption feature around λ = 942 nm. With conventional pump sources such as flashlamps, the threshold is very high. Only with the emergence of powerful InGaAs laser diodes that emit at 942 nm has Yb:YAG become a highly important laser medium of highest quantum efficiency: the photon energies of emission and pump are in the ratio of 942:1030, corresponding to 91.4%. The energy level diagram differs somewhat from Nd: the upper laser level $^2F_{5/2}$ represents a manifold spanning about 300 cm^{-1}. The lower laser level is represented by one line within the $^2F_{7/2}$ state 612 cm^{-1} above the ground level. As the thermal energy at room temperature corresponds to 200 cm^{-1}, the lower laser level is thermally populated (5.5% at room temperature), making the laser a quasi-three-level system with disadvantages somewhat milder but similar to those descriped for the ruby laser. Only at high pump energy density can efficient operation take place (typically 10 kW/cm^2, compare Fig. 1-23).

In practical application, Yb:YAG has to be cooled well to provide high efficiency. As the pump band has 18 nm width, this represents a relaxed specification for the precision of the emitted wavelength of the pump diodes (temperature-dependent). The long fluorescence lifetime of 951 µs allows efficient energy storage. The broad upper laser level provides enough bandwidth to support much shorter pulse durations than Nd:YAG (~ 100 fs). As a consequence, this laser is the source of commercial kW cw radiation for materials processing (such welding). It also is employed more and more for ultra-short pulse generation in the ps and sub-ps regime – representing exactly the temporal range of optimum pulse durations for dental hard tissue preparation.

Detail 1-18.
Parameters of Nd:YAG and Yb:YAG lasers.

Nd:YAG	Yb:YAG:
Doping density $N = 1.4 \cdot 10^{20}$ cm^{-3} ≅ 1% at	5.5% at
Most important pump wavelengths: λ = 750 and 810 nm	λ = 808 nm and 943 nm
Most important transitions from $^4F_{3/2}$: → $I_{9/2}$: λ = 0.90 µm, rel. intensity 0.25 → $I_{11/2}$: λ = 1.06 µm, rel. intensity 0.60 → $I_{13/2}$: λ = 1.35 µm, rel. intensity 0.14 → $I_{15/2}$: λ = 1.7–2.1 µm, rel. intensity " 0.01 Four-level system	$^2F_{5/2}$: → $^2F_{7/2}$: λ = 1.03 µm Quasi-three-level system
Data of YAG crystal: Melting point 1970 °C Knoop hardness 1215 density 4.56 g/cm^3 thermal expansion coefficient (10–250°C): (100) 8.2·10^{-6} °C^{-1}, (110) 7.7·10^{-6} °C^{-1}, (111) 7.8·10^{-6} °C^{-1} index of refraction 1.82 (bei 1.0 µm)	

1.5.8 Holmium and Holmium-Thulium lasers

The Ho^{3+} ion, which is also one of the group of rare earth ions, can be implemented in basically the same host crystals or glasses as Nd^{3+}, following similar considerations; the same idea will hold for Er^{3+}. The emitted radiation at 2.1 µm is considered to be safe for the eyes; to be sure, it can propagate nearly unattenuated through the atmosphere, but it penetrates only 0.1 mm into the cornea of the eye and hence does not reach the retina[*124].

The energy levels of Ho^{3+}, relevant for a principal understanding, are illustrated in Fig. 1-39

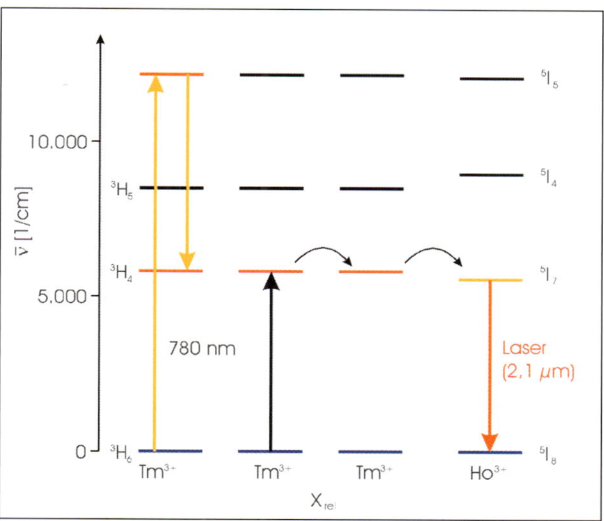

Fig 1-39 Energy levels of Tm^{3+} and Ho^{3+} representing a classical example for cross relaxation as a process for increasing pump efficiency. The 2.1 µm radiation was considered at one time to be relevant for dental applications; ν, wave number, X_{rel} ,cross relaxation.

(right column): the laser transition takes place between $^5I_7$ and $^5I_8$ which represents also the ground level; hence this laser is a three-level one, with properties sufficiently discussed above. As a consequence, at room temperature it can work only in pulsed mode with pulses up to 500 mJ. Q-switched operation is also possible. At the temperature of liquid nitrogen (–196°C) cw operation can also be achieved.

Traditionally, the Ho:YAG laser is flashlamp pumped, exciting first the upper ^5I levels, from where the upper laser level becomes populated, with a lifetime τ_2 = 8.5 ms. Following modern developments, diode pumping can also be successful if co-doping with Tm^{3+} is employed as an auxiliary feature (see the three left columns in Fig. 1-39): Tm^{3+} can absorb the pump radiation at

*124 The problem of eye safety of laser radiation is created by the focusing properties of the eye as an "optical instrument". Intensities at the cornea and at the retina (these can reach up to 1.5 µm radiation, at least with attenuated power may be in the ratio of 1:10^5!

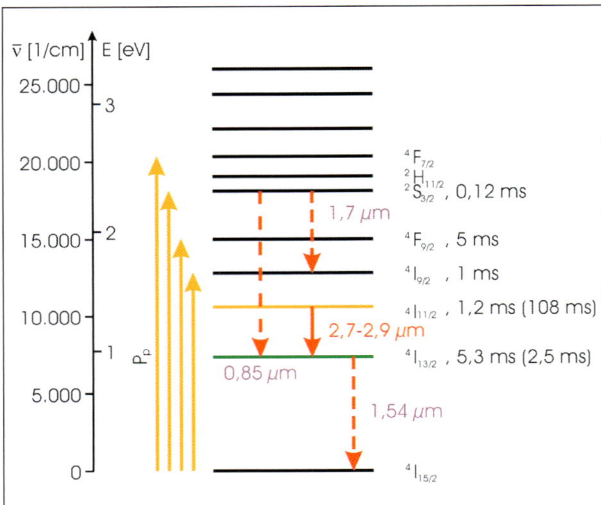

Fig 1-40 Energy levels as well as pump and laser transitions of Er^{3+} in YALO, YAG, YSGG, YLF: four-level system indicated by the corresponding color code. The lifetimes indicated refer to YALO/YAG. The wavelengths 2.7–2.9 μm are presently the ones most used in cavity preparation; $\bar{\nu}$, wave number or E, energy on the ordinate; P_p, optical pumping.

780 nm provided by well-developed GaAlAs/GaAs diode lasers. In the co-doped Tm,Ho:YAG crystal a Tm-Tm cross relaxation takes place populating Tm $^3H_4$ levels, which is explained in the easiest way by the graphics in the figure 1-39. By means of additional Tm-ions, all of them coupled by the crystal lattice, the excitation energy reaches the Ho $^5I_7$ level to be inverted for laser operation.

For some time in laser dentistry, great things were expected of the Ho laser. In contrast to the Er laser, the 2.1 μm radiation of the Ho laser can be directly absorbed by dental hard tissue without the interaction of water. Especially with respect to enamel, which has the lowest water content, this aspect was considered to be advantageous. Practical experience, however, has revealed major problems of heat deposition associated with the application of this laser, which finally caused the clinical and commercial interests to fade away.

1.5.9 Erbium and Erbium-Chromium Lasers

The interest in the Er^{3+} laser is based on the wavelengths it can emit, i.e., λ = 1.54 μm and λ = 2.7–2.9 μm. The former coincides nicely with the absorption minimum of optical silica fibers, allowing long-range optical communications incorporating optical amplifiers.[*125] The latter wavelength coincides nicely with the peak of water absorption. As water is contained in every biological tissue, efficient interaction and dense optical energy deposition is guaranteed.

In the case of crystalline Er-lasers, the host crystals are usually YAG, YALO (yttrium aluminum oxide – $YAlO_3$), YSGG (yttrium scandium gadolinium garnet – $Y_3Sc_2Ga_3O_{12}$) or YLF (yttrium lanthanum fluoride – $YLiF_4$). Usually, doping is relatively high, i.e., about 50% of the Y ions in YAG are replaced by Er ions. The corresponding level scheme is depicted in Fig. 1-40, including the potential pump and emission wavelengths.

The "3-μm-Er:YAG" laser can be pumped, just like other solid-state lasers, by flash or arc lamps as well as laser diodes. All the absorbing levels, starting from $^4I_{9/2}$ upwards, are split into sub-levels, so that in every case bands of ~ 5 nm are to be excited. For this radiation emitted by transitions between $^4I_{11/2}$ and $^4I_{13/2}$, representing four-level operation, it is remarkable that the lower level has a longer lifetime, τ_1 = 5 μs, compared to the upper one. This prevents cw emission, and requires pump pulses of fast rise times. Before the next pulse can be generated, the lower laser level must be empty. Besides simple decay processes of the upper level, energy exchange processes with neighboring ions can also take place. This complicates the transfer of pump energy to the relevant levels of operation. Typical pulse energies of

*125 These are sections of silica fiber of ~ 30 m length with an Er^{3+}-doped core which can be pumped by diode lasers.

Er:YAG lasers are 10 to 100 mJ. In cases where higher energies are required, amplifiers have to be employed. Generally, e.g., Er:YSGG offers no real advantage, although it reveals a somewhat higher gain, but at a slightly changed wavelength that, unfortunately, deviates to a small extent from the maximum absorption of water.

In medical applications, and especially in dentistry, the Er lasers represent highly developed commercial lasers with very high yield and efficiency in tissue removal. For dental hard tissue ablation, this is currently the type of laser most often used.

1.5.10 Carbon Dioxide Laser

As the sequence of sub-sections is organized with rising wavelength, the CO_2 laser is the last in the list of special lasers discussed. Compared to the solid-state lasers explained above, it is very different with respect to its gaseous medium, its long wavelength emitted from molecular vibrations and its pump mechanisms which are mostly based on gas discharges. In a way, it somewhat resembles the masers, which were developed before lasers.

The CO_2 laser is one of the oldest lasers[*126] and one of the most important, especially for industrial applications in materials processing such as cutting and welding[*127]. Thereby its high efficiency of 10–20% plays a major role, which can only be surpassed[*128] by modern solid-state lasers such as Yb:YAG. There are, however, models of little power on the 1-W level that are employed for some dental bleaching processes. More often, in medical applications, the 10-W power range is observed.

The CO_2 molecule symbolically shown in the insert of Fig. 1-41 consists of a linear arrangement[*129] of three atoms with the C atom lying in the middle; (a) represents a bending oscillation, and (b) symmetric and (c) asymmetric stretching oscillations. They are the source of three groups of rovibrational modes labeled *(010)*, *(100)*, *(001)*, respectively. The resulting laser transitions can be observed in Fig. 1-41. Similar to the HeNe laser, the laser medium consists of more components than just CO_2: $CO_2 + N_2 + He$ (60 to 80%). N_2 becomes effectively excited by e^- impact in a discharge and it can also store this energy[*130] for some time, finally transfering it via non-radiative collisions[*131] to the CO_2 molecules. Helium is not directly involved in the lasing process. Its function is to increase pressure inside the discharge tube and stabilize it. Furthermore, it reduces the gas temperature and empties the lower laser level by collisions. There are many details within the interaction of the various rotational and vibrational levels, which are beyond the scope of this text. The same applies to the various versions of CO_2 lasers called (i) laser with slow axial gas flow (the very one being illustrated in Fig. 1-42), (ii) sealed-off laser[*132], (iii) waveguide laser (ideal for low power[*133]), (iv) laser with fast longitudinal or transversal gas flow (kW), (v) transversal atmospheric pressure (TEA) laser (μs to ps pulses), and (vi) gas dynamic CO_2 laser.[*134]

*126 First published by Q. Patel et al. (1964).
*127 In this case high cw energy models emitting up to 100 kW are available.
*128 Of course, the efficiency of diode lasers may be even higher. They may also be assembled as stacked arrays emitting also in the kW range. The brightness, however, remains many orders of magnitude behind and allows only soldering or localized heating treatments in industrial manufacture.
*129 Be aware that the H_2O molecule also consisting of three atoms is non-linear (angle 105°) due to the background of its dipolar nature which is the reason for the many special properties of water making it essential for life.
*130 Molecular N_2 has no permanent dipole moment. Therefore optical transitions between vibrational levels of the same electronic state are forbidden leading to metastability which acts as an energy storage mechanism.
*131 A small energy difference of the order of thermal energy (25 meV at RT) can always be added or removed in this case according to the velocity distribution in a gas.
*132 In this case, dissociation products of the gas discharge such as CO and O_2 can be chemically removed by small additions of H_2O, H_2 or O_2 via catalysts (Pt or Ni at 500°C).
*133 Consisting of BeO or Al_2O_3 capillaries of typically 1 mm diameter; power ≤ 1 W.
*134 Different from all other versions: inversion is generated by rapid expansion of hot gas mixture.

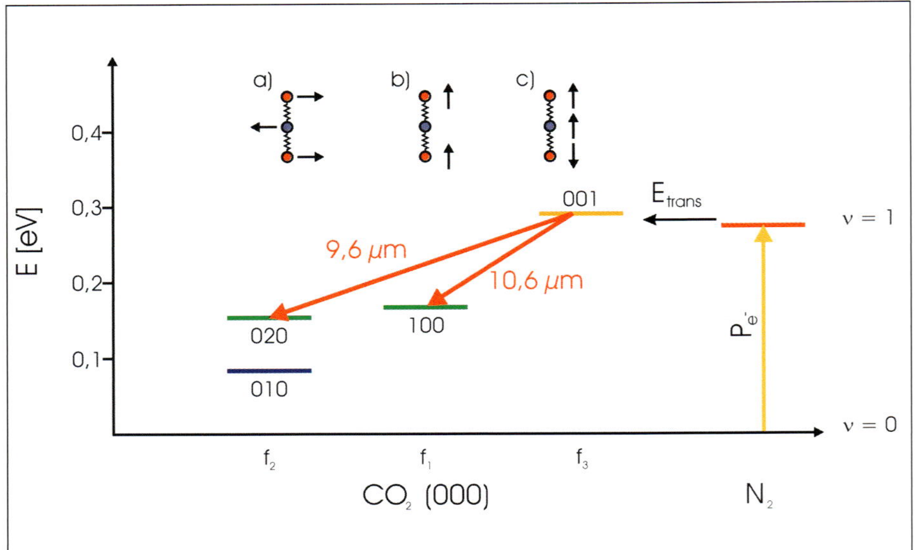

Fig 1-41 Vibrational energy levels of CO_2: forming a four-level system (observe the characteristic color code). The excitation energy is transferred non-radiatively via N_2 to CO_2; *E*, energy; E_{trans}, energy transfer; P_{e^-} electron impact. The small insert shows the three possible modes of vibration of the CO_2 molecule labeled (a), (b) and (c).

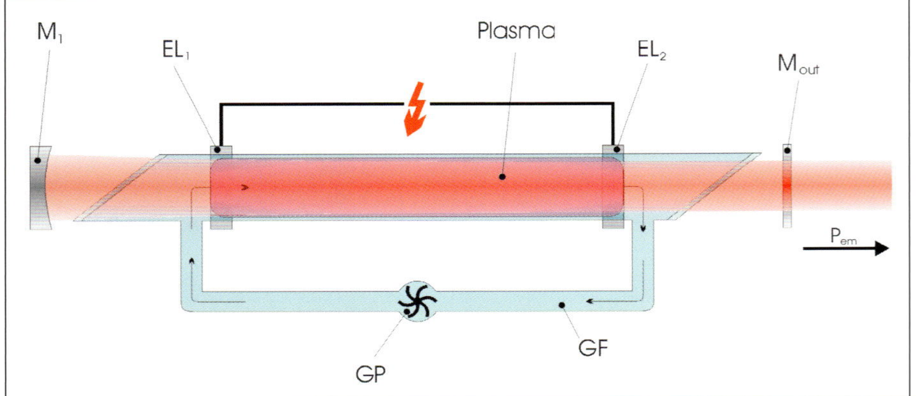

Fig 1-42 CO_2 laser discharge tube: revealing typical Brewster window arrangement for gas lasers; M_1, M_{out}, laser mirrors; *P*, plasma; EL_1, EL_2, discharge electrodes; *GP*, high speed pump; *GF*, gas flow; P_{em}, emitted laser power.

In Fig. 1-42, variant (i) is illustrated revealing all typical features of a gas laser: Brewster windows, gas discharge, enforced cooling, and removal of dissociation products via gas flow. In addition, modern versions may contain mirrors acting as windows. In this case, the adjustment during manufacture must be precise and final. Such CO_2 lasers can be cheap, reliable, compact and efficient, major prerequisites for commercial and medical application.

1.6 Textbooks and References

1.6.1 Textbooks

Dinstl K, Fischer P L: Der Laser, Grundlagen und klinische Anwendung. Springer Verlag Berlin, Heidelberg, New York 1981 (ISBN 3-540-10654-5)

Eichler J, Eichler H J: Laser. 5., aktualisierte Auflage. Springer Verlag, Berlin, Heidelberg, New York 2003 (ISBN 3-540-00376-2)

Koechner W, Bass M: Solid-State Lasers. Springer Verlag, New York, Berlin, Heidelberg 2003 (ISBN 0-387-95590-9)

Miller J L, Friedman E: Photonics Rules of Thumb, Optics, Electro-Optics, Fiber Optics, and Lasers. McGraw-Hill, Boston 1996 (ISBN 0-07-044329-7)

Mollwo E, Kaule W: Maser und Laser. 2. Auflage. BI Hochschultaschenbücher, Bibliographisches Institut, Mannheim 1968

Reider G A: Photonik, Eine Einführung in die Grundlagen. Springer Verlag, Wien, New York 1997 (ISBN 3-211-82855-9)

Svelto O: Principles of Lasers. 3rd Edition. Plenum Press, New York, London 1989 (ISBN 0-306-42967-5)

1.6.2 References

Just a few key or recent overview references are provided in this textbook chapter.

1. Maiman T H: Stimulated Optical Radiation in Ruby Masers. Nature 187: 493, 1960
2. e.g. Schawlow A L, Townes C H: Infrared and Optical Masers. Phys Rev 112: 1940–1949, 1958
3. Einstein A: Zur Quantentheorie der Strahlung, Physikalische Z 18: 121–128, 1917
4. Einstein, A: Über einen die Erzeugung und Verwandlung des Lichtes betreffenden heuristischen Gesichtspunkt. Annalen der Physik 17: 132, 1905
5. Göppert-Mayer M: Über Elementarakte mit zwei Quantensprüngen. Annalen der Physik 9: 273, 1931
6. Apolonski A et al.: Controlling the phase evolution of few-cycle light pulses. Phys Rev Lett 85: 740–743, 2000
7. Wintner E: Ultra-short pulse solid-state lasers and modern applications. Proc. SPIE 4752: 1–12, 2002
8. Brabec T, Krausz F: Intense few-cycle laser fields: Frontiers of nonlinear optics. Rev Mod Phys 72: 545–591, 2000
9. Fercher A F, Drexler W, Hitzenberger C K, Lasser T: Optical coherence tomography – principles and applications. Rep Prog Phys 66: 239–303, 2003
10. Strassl M, Kasenbacher A, Wintner E: Ultrashort Laser Pulses in Dentistry. J Oral Laser Appl 2: 213–222, 2002

2 Laser Safety

F. Beer, M. Straßl, J. Wernisch

2.1 Introduction

The aim of this chapter is to focus on the properties, effects and especially on the dangers of laser and LED radiation and to introduce several protective arrangements.

Lasers are excellent tools, but they also bear a very high risk for severe injury and damage. Laser radiation mainly endangers eyes and skin. Especially for the eye the retina, cornea and the lens are concerned. Damage of the retina usually cannot be repaired. Thus, just a slight carelessness can destroy the vision affected for the rest of life.

The second affected organ is the skin, although it is much less sensitive than the eye and damages occur only at higher energies.

Hence, the high risks require suitable protective measure; their strict observation is the responsibility of the employer and thus of the management. In the case of medical professions it is the duty of the surgery owner or the head of a department.

The requirement to control and verify the correct implementation of the necessary protective arrangements necessitates an intensive safety education.

The risks and protective arrangements treated in this chapter are valid for laser and LED radiation. Basic information on laser light, basic optics and the laser – tissue interaction are contained in other chapters of this book.

It shall be remarked once again that the impact of laser radiation on biological tissue depends not only on the radiation properties (e.g. wavelength, intensity or irradiation time), but also on the irradiated tissue. Its optical and thermal properties determine the absorption, reflection and transmission characteristics of the applied radiation.

One very important factor in this regard is the spectral coefficient of absorption; indicates the fraction of energy being absorbed when penetrating a layer of a certain thickness. For biological tissues, however, the knowledge of the absorption coefficient alone is not sufficient to describe the behavior of the penetrating radiation, since several additional factors like scattering and reflection being classed under the general term of remission determine its actual distribution and backscattering properties.

The remission parameters also depend on the wavelength of the applied radiation. Thus the optical properties of the tissue determine the extent and the form of the coagulation zone.

2.2 Maximum Permissible Exposure

The maximum permissible exposure values (MPE-values) are limiting values that have been determined in experiments just as have other chemical or physical influence factors. As different body tissues have different sensitivities to light irradiation, the MPE-values are defined separately for skin and eyes. Their physical units are W/m^2 and J/m^2.

The values are generated out of animal experiments under consideration of the different anatomical properties and additional safety factors, thus reliably preventing damage if the incoming radiation is below the specified limits.

The specified MPE-values always are determined by national standards.

2.3 Laser Classes

Laser devices have to be classified by the manufacturer according to their hazard to enable the user to choose the right protective arrangements. The different laser classes are defined in the international laser safety standard IEC 60825-1 and in the European standard EN 60825-1 (Fig 2-1).

If there are modifications of the laser device implemented by the user, an evaluation of the actual hazard has to be performed and a new classification has to be done if necessary.

The classification of the laser is done always by assuming the worst-case hazards:

- The user uses a magnifying glass or other optical device
- Minimal distances during measurement
- Longer exposure time than usual
- Consideration of foreseeable failures
- No consideration of the user's actual training

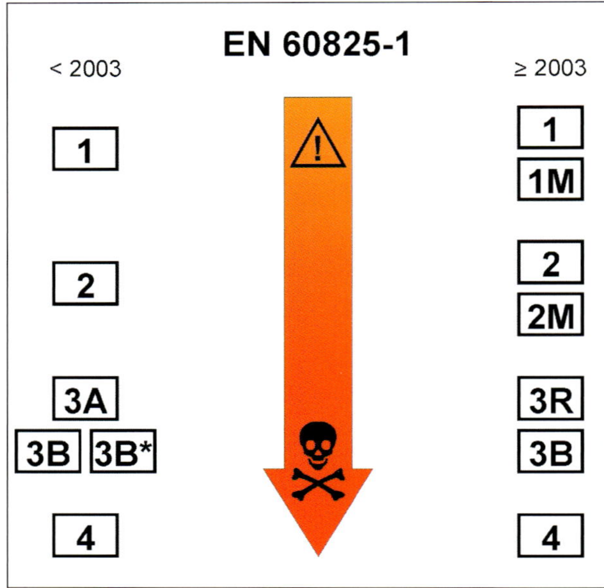

Fig 2-1 Summary of the six old (valid until 2003) and the seven new laser classes (valid since 2003) according to the European standard EN 60825-1. The same graphical level of the classes indicates a comparable safety hazard. The danger rises with rising number of the laser class.

2.3.1 Class 1

Safe laser devices are referring to Class 1. These devices either have a very low output power that remain under the MPE-values even at long irradiation times or, if they have high output power, they are fitted with a protective housing that prevents the radiation from emerging to the outside under all normal operating conditions. Thus, even lasers normally being devices of higher classification can be classified as class 1 devices.

Condition: below 40 µW in the blue, 400 µW in the red spectral range.
Examples: range finders, CD-Players.
Protective Arrangements: none.
***Warning:* none.**
Remark: The new laser safety standards define a new class for laser devices being safe for the naked eye but bearing safety hazards for the use of optical instruments called class 1M ("M" meaning "Magnifying Instruments").
***Warning:* "Laser Radiation. Do Not View Directly With Optical Instruments. Class 1M Laser Product."**

2.3.2 Class 2

Class 2 is only defined for visible wavelengths (λ = 400-700 nm). Natural reactions of turning away (e.g. shutting of the eyelid, time: approx. 0.25 s) are sufficient protection for the eye. The output power of the laser devices is low enough to cause no damage within this time span.

Thus, laser devices of class 2 are safe as long as the reflex of turning away is not suppressed (e.g. intended looking into the beam) or affected (e.g. by medicaments, drugs, etc.).

Condition: For cw lasers, the output power has to be below 1 mW (with an assumed diameter of

7 mm for the iris an average intensity of about 25 W/cm^2 is achieved on the cornea according to the corresponding MPE-value).

Examples: laser pointer, targeting lasers.

Protective Arrangements: none.

Warning: **"Laser Radiation. Do Not Stare Into Beam".**

Remark: The new laser safety standards define a new class for laser devices being safe for the naked eye up to 0.25 s exposure time but bearing safety hazards for the use of optical instruments called class 2M ("M" meaning "Magnifying Instruments").

Warning: **"Laser Radiation. Do Not Stare Into Beam Or View Directly With Optical Instruments. Class 2M Laser Product."**

2.3.3 Remarks on laser classes 1M and 2M

"M" means "Magnifying Instruments". Lasers of these classes are safe for the naked eye but can be dangerous if optical instruments such as magnifying glasses or telescopes are used. In these cases the MPE-values can be exceeded, and this can damage the eye even with short irradiation times. As such instruments focus a larger light intensity into the eye, the rise of the exposure is evident.

2.3.4 Class 3A (old class)

In the new laser safety standards this safety class is replaced by the new classes 1M and 2M.

The exposure is similar to class 2 in the visible range and similar to class 1 in the invisible ranges as long as no magnifying instruments are used. If using such optical instruments are used, damage can occur even within 0.25 s as aresult of focussing. The reflex of turning away is no longer sufficient protection.

Condition: Output power below 5 mW and intensities below 25 W/cm^2 for the visible range, five times the limits of class 1 in the invisible range as long as the MPE-values are not exceeded.

Examples: lasers for measurement, lasers for building grounds.

Protective Arrangements: Laser protective eyewear, attenuation filters, organisational protective arrangements, training of the users. Necessary if the use of optical instruments has to be assumed.

Warning: **"Laser Class 3A (or 1M, 2M): Do not stare into the beam (3A, 1M), also when using optical instruments (3A, 2M)."**

2.3.5 Class 3B

Eyes are endangered, even skin in special cases. Damage can occur even at very short irradiation times. The reaction of turning away is no longer sufficient protection, and even accidental irradiation is dangerous (inside the danger zone) for the direct or specular reflected beam. In most cases there is no risk for diffuse reflection or irradiation of the skin.

Condition: Output power < 0,5 W (UV-A to far IR). The thresholds for UV-B or UV-C are much lower.

Examples: Lasers for measurement, laser shows and alignment.

Protective Arrangements: Safety precautions for the danger zone (boundary, laser protective eyewear), training, laser safety officer.

Warning: **"Laser Radiation. Avoid Exposure to Beam. Class 3B Laser Product."**

2.3.6 Special Class 3B (old classification)

Remark: in the new laser safety standard EN 60825-1 this class is renamed "Class 3R".

Laser devices in the visible range belonging to class 3B, but with output powers < 5 mW are excepted from all technical and organisational

requirements. Even through the MPE-values may be exceeded, the output power is still very low, and this reduces the risk for damage by accidental and short time irradiation to a very low level. Such lasers typically are used as alignment lasers in technical applications and research and as a pilot beam in medical applications.
Conditions: Adequate training of the user is assumed to be sufficient as long as irradiation of persons is improbable.
Examples: targeting lasers, lasers for measurement, lasers for building sites, etc.
Protective Arrangements: training of the user, laser safety officer.

2.3.7 New Class 3R

("R" means "relaxed"). The new class 3R can be seen as the junction between the practically safe Class 2 and the dangerous Class 3B with regard to eye hazards. Even when the limit is exceeded by up to 5-fold, a real hazard arises only at an irradiation time of several seconds; this has been proved by several studies and reports of accidents. It is important that lasers of class 3R are only operated by persons who have been instructed about the residual risks. Other safety precautions are not necessary.

Conditions: 5x output power of Class 2 in the visible range is not exceeded, maximum 5x output power of Class 1 in the invisible ranges.

	① (t>>)		② (t<<)		③	④
1	✓	✓	✓	✓	✓	✓
1M	⚠	✓	⚠	✓	✓	✓
2	⚠	⚠	✓	✓	✓	✓
2M	⚠	⚠	⚠	✓	✓	✓
3R	⚠	⚠	~	~	✓	✓
3B	⚠	⚠	⚠	⚠	~	~
4	⚠	⚠	⚠	⚠	⚠	⚠

Fig 2-2 Synoptic table of the hazards caused by the particular laser classes: ① at permanent irradiation, either with optical instruments (left column) or for the naked eye (right column); ② brief irradiation, with optical instruments or the naked eye; ③ for diffuse reflection and ④ for irradiation of skin. Legend: green check mark = safe, orange swung dash = low risk, warning sign: high hazard.

Examples: targeting laser, laser for measurement, laser for building sites, etc.
Protective Arrangements: training of the user, laser safety officer for lasers in the invisible range.
***Warning:* λ = 400–1,400 nm: "Laser Radiation. Avoid Direct Eye Exposure. Class 3R Laser Product." All other wavelengths: "Laser Radiation. Avoid Exposure To Beam. Class 3R Laser Product."**

2.3.8 Class 4

For output powers > 0.5 W. Eye and skin are endangered even at diffuse reflection. Fire hazard for flammable materials in the beam path.
Conditions: Output power > 0.5 W.
Examples: Lasers for material processing, lasers in medical therapeutic use.
Protective Arrangements: technical protective arrangements for the danger zone, laser safety officer, training of the users, consideration of fire hazards.
***Warning:* "Laser Radiation. Avoid Eye Or Skin Exposure to Direct or Scattered Beam Radiation. Class 4 Laser Product".**

2.4 Secondary Hazards

Primary hazards are directly caused by the laser beam, like the endangering of skin or eyes discussed above. Secondary hazards are in causal connection with the operation of the laser, but mainly independent of radiation characteristics.

2.4.1 Common Hazards

2.4.1.1 Mechanical Hazards

Mechanical hazards are particularly caused by mechanically moved parts such as industrial robots, parts operated by them and automatic door locks. Special hazards can be caused by high pressure in tubes and low pressures in the laser cavity.

- *Tubing:* Gas tubes usually are under pressure. Hence, they should be mechanically secured to avoid uncontrolled lashing in case of burst.
- *Laser Resonator:* In the CO_2 laser, glass tubes are used in the resonator very low. At the pressures operational they may implode if incorrectly mounted. Also during exchange service of flashlamps (high-pressure lamps) used with solid-state lasers there is the danger of an explosion.

2.4.1.2 Electrical Hazards

The CE-Sign signifies that the construction of the device is safe. Subsequent alterations to the device can affect the electrical security.

Each laser device needs a very strong power supply due to its low plug efficiency (e.g. a 800W Nd:YAG-laser needs a plug power of 25.000 kW) requiring an adjustment of the fuses and wires for the current supply. Further, in flashlamp-pumped laser units, condensers with very high capacity can carry a charge for some time after the device has been turned off.

If an external cooling-water circuit has to be installed, a close contact between water and power lines should be avoided.

2.4.1.3 Chemical Hazards

Chemical hazards are mostly caused by the materials used in laser construction.

- For excimer lasers toxic flourine and chlorine are used as laser medium. Thus, the gas containers have to be stored under secure conditions, e.g. in gas-proof cupboards with passive air ventilation. All connections of the gas tube system have to be examined carefully. In case of gas leakage, a gas mask has to be stored within reach. Modern excimer lasers mostly have the gas supply already integrated in their sealed housing.
- Most dyes of dye lasers are toxic or neurotoxic substances. Widely used dyes are rhodamine and coumarine. During dye exchange the recommendations of the manufacturer must be followed. Contact with skin and inhaling of the released vapors must be avoided. Used dyes have to be disposed of according to national and local rules and regulations.
- The laser tubes of Ar^+- and Kr^+-lasers contain highly toxic beryllium. Thus, these tubes have to be handled with special care.
- Dusts from broken ZnSe lenses (transparent material for CO_2 lasers) are toxic. ZnSe dust has to be collected while wearing protective goggles, gloves, protective clothing and breathing mask. Disposal has to be carried out according to national and local rules and regulations.

Hence, opening of laser cavities should not be done by the user himself but left to the service personnel or the manufacturer.

2.4.1.4 Fire Hazard

Flammable materials represent a fire hazard during operation of lasers with high output power, mainly because of flammable material in the beam delivery system, on the operation area and in the surrounding area.

Beam Delivery System: Potential danger occurs when the beam axis has been changed by alignment work if the beam directly or indirectly hits cooling tubes (e.g. from guiding mirrors) or the housing of the optical path. Even fracture of optical fibers or the wrenching of their connection plugs can allow laser radiation to escape.

Operation Area: endangered objects in this region are:

- cooling tubes or supply devices on the laser head
- objects in the vicinity of the operation site such as paper rolls and cleaning agents or solvents.

Surrounding area: Special onsideration must be given to the combustibility of inspection windows, sealings and the paint on the housing. Another critical device, although mostly situated further away, is the filtering installation. Fire can occur if the wrong combination of filters and exhausted particles is chosen, e.g. aluminum can cause sparking in and electrostatic filters, thereby constituting on acute fire hazard.

Directly and indirectly reflected laser radiation has the highest potential for danger, especially in 3D working stations if the beam is directed horizontally or vertically by accident, thus propagating freely into the room. For very high-powered lasers, even is a diffuse reflected radiation fire hazard.

Further, high reflection might occur during treatment of metallic materials such as aluminum, copper and brass or amalgam. Sparking of the processed material also represents a fire hazard, thus endangering even flammable material not in the operation site, especially synthetics, clothes, wood and alcoholic fluids.

2.4.1.5 Specific Hazards

Plasma: Laser light generation in gas lasers as well as laser welding produces plasma. Physical plasma is a gas mixture containing ions and free electrons. Laser welding and conventional welding both produce a bright welding plasma emitting intense ultraviolet and short-waved blue light. This emission is called secondary radiation; prolonged exposure can cause retina damage, inflammation of the cornea and even erythema.

Working processes: If powders are applied, aerosols occur and have to be exhausted and filtered. Just as for dusts and vapours, the MAC-values have to be considered. Unused powder has to be collected by suitable devices (dental laboratories!)

Programming: The programs of 3D-working station (robots, multi-axis-machines) have to ensure that the beam shutters cannot open during positioning of the laser head. For test runs a workpiece has to be mounted. In both cases free propagation of the laser beam could occur.

Adjustment work: Most of the reported laser accidents happened during adjustment tasks! Usually these tasks have to be performed at the opened laser device. As mirrors have to be adjusted during these works, attention has to be paid that

- The beam is not reflected onto the delivery system.
- No parts of the body or tools reach into the optical path.
- Only the minimal necessary power is applied.

CO_2 lasers: Particular HF-stimulated CO_2 lasers create ozone around the resonator, irritating eyes and airways. Thus, the resonator has to be capsuled in a sealed housing or a suitable ventilation has to be installed.

2.4.2 Vapours and dusts

Usually the emission of vapours and dusts during material processing is lower than with other thermal methods. Particularly for laser cutting this can be explained by the much smaller cutting widths. Nevertheless, the emerging gases, vapours and dusts can not be neglected.

The emissions can be divided into

a) irrespirable dusts and vapours
b) respirable dusts and vapours (aerodynamic diameter < 10 µm)
c) gases

Irrespirable dusts and fumes represent no hazard for the user but should be avoided in order to protect of the optical devices of the laser apparatus.

Respirable dusts and fumes carry a high health risk for the user, particularly carcinogenic or toxic substances.

Their absorbance mainly is performed by respiration. Deposition occurs during inspiration as well as during expiration, with the interior surface of the respiratory tract presenting an area of 80–100 m^2 for the settlement of particles.

Dust is produced by separation of solid matter, fumes by thermal and/or chemical processes. For evaluation of the health hazards not only effects of the contaminant but also its concentration, the exposure time and most of all the size of the particles have to be considered.

Dusts, gases and fumes are distinguished by their effects driving the limits for the MAC:

a) *lung stressing substances:* inert fine dusts or fumes that are not toxic or carcinogenic but deposit in the lung, thus impeding oxygen exchange.
b) *toxic substances:* all toxic gases, fumes and dusts; these can affect various organs and can use acute or chronic diseases.
c) *carcinogenic substances:* their handling requires special care. They are divided into the three subclasses A1, A2 and B:
   - *A1:* Substances definitely categorized as carcinogenic, e.g. benzene, nickel.
   - *A2:* Substances that have been categorized as carcinogenic only in animal experiments, e.g. butadiene, cobalt and its derivates.
   - *B:* Substances under strong suspicion for carcinogenic potential, e.g. formaldehyde, pyrolysis products from organic materials (dentistry!).

2.4.2.1 Metals

Exposure to the emissions caused by the cutting of metals is only of secondary importance in dentistry but for the sake of completeness has also to be discussed.

During cutting of stainless steels, chromium and nickel are set free. Nickel and all its derivates definitely are carcinogenic, whereas for chromium only Cr VI is dangerous.

In all studies the particles showed a diameter between 0.042 µm and 0.35 µm, thus requiring filters for particles of < 1 µm diameter.

2.4.2.2 Organic Matters

Particle diameters are between 0.07 µm and 0.25 µm, comparable to metals. The diameters tend to decrease with increasing generation of gaseous pyrolysis products.

a) *concentration of hydrocarbon*: Studies show that substances with a high aerosol rate deliver less gaseous hydrocarbons. Polymers have a very high hydrocarbon emission.
b) *Concentration of carbon monoxide*: processing of polycarbonates cause the highest CO concentration of about 50 mg/m^3. Polyamide causes about 25 mg/m^3.
c) *Carcinogenic substances*:
   - polycyclic aromatic hydrocarbons
   - benzene
   - carbonyl derivates
   - phenol

2.5 Protective Measures

The protective measures introduced in this chapter follow the international standard IEC 60825-1 and the European standard EN 60825-1. The prescribed measures always describe the minimum safety requirements to be fulfilled.

Although the introduced proceedings are highly recommendable in any case, it has to be explicitly noted that the national rules and regulations for safe operation of a laser device differ from country to country.

2.5.1 Laser Protective Eyewear

The standard EN 207 (following up the DIN) requires a safety level for protective glasses whereby not only the laser radiation is attenuated to MPE-values, but the filter material withstands the specified laser power. Hence, e.g. normal spectacles offer no protection against CO_2 radiation as often wrongly believed: in fact the glass absorbs the radiation, but due to the instantaneous heating it would splinter immediately and endanger the eye mechanically.

The filter's transmittance T(λ) only has to reduce, visible the specified wavelength to the MPE-value without strong suppression of the other; only then can normal work be carried out while the goggles are worn. The resistance of a filter against laser radiation is analyzed by examining if the optical density persists at least for 10 s, as this should be enough time for the weaver to leave the danger zone. For pulsed lasers the requirement is to withstand 100 pulses. By passing the test, the laser goggle not only has an optical density of e.g. 5, but also the protective grade 5.

Thus, laser goggles are not designed for prolonged looking into the direct beam, but only for accidental irradiation!

For high protective level it is usually not the optical density that causes problems for the manufacturer, but the resistivity against high intensities. Hence, a protective level of 5 means that the optical power density is at least 5 and that the filter withstands the maximum power density this filter may be exposed to. Further, EN 207 requires that:

- the goggles must transmit at least 20% of the visible radiation, otherwise the manufacturer has to inform about it in written form.
- the goggles must not lose their protective grade even at longer UV irradiation.
- the goggles have to keep their protective effect even at higher temperatures (55°C) and high humidity
- wavelength and protective grade must be specified on the goggles.
- the instructions for use (in the language of the country it is distributed in) have to contain all the relevant specifications of the goggles.

2.5.1.1 Labeling

EN 207 demands the following scheme for labeling laser goggles:

DIR: operation mode
1060: wavelength (λ) in nm
L6A: protective level
RH: sign of the manufacturer
DIN: testing standard

Operation modes (simplified): The letters come from the German standard and have to be verified for the specific languages. Table 2-1 shows a simplifyied chart of operation modes. All tested operation modes have to be declared. In any case, all goggle have to be tested for cw. If no operation mode is shown at all, the goggles can be used for cw.
Wavelength: Written in nm; also the indication of ranges is possible (e.g. 600-800 nm).

Table 2-1 Operation modes for labelling laser protective eyewear.

OPERATION MODES (SIMPLIFIED)		PULSE DURATION
M	mode-coupled lasers	$<10^{-9}$ s
R	Q-switched lasers	from 10^{-9} s to 10^{-7} s
I	pulsed laser	from 10^{-7} s to 5×10^{-7} s
D	continious-wave lasers	from 0.1 s (if 315 nm–1400 nm, then > 0.5 ms)

Warning: the wavelengths 1064 nm (Nd:YAG) and 10,600 nm (CO_2) can easily be confused! Goggles only for CO_2 radiation do not protect against Nd:YAG radiation!

Protective Level: Defined as discussed above.

According to wavelength and operation mode, different protective levels can be indicated:

- e.g. for different ranges of wavelengths:
  - λ = 570–620 nm L5A RH DIN
  - λ > 620–900 nm L4A RH DIN
- e.g. for different operation modes:
  - D 1060 nm L5A CZ DIN
  - IR 1060 nm L3A CZ DIN

The required protective grade for a certain laser unit has to be written in its handbook. In case of doubts a higher protective grade is the better choice.

Many goggles also are marked with the CE sign. The requirements for the CE are not as strict for several aspects as a survey according to EN or DIN 207. E.g. for the CE certificate only a prototype has to be tested, whereas for a survey according to EN/DIN 207 recurrent random tests have to be done during manufacturing.

2.5.1.2 Directions

Protection of the Eyes. If a free propagating laser beam is operated, protective eyewear should be worn on plinciple; the same is true when optical instruments such as microscopes are used during laser application.

When laser goggles are used it is important to check wheater they are suitable for the operated wavelength. The necessary protective grade, e.g. L3 or L5, can be calculated. For practical use the goggles with the highest protective grade should be purchased, (as far as of the distributors supplies permit). Further, the permitted operation modes have to be checked.

It should be ensured that the goggles transmit sufficient visible light apart from the laser wavelength. Hence, no broad-band filtering systems absorbing many wavelengths, thus transmitting almost no visible light, should be purchased.

A strong decrease of transparency reduces safety during work and increases the risk of accidents, especially due to reducing the visibility of illuminated warning signs, controls etc. Thus, a clear sight of controls has to be assured during use of protective eyewear! Before EACH use, the goggles should be checked for faults. Scratches, cracks or discolorations reduce safety. Defective goggles never must be used.

Another important point is the comfort during use: goggles with glass filters are heavy, and goggles are mostly more uncomfortable to wear than spectacles or wraps. Wraps are usually also are suitable for persons wearing glasses. A new development is systems where reflection layers are sputtered on plastics, thus allowing high protective grades at low weight.

Windows. The Laser Safety Officer has to consider the estimated irradiation time for windows and shieldings by means of a risk analysis. The windows have to withstand the expected irradiation time.

Usually, normal glass provides sufficient protection for wavelengths over 4 µm. Lasers with shorter wavelengths (e.g. Nd:YAG) can reach into neighbouring rooms. For these wavelengths, windows and shieldings have to be covered with absorbing materials.

In this regard, it also has to be assured that the beam axis does not hit windows and doors. If possible, it should not be at eye level (110 to 172 cm), althrough this is sometimes of difficult to manage.

Reflecting Surfaces. Reflecting surfaces not only reflect laser radiation; in some cases they can even focus it. Thus, the laser safety officer has to make sure that reflecting surfaces are avoided in the working range.

In dentistry the use of matt finished instruments and a suitable covering of reflecting surfaces in the mouth (metallic fillings, etc.) is recommended.

2.5.2 Organizational Protective Arrangements

Nomination of a Laser Safety Officer (LSO). The LSO on the one hand has the duty of training the employees and on the other hand has to set the rules govening access to the laser zone.

If only laser devices of class 1, 1M, 2, 2M or 3R (visible) are operated, no LSO is necessary (3R invisible requires one). Nevertheless, it is strongly recommended that one of the staff is briefed with the basic safety aspects for these laser classes.

2.5.3 Technical Protective Arrangements

2.5.3.1 Constructive Protective Arrangements

All surfaces in rooms where lasers of class 3B and 4 are operated should have a matt and diffuse reflecting finish to avoid specular reflection. For CO_2 lasers the roughness should be more than 40 µm, for Nd:YAG lasers more than 4 µm in depth. Special care has to be taken with enameled surfaces on metallic structures (office equipment!), because simple lacquers cannot withstand the laser radiation.

Materials containing Si-O_2 (ceramics, tiles, plaster) have a reflection band at roughly 9 µm. Common glass surfaces reflect about 8% of the incoming radiation, increasing to almost 100% at grazing incidence. Here, special care has to be taken, as these reflections are specular.

Walls in the operation zone should be constructed of bricks, limestone or concrete. Solid masonry is recommended to avoid penetration by laser radiation in case of a failure until it has been discovered and stopped.

2.5.3.2 Protective Arrangements in the Laser Devices

The user can verify that the required technical protective arrangements are included in the laser device by checking that it has the related seals for approved safety. Furthermore, a manufacturer is only allowed to place a CE sign for his device if, within the scope of a risk management, he has assessed and analyzed all foreseeable hazards for normal operation and in the case of damage, and demonstrably has implemented the requisite protective arrangements for protection of the user and other persons in the endangered zone. In this context the user should know that for some assessed hazards it is a sufficient implementation of protective measures to inform the user to behave according to the operating instructions, since for some cases technical protective measures cannot help (e.g. delivery of ionizing radiation after severe damage of the device due to handling malpractices). Hence, the required behaviour according to the operating instructions always has to be observed. Otherwise, the full liability for damages to persons or equipment rests with the operator of the device.

For lasers of class 2 to 4, safety interlocks have to make sure that unintended radiation always is prevented. This is especially required for electromagnetic glitches etc. as triggers.

A constructive arrangement against unwanted redirection of the beam is its defined guidance through protective housings or optical guiding components. Foreseeable failures such as spring fracture or loosening of mounting parts may not lead to critical failure of the whole construction.

Another protective measure pertaining to an apparatus are the electrical interlock switches on manipulation flaps and doors, as well as the key-lock. When starting the laser with the key-lock, a warning sign for radiation emission has to be implemented.

2.6 Standards and Legal Rules

Again it has to be stated that the standards and legal rules are slightly different for each country. The Austrian rules and standards will be discussed here as an example (all the authors of this chapter are from Austria). The actual regulations for each country have to be obtained from the national professional organizations.

2.6.1 Laser Safety Officer

According to ÖNORM ÖVE EN 60828-1 and ON Rule ONR 1960825-8 a laser safety officer (LSO) has to be nominated by the responsible operator, if a class 3B or class 4 laser is operated in an institution. The LSO has to attend a special course. For Austria, contents and duration of the course is regulated by ÖNORM S 1100.

2.6.1.1 Responsibilities and duties of the Laser Safety Officer

The main task of the LSO is support and advice for the responsible operator concerning protective arrangements and safe operation of the laser devices.

The specific tasks of the LSO are:

a.) Performance of hazard analysis in the rooms where the lasers are operated, comprising the definition of the danger zone. This shall be done according to risk management.
b.) Advice for the responsible operator and for the supervisors of the laser areas for safety aspects, purchase and starting of laser devices and arrangements concerning occupational medicine.
c.) Choice of the personnel-protecton equipment.
d.) Cooperation in laser safety education for employees working with laser devices or in the laser control areas concerning hazards and protective arrangements.
e.) Cooperation in examination and official acceptance of laser devices according to national rules and regulations. Assurance that maintenance and service of the devices is performed only by trained workers to do this.
f.) Scheduled checks that the prescribed protective measures are being observed, e.g. wearing of personnel protective equipment, installation of protective screens and warning signs, standardized work methods and procedures for adjustments.
g.) Information of the responsible operator and the supervisors of the laser areas on defects and failure of laser devices.
h.) Investigation of all accidents and incidents involving lasers, were and forwarding of all relevant information on preventive actions to all involved persons including the safety officer.

Additional tasks can be:

a.) decisions on technical and operational protective measures
b.) advice of employees working with lasers or supervising them
c.) preventing the use of lasers if necessary
d.) Contacting authorities and keeping in touch with them

Here it has to be especially noted that responsibilities of the LSO simply have the character of so-called expert responsibilities. Thus, the management is never and in no case excused from its duty of care and its responsibility for the safety of the employees. As long as e.g. the owner of a dental practice himself undertakes the training for the LSO, there is no doubt of the undivided responsibility of his person for the safety of his employees. But as soon as another person is nominated and trained as LSO, as often happens e.g. in clinical departments, this person can be held responsible only if his duties were not properly fullilled: e.g. choice of insufficient protective clothing (including eyewear), no annual training of the concerned persons, no information on required constructional measures (coating of windows, interlock switches, etc.), no regular checks of odherence to the rules for safekeeping of the keys, and so on.

But as the LSO usually has no authority to issue directives against the management or the head of the department, he is not responsible for neglected protective measures (e.g. no installation of interlock switches, purchase of personnel-protection equipment of only poor grade (e.g. for economic reasons)) as soon as he can prove in any way that he had asked for sufficient measures.

2.6.2 Legal Scope

Usually standards have no legal character but are rules for technical demands. But standards can be explicitly cited in rules and regulations, thereby becoming authoritative.

Recommendations for users that are published by standardization organizations have no legal character, because the behavior of users cannot be standardized. Thus they are handled as rules or recommendations.

At the moment there is no law in Austria regulating laser safety for the user, except laser pointers (BGBl. II Nr. 321/1999) and laser weapons (BGBl. I Nr. 4/1998), but there are several laws for general occupational safety.

Remark: in Germany the rule for accident prevention BGV B2 (former VBG 93) of the German employer's liability insurance association is applied. This provision is based on EN 60825-1 and prescribes several mandatory rules for the user.

2.6.3 Behavior in the Case of Incidents and Accidents

The LSO has to be informed immediately about incidents and accidents caused by laser devices. There should be no further use of the laser device concerned until the investigations of the incident are closed and appropriate measures have been taken to avoid further accidents or incidents.

The LSO should work out recommendations based on the investigations to avoid further events of this kind and should forward them to the responsible operator at least to the following persons or departments:

- all other LSOs of the institution
- the technical department (e.g. the technical service center)
- all laser users

2.6.3.1 Report Procedure According to ON Rule ONR 1960825-8

In a case in which an accident must be assumed involving a laser device, the LSO has to write a report of the relevant circumstances containing at least:

a.) A summary of the circumstances of the incident leading to injury:
   1) date, location and time of the incident
   2) names and tasks of all involved persons
   3) details of the accident as described by the injured person
   4) factors that obviously contributed to the incident
   5) recommendations of the LSO to avoid a recurrence
   6) obvious or presumed nature of all injuries.

b.) If necessary, a written statement from all involved persons (including the LSO, and if possible, who are the laser user and/or operator) being able to give relevant information regarding the incident

c.) Medical reports for all injured persons.

d.) Complete data of the laser product, especially of state and settings of the device and accessory immediately after the incident.

e.) A list of devices and accessories that were used during the incident including, sufficient information for their recognition.

2.6.3.2 Evaluation

The health and safety guidelines of the employee safety law demands an evaluation of all workplaces concerning possible danger. Further information can be found e.g. on the Internet at www.eval.at which includes details of a multimedia CD ROM about this topic.

An evaluation scheme could contain the following aspects (for more detailed schemes see guidelines):

- definition of the evaluated area (department, location)
- description of the workplace in the laser control areas (activities)
- description of the laser device (i.e. the tools and supplies for work)
- laser class
- wavelength
- output power (according to accessories)
- accessories
- identification of the hazards and the risk
- damage of the retina
- Nominal Hazard Zones (NHZ, usually information from the manufacturer)
- fixing of the protective measures (see chapter 2.5)
- documentation (health and safety protection documents)

The documents of the evaluation have to be updated regularly!

Acknowledgement:
The present chapter is largely based on the script “Lasersicherheit in Industrie und Technik”, 2003, by Dr. Georg Vees, Austrian Research Centers Seibersdorf.

3

Cavity Preparation

A. Moritz, U. Schoop and M. Straßl, E. Wintner

3.1 Overview

3.1.1 Development of the Laser-Assisted Cavity Preparation

Soon after the realization, by Maiman, of the first ruby laser in 1960, the exploration of new ways of using the tool in medicine started. From the outset there was interest in the preparation and conditioning of dental hard tissues: Already in 1964, Stern and Sognnaes[1] first experimented on hard tissue ablation with a ruby laser. Since that time, it has become the most explored field in laser dentistry. In recent years it has become recognized by the media and public through descriptions such as pain-free treatment and minimal invasive therapy. Because of that it is necessary to have a clear picture of the possibilities and advantages of this therapy and also the limits and risks, irrespective of all advertising and commercial interests.

The first trials by Stern and Sognnaes with the ruby laser were not very successful: the ruby laser showed the expected ability to ablate dental hard tissue, but the treatment led to a marked rise in temperature in the surrounding tissue, and recognizable damage was observed.[1,2] Similar results were seen for the Nd:YAG- and the CO_2-laser in 1965.[3] These results were later confirmed in the 1980s.[4,5] Additionally, the holmium laser, that was

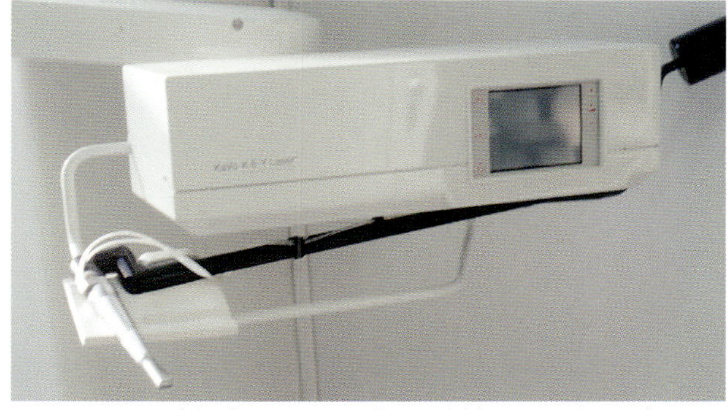

Fig 3-1 One of the first commercially available Er:YAG lasers for preparation of dental hard tissue. In this the source of radiation and power supply were separated. Fibers for this wavelength were not yet sufficiently developed for routine use.

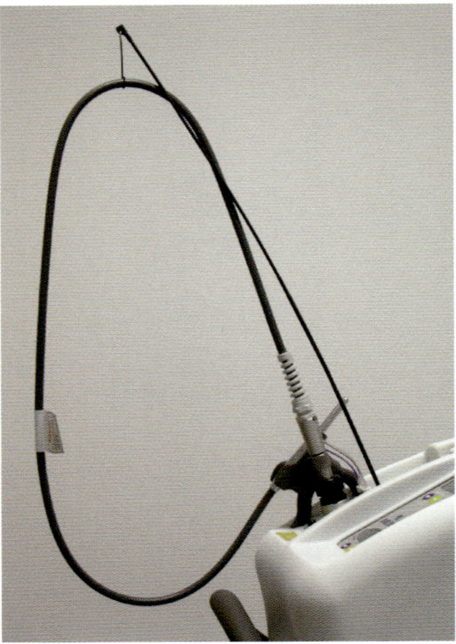

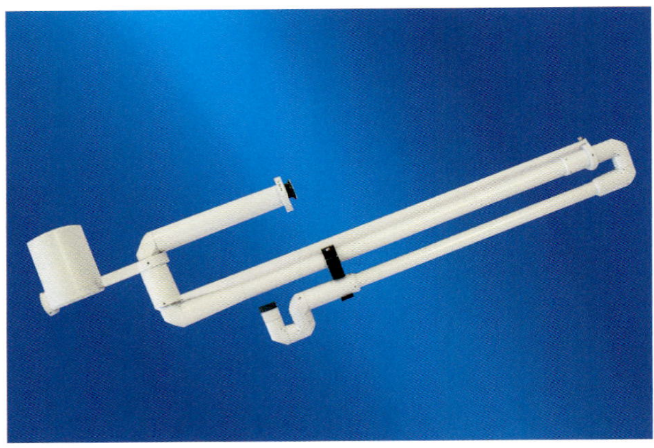

Fig 3-2 und 3-3 In today's generation of devices, fibers are provided for beam delivery. Fig 3-2 (left) shows a fiber-based delivery system, Fig 3-3 (right) a modern articulated arm.

studied later, showed similar effects.[6] In all these systems massive thermal side effects led to dangerous temperature rises in the pulp as well as to micro cracks and carbonization (CO_2, Ho:YAG). Therefore, all these laser types were abandoned for the preparation of dental hard tissue.

The reason for the negative results is the direct thermal side effect of the explored wavelength on the dental hard tissue, which leads to a high temperature within the tooth. With the ruby and Nd:YAG laser, deep penetration of the radiation also leads to transport of heat to the pulp.

To establish a clinical preparation of dental hard tissue, an ablation mechanism with a small penetration depth had to be found. This would lead to a lower temperature rise in the surrounding area and give the chance to control the temperature.

Wavelengths suitable for this were found with the excimer laser within the ultraviolet range[7,8] and the erbium laser within the infrared range[9,10]. For both the excimer laser and the Er:YAG laser it could be shown that with the right laser parameters the thermal side effects were small.

Since the excimer laser showed only a restricted ability in clinical use, mainly because of ablation and technical reasons (see Section 3.3), the erbium-based laser systems (Er:YAG and Er,Cr:YSGG) have become standardized treatment tools for dental hard tissues.

Besides the development of small devices, suitable for mass production for use in clinic and practice, the science of dental hard tissue treatment in the last few years has focused on limiting the damage to the surrounding tissue. This has been accomplished mainly through the correction of irradiation parameters. Therefore, totally new ablation techniques were established in the 1990's.[11–13] Through the use of ultra-short pulsed laser systems of other wavelengths, with pulse durations of pico- or femto-seconds, the thermal and mechanical stress was reduced. For the first time this enabled preparation without the necessity for water-cooling. Further advantages are the possibility of precise preparation with a high selectivity for caries. A closer look at these new ideas and techniques is taken in section 3.4.5 of this chapter.

3.2 Technologies for Cavity Preparation

3.2.1 Indication-specific Problems

The primary indication for dental hard tissue treatment is the removal of tissue parts changed due to caries. Conventionally, mechanical methods are used which allow a more or a less selective removal because of density differences between the regular and changed material.

A few decades ago the "extension for prevention" theory postulated by Black was mainly used in dentistry. However, a change of thought took place. Over the years minimal invasive treatment (micro-preparation), where the healthy dental hard tissue is saved, gained importance. Today, the selective removal of carious lesions combined with the very small loss of unaffected tissue is often requested. With the development of a variety of adhesive filling materials, the first step towards this was taken. Through the direct adhesion of the composites with the dental hard tissue, it is even possible to work with very irregular cavities and undercuts. This allows the form of the cavity to closely match the extent of the lesion. A departure from Black's preparation concept, from the filling aspect, is consequently possible nowadays.

The second main condition for allowing a maximum conservative preparation is a suitable tool, which enables the selective removal of the affected tissue.

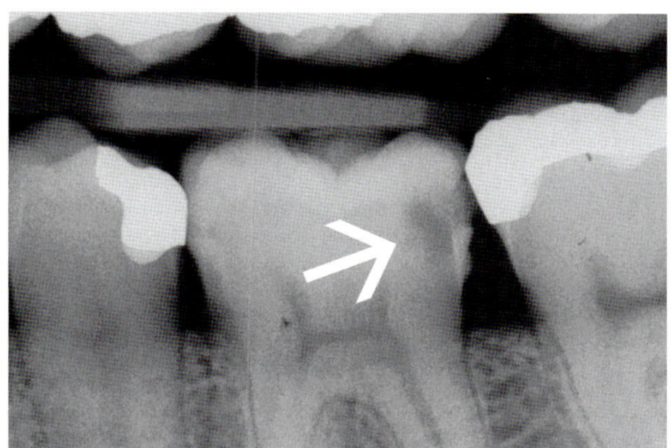

Fig 3-4 Typical carious lesions starting from the distal approximal contact of tooth 36. Introral X-ray picture, bite-wing technique.

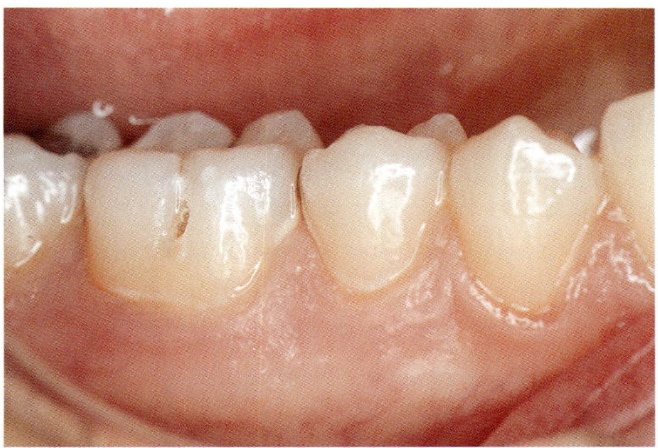

Fig 3-5 Contact point decay at tooth 36, clinically hard to recognize. Following today's doctrine a wide preparation according to the preparation concept of Black (extension for prevention) is no longer indicated.

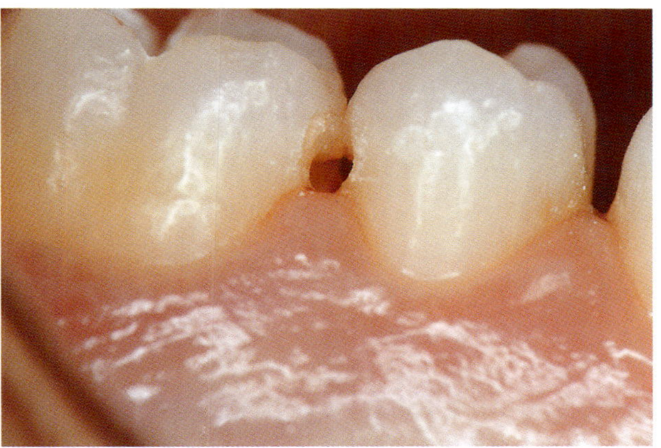

Fig 3-6 The carious lesion should be removed by micro-preparation, saving as much sound tissue as possible. In this case preparation was executed with a laser.

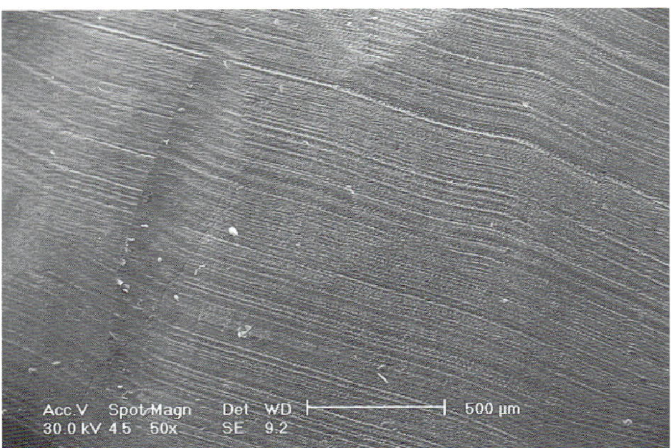

Fig 3-7 Electron micrograph of enamel surface after preparation with a diamond drill at low magnification (50x).

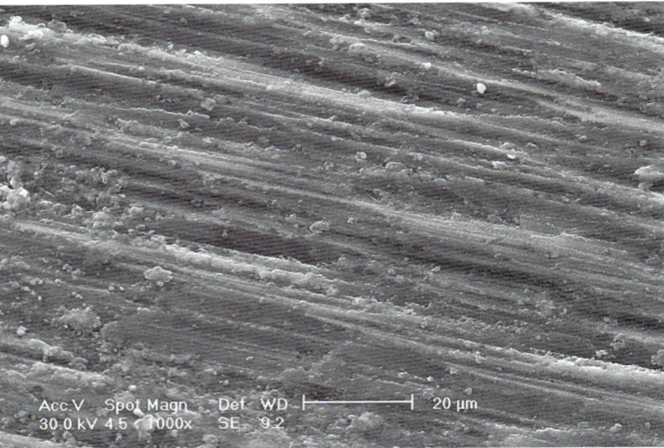

Fig 3-8 At higher magnification (1000x) the smear layer is visible, which has to be removed by cleaning with EDTA or ethanol after conventional preparation.

3.2.2 Conventional Methods – Rotating Instruments

The development of dental turbines and angle pieces has proceeded rapidly in the last few decades. Speeds of 200,000 revs/min or more, allow a quicker and less painful removal than 20 or 30 years ago. The high speed, the multi-edged tools and fine diamond grinding pieces have led away from the classical drilling procedure, to a more or less grinding form of tissue removal. Through this, a more precise and minimally invasive cavity preparation is facilitated. Furthermore, the smaller vibrating effect of these finer cutting tools combined with efficient cooling techniques, e.g., threefold water spray, lead to a reduced sense of pain. However, the ache caused by pressure, vibration and temperature can never totally be prevented and therefore anesthetics still have to be applied.

The variety of rotating tools and angle pieces also allows the dentist fine adjustment of the tool. Combined with variable rotation speeds, the tool can better meet the needs of the preparation. A quick and efficient preparation and finishing of the cavity is thus possible. Another advantage of using rotating instruments is the possibility of shaping a very precise cavity form. This can be achieved due to the geometrically exact form of the cutting tools as well as the tactile feedback during the preparation.

Despite the general advantages of the rotating tools, certain limitations in their use exist. For instance, caries-selective and minimally invasive excavation is not possible with such instruments. Furthermore, during treatment a 1–5 µm thick smear layer is formed and has to be removed before new adhesive techniques can be applied.

Detail 3-1. Temperature development and hygienic aspects of rotating instruments.

One of the main problems is the heat developed during the cutting process. In some studies temperatures of 700°C to 900°C were found. Temperature is mainly related to the cutting speed, the applied pressure and the sharpness of the drill. Since these factors are only partly controllable, as described above, an effective cooling procedure is of major importance. Results indicate that with ineffective cooling, temperature rises of up to 15°C can be reached in the pulp. The critical temperature rise lies at about 5.5°C, at which a high percentage of the pulp cells are killed[14].

The development of the dentin wound has extensive influence on the vitality of the pulp: with every mm^3 removed, about 40,000 odontoblasts

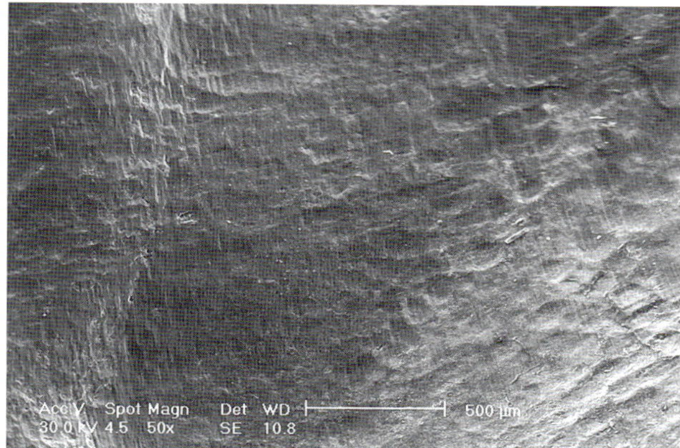

Fig 3-9 Electron micrograph picture of human dentin after preparation with carbide bur, at low magnification (50x).

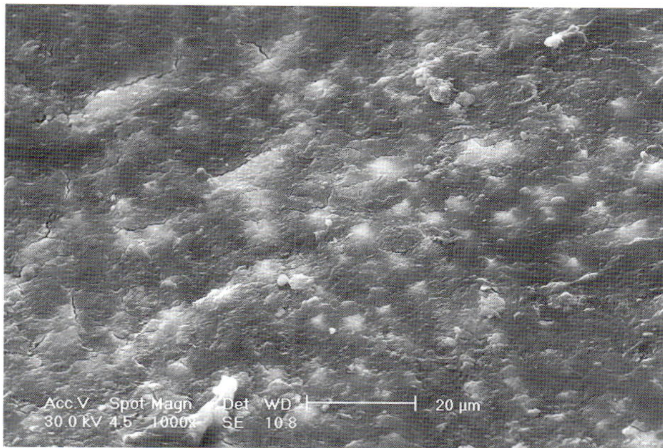

Fig 3-10 Electron micrograph picture of human dentin after preparation with carbide bur at higher magnification (1000x), smear layer is visible, as well as the therefore closed dentinal tubules and cracks.

can be destroyed. In the case of excessive temperature rises, a pulpitis or necrosis can result. The reasons for this can be too high a contact pressure or insufficient cooling, such as in the shade of the cavity edge where the water spray cannot reach. In deep cavities the danger of bacterial infection of the pulp through invisible micro cracks is also present.

Kerschbaum and Voss found, in a study in 1979, that 9% of examined capped teeth are no longer vital[15]. In a long-term study in 1981[16], they reported loss of vitality in capped teeth stood at 4% after 5 years and 15% after 10 years.

A too-high rise in surface temperature leads to a significant weakening of the surrounding enamel. The hardness under the heated area can be reduced by up to 20% at a depth of 550 µm. The surrounding enamel can also be softened by up to 10%. Additionally, the induction of micro cracks of 20 µm in depth is possible.[12]

One further potential danger can be the injury of the surrounding soft tissues through bad practice. In this case it is more likely that abutting hard tissues, such as neighbouring teeth, can be damaged. Between 1998 and 2003, Lussi et al.[17,18] found that after proximal preparation, neighbouring teeth were damaged in 95% of cases.

From the hygienic point of view, the use of water or aerosol sprays has to be looked at critically because of the possibility of infection. It is known that spray from the oral cavity can be sucked back into the device, thus contaminating it. There are two ways this can occur. Firstly, the spray media, water and air, can contaminate when sucked back into the device. Secondly, ambient air can be sucked into the device through the bearings gaps in the head piece of the device. Contamination with the spray media can be prevented by installing a non-return valve that prevents dripping. The water stops after a very short distance because of the valve, so stopping germs entering the device.

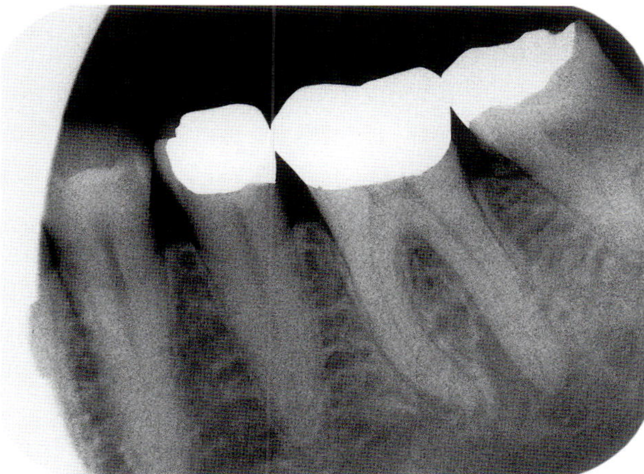

Fig 3-11: Introral X-ray. Eight months after definitive maintenance of tooth 25 with a technically faultless metal/ceramic crown, a periapical lesion is radiologically detectable. The preparation done with conventional rotating instruments had led to necrosis of the pulpal tissue.

The sucking in through the bearing gaps can be explained by the fact that, at high speed, pressure develops. This causes the surrounding air to be sucked in. At full speed, overpressure in the turbines and the angle piece equals the under pressure, thus preventing air from being sucked in. When the turbines slow down the pressures become unequal and air – and possibly germs – can enter the device. When the device is next used, any contaminants can be sprayed out again. Consequently, there is a possibility for cross contamination between patients if no adequate sterilization procedure is followed. Angle pieces are usually not as much affected since the drills usually slow down very quickly. A bigger problem is with turbines because the rotors can take up to 5 seconds to stop rotating. This problem is one that dentists are usually unaware of, but safety requirements of the industry are focusing on solving this problem.

In many high-end devices, or at least in leading companies, this problem has been solved through the installation of a so-called back-suction-preventer. In the low-cost market range, these technologies are rarely found.

3.2.3 Kinetic Cavity Preparation – KCP

Kinetic cavity preparation uses a high-speed particle stream instead of rotating drilling and grinding tools for removal of material. Similar to sandblasting, aluminium-oxide particles are used. From a reservoir, the particles are swept along in an air stream that leads through a tube to the hand piece where it is finally directed onto the preparation area. Through the collision of the particles with the surface, small fragments are torn out and an ablation process results. The pressure of these systems lies between 5 and 15 bar. The diameter of the spherical particles is 10–50 µm.

This preparation technique allows a very fine ablation and therefore the forming of a lesion-specific cavity form. Through the difference in density of healthy and carious material, the selectivity of this method is comparable to the rotating instruments. A further advantage of this method is the micro-retentive pattern on the cavity walls that enhances the bonding of the adhesive material and the tissue. Furthermore, the smear layer that is typical for preparation with rotating instruments does not occur here and the use of acid etching techniques with their occasional unfavourable side effects is not necessary[19].

One disadvantage of the method is the development of massive particle dust clouds. Therefore, special arrangements have to be made to avoid the inhalation of the dust by the patient, the doctor and the assistant (e.g., rubber dam and good suction).

3.2.4 Preparation Lasers

In laser preparation, intensive electromagnetic energy (light energy) is used for ablation of the tissue. Depending on the wavelength of the laser light, the ablative effect can be based on chemical or thermal effects (photochemical or photothermal ablation, see section 3.4).

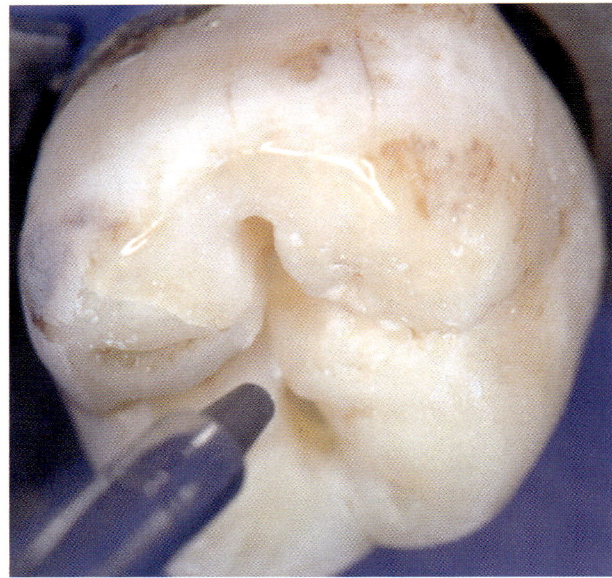

Fig 3-12: Kinetic cavity preparation.

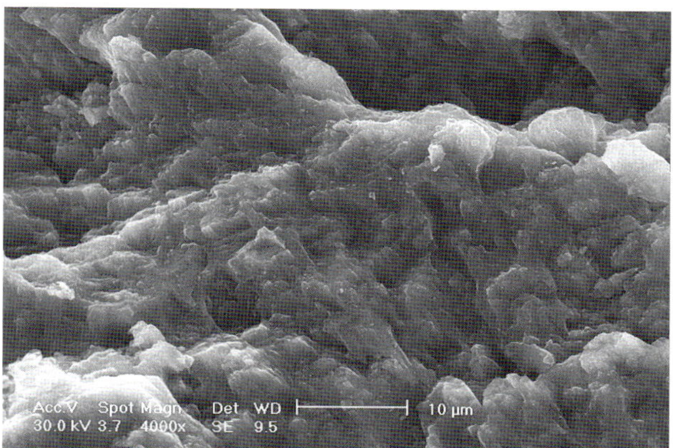

Fig 3-13a Electron micrograph (4000x) of an Erbium laser preparation in human enamel. At this high magnification the micro-retentive pattern at the surface is clearly seen. Due to the kind of ablation there is no smear layer present.

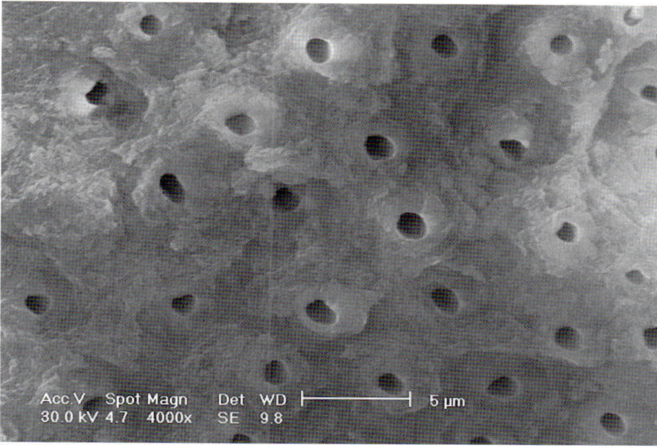

Fig 3-13b: Electron micrograph of an Erbium laser preparation in human dentin. The surface is relatively rough and therefore provides good retention for adhesive filling materials. There is no smear layer visible and the dentinal tubules are open. This facilitates penetration of composite for further increase of mechanical adhesion (orig. 4000x).

The differential absorption of laser light by materials with different consistencies results in higher or lower ablation rates. This explains the selectivity of laser ablation.

As with the KCP, the laser is not combined with any geometrical cutting form. This gives the opportunity to follow the carious lesion and have a maximally conservative preparation.

As previously mentioned, the erbium-based systems became widely accepted for preparation of dental hard tissues. Through their specific ablation mechanism (see section 3.4.1), they cause a micro-retentive pattern in the walls of the prepared cavity. This enhances the adhesion between the composite material and the cavity. This allows the use of adhesive materials without etching techniques and excludes the possible side effects. These include over-etching, danger of injury, toxicity for the pulp as well as pain resulting from acid remaining in the dentin tubules (for more see section 3.3).

Besides the preparation of the dental hard tissue for caries treatment, the erbium laser can also be used to prepare a fissure sealing (Figs 3-15a–d).

Here the use of the correct parameters is especially important. Specifically, the pulse energy should be as small as possible to prevent changes to the structure of the tissue[20]. One of the problems of laser preparation tools is that metallic fillings made of amalgam and noble metals cannot be removed. On the one hand, the fillings reflect the light strongly thus preventing efficient interference with the material. On the other hand, poisonous vapour can develop (e.g., mercury from amalgam[21]). However, phosphate, carboxylate, glass-ionomere cements, polyketones and composites can be easily removed with this method.

Difficulties can also occur during preparation of crown stumps or box preparation for inlays. Except for the use of the ceramic adhesive technique, the cavities have to be reworked with an ultrasonic device with a precision attachment (see also sections 3.7.4 and 3.7.5). This is because of the uneven form of the cavity (Fig 3-14), which has to be reformed for the inlay, and to achieve the necessary gap width. Preparation techniques like parallelization, the formation of plane boxes, and the correct preparation margins are limited by the production of rough margins and irregular cavity walls. For the preparation of suitable surfaces for Maryland bridges, ceramic inlays or similar works with adhesive materials,

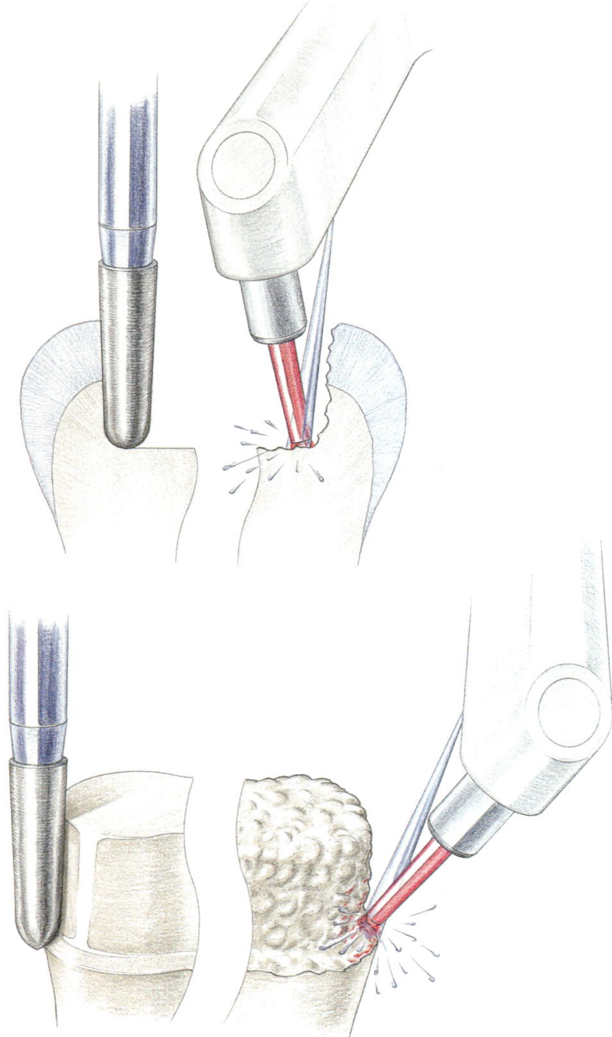

Fig 3-14 Difficulties in preparations with erbium lasers: geometrical precisely defined shapes. Whereas in cavities there are no disadvantages with regard to modern composite techniques, it is not possible with today's available laser systems to achieve precisely finished surfaces such as are necessary when grinding a tooth for a crown.

the laser offers the advantage of producing a retentive pattern for a strong adhesion by composite cementation.

The ablation speed of the laser is much slower compared to the rotating instruments. The difference can already be seen in the power applied (turbines: about 15 W, laser: 6 W). Clinical studies and routine use show a laser preparation requires about 1.3 times longer to finish. Of course, the ablation rate of the laser can be improved up to a certain level by accelerating the pulse energy. Different studies show a considerable increase of the ablation rate under laboratory conditions when the pulse energy is increased. However, every increase above the optimized parameters leads to a decrease in the thermal safety of the pulp and the structural integrity of the residual tissue (for further information see section 3.4.3).

With an increase of the pulse energy over the optimized minimal parameters, the generation of excessive microcracks in the dental hard tissues is possible (see also in Figs 3-16 and 3-17). To be able to use the advantages of the laser and protect the patient from damage, the option of a longer preparation time with optimized parameters must be taken.

One of the very interesting, typical properties of the erbium lasers is the additional bactericidal effect (see the chapters "Lasers in Endodontics", and "Lasers in Periodontology"). This feature is already well known in very strong thermal interactive systems. Examples include the CO_2, Nd:YAG and diode laser. It is interesting to note that the radiation of the erbium laser shows a bactericidal effect, even though it has the lowest thermal side effect within the hard tissue. The reason for this is the same effect that also leads to micro-explosions: since the 3 μm radiation is strongly absorbed by water it also leads to a heating effect of the cell liquid. The bacteria are therefore severely damaged and lose the ability of multiplication or are even destroyed. With good edge sealing and accurate filling, prevention of secondary caries can be strongly expected (see Figs 3-15).

As mentioned, the thermal stress on the residual tissue by the erbium laser is small compared with

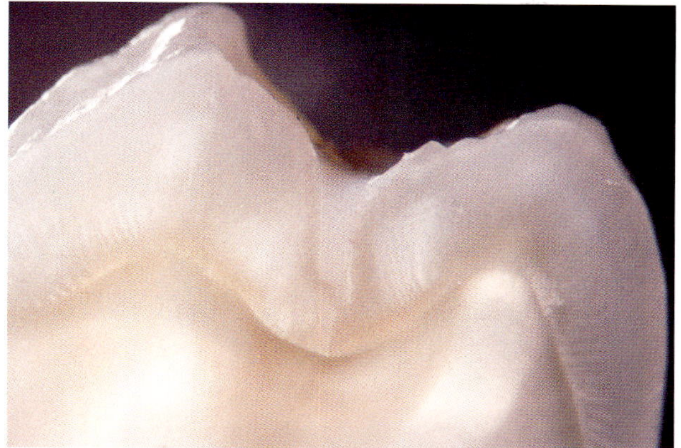

Fig 3-15a–c Histological picture (15a) and SEM picture of fissure sealing (15b, 400x, 15c, 1600x). The perfect interconnection between dental tissue and sealing material after laser preparation is clearly visible (pictures courtesy of W. Sperr).

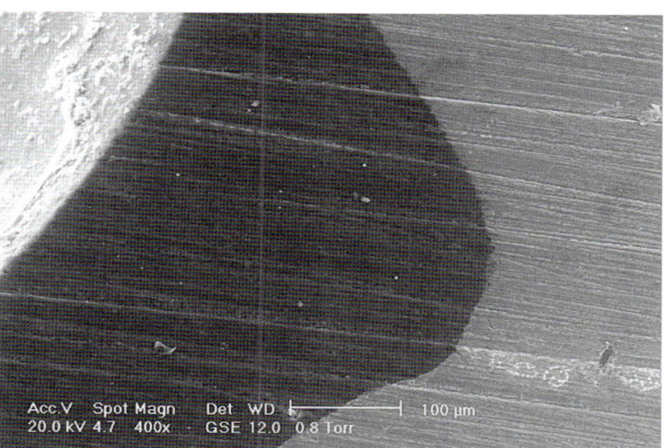

Fig 3-15b

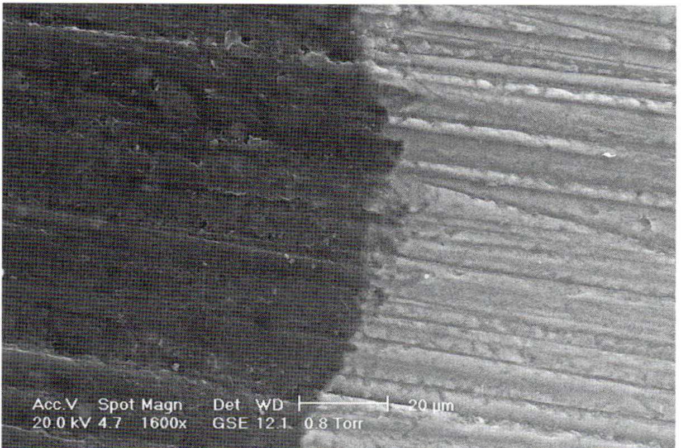

Abb. 3-15c

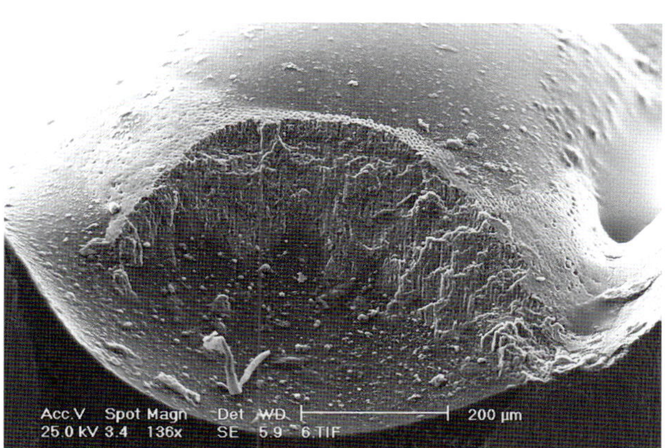

Fig 3-15d Example of a laser prepared fissure, which has not been completely sealed. The prepared cavity edge is discernible.

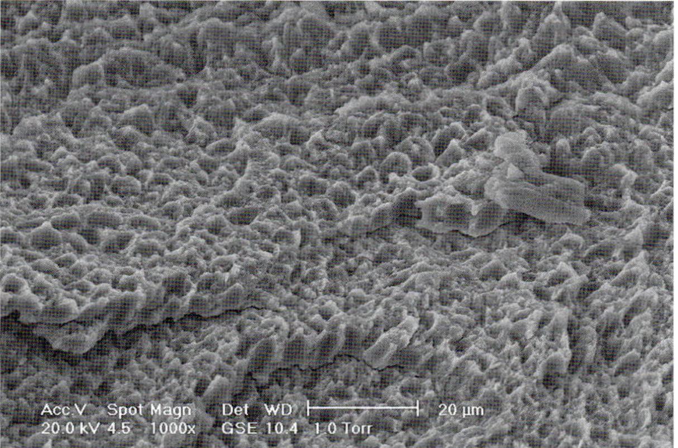

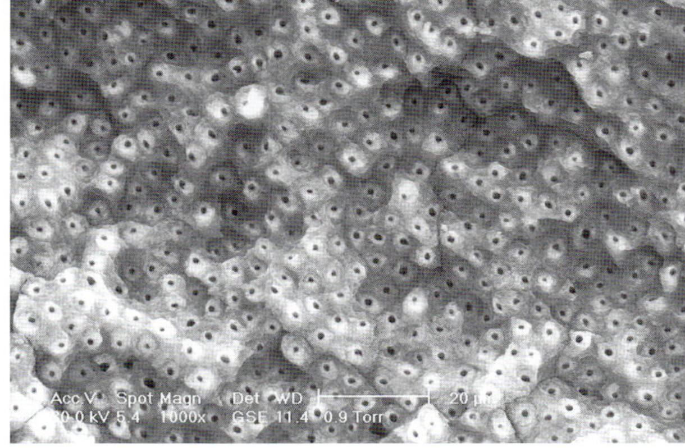

Fig 3-16 und 3-17 Electron micrograph of cracks in enamel (Fig 3-16 left, magnification 1000x) and dentin (Fig 3-17 right, magnification 1000x), which can occur easily at a too-high pulse energy. According to measurements by Frentzen they can reach up to the dentin/enamel interface.[22,23]

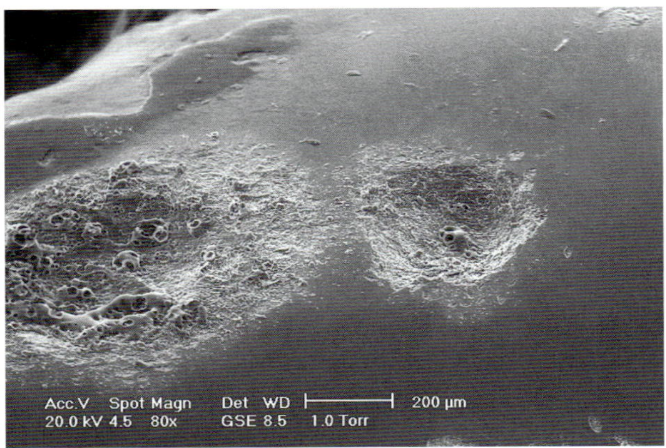

Fig 3-18 Already at low magnification (80x) melted and re-crystallized dental hard substance can be seen.

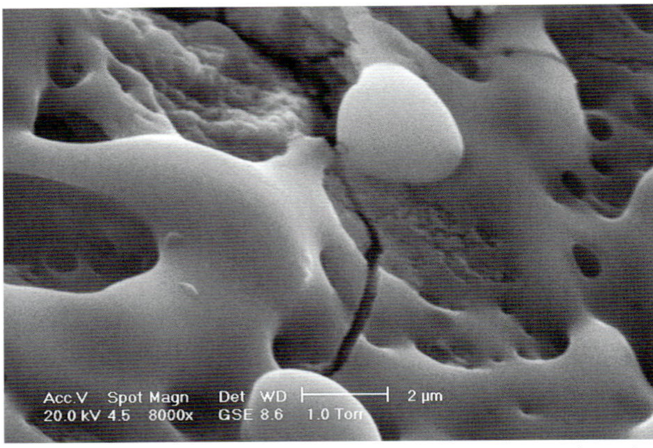

Fig 3-20 At the highest magnification (8000x) numerous cracks and melted or re-crystallized hard tissue is observable.

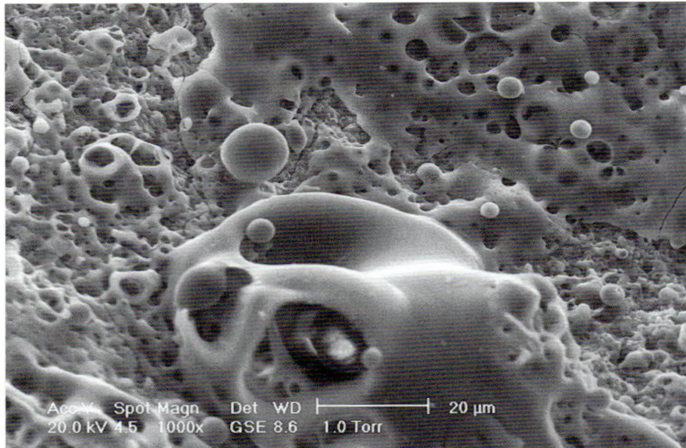

Fig 3-19 The higher magnification (1000x) makes this even clearer. Moreover, enamel cracks are visible.

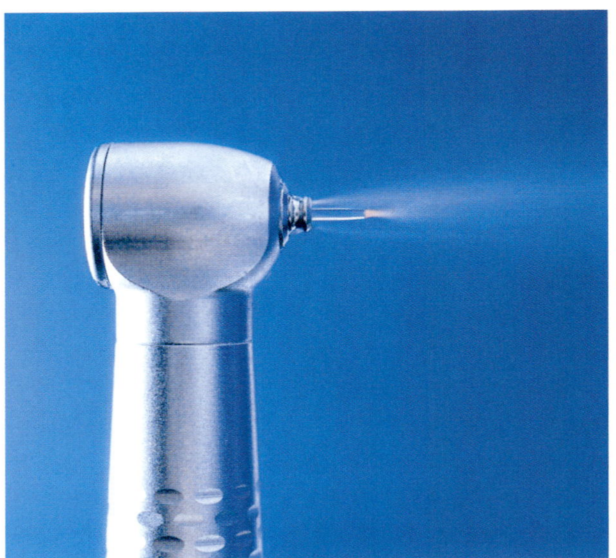

Fig 3-21 Hand piece of an Er,Cr:YSGG laser providing sufficient water cooling.

other wavelengths (also see section 3.4). However, it is still too high to refrain from cooling (for instance with a water spray). Therefore, the laser-supported hard tissue preparation is similar to the conventional methods with the danger of inducing iatrogenic pulp damage through hyperthermia. If the preparation were to be accomplished without water cooling (see Figs 3-18 and 3-19) there would be a high risk of severe damage to dental hard tissues (melting, craters, cracks and carbonization).

The burden of radiation that can be tolerated by the pulp is mainly related to the conduction of the heat by the hard tissue. Therefore, it is highly influenced by the pulse duration and the form and shape of the applied pulses.

Since every company producing laser instruments sets the parameters at different levels, there can be big differences between devices.

The basic principles thereto will be discussed in section 3.3.2.

In comparison to the rotating instruments, the laser has one major advantage. Laser treatment is contact-free, thus allowing direct cooling of the area with a water spray. Hence, it is only dependent on the construction of the hand piece as to whether the water spray can reach the area as easily as it does with the drill, or if it can be blocked out by cavity edges or overhanging cavity walls. If the spray comes in a diagonal direction from the region of the instrument's neck, as is the case for conventional hand pieces, the cooling stream can easily be disrupted by leaning edges. If the water is delivered close to the application window or the sapphire tip, a blocking-out is hardly possible.

From the patient's perspective the laser has met with positive acceptance primarily due to contact-free treatment as compared to rotating instruments. Additionally, because of the absence of pressure and temperature pain, anesthesia can often be omitted. This is especially useful when treating traumatized people and children, as a calmer treatment procedure can be followed. Also, the absence of the drilling sound is appreciated[24].

3.3 Laser-supported Cavity Preparation

3.3.1 Er:YAG and Er,Cr:YSGG Lasers

As was mentioned at the beginning of the chapter, use of the erbium-based systems (Er:YAG, Er,Cr:YSGG) has been established in the last few years. For various technical, physical and medical reasons, they are used for treatment of dental hard tissues. The basic principle of how laser light is generated has already been discussed in chapter 1 "basics of laser physics".

The advantage of the erbium wavelength is that it is better absorbed by water than by the dental tissues (see Fig 3-26). Since the enamel and the dentin consist of a relatively high percentage of water, the laser has a very low penetration depth.

The strong absorption property of water is used to hold down the development of heat during ablation: since water absorbs the laser radiation better than the dental hard tissue, the temperature rise of the tissue is relatively low during ablation. The water reaches its boiling point and causes a micro-explosion in the tooth. This divides the surrounding tissue into very small pieces and at the same time blows them apart. Since the explosion occurs in the water, we call this method water-induced ablation. Further details of this mechanism, the advantages, disadvantages and limits are discussed in section 3.4.

Since some conduction of heat can not be avoided, even though most of the radiation is absorbed by the water, a water-spray has to be used for cooling (see temperature development without cooling, Fig 3-51 and section 3.1.2.4).

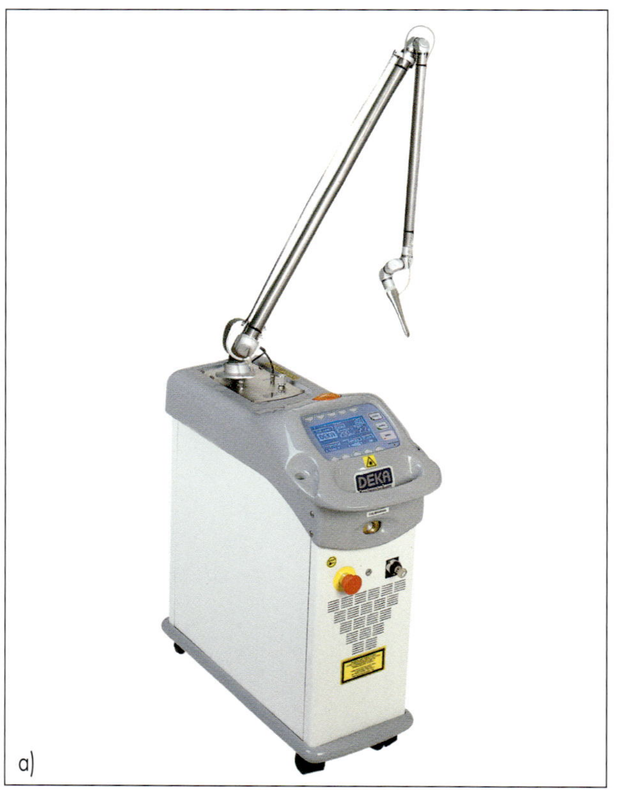

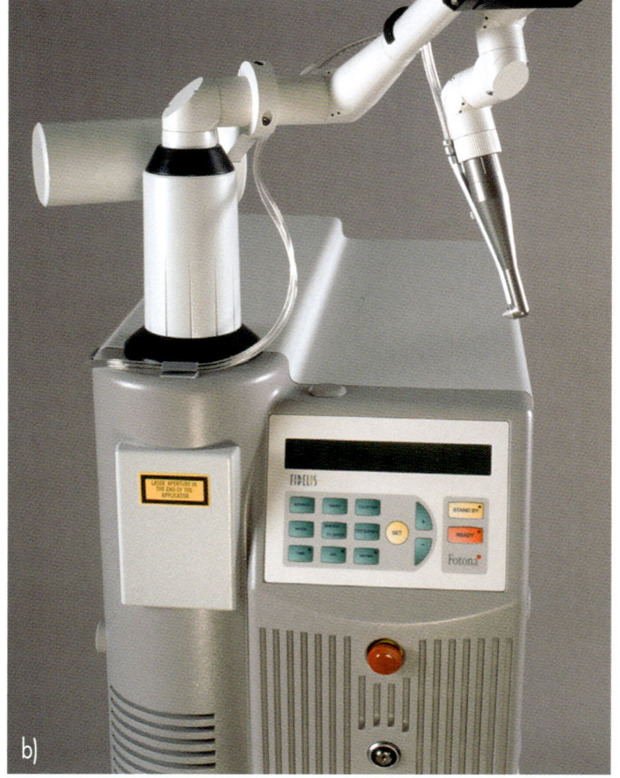

Fig 3-22a and b Examples of Er:YAG laser units.

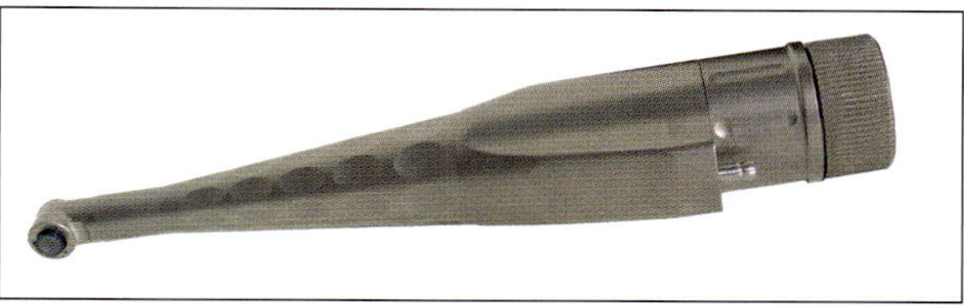

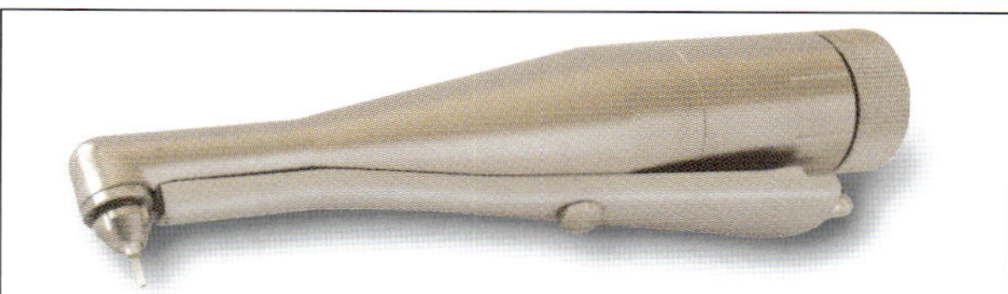

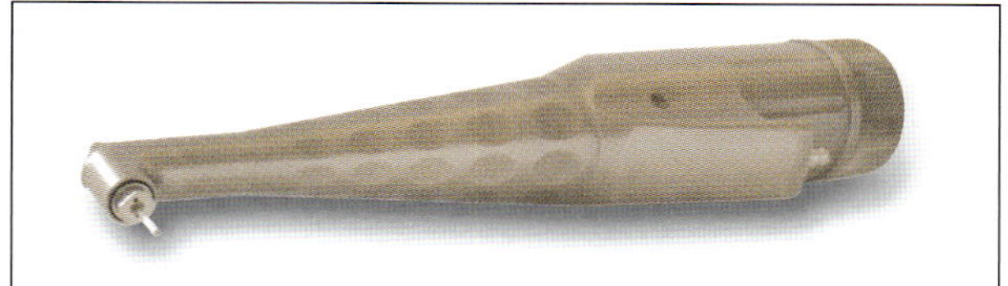

Fig 3-23a to c Hand pieces of an Er:YAG laser; top with window, in the middle and bottom with fiber tip.

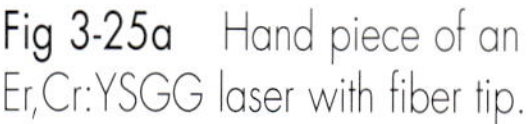

Fig 3-25a Hand piece of an Er,Cr:YSGG laser with fiber tip.

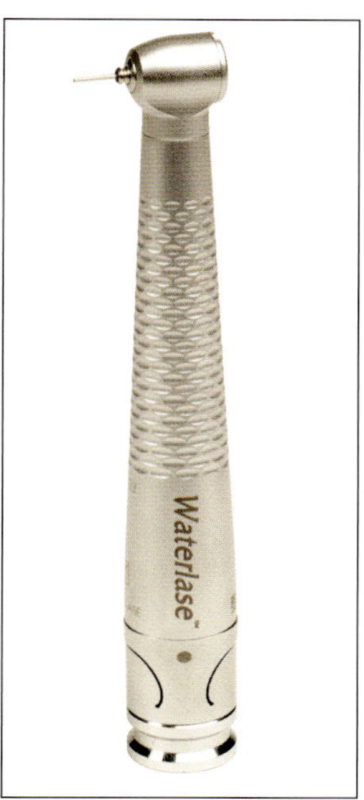

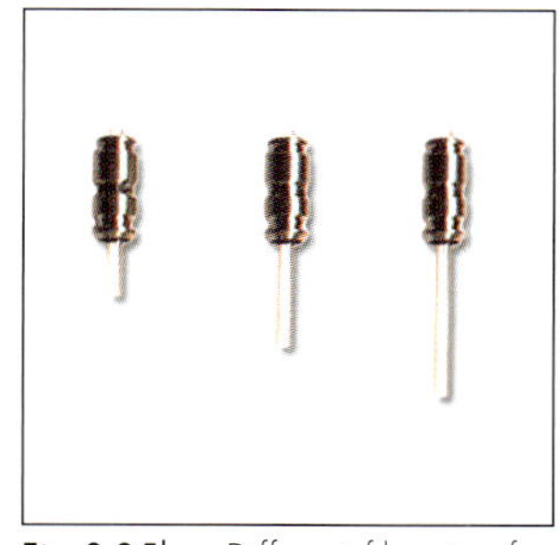

Fig 3-25b Different fiber tips for an Er:YSGG laser.

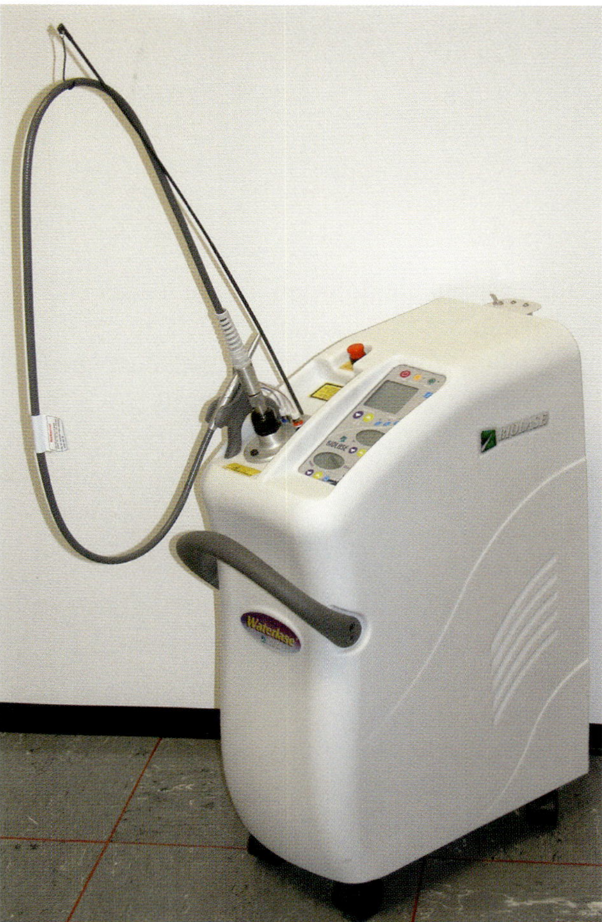

Fig 3-24 Example of an Er,Cr:YSGG laser system.

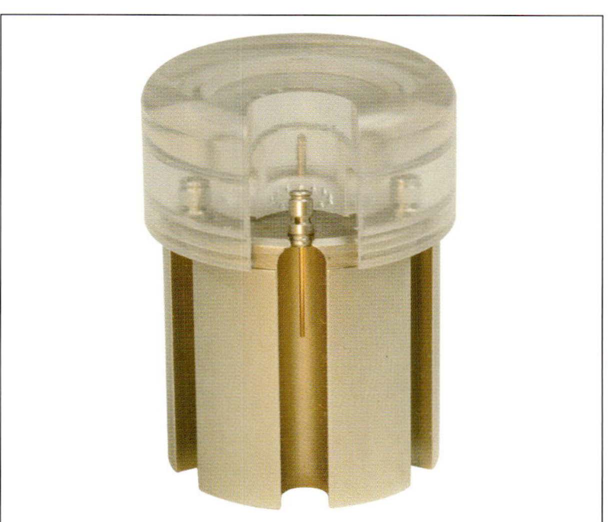

Fig 3-25c Tip holder.

Through an adequate amount of spraying, thermal damage of the pulp can nowadays be avoided.[25–27] Since the conduction of heat is highly dependent on the pulse duration and the form, the amount of water spray does not only vary from system to system but also during the treatment itself (see section 3.4). If not enough spray can be applied (e.g., because of blocking out by cavity edges) there is always the danger of pulp damage.[23]

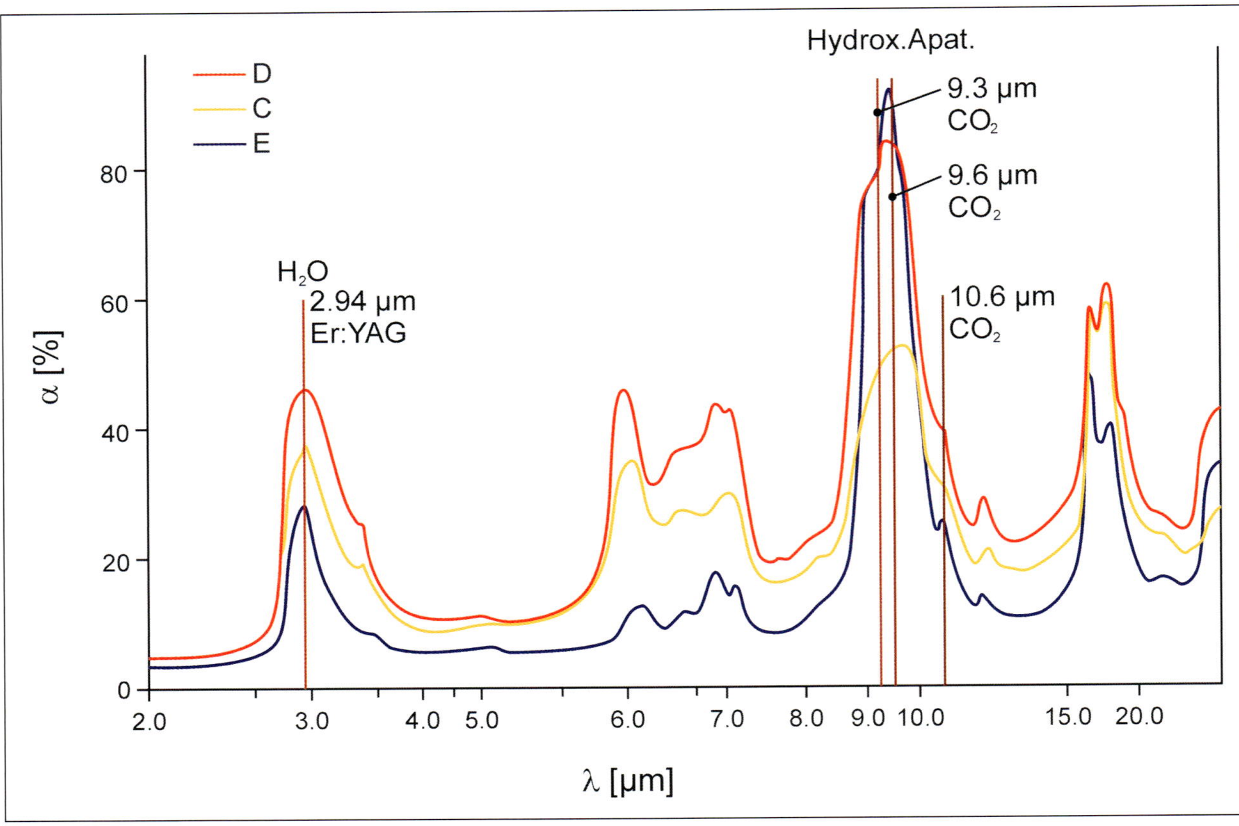

Fig 3-26 Absorption spectrum of dental hard tissues related to different laser wavelengths.
D = dentin, C = cement, E = enamel, λ = wavelength, α = absorption

Contrary to earlier studies, no immunohistochemical differences between laser- and conventionally-treated pulps have been shown.[28] Moreover, the positive effects of the laser on the regeneration of the pulp have been discussed.[29,30]

The contradiction between the studies by Tanabe and Inoue, even though they both used the same brand of laser on rat molars, can be explained by the fact that Inoue only found changes using electron microscopy. Tanabe, on the other hand, only looked using a light microscope. Additionally, it has to be mentioned that pulse durations of 50 ms used by Inoue are too long for a preparation with low thermal burden. They are much longer than the pulse duration of 80–250 µs used nowadays (see detail 3-4, section 3.4.2.2.1). Results like these show how dependent a successful laser preparation is on accuracy, practice and education of the treating doctor: only if the user has an overview of the basics and the background of this technology will he be able to prevent any damage, such as that described by Inoue, from becoming pathological. As a basic requirement, the preparation has to be performed with an optimized device using the "Method of minimal pulse energy" according to the manufacturer's instructions (see section 3.4.4). The reason is to work with the minimal potential of collateral damage.

Fig 3-27a and b Graphic depiction of water-induced ablation.

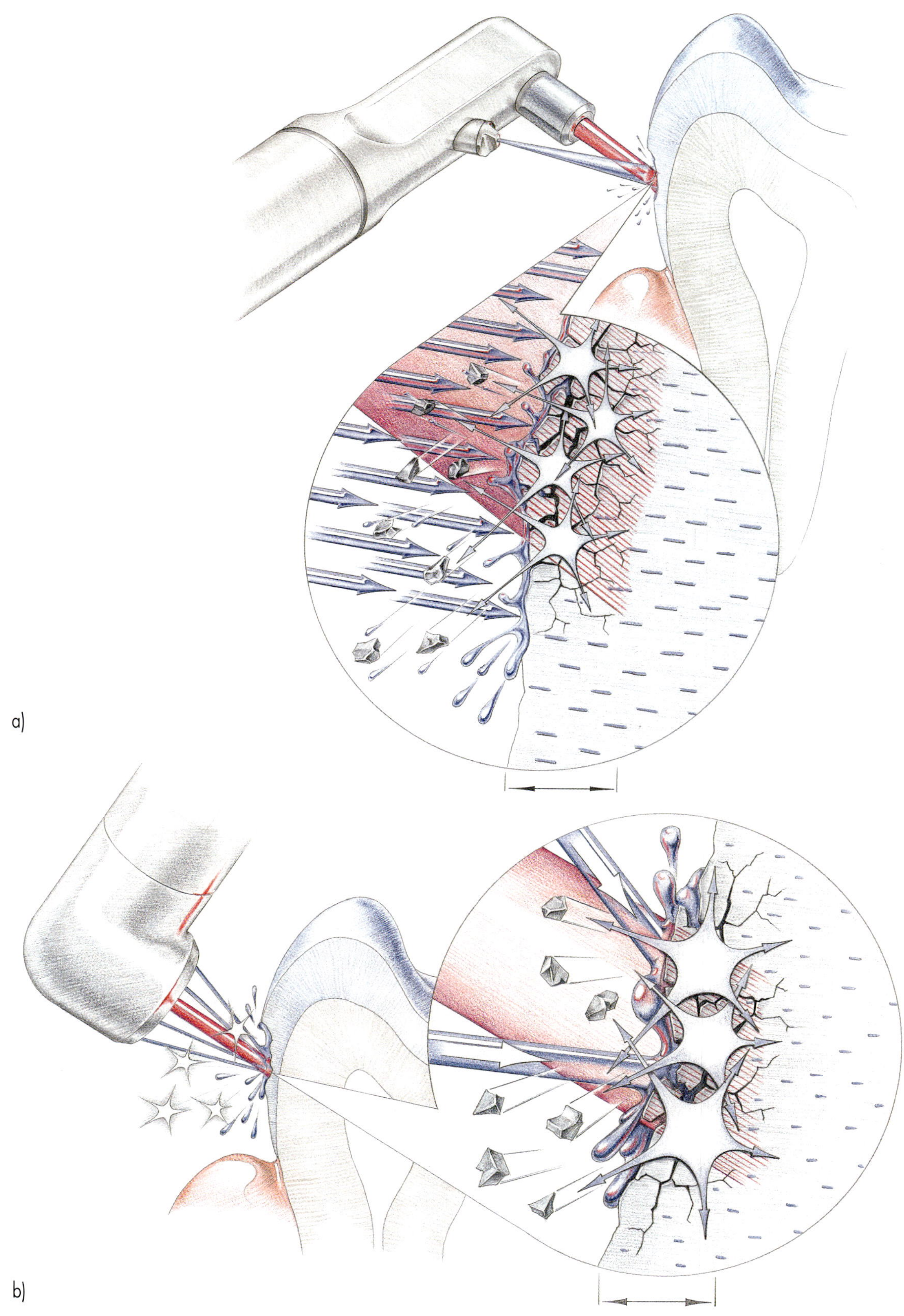
a)
b)

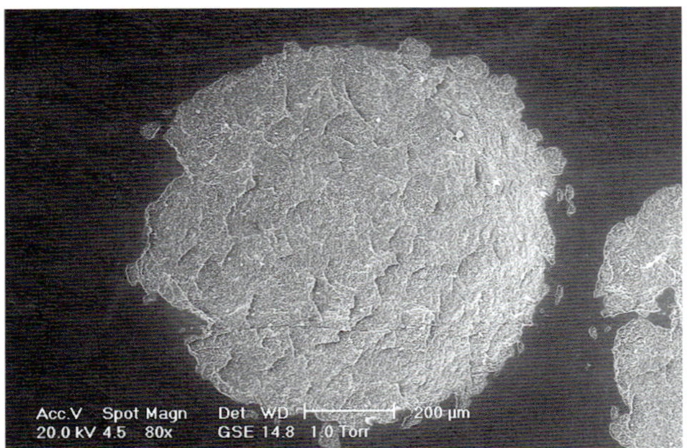

Fig 3-28 Enamel surface after a laser pulse (orig. 80x, fiber diameter 400 µm, pulse energy 400 mJ).

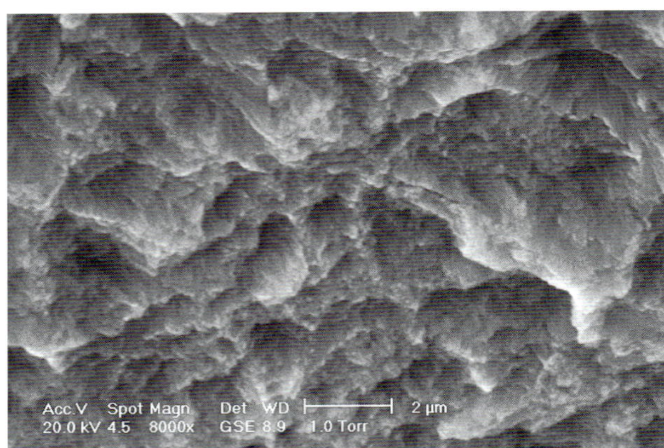

Fig 3-30 Detail from Fig 3-28 (orig. 8000x, fiber diameter 400 µm, pulse energy 400 mJ).

3.3.2 Surface Characteristics of Laser-prepared Cavities

The following series of electron micrographs shows the effect of erbium-based laser systems on dentin and enamel surfaces. The ablations in Figs 3-28 to 3-34 were prepared with an Er:YAG laser. The hand piece was moved so fast that the individual pulses were beside one another. Hence, each ablation illustrated was produced by a single pulse.

Fig 3-28 shows in overview an ablation crater after one pulse. The crater has a diameter of about 1 mm. The roughness of the cavity ground and the typical uneven ablation edge are easily visible. In the ablation pattern the typical shards of the enamel prism layers are clearly recognizable.

Fig 3-29 shows a detail of the ablation area of Fig 3-28. Here, the sites of fracture of the particles thrown out during ablation can be seen. The sites of fracture follow the facets and edges of the enamel prisms. Through their irregular course the microretentive pattern of the laser cavity is produced in the enamel.

Fig 3-30 shows a close-up view of a fracture in the enamel. It can be seen how the roughness of the site of fracture extends into the microstructure even at a magnification of 8000. Therefore, a large adhesive surface is available for bonding with filling materials.

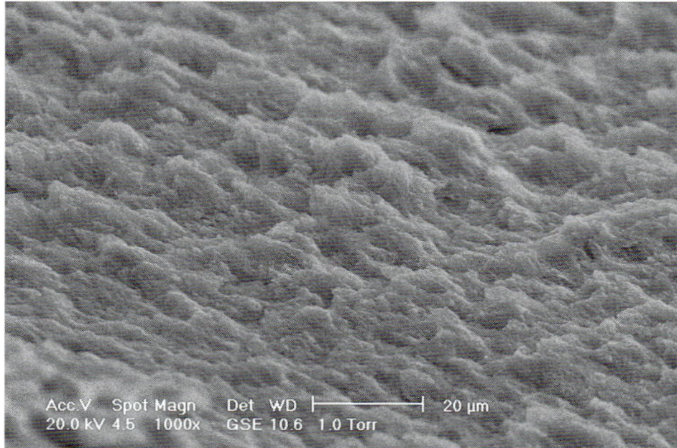

Fig 3-29 Detail from Fig 3-28 (orig. 8000x, fiber diameter 400 µm, pulse energy 400 mJ).

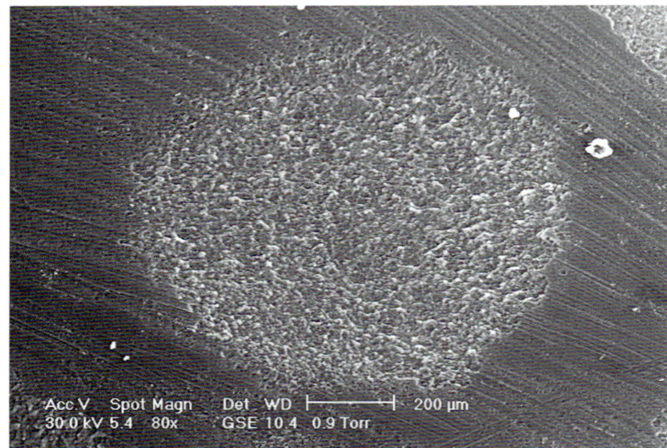

Fig 3-31 Dentinal surface after laser pulse (orig. 80x, fiber diameter 400 µm, pulse energy 400 mJ).

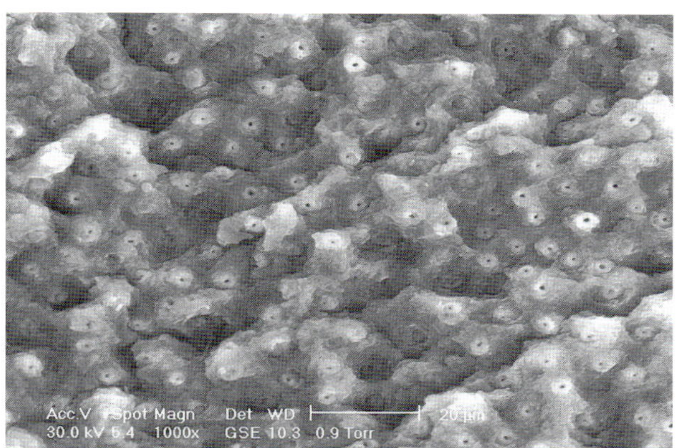

Fig 3-32 Detail from Fig 3-31
(orig. 1000x, fiber diameter 400 μm, pulse energy 400 mJ).

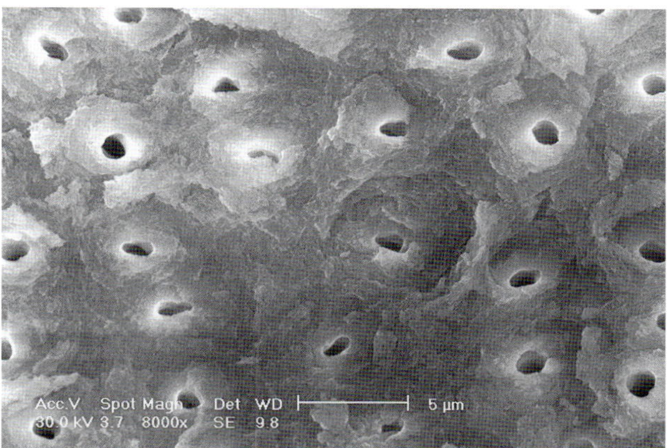

Fig 3-33 Detail from Fig 3-31 (orig. 8000x, fiber diameter 400 μm, pulse energy 400 mJ). Clearly visible is the peritubular dentin, which remains in "chimney-like" structures after laser ablation.

Fig 3-31 shows the ablation crater of one pulse in the dentin in an overview. The crater has a diameter of 0.8 mm. Again, the roughness of the cavity ground is easily visible, but in dentin the shard-like character is missing. The ablation edge is less irregular than in enamel because dentin is less brittle.

Fig 3-32 shows a detail of Fig 3-31. Here the open ends of the dentin tubules are clearly visible. Unlike enamel, the dentin has no shards, but rather soft edges at the sites of fracture. This picture shows the typical retention pattern in the dentin.

Fig 3-33 shows a close-up picture of the open dentin tubules. The strong micro-roughness of the ablated dentin is again visible. Also, the difference of density between the peritubular and the intertubular dentin can be seen: the peritubular dentin is harder and therefore the intertubular dentin is ablated more extensively. The dentin tubules protrude into the preparation area like chimneys. The open dentin tubules offer a good key for the bond between filling and dentin. The liquid bonding material can penetrate them deeply and so form a firm anchoring in the hard tissue of the tooth

Fig 3-34 shows an overview of a cavity prepared with numerous pulses. It leads from the enamel into the dentin. Here, the rough enamel area with shard-like delaminations is in the foreground. The enamel-dentin border is visible as a transverse crack accross the back wall of the cavity. Through dehydration of the samples in the vacuum of the electron microscope the dentin evaporates more than the enamel because of the higher percentage of water. Often a separation of the layers can be observed.

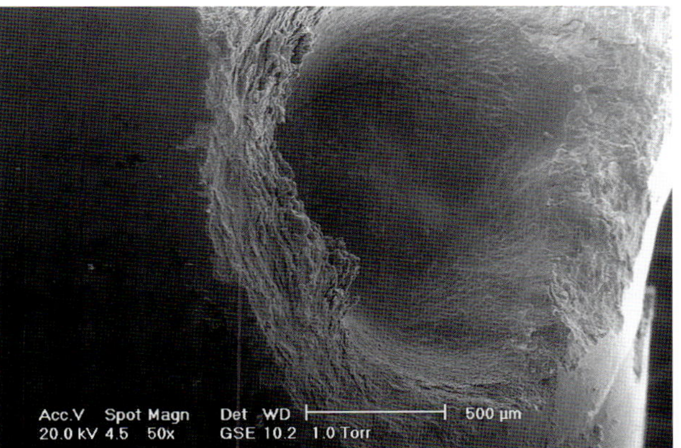

Fig 3-34 Cavity prepared with laser in enamel and dentin. (orig. 50x, fiber diameter 400 μm, pulse energy 400 mJ).

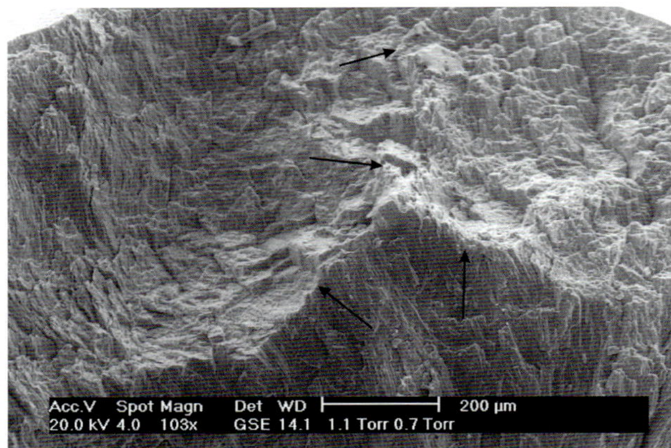

Fig 3-35: Preparation in enamel (orig. 103x, fiber diameter 600 µm, pulse energy 300 mJ). Picture courtesy of W. Sperr.

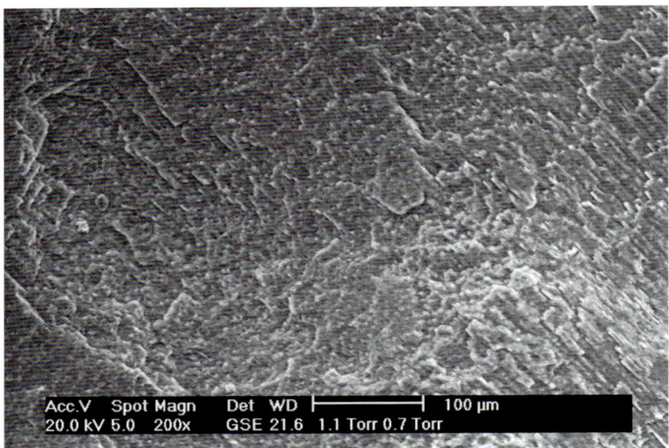

Fig 3-37 Dentin surface after Er,Cr:YSGG laser preparation (orig. 200x, fiber diameter 600 µm, pulse energy 300 mJ).

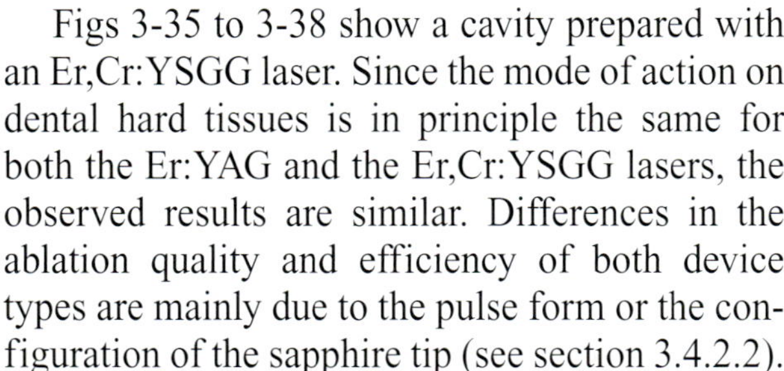
Figs 3-35 to 3-38 show a cavity prepared with an Er,Cr:YSGG laser. Since the mode of action on dental hard tissues is in principle the same for both the Er:YAG and the Er,Cr:YSGG lasers, the observed results are similar. Differences in the ablation quality and efficiency of both device types are mainly due to the pulse form or the configuration of the sapphire tip (see section 3.4.2.2).

Fig 3-35 shows a cavity preparation with numerous pulses in enamel. As seen in Fig 3-34 and the following pictures, a micro-retentive pattern through the rupture along the edges of the prisms is recognizable. Furthermore, the ablation edges of the individual pulses can be seen (arrows). At the top of the picture are sections of a sharply defined border of the preparation.

Fig 3-36 shows the fine structure of the laser-prepared enamel surface with details of its micro-retentive pattern.

Fig 3-37 shows the dentin surface of an Er,Cr:YSGG cavity at 200x magnification. As already observed with the Er:YAG cavity, a micro-retentive pattern is visible. It differs in form from the shard lines of the enamel pattern.

Fig 3-38 shows a magnification of the dentin surface. Again, open dentin tubules are visible. The structure of the cavity surface looks different than in Fig 3-17 since there they stand rectangular to the surface. Here the tubules stand perpendicular.

How strongly energy density can influence ablation can be seen in Figs 3-39 to 3-41. Here,

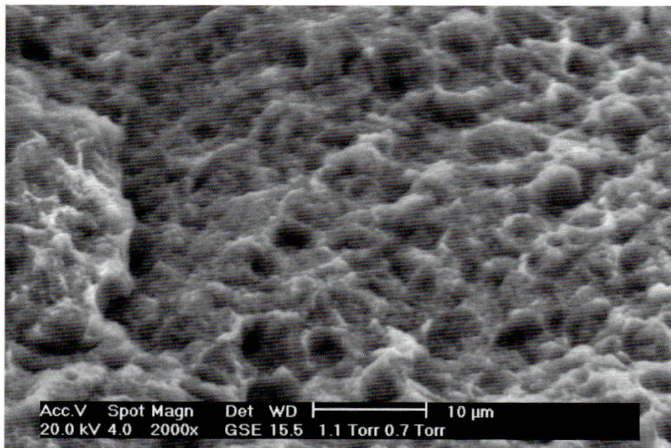

Fig 3-36 Detail of the enamel surface of the cavity of Fig 3-35 (orig. 2000x, fiber diameter 600 µm, 300 mJ).

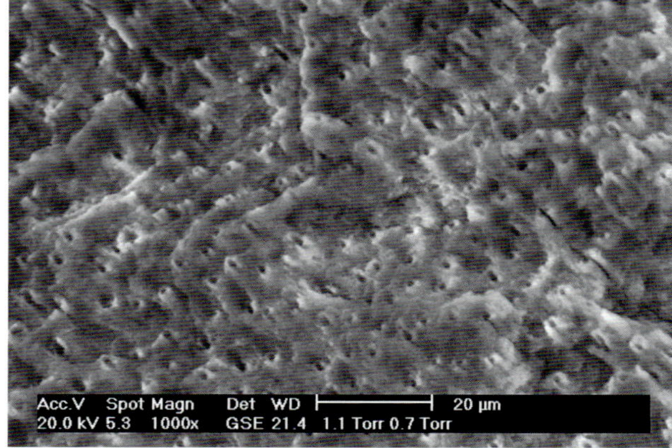

Fig 3-38 Dentin with open tubules (orig. 1000x, fiber diameter 600 µm, 300 mJ).

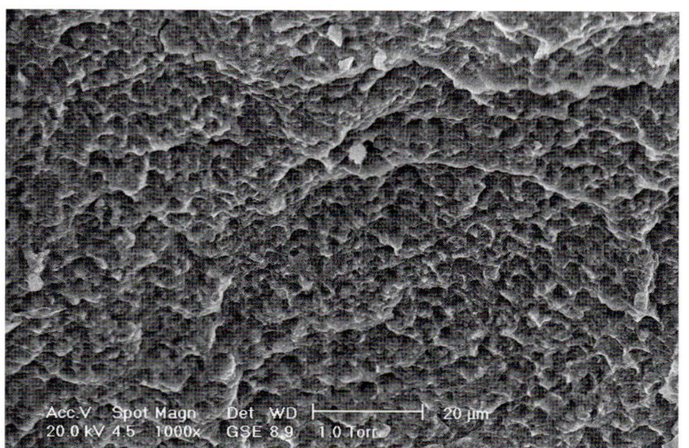

Fig 3-39 Preparation with a fiber diameter of 500 µm (orig. 1000x).

enamel of the same tooth has been irradiated with the same parameters but with different tip diameters.

With the enlargement of the diameter, the intensity on the surface decreases, since the pulse energy spreads to a bigger surface.

The most obvious differences can be seen in the SEM-pictures with 500, 800 and 1000 µm fiber diameter. Here, the area difference is also the biggest (2.56-fold from 500 to 800 µm and only 1.56-fold from 800 to 1000 µm). Ablating with the 500-µm-tip causes the retention pattern to have smaller structures and to go deeper, whereas with the 800 and 1000 µm tips, the pattern is shallower and more even, which corresponds to the decreasing intensity.

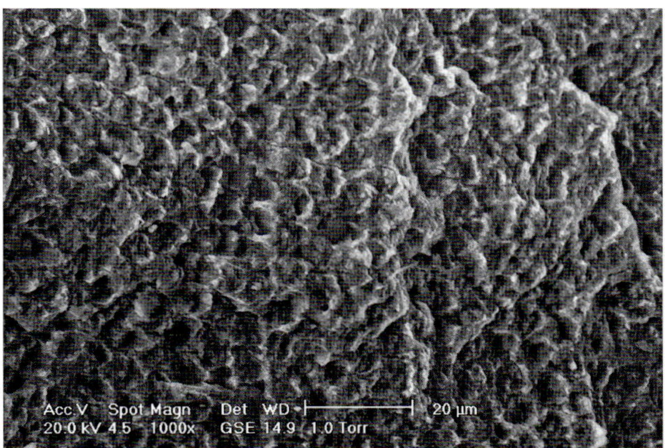

Fig 3-40 Preparation with a fiber diameter of 800 µm (orig. 1000x).

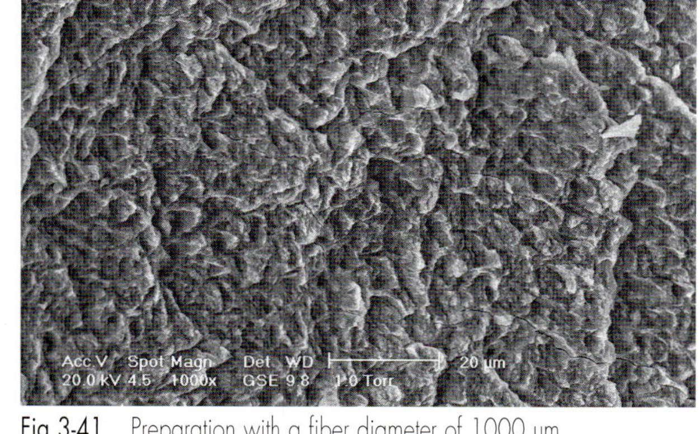

Fig 3-41 Preparation with a fiber diameter of 1000 µm (orig. 1000x).

3.3.3 Adhesion and Margin Tightness of Laser-prepared and Adhesive Techniques-treated Cavities

The adhesion of composites in laser-prepared cavities, and hence the question of the quality of the micro-retentive patterns through laser ablation, are of significant importance for conservative dentistry. Even though many studies into this topic have been carried out, much controversy remains.

One reason might be that these studies do not follow any standardized procedure and the results are therefore hard to compare. Another reason could be the kind of composites used and the way they were used. It is well known that composites shrink differently while curing if they are used in bulk or in layers. Although this factor has nothing to do with the laser preparation it has a big impact on the result. Furthermore, the self-etching composite leads to a worse result because of the lack of a smear layer after the laser preparation, which the composites need chemically. Therefore, all studies in this field have to be looked at very carefully – positively as well as negatively to filter out the factors that can affect the overall result. The very fact mentioned above, that the applied tip diameter has a decisive influence on the retentive

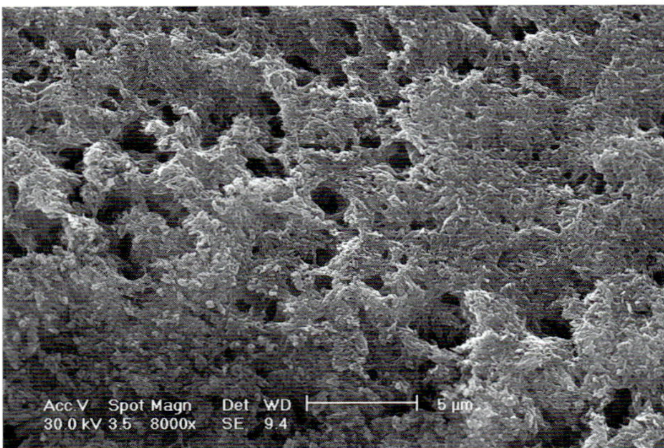

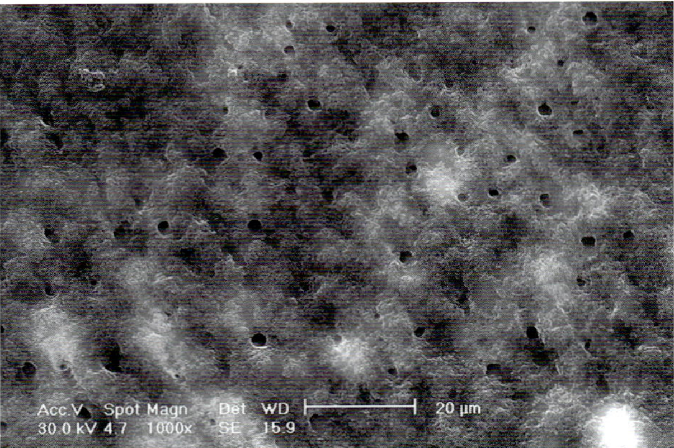

Fig 3-42 and 3-43 Conventionally etched enamel (Fig 3-42 left) and dentin surface (Fig 3-43 right). The micro-retentive patterns in enamel and the open tubuli in dentin are reminiscent of the surface structures after laser irradiation.

pattern, illustrates the different prerequisites for a comparable evaluation of individual studies (see Fig. 3-39 to 3-43).

A representative overview of the literature and practical experience indicates that stable fillings with a sufficient marginal tightness can be produced in laser-prepared cavities. Consequently, accuracy and a "best practice" procedure for the preparation and application of the filling material are necessary.

For the interested reader, a detailed summary of the most important publications on this topic can be found at the end of this chapter.

A number of studies[19,31] have compared the adhesive power of composite restorations on enamel and dentin surfaces treated with conventional preparation and acid-etch techniques, KCP and three different laser systems. Here, adhesive power for the Er:YAG laser was equal to or even better than the usual acid-etch technique.

In contrast to that, in another study[32] the adhesive power after enamel preparations that were done with an Er,Cr:YSGG laser was not as good as with the usual methods.

A study by De Munck et al.[33] also concluded that the laser-prepared cavities give less bonding for adhesive materials than conventionally prepared and etched ones. Similar results were found during examination of the adhesive power of dentin prepared Er:YAG laser.[34] The adhesive power was significantly lower than with conventional treatment. The authors attributed this to a modified dentin layer, developed through irradiation.

The majority of the authors, however, find that the roughness produced with the laser at least equals the acid-etched.[35–37] The adhesive power of composite materials is also at least as good.[38–43]

In a recent study, Staninec et al.[44] looked at the effects of the Er:YAG and the 9.6 µm CO_2 laser radiation on the enamel surface. They started from the hypothesis that the presence of a water film would prevent a calcium phosphate phase from building up. This phase seems to lower the adhesive power of the filling material. The enamel surface was laser-irradiated and inspected with SR-FTIR (synchrotron radiation-Fourier transform infrared spectroscopy) and light microscopy. Additionally, shear strength tests have been done. The authors concluded that an additional acid etching is not necessary. A thick water film is, however, required during treatment. This is necessary for cooling in anycase.

Furthermore, there are controversial opinions about the morphological and structural changes, in vivo, of the dental hard tissues that are exposed to the laser beam. The results are difficult to categorize. The different operational parameters, localization and study design preclude reliable comparison among studies concerning the morphology and the change of composition.

There are still few reports on the compositional changes of dental hard tissues and micro-hardness of the cavity floor prepared by Er:YAG laser irradiation. Hossain et al.[45] performed a study to compare the compositional changes of human dentin and Knoop hardness of the cavity floor prepared by Er:YAG laser irradiation with that of the conventional bur cavity. They found that the quantities of Ca (weight %) and P (weight %) were increased significantly in the laser cavities, but no significant differences were found between the Ca/P ratio and the Knoop hardness number of laser and bur cavities. The results of SEM observation revealed that the lased cavity surface was irregular, and there was also the absence of a smear layer; the orifice of dentinal tubules was exposed. This led them to conclude that the Er:YAG laser device produced minimal thermal-induced changes of dental hard-tissue compositions and did not cause changes in the Ca/P ratio and Knoop hardness compared to the bur cavities.

Maintenance of pulpal health is a critical prerequisite for successful application of lasers in the hard-tissue management of vital teeth. Nair et al.[46] investigated the short- and long-term pulpal effects of cavity preparations in healthy human teeth using an Er:YAG laser. They relied on light and transmission electron microscopy for results and found that in the short-term group most of the laser-drilled teeth did not reveal any pathological changes in the pulp-dentin complex. The teeth under long-term observation revealed distinct apposition of tertiary dentin (TD), lined predominantly with cuboidal cells on its pulpal aspect. These results allowed them to conclude that the Er:YAG laser is a pulp-preserving hard-tissue drilling tool when used with the specific energy settings and emitting radiation at a wavelength, λ, of 2.94 μm.

An interesting and useful study to observe and measure the morphological changes that occur in the hard tissue after the application of an Er:YAG laser was made by Shigetani et al.[47] Another objective of this study was to evaluate and compare the duration of application of both the laser apparatus and a conventional cutting device. In this study, from freshly extracted teeth was carious tissues were used. The morphological changes in hard tooth structures produced by Er:YAG laser irradiation were examined by using a SEM and a laser scanning microscope. The results showed that appropriate laser irradiation was 100 mJ/pulse for dentin, and 200 mJ/pulse for enamel. Also, the quality of laser scanning microscopic images was superior to that achieved by SRM imaging due to the damage caused by the necessary pretreatment of the specimens. The time taken to remove carious enamel by laser irradiation was slightly longer than with the rotary cutting device; however, no differences between the two methods were observed in terms of duration and results of carious dentin removal.

In addition to the adhesive power reached, the sealing of the restoration is also interesting. Numerous authors have been concerned with these problems but have found different results.

Shigetani et al.[48] established the usefulness of Er:YAG in cavity preparation in their evaluation of marginal leakage of composite resin restoration from cavities prepared by Er:YAG laser. The dentin surface was assessed after laser irradiation was performed by LSM; the cut surface showed a rough texture similar to scales, and exposed dentinal tubules lacked striations and the smeared layer formation that were observed when using a rotary cutting device. Leakage tests revealed no significant differences in the marginal seal for either enamel or dentin between cavities prepared by Er:YAG laser irradiation and when using an air-turbine. Thus, the usefulness of cavity preparation by Er:YAG laser irradiation in composite resin restoration was suggested.

There have been few reports on microleakage from cavities prepared by Er:YAG laser irradiation. Gonzalez Bahillo et al.[49] performed scanning electron microscopy (SEM) in order to compare the surfaces of cavities prepared using laser with those prepared conventionally, and to measure the degree of leakage through both enamel and cementum. They analyzed samples that were laser treated, laser treated and acid etched and those prepared with conventional methods. On analyzing the tooth enamel, the amount of leakage was found to be similar in the two groups treated with lasers, whilst the samples prepared conventionally were found to be more prone to leakage. On analyzing the cementum, the conventionally prepared samples appeared to display surfaces that were more conducive to the adhesion of the materials used in obturation (although this difference was not strictly significant), and this might explain the relatively low levels of leakage. Thus, the use of acid etching in conjunction with both conventional and laser cavity preparation improved the adhesion of the materials used in obturation to enamel surfaces.

Matsumuto et al.[50] also did a study, on the same lines, to investigate cavity surfaces morphologically, and to compare microleakage at cavities prepared by Er:YAG laser after composite resin restoration versus conventional mechanical treatment in human primary teeth in vitro. Their results were consistent with the ones mentioned; they, too, observed micro-leakage at cavities prepared by laser to be significantly less than after preparation by bur. Additionally, SEM observation showed that, compared with the relatively flat appearance of cavities prepared by bur, cavity margins prepared by laser were irregular but there was almost no smear layer at the cavity walls. With the help of the dye penetration, they concluded that the irregular cavity surfaces prepared by Er:YAG laser afforded better adhesion and sealing than did those prepared by mechanical bur.

A study by Armengol et al.[51] compared microleakage at enamel/composite and dentin/composite interfaces following Er:YAG laser, Nd:YAG laser, or acid-etch preparation. The results showed that irradiation with Er:YAG and Nd:YAG lasers did not produce a good seal; mean micro-leakage was observed to be greater than with acid-etch and statistically comparable to that of control cavities (Kruskal-Wallis test).

Ishizaka et al.[52] concluded from their studies that the Er:YAG laser irradiation of dentin probably denatures the organic part of the hard tissue.

Corona et al.[53] found a significantly laxer marginal seal at restorations prepared with Er:YAG laser compared to conventional fillings in a colour penetration test. Similar results were found in other studies.[51,54,55]

Despite advantages in terms of mechanical durability, Ceballo et al.[56] observed a laxer marginal seal at composite restorations prepared with an Er:YAG laser. Therefore, Gutknecht et al.[57] recommend the etching of laser prepared cavities.

Rocca[58] and Bertrand et al.[59] stated in their studies of marginal tightness: when dentin is prepared with an Er:YAG laser under water cooling, the surface is free of smear layer. The intertubular dentin is partially removed owing to the larger water content in its composition. Conversely, the Er:YAG laser is less effective on peritubular dentin and does not enlarge the tubule orifices; the laser irradiated surfaces have a microcrater-like appearance. The resin monomers can penetrate into open dentinal tubules and the subsequent polymerization allows formation of resin tags. However, hybridization does not occur either for the dentin surface or for the tubule orifices.

When etching with 35% phosphoric acid gel is applied to the irradiated dentin, the acid partially removes the highly mineralized peritubular dentin, decalcifies the underlying dentinal structures and opens the dentinal tubules, which acquire a funnel-shaped appearance. The bonding agents should effectively seal the dentinal surface and the dentinal tubule orifices to prevent postoperative sensitivity and protect the pulp.

Depending on the filling material, good results can be achieved. So Hossain et al.[45] discovered that with the Er:YAG laser and composite fillings a similar sealing effect can be found in comparison to conventionally prepared and etched restorations – or even a better marginal seal[60] .

Other studies, by Shigetani et al.[48], Khan et al.[61] or Niu et al.[62] recommended the Er:YAG laser as a perfect support for preparation.

Roebuck et al.[63] showed dependencies between the laser energy used and the tightness of the

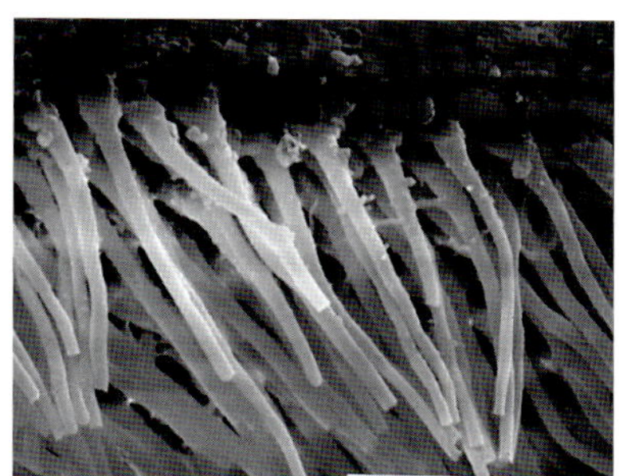

Fig 3-44 Dentin surface prepared with a round carbide bur then etched with 35% phosphoric acid gel for 15 seconds (2000x). The hybrid layer was 5 to 6 µm thick. A funnel-shaped configuration of the resin tags at their base was visible. The resin tags exhibited a smooth texture. (Figure courtesy of Bertrand and Rocca).

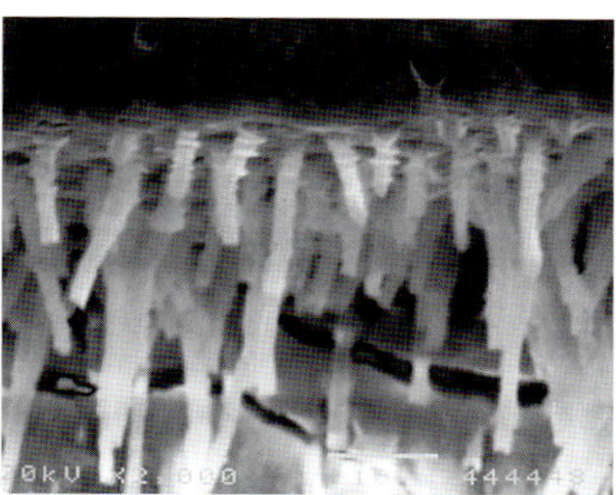

Fig 3-45 Dentin surface prepared with Er:YAG laser at 500 mJ/pulse and 10 Hz (fluence: 44 J/cm^2), under water cooling (2000x). No hybrid layer was visible. The resin tags were directly connected with the composite resin. They showed a regular cylindrical shape with no bulge at their base. They seemed to be less bulky. (Figure courtesy of Bertrand and Rocca).

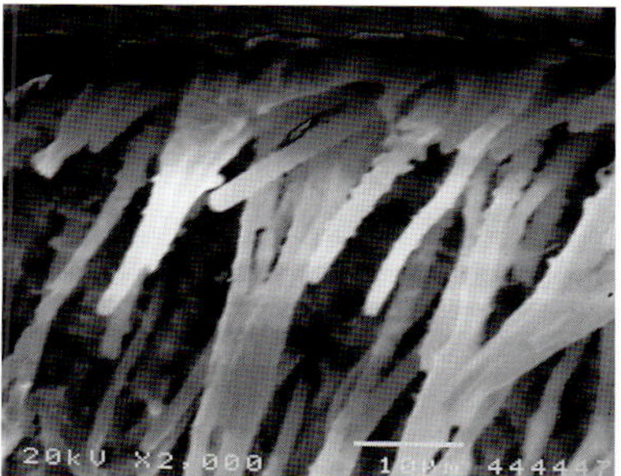

Fig 3-46 Dentin surface prepared with Er:YAG laser at 500 mJ/pulse and 10 Hz (fluence: 44 J/cm^2), under water cooling then etched with 35% phosphoric acid gel for 15 seconds (2000x). The hybrid layer was 5- to 6-µm thick. A funnel-shaped configuration of the resin tags at their base was visible. The resin tags exhibited a rough texture. (Figure courtesy of Bertrand and Rocca).

applied fillings; however, they attributed an overall high preparation quality to the Er:YAG laser. Likewise for ionomer materials, the Er:YAG laser gives equal performance in terms of sealing[64].

Niu[62] showed that class V cavities can be created with Er:YAG systems and leave few edge cracks. Color penetration tests confirmed these microscopical results.

In a clinical study, Dostalova et al.[65] described that the quality of the filling therapy after Er:YAG-laser preparation is equal to the conventional preparation techniques.

In conclusion, the study design concerning an investigation of the bonding characteristics of laser- and conventionally-etched cavity surfaces will be presented.[19]

Fig 3-47 Conditioning of the embedded sample with etching gel for the classical preparation.

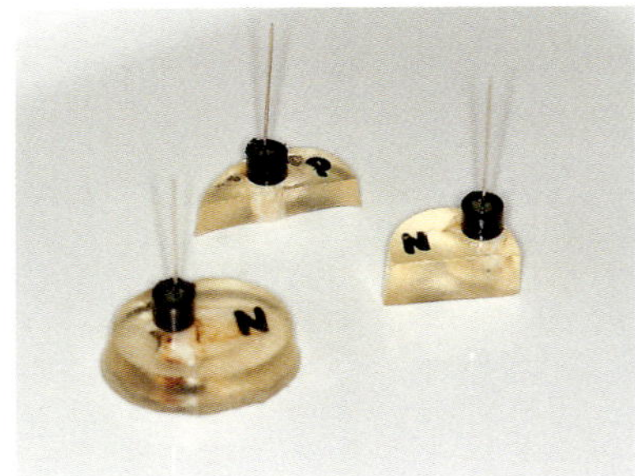

Fig 3-48 Application of the composite material with embedded needles.

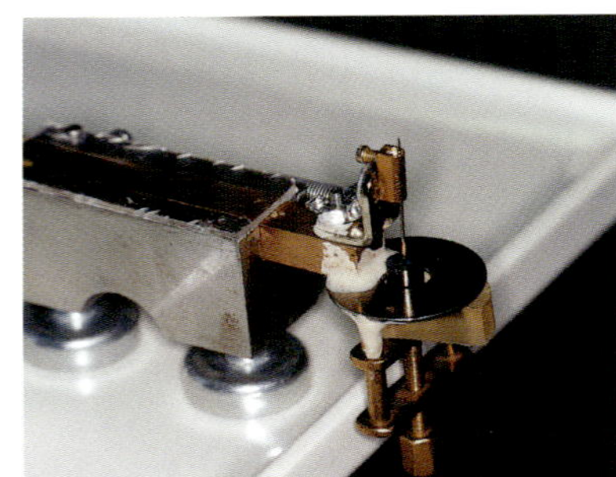

Fig 3-49 Completed samples before the tear strength tests.

3.3.3.1 Example: A Study to Evaluate the Bond Strength of Composite Restorations in Connection with Laser-assisted Cavity Preparation

The aim of the study was to assess the shear- and tear-bond strength for composite restorations after laser preparation in comparison with conventional preparation. For the assessment, teeth were embedded in synthetic resin. Subsequently, a defined area of dentin or enamel was exposed through grinding, and conditioned with several techniques (phosphoric acid, maleic acid, different laser wavelengths and KCP).

Then the composite material was applied to the conditioned area using a hollow mold. For conducting of tear-bond-strength tests, needles had to be embedded in the composite body.

The completed samples were fixed to a calibrated testing device and the bond strengths were evaluated. The results for dentin and enamel are depicted in Table 3-1 and 3-2. In the case of enamel, the values achieved by the Er:YAG laser were comparable with those reached by etching with phosphoric acid; in dentin they were far superior.[19,31]

Table 3-1 Adhesion values for enamel.
Black bar: acid etching
Coloured bars: Er:YAG laser at different settings
Gray bars: Other laser systems at different settings

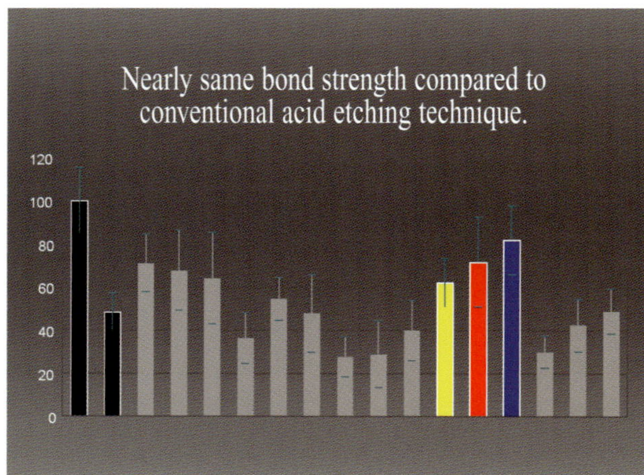

Table 3-2 Adhesion values for dentin.
Black bar: acid etching
Coloured bars: Er:YAG laser at different settings
Gray bars: Other laser systems at different settings

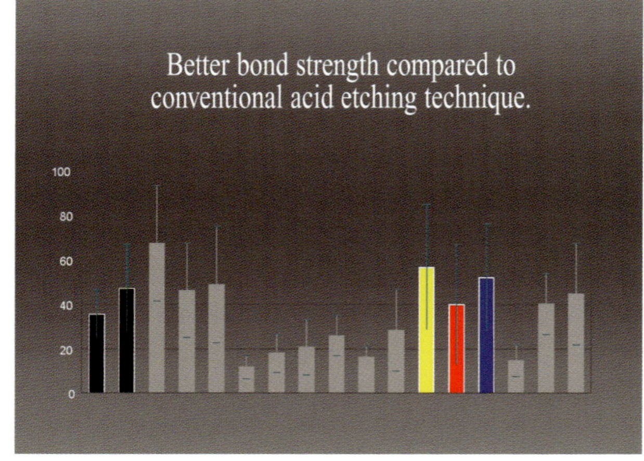

3.3.4 Caries-preventing Properties of Laser-prepared Cavities

Laser preparation nowadays is said to have a caries preventive effect. To date, it has been shown in vitro that, with the argon-, Nd:YAG, and CO_2 lasers, an improvement of the surface can be reached through irradiation of the dental hard tissue. Through solubility testing it can be proven that enamel that is irradiated in vitro with low energy shows a significantly higher acid resistance than enamel that is untreated or treated only with fluoride preparations. Some studies found that the Er:YAG laser can also be used for caries prevention (see chapter 5).

For the induction of such a structure modification that possesses preventive properties, a significant temperature rise must be produced on the tooth surface. For this reason, the question arises whether such a superficial temperature rise can be achieved when the necessary cooling spray is used.

Therefore Apel et al. assessed the progression of the demineralization front in "best-practise"-prepared Er:YAG- and Er,Cr:YSGG-cavities in comparison to conventionally prepared ones[66]. Whereas in this study no differences between the two laser wavelengths could be found, the demineralization front in the applied caries model had progressed by ~170% in comparison to the control group.

Thus, using erbium lasers, no advantages for the prevention of secondary caries can be expected. The reasons for the significantly inferior result of the laser-prepared cavities and the impacts in vivo still have to be investigated. Nevertheless, the findings support the already described (section 3.2.3) necessity of a careful adaptation of the filling materials in relation to the laser cavity to grant optimal marginal tightness.

3.4 Mechanisms of Ablation

3.4.1 Overview

The usual mechanisms that lead to ablation or decomposition of biological materials are photochemical, thermal or plasma-mediated[67]. Whereas the first mechanism is typical for ablation at very short wavelengths (UV, provided by excimer lasers), the last mostly refers to very high energy densities in the irradiated area and thus is very independent of the applied wavelength.

Photochemical ablation was found not to be very effective in dental hard tissues for practical reasons, and lasers for plasma-mediated ablation are only now in a state of development for a broad market application.

Hence, in this section we will only consider thermal ablation, and here again just pulsed ablation achieved by lasers in the 3 μm range (i.e., the Er:YAG and the Er,Cr:YSGG lasers), as they represent the most commonly used laser systems nowadays for dental hard tissue removal. Plasma-mediated ablation as a technology of the near future, from today's point of view, will be treated in the section on future perspectives at the end of this chapter.

Detail 3-2.
Thermal ablation and wavelength dependence of absorption

Generally, thermal ablation means that the energy delivered by the laser is coupled into the irradiated material by an absorption process yielding a temperature rise there. Several consecutive mechanisms then lead to ablation. Therefore, an absorptive component has to be present in the irradiated material that converts the incoming energy in a very efficient way into a temperature rise of the material. After a certain temperature is reached, melting, vaporization or sublimation of the irradiated material can be achieved that allows its removal.

The removal is done either by ejection via expansion of the heated material (i.e., by using the deposited energy in the heated volume) or by applying an additional fluid jet to blow it out (the latter is mostly used in material processing such as cutting of metallic blanks, not in medicine). However, depending on the material, or rather on constituents of biological tissues, different wavelengths are predestined for their processing and the most suitable laser has to be chosen. (For more detailed information see detail 3-3 and section 3.4.2.2.4 in this chapter.)

Looking at the ablation process caused by pulsed laser radiation in the 3 μm range, the main absorbing constituent in hard dental tissue is the embedded water. Its maximum absorption peak in the infrared is situated around this wavelength (2.94 μm at room temperature and slightly smaller wavelengths at higher temperatures[67,68]) and therefore fits exactly to the Er:YAG (λ = 2.94 μm) or the Er,Cr:YSGG lasers (λ = 2.79 μm).

The absorption of water in this range is so high that scattering and the absorption of other tissue components can be neglected as a first approximation. Thus, when irradiating dentin or enamel by a laser pulse with sufficient pulse energy, the water embedded in the tissue is heated up very rapidly above the boiling point. This causes a micro-explosion leading to mechanical decomposition of the tissue and blowing out of the generated small particles (spallation).

In this way, an ablation threshold describing the minimal pulse energy for removal of material can be defined.

This process of ablation has been studied by various scientific groups and nowadays is very well understood.[69,70]

Detail 3-3. Mechanism of absorption of light in the 3 μm range by water.

The energy absorbed by a certain material out of an irradiating light beam very often is converted into heat. This especially applies for light in the IR range at energy densities that cause no nonlinear effects in matter.

For a better understanding of the absorption process, we have to make a short digression into quantum physics:

As we know, matter can be brought into an excited state by energy transfer. The input energy is absorbed by the single atoms or molecules, which are able to store it for a certain time. Hence, in this state the particles have a higher energy, i.e., they populate a higher energy level.

The single energy levels are discrete and quantized. That means they have a certain energetic distance and do not overlap in the simplest case. When they get excited, the particles can populate only these energy levels and no states in between. Hence, if a particle is to be excited, the exciting energy at least has to be similar to the energy difference between two adjacent levels. Otherwise the particle remains in its ground state (all-or-nothing principle). The single energetic states of a particle can be manifested either as different orbits of electrons in atoms (= electric states) or in different kinds of rotation or vibration in molecules.

Also, the energy of the irradiating light is quantized. One light quantum is called a photon. As mentioned above, for an excitation the photon energy has to fit to the difference between two energy levels. As the photon energy is coupled to the wavelength, the ability for absorption for a certain matter depends on the wavelength of the irradiating light (see also chapter 1).

In the case of water, light is absorbed by the H_2O molecule, thereby changing its rotational and vibrational states. The increase of energy in the molecule leads to a change in the length and the eigenfrequencies of the OH-bonds.[67] After a certain lifetime the molecule drops down again to its ground state and releases the absorbed energy. This action is called recombination.

If thereby no radiation is emitted, as in the case considered here, the released energy remains in the volume via several steps, and, is converted into a temperature distribution in the water.

The change in the eigenfrequencies of the vibrating molecule due to temperature increase means a change in the energy gaps between the single energy levels, thereby causing a shift of the absorption maximum to shorter wavelengths as considered for water in section 3.4.2.2.4.

3.4.2 Physical Factors Influencing Ablation Efficiency and Quality

There are several physical factors that affect the efficiency and quality of ablation and its implication for the remaining tissue. Here we can distinguish between two main types: the material properties and the properties of the irradiating laser light.

We can influence only the latter, whereas the former properties are determined by nature. Both types contain a number of single factors, such as:

1. relevant material properties for biological hard tissues:
   - coefficient of absorption (α)
   - reflectivity of the tissue surface (R)
   - specific heat capacity (c_p) of the absorbing constituents in the tissue
   - capability of heat conduction (thermal diffusivity κ) in the tissue
   - distribution of water within the tissue

2. properties of the laser light:
   - wavelength (λ)
   - pulse energy (E_p)
   - pulse duration (τ_p)
   - temporal beam profile (pulse shape)
   - spatial beam profile (TEM modes).

The main physical factors that refer to the ablation efficiency and, most important, to the quality of ablation (i.e., the best possible absence of collateral damage), are: pulse energy, pulse duration, spatial and temporal beam profile, wavelength and the spatial distribution of water within the matter.

Before we consider their mutual interaction, we have to take a short look at the meaning of the single factors to be discussed in the following sections.

3.4.2.1 Material Properties

The *coefficient of absorption* α *[cm^{-1}]* describes how strongly the radiation is absorbed in a medium (the decay is exponential). The optical penetration depth is the reciprocal of the absorption coefficient and describes at which depth of penetration the energy density of the incoming radiation has dropped to $1/e$ of the surface value.[67]

The *reflectivity R [%]* describes how much intensity is reflected at the interface between a material with low optical density and a material with high optical density, as, for example, occurs at the interface between air and dental hard tissue.

The *specific heat capacity* c_p *[J/kg K]* of a material describes the amount of energy it takes to heat up 1 kg of the material for 1° Celsius (properly 1 K in SI terms). The temperature change in any substance is a measure of the change of its intrinsic energy. Thus the specific heat capacity connects the laser energy deposited in the tooth to the temperature rise induced thereby in the affected volume.

The *thermal diffusivity* κ *[cm^2/s]* describes the capability of the material for heat conduction. As we always heat up just a small volume in the whole tooth by laser irradiation, the heat induced immediately starts to flow into the colder regions. The thermal diffusivity characterizes the velocity of this heat flux.

The distribution of water in the tissue refers to the fact that for thermal ablation in the 3 µm range the main absorbing constituent in dental hard tissue is the embedded water and so its local concentration plays an important role in ablation efficiency.

3.4.2.2 Factors Influencing the Efficiency and Quality of Thermal Ablation

3.4.2.2.1 Pulse Energy and Pulse Duration

As described above, explosive ablation needs a tissue constituent that can be heated up very rapidly by light absorption and causes cracking and erosion due to its rapid expansion, like the embedded water in the case of dental hard tissues. For the most effective erosion, the phase transition of water into vapor must be initiated; this will yield a strong volume increase, simultaneously blowing out the generated particles. Thus, a sufficient amount of energy has to be provided by the laser pulse.

However, the required amount of pulse energy depends on several factors: predominantly, it depends on the size and specific heat capacity of the volume to be heated up. But, as heat transport causes losses of energy from the heated volume to the surrounding tissue, it is easy to imagine that the same amount of energy delivered by a longer laser pulse will yield a lower temperature but a larger heat-affected volume than delivered by a shorter laser pulse. Hence, the ablation threshold in terms of pulse energy E_p is always a function of the pulse duration as it describes the minimum energy that is necessary to cause ablation of the heated volume.

Thus, as pulse duration significantly influences heat distribution in the tooth, it plays an important role in ablation efficiency and quality (for more information see detail 3-4).

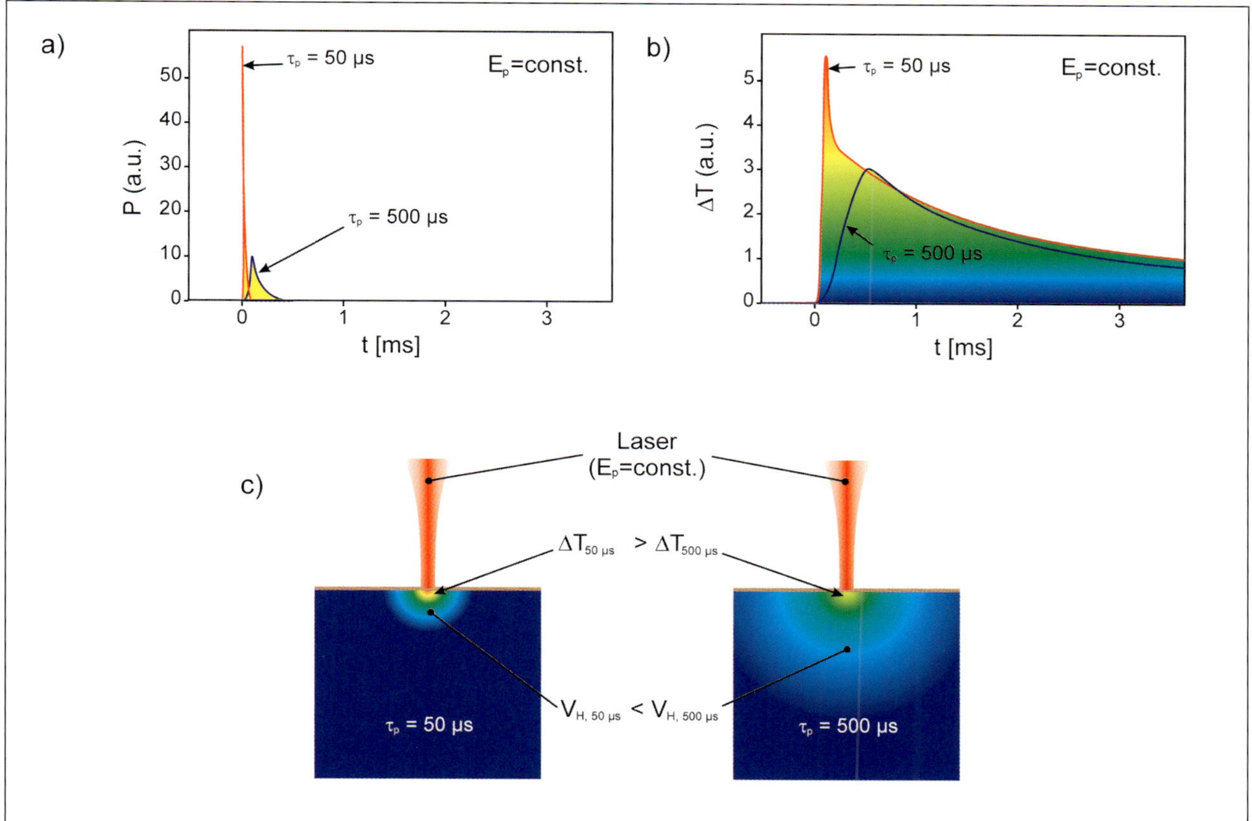

Fig 3-50 Heat distribution in the tissue for the same pulse energy E_p at different pulse durations τ_p:
(a) The pulse energy E_p (the yellow area underneath the temporal pulse evolution) is constant. As power is energy per unit time, the peak power P of shorter pulses is higher than of longer ones if E_p is held constant.
(b) The temperature rise ΔT induced in the irradiated volume is much higher for the shorter pulse.[70]
(c) As less heat can be transported to the surrounding tissue via heat conduction during the short period of time, the energy remains confined thus in a smaller heated volume V_H.

Detail 3-4. Energy distribution and spatial heat confinement in the irradiated tissue

Irradiation by a laser pulse induces a temperature gradient in the material (higher temperatures at the surface than in underlying layers). Thus, the heat tends to flow to colder regions. The velocity of this heat transport is determined by the temperature difference between the hotter and colder region as well as by the ability of the material to heat. The magnitude of the heat transport is characterized by the time it takes to reduce the temperature in the laser-heated volume roughly by one-half, called the characteristic thermal relaxation time τ_{rel}[71,72]:

$$\tau_{rel} = \Delta x^2 / 4\kappa$$

where $\Delta x = 1/\alpha$ is the optical penetration depth characterizing the thermal gradient length, α is the absorption coefficient of the tissue and κ is the thermal diffusivity. With κ typically being ~4.7×10^{-3} cm^2/s for enamel and α being ~10^4 /cm[71], the thermal relaxation time is:

$$\tau_{rel} \sim 0.5 \text{ µs (enamel)}.$$

To achieve a good spatial confinement of the temperature rise during pulse exposure, the pulse duration τ_p should be equal to or less than the thermal relaxation time τ_{rel}[67]:

$$\tau_p / \tau_{rel} \leq 1$$

hence yielding an optimum pulse width τ_p of about 0.5 µs.

Of course, if we talk about spatial confinement of energy within this temporal regime, it does not mean that there is no heat transmitted into the surrounding lattice. But as the amount of deposited pulse energy stored in the spalled particles is removed together with them during ejection, less energy penetrates into deeper layers the more it stays spatially confined.

Since typical pulse widths of commercially available free-running pulsed Er laser systems for medical applications are around 140–150 µs, significant heat transfer into the remaining material has to be taken into consideration.
There are several reasons the spatial extent of the heating should be held as low as possible: firstly, the heating of the pulp has to be restricted to a rise of less than 5°C[14]. Secondly, the available pulse energy should be used in the most efficient way, i.e., heating up the smallest possible volume to achieve the highest expansion of the embedded water. The influence of the pulse duration on the resulting surface temperatures is discussed in Fig 3-53.

The smallest achievable heated volume depends on the absorption length $\Delta x = 1/\alpha$ of the irradiated tissue. For usual laser systems with pulse durations around 140–150 µs, significant heat conduction into deeper layers during cavity preparation has to be taken into account (see detail 3-4).

This implies that below a certain depth the deposited energy is not sufficient any more to cause efficient evaporation of the embedded water and hence the tissue cannot be ablated any more via spallation. As a matter of fact, this energy cannot be removed together with ablation products that are ejected. Hence a coolant jet such as a water spray has to be applied to keep the temperature in the remaining tissue at an acceptable level. Hibst and Keller have shown that a certain amount of water spray can cause such a decrease[69], but also that too much water will inhibit ablation efficiency (see Figs 3-51 and 3-52).

The strong decrease in ablation efficiency depicted in Fig 3-52 is due to the absorption of the laser light by the cooling water spray: as the amount of water sprayed on the treated surface increases, more water droplets will absorb the incident laser light, thus reducing the energy available for tissue penetration.

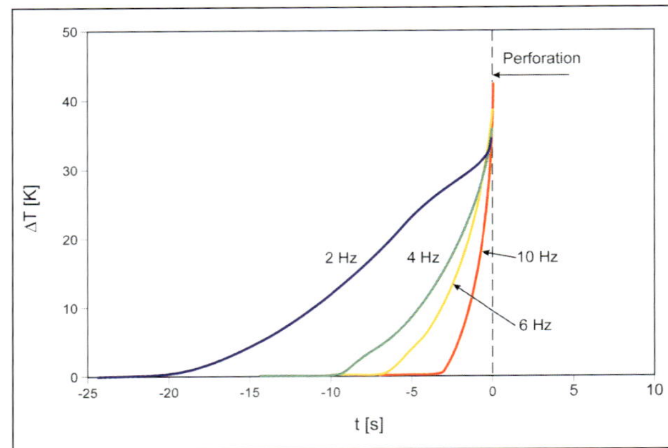

Fig 3-51 Temperature rise ΔT after several pulses on the back of a 3-mm-thick dentin slice without the application of coolant[69], recorded for different pulse repetition rates: E_p = 200 mJ, time is normalized on the time of perforation.

The necessary amount of spray of course depends on the pulse energy and the tissue constitution. Thus, an experienced user can influence considerably the ablation efficiency with simultaneous sufficient cooling by adjusting the amount of water-spray.

3.4.2.2.2 Temporal Beam Profile (Pulse Shape)

In addition to the duration, also the temporal shape of the delivered laser pulse has a strong influence on the ablation efficiency. It plays an important role for the spatial confinement of temperature rise discussed in section 3.4.2.2.1.

For rapid vaporization of the water and small penetration depth of the applied heat, a very steep leading edge of the incoming laser pulse is necessary. The steeper this rise, the faster the temperature rise, allowing an efficient spallation of the

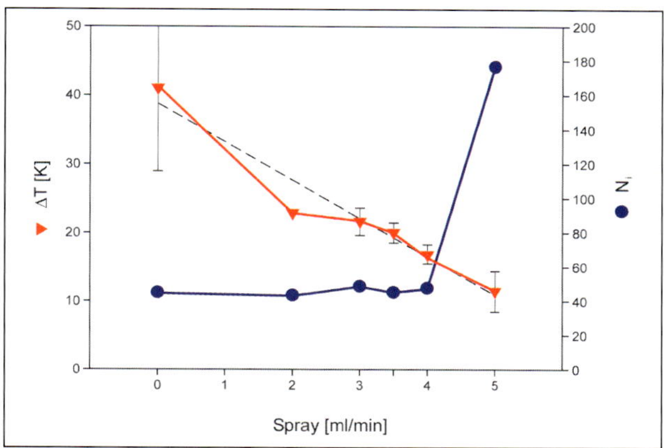

Fig 3-52 Maximum temperature rise and ablation efficiency (prop. $1/N_p$) at different fluxes of applied water spray. The number of pulses N_p indicated on the right scale was necessary to achieve the perforation of a 3-mm-thick dentin slice. Temperatures were measured at the back of the slice.[69]

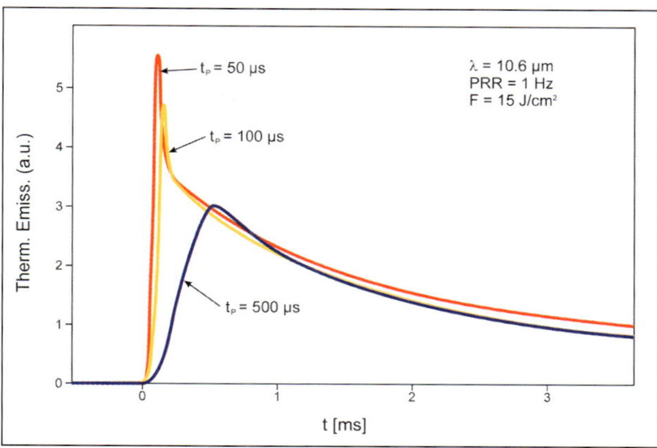

Fig 3-53 Pulse-width τ_p dependence of the thermal radiation for constant fluence F (= energy on the irradiated area) and PRR (pulse repetition rate) in enamel.[71]

material. The trailing edge of the pulse helps to penetrate deeper into the tissue, thus increasing ablation depth, but also is mostly responsible for the remaining sub-ablative energy densities in these layers. Figures 3-54 to 3-56 show some of these temporal pulse shapes.

The influence of pulse duration in the µs-regime on the thermal radiation of the irradiated surface, indicating temperatures reached in the volume, is shown in Fig 3-53.

As can easily be seen, the sharp initial peak of the thermal surface emission flattens for longer pulse durations. Its high initial temperature at short pulse durations shows the emission of the plume of ablated volatile tissue components, indicating high temperatures reached in the outermost layers close to the surface before ablation.

From this it can be found that a very steep rise of the laser plays a crucial role for a good ablation efficiency of a free-running pulsed laser whose pulse durations are longer than the thermal relaxation time τ_{rel}. According to this, a pulse shape like the one depicted in Fig 3-54 represents the best solution out of the options shown in Figs 3-54 to 3-56.

3.4.2.2.3 Spatial Beam Profile (TEM Modes)

To cause ablation, pulse energies mostly far above the ablation threshold are used. In this case, influences of the spatial beam profile can be neglected generally. But, if in special cases where working at the lowest possible influence on residual tissue is required (e.g., near the pulp), energy settings just slightly above the ablation threshold will be chosen. Under these conditions one has to consider that the ablation threshold may drop by more than 50% if the laser emits no Gaussian beam profile but one of higher order[73] (for more detailed information about TEM modes see chapter 1 about basic physics in this book).

Usually, the energy density on the irradiated area is calculated by dividing the pulse energy by the area of the irradiated spot, thus assuming constant spatial power distribution. In a strict sense this is only correct for very special types (so called "flattop-profiles", mostly emitted by excimer lasers). But working with this kind of definition is still correct if it can be assumed that the emitted beam profile is always the same. In a kind of unwritten convention this usually is presumed in the interpretation of given values, e.g.,

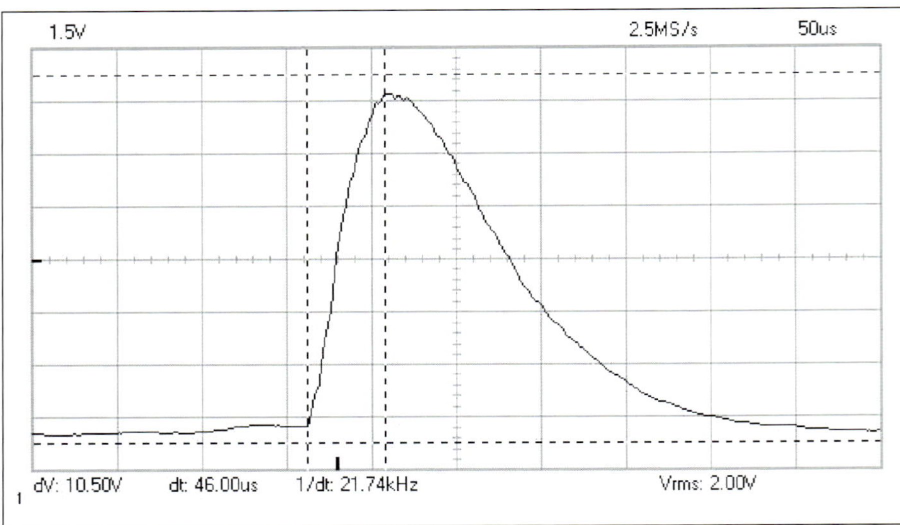

Fig 3-54 Temporal pulse shape of an Er,Cr:YSGG laser.

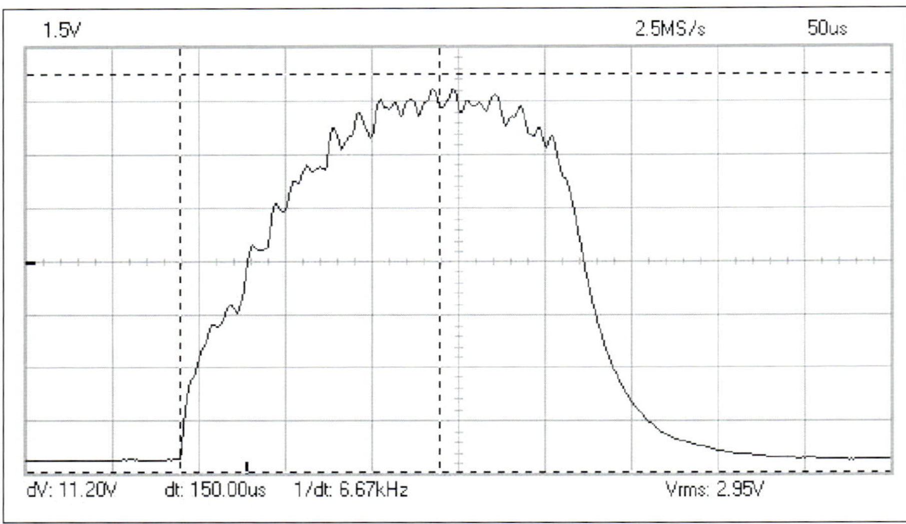

Fig 3-55 Temporal pulse shape of an Er:YAG laser.

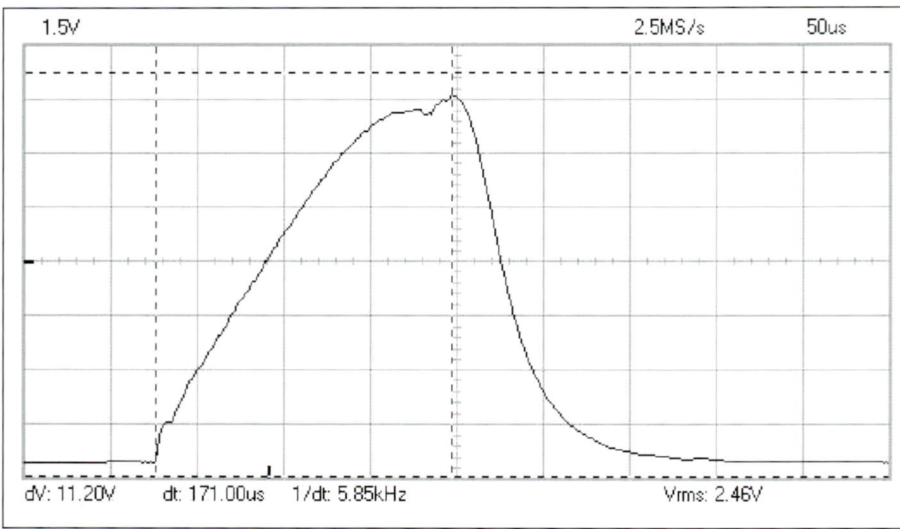

Fig 3-56 Temporal pulse shape of a second Er:YAG laser.

the ablation threshold. Normally, it is measured with a laser whose spatial beam profile corresponds to the TEM_{00} "fundamental mode", i.e., a Gaussian beam profile[73] (see Fig 3-57).

Nevertheless, especially if values from the literature are to be used for critical cavity preparations, the beam profile of those values should be ascertained employed for measurement present. If it corresponds to the one of the laser employed for the present measurement, this factor will be of no further influence on the reproducibility of the reported values. If it is not possible to find out the TEM-Profile, looking for the name and type of the laser used might help. In any case, it is recommended to perform some preliminary experiments on an extracted tooth to ensure absence of damage before clinical application.

Anyway, if ablation thresholds are to be determined, detection of the beam profile is inevitable.

The energy distribution can be measured either by very sophisticated devices or, if merely qualitative information is required, by irradiating thermal paper with low energy densities. In this case, areas with high intensity levels will darken while those with low energy densities will show several shades of gray. A good resolution can be achieved if with a divergent beam, the paper is placed at some distance from the outcoupling area of the delivery system (i.e., several cm after the focal plane if the beam is focused by a lens or at a sufficient distance if it is coupled out of a fiber).

The same TEM patterns can also be seen on ablated surfaces when using pulses with energies just a little over the real ablation threshold (see Fig 3-59).

Of course, as the TEM modes are caused by properties of the resonator, they only have an influence on the ablation quality in laser systems with a lens-based delivery system, such as an articulated arm, because the beam profile stays unchanged during transformation through a lens.

When using a laser system with a fiber-based delivery system, the initial TEM mode structures of the resonator are homogenized during their travel through a fiber of length ~1 m, as a result of the transit time dispersion of the light[73], thus leading to a quasi-Gaussian distribution at the distal end of the fiber.

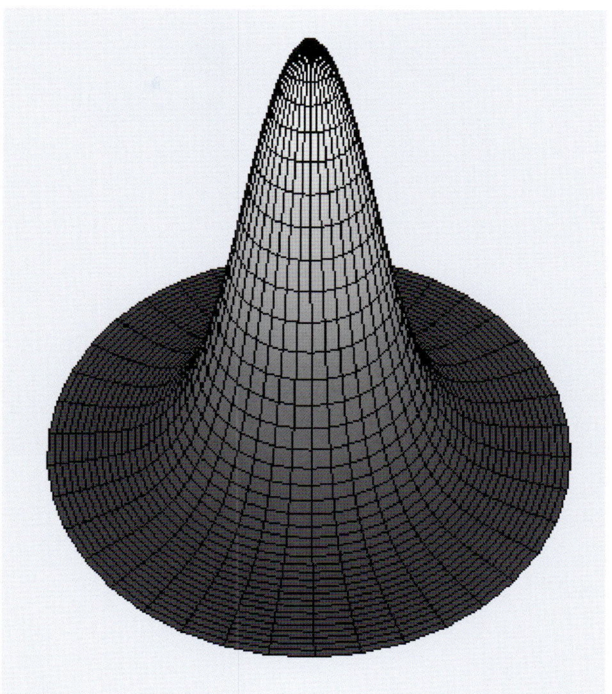

Fig 3-57 TEM_{00} mode (Gaussian beam profile).[73] (Figure from J. Meister, Aachen, Reprinted with permission.)

However, also lasers with fiber-based delivery systems, as in most of the commercially available 3 µm systems, may not be free of intensity profiles highly deviating from the ground mode: the

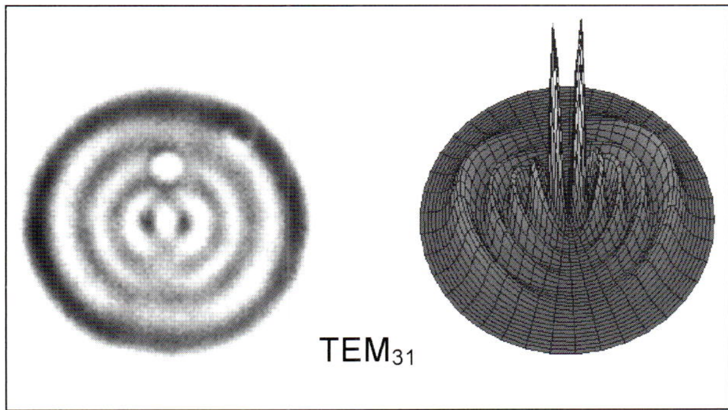

Fig 3-58 TEM_{31} mode visualized with thermal paper and calculated by solving the Laguerre polynomes for a special resonator geometry[73]. The white spot in the left visualization is an artifact caused by a dust particle in the beam delivery system. (Figure from J. Meister, Aachen, Reprinted with permission.)

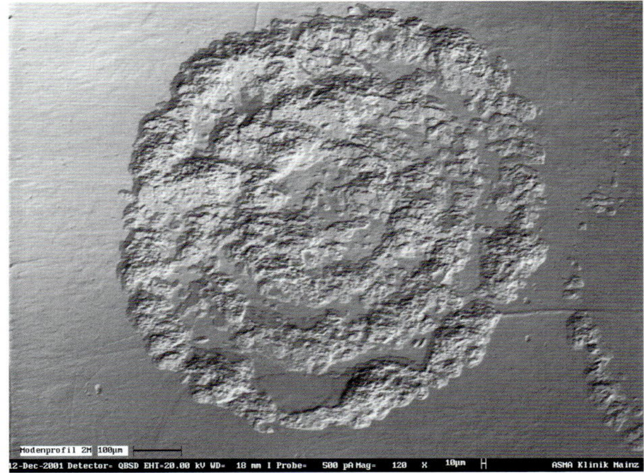

Fig 3-59 Ablation pattern of the beam profile shown in Fig 3-56.[73] (Figure from J. Meister, Aachen, Reprinted with permission.)

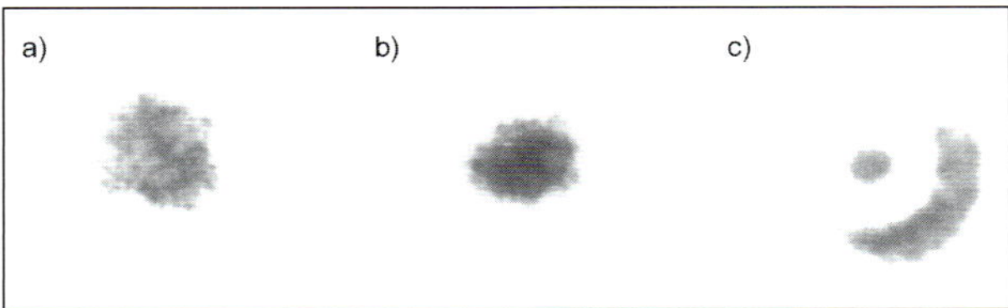

Fig 3-60 Intensity patterns of round tips:
(a) out of the distal end of a 400-µm fiber,
(b) out of a cylindrical tip with 600-µm distal diameter,
(c) out of a conical tip with a 400-µm distal diameter.

quasi-Gaussian beam profile can be maintained only when the emitted light is focused by a lens onto the target. But these "non contact" hand pieces have the disadvantage that there is no tactile response to the operator, so that it is very difficult to maintain the correct working distance (in almost all cases about 12 mm, corresponding to the length of a dental drill).

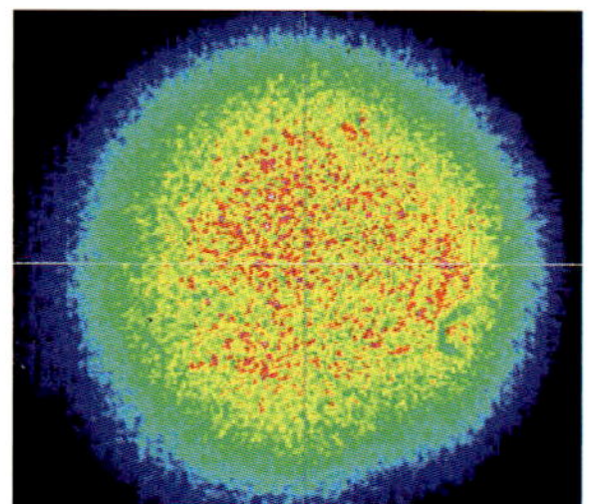

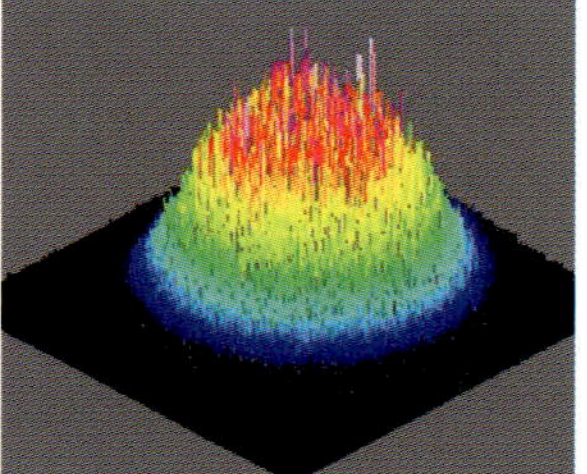

Fig 3-61a and b Distribution of intensity of a laser beam coming out of a sapphire tip, measured with a CCD-Chip.
(Fig 3-61a two-dimensional, Fig 3-61b three-dimensional.)

If contact hand pieces are used, the laser radiation propagating out of the fiber is deflected and focused and transmitted through a second, distal waveguide, mostly implemented as a sapphire tip. Depending on the quality of this coupling and the shape of this tip, the quasi-Gaussian beam profile can be destroyed again, thus leading to very special intensity profiles (Fig 3-60 and 3-61).

The question wheter the variation of the spatial distribution has other influences on the quality of ablation, additional to the change of threshold, will be part of further investigations.

3.4.2.2.4 Dependence of Absorption on Wavelength and Reflectivity of the Tissue Surface

As already discussed above, the absorption of optical radiation in matter depends on the applied wavelength. So, e.g., the absorption coefficient of water in the infrared has its highest peak at 2.94 µm at room temperature. This is commonly one of the first facts one may find out when engaging in appropriate laser treatments. But it is less well known that in the case of water the absorption peak is extremely reduced at higher temperatures and additionally shifts to lower wavelengths at high irradiation densities such as those used in pulsed laser ablation[67]. So it can be deceptive simply to look up an optimum wavelength for a certain absorber in an absorption diagram without considering temperature and laser intensity.

The absorption coefficient of several types of tissue recorded under room conditions are shown in Fig 3-62. As depicted in Fig 3-63, the absorption coefficient of water for pulsed Er:YAG (λ = 2.94 µm) and Er,Cr:YSGG laser radiation (λ = 2.79 µm) drops for higher energy densities (i.e., at higher intensities) in the irradiated volume. The initially (i.e., at very low irradiation densities) very high absorption coefficient α of water for λ = 2.94 µm drops monotonically for higher irradiation rates. The absorption coefficient for λ = 2.79 µm initially is just ~38% of the corre-

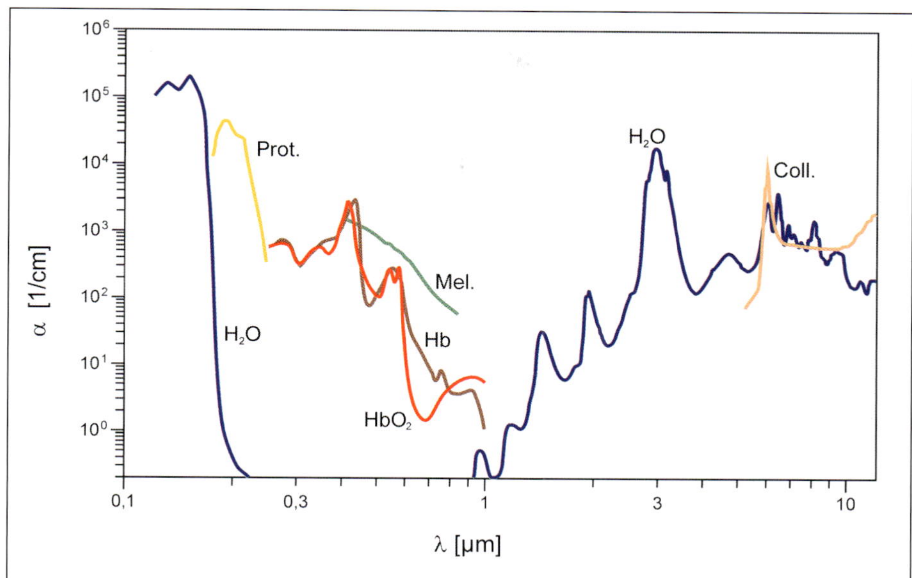

Fig 3-62
Absorption coefficient of several types of tissue recorded under room conditions[67]. Prot., = protein; Mel., = melanin; Coll. = collagen.

sponding value for λ = 2.94 μm, but it stays constant over a long range of deposited volumetric energy density before it starts to rise and overcome Er:YAG absorption at high irradiation densities.

This indicates that for high volumetric energy densities the absorption coefficient not only decreases but also its maximum shifts to the lower wavelength. Hence, when considering the energy density transferred into the irradiated matter, one has to be aware of a much deeper penetration depth due to the reduction of the absorption coefficient than would be estimated by well-known absorption diagrams like Fig 3-62.

Surface reflectivity representing a determining effect for energy deposition in the tissue also has to be considered.

Reflections at the surface reduce the amount of energy coupled in. Their magnitude depends on

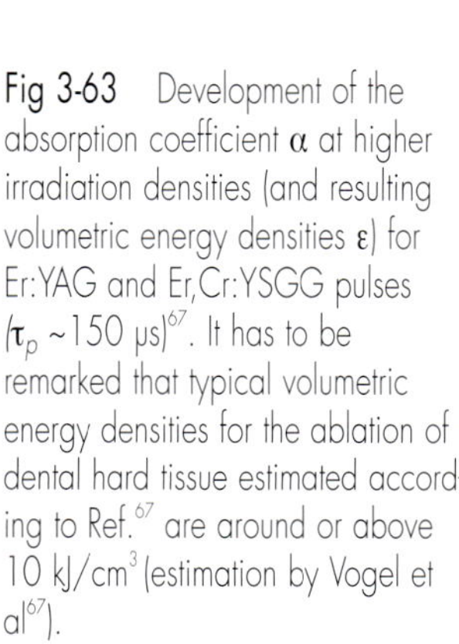
Fig 3-63 Development of the absorption coefficient α at higher irradiation densities (and resulting volumetric energy densities ε) for Er:YAG and Er,Cr:YSGG pulses (τ_p ~150 μs)[67]. It has to be remarked that typical volumetric energy densities for the ablation of dental hard tissue estimated according to Ref.[67] are around or above 10 kJ/cm³ (estimation by Vogel et al[67]).

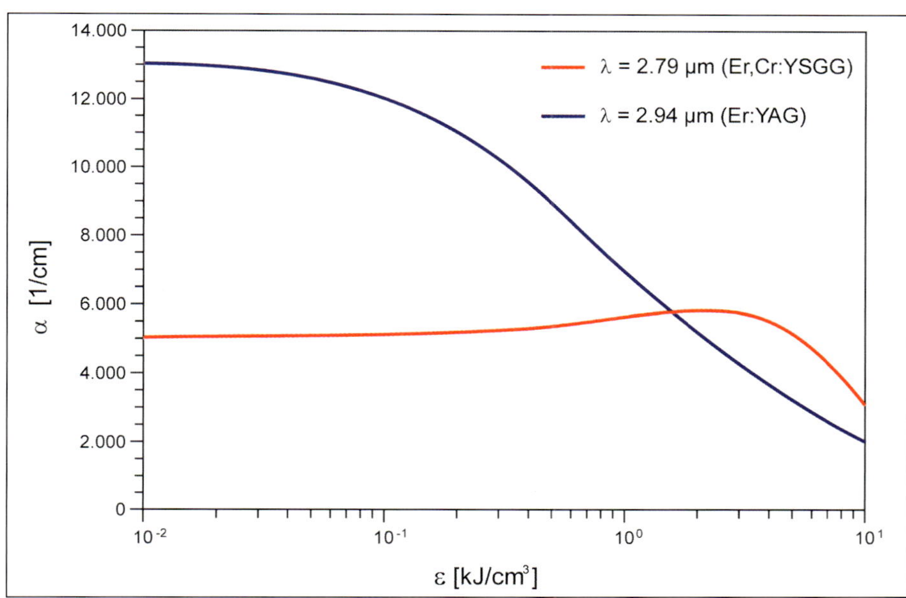

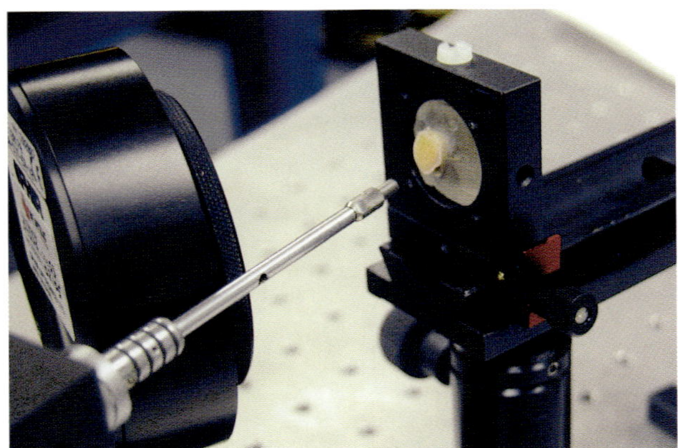

Fig 3-64a Set-up for the reflection measurement in dentin: a molar with the crown cut off is fixed to a device on the right-hand side. On the left, the delivery system can be seen, which delivers the energy to the tooth. The reflected portion is captured by detectors and evaluated.

the color of the tooth and the physiological state of the tissue as well as on the roughness of the irradiated area. On average, surface reflectivity of polished dentin is about 1.6%, depending on its physiological state. Of course, for the practitioner, the reflectivity of the surface need not be especially considered, as, in the published parameter sets for tissue processing, it is always automatically taken into account. He should, however, be aware of the amount of the laser energy reflected during irradiation, which plays a role in laser safety.

3.4.2.2.5 Distribution of Water in the Tissue

As the water content of tissue is one of the most important factors for ablation efficiency, tissue layers with less embedded water will yield less ablated volume per unit time in the 3 μm range. This is one reason why enamel needs much more pulse energy than, e.g., dentin for acceptable processing speeds.

The water content of healthy enamel is about 12 vol.%, that of healthy dentin about 24 vol.%[70]. The water content of carious tissue is much higher than in healthy tissue, but it differs significantly with the kind and the physiological state of the carious lesion. Since we can assume that, the higher the water content in the tissue, the higher the ablated volume, there is a certain selectivity for higher ablation rates at carious regions.[74]

This assumption also shows that with increasing dehydration of the tooth during treatment, the ablation efficiency will drop. So the applied water-spray has not only the task of cooling the tooth down to safe temperatures, but also to increase the absorption again to initial values.[74]

The role of dehydration in ablation efficiency and collateral impact on the remaining tissue can be reconstructed by performing a little experiment on a freshly extracted tooth.

Immediately after extraction the physiological state of the tooth, especially the water content, is approximately unchanged the in-vivo state. Thus, ablating it in vitro with a normally used set of parameters for cavity preparation, one will find nearly exactly the same values of efficiency and surface structure as in a normal in vivo preparation. Afterwards, the tooth is stored under ambient conditions, i.e., in air without any artificial moisture, for 15–20 min. When processed with the same parameter set after this time, the tissue will show decreased ablation depth and increased melting, carbonization and sometimes even micro-cracks.

3.4.3 Physical Limitations for Present-day Laser Systems

Even the physically simple free-running pulsed laser systems, mostly used in dental practices, represent highly sophisticated devices for material removal compared to conventional systems like rotating instruments. Thus, as we have shown in the previous sections, one has to consider several physical conditions to achieve the best possible results for the patient.

As in every technology, unprofessional handling can cause more harm than benefit. Therefore, we shall now take a look at the physical limitations that occur with the present-day laser systems and how they can be minimized. Section 3.4.5 is an outlook on a possible future perspective and how the limitations mentioned here could be reduced or even eliminated.

Detail 3-5. Free-running laser systems.

Here the term "free running" for a pulsed laser system will be described briefly, because it plays an important role in the limitations described further below.

In laser physics there are several possibilities to produce pulsed laser radiation (see chapter 1). One of them is pulsing the pump irradiation. Thus, at the beginning of the pulse a very high population inversion in the laser medium can be achieved, allowing peak powers of the laser pulse far above the cw mode. By employing the control electronics of the pump source, several pulse durations can be set. For technical and physical reasons these pulse durations have a lower limit. For flash lamp pumped solid-state systems (e.g., typically Er:YAG and Nd:YAG lasers for medical purposes) this limit is around 50–90 µs. Similar values are achieved for systems pumped by the quasi-cw laser diodes usually applied. To get even shorter pulses, quality switching (Q-switching) or mode locking would have to be employed forcing the pulse into shorter temporal regimes. Hence, lasers without such expensive devices are called "free running".

Generating micro-explosions for ablation means induction of shock waves in the remaining tissue. If this happens to very brittle materials, as enamel and dentin are, micro-cracks reaching far into the tissue can be caused. So, on the one hand, a very high pulse energy means higher ablation rates, but on the other hand, if it is too high, it will penetrate deeper into the tissue. In addition to warming this region, it will cause microcracks because the energy is no longer sufficient to evaporate enough water for a complete delamination of these layers. Hence, usable pulse energies have an upper limit. According to this, inhibition of crack formation in dentin reported by many authors will be achieved only if the given limits are not exceeded. Thus, the ablation rate clearly has an upper limit.

A rise in temperature in the tooth also limits the ablation speed. It has to be ensured that the energy remaining in the matrix after spallation can be removed, otherwise the pulp overheats. For temperature development the average power delivered is more important than the pulse energy, as the former describes the energy delivered per unit time. The cooling capability (i.e., capability for energy removal) of the water-spray is also a function of time and is limited by the amount of water applicable per unit time (see section 3.4.2.2.1). If the energy remaining in the matrix is higher than the energy removed, temperature will increase. In this context, it has been reported by many dentists, that above an average power of 5–6 W patients start to feel significant pain.

From all of the above, we can draw the following conclusion for an optimized laser system for dental hard-tissue ablation.

3.4.4 Conclusion for the Specifications of Laser Systems Optimized for Minimal Collateral Effects on Dental Hard Tissues

The central conclusion from the previous considerations is the demand to perform ablation with the lowest possible energy ("Method of Minimal Pulse Energy"). Any energy coupled into the dental hard tissue that exceeds the absolute necessary minimum will cause unnecessary damage.

The first step in this direction is the application of very short pulse durations to achieve the spatially best possible confined energy distribution.

For the free-running laser systems, the lower limit for the pulse duration is around 50–90 µs. That means that such laser systems will not be able to cross this limit unless they have special features such as, e.g., a Q-switching device (see also Detail 3-5). So, if a laser system shall be employed for hard tissue ablation, its pulse duration should be at least very near to the achievable minimum.

Recently, a new technology providing shorter pulses than the usual pulse durations became available. With these short pulses, having a pulse width of 50 µs, the ablation rate could be enhanced by 20% compared to 100-µs pulses.[75]

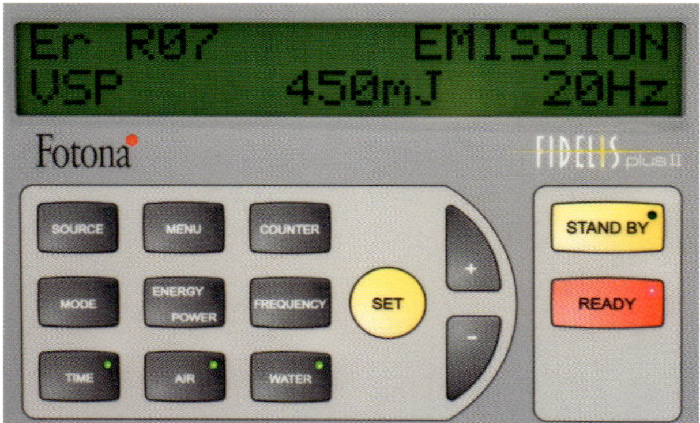

Fig 3-64b Display of a laser system with adjustable pulse duration. VSP, means "Very Short Pulse".

Detail 3-6. Pulse duration and spatial confinement in practice

At this point, it has to be noted explicitly that the required short pulse durations are of primary interest where lasers for dental hard-tissue treatment are concerned. The physically exceptional position of teeth is caused by their anatomy: normally, in strong vascularized tissues externally applied heat can be removed by the blood stream up to a certain amount, to prevent the tissue from possible damage. Such heat removal is impossible in the tooth as the small vessels embedded in the pulp just cannot transport enough blood to cool down the tissue efficiently. This is the reason why especially in dental applications the heat remaining in the tissue has to be reduced to an absolute minimum to prevent necrosis.

In soft tissues the situation is somewhat different. Here, in many cases the application of remaining heat is desired to induce sealing of the opened vessels and the other tissue via coagulation to prevent bleeding and provide a protection against wound infection. Thus, longer pulse durations up to quasi-cw and cw-lasers are absolutely desired and necessary. Via regulation of the pulse duration and the pulse repetition rate it is even possible for the user to determine the depth of the coagulation zone to find the optimum between secure sealing of the wound and healing time due to the thickness of the denatured areas.

In addition to the pulse duration, the rise-time of the pulse plays a very important role for the spatial confinement of energy in the tissue. The benefit of a very steep slope is a high ablation speed with less energy remaining in the lattice. As the amount of applicable water spray is limited on account of its influence on ablation efficiency, as discussed in chapter 3.4.2.2.1, the rise-time is more important than generally assumed.

The pictures of our measurements of the temporal pulse profile show that the leading edge of the investigated Er,Cr:YSGG laser pulses is very steep (Fig 3-54). It has the additional advantage that the wavelength fits to the shifted absorption maximum at high energy densities. From these data, very good ablation efficiency can be expected.

The Er:YAG laser investigated in Fig 3-55 shows a rather poor rise of the first pulse peak, so no premium ablation efficiency will be reached. The Er:YAG laser in Fig 3-56 shows a very similar pulse profile to Fig 3-55, thus an ablation efficiency of the same order of magnitude can be estimated. In contrast to the laser in Fig. 3-55, the pulse subsides much faster after the maximum. This might bring advantages regarding the heating of the tooth, but this effect can be quickly cancelled by selection of pulse energies that are too high. For a direct comparison of both systems, a test for the ablated volume per unit time would have to be performed together with an exact measurement of the delivered pulse energy.

From the device-related point of view, a very simple set-up of the laser unit turned out to be the most advantageous and reliable. But of course this also means a reduction of parameters that can be adjusted by the user.

Necessary or advantageous parameters for adjustment are: pulse energy (or the average power) for adjusting the laser power to the treated tissue, the amount of the water-spray (see Fig 3-53 and sections 3.4.2.2.1 and 3.4.2.2.5), and, for some kinds of therapy, the decrease of the pulse repetition rate for further reduction of the thermal impact on the tissue and the resulting pain sensation. Adjustment of the pulse width to longer durations is only suitable when soft tissue has to be treated.

Nearly all manufacturers implement the mentioned features in their units, although none of them provides all of them simultaneously or in sufficient form. Often some of the controls are not included for technical reasons. Thus it is up to the user and his experience to choose the device that fits best to his needs.

But beside all the technical considerations one should not forget the most important influence on ablation quality: the user himself. He has to bring the right prerequisites to perform well on the patient. It is an often-confirmed matter of fact that an experienced operator can achieve much better results with an average tool than an inexperienced could with the best.

That means that it is highly recommended to someone who wants to start up with laser applications to attend courses and workshops with experienced tutors to learn about the basics of practical laser application to prevent avoidable mistakes.

3.4.5 Future Perspectives

3.4.5.1 Requests for Improved Ablation Techniques and Laser Systems

In the last two sections we have discussed the best fitting parameters for the ablation of dental hard tissue, and also the physical limitations of the commercial laser systems nowadays available for these purposes.

Our most important concern was to perform ablation with the lowest possible energy and with pulses as short as possible to induce the lowest possible collateral damage. The central point therein is to leave as low an energy level as possible within the residual tissue.

However, the systems available today exceed the maximum allowed pulse length $\tau_p \leq \tau_{rel}$ sometimes by 300–400 times (150–200 μs instead of 0.5 μs) and the necessary heating of the mediator water will cause heat transport into the postablative remains.

Hence, we can regard the thermomechanical ablation process we have applied until now to be also part of the "limiting problem" for reliably damage-free preparation of teeth. This means that we have to find another kind of ablation process that must be able to ablate the material via direct impact on the hard tissue components without generating thermal damage. (For example, holmium laser radiation is absorbed directly by the dental hard tissues, but as a result of the long pulse duration of the systems in the free-running or Q-switched mode it causes more thermal damage than erbium lasers.)

So we can sum up that an ideal process for dental hard tissue ablation should have the following properties:

- no crack formation in the remaining tissue
- no heat transport into the residual tissue
- no shock wave delivery into the tooth
- no adverse effect of heat or high energetic radiation on the pulpal soft tissue.

As an additional benefit it would be appreciated if the ablation could be very precise, as the actual laser-prepared cavities mostly have an irregular shape thus not allowing the whole range of filling techniques such as inlays, onlays or overlays, to be applied.

3.4.5.2 Candidates for Ablation with Low Collateral Damage

As stated at the beginning of this chapter, there are two other mechanisms of ablation that can be used for precise material removal: ablation by excimer lasers with wavelengths in the ultraviolet range and the application of ultra-short laser pulses in the near infrared region.

Ablation with excimer lasers was found not to be suitable for dental hard tissue treatment, beause they have very low ablation rates per pulse together with very low pulse repetition rates. Although the character of photochemical ablation does indeed permit very precise ablation, the high costs of these laser systems for purchase and operation, together with their complicated handling and maintenance, decrease their usability in everyday practice. Due to this and the carcinogenicity of several UV-wavelengths, these systems have not found their way into the dental laser market during the past 15 years. Ablation by ultra-short laser pulses seems to be a very promising approach, since this relatively new technology bears a high potential for a fast, precise and nearly damage-free material processing, also for broad industrial applications. As this approach has proved its applicability also for dental hard tissue treatment in recent years, we will discuss it in more detail in the following sections together with an estimation of its benefits and present limitations for a broad application in dental clinics or practices.

3.4.5.3 Ablation by Ultra-Short Laser Pulses – from Thermal Ablation to Plasma-Mediated Ablation

Before we can start the discussion about the suitability of ultra-short laser pulses for dental applications, we have to take a look at what ultra-short laser pulses actually are and how they interact with material.

Ultra-short laser pulses are pulses with durations in the time regime of several tens of ps (picoseconds, (1 ps $= 10^{-12}$ s) down to some fs (femtoseconds, (1 fs $= 10^{-15}$ s) or even below. As these time regimes cannot be imagined easily, a little illustration for better representation should be given: 1 ps (= 1000 fs) compared to 1 s represents the same relation as 1 s to 31,709 years. Or another way round: if we assigned the period of 1 ps to the length of 1 mm on a time scale and we delivered 10,000 pulses per second (= a pulse repetition rate of 10 kHz), the distance between two subsequent pulses would be 100 km.

Detail 3-7. Present records for shortest pulse widths

The present record for shortest pulses in the wavelengths of the electromagnetic spectrum that can be described as light is around 4.5 fs, held at the Photonics Institute of Vienna University of Technology; 4.5 fs is a time period wherein light oscillates a little less than 2.5 times (see basic laser chapter).

The present record for the shortest pulses in the electromagnetic spectrum except gamma radiation is also held by the same research institution with a pulse width of 550 as (attoseconds, (1 as = 10^{-18} s), but, owing to physical limitations, at very short wavelengths.

Why do ultra-short laser pulses yield such a precise and damage-free ablation?

The ablation threshold of a material (i.e., the required pulse energy for ablation) falls significantly with decreasing pulse length[76]. This means that less energy per pulse has to be applied to cause ablation. Hence, there is less energy to produce collateral damage. But it is decisive that almost no heat transfer to the surrounding matter can take place if the pulse durations are short enough. Regarding this, sufficiently short pulses for the treatment of dental hard tissues have durations around 1 ps, since the time constant for photon-phonon coupling for these materials (i.e., the transfer of photon energy to vibrations of the lattice and finally into heat) can be estimated as ~1 ps[77].

Hence, it is very interesting to use these ultra-short pulses for the treatment of biological tissues where only small or even no heat-affected zones can be tolerated (e.g., neurology, ophthalmology and, of course, the preparation of teeth).

The decrease of the ablation threshold at short pulse lengths is caused by the high power densities that can be achieved: the shorter the duration of a pulse with a certain pulse energy can be made, the higher is the achievable peak power of the pulse (see Fig 3-65).

If these high peak powers are combined with a sufficient focusing of the beam, very high power densities can be generated at an irradiated surface (up to several TW/cm^2).

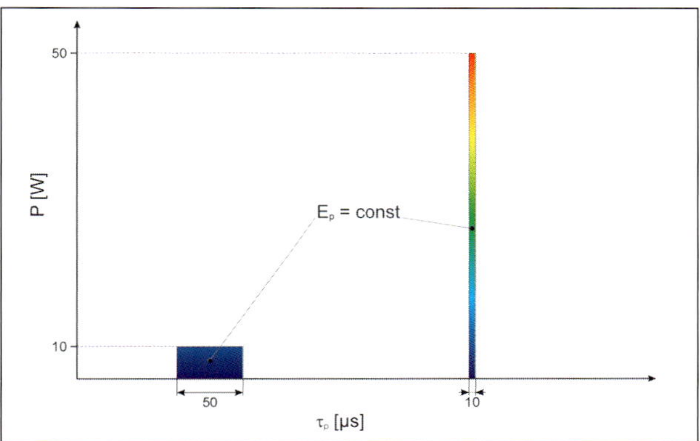

Fig 3-65 Development of the peak power *P* of a laser pulse by alteration of the pulse duration τ_p at constant pulse energy E_p (= rectangle area).

Thus, an ablation mechanism completely different to the thermomechanical stress generation occurs: the plasma-mediated ablation.

In this intensity range the power densities generated on the surface of the irradiated material are so high that nonlinear processes (see chapter 1) are initiated. These allow the generation of a thin layer of plasma in the irradiated zone. This plasma layer absorbs nearly all the energy contained in the laser pulse.

When matter is in the plasma state, the single atoms have overcome the material bonds and can move freely in the affected volume.

Owing to the laws of thermodynamics, the plasma expands rapidly and blows itself out. Since the pulses are so short, there is nearly no time for heat to flow into the surrounding lattice, as the irradiating energy is "switched off" again before significant heat transport can take place. As the plasma is completely removed by the blowing out process and the heat transport is nearly negligible, practically all the energy deposited in the matter is removed again during the ablation process from the lattice, thus yielding almost no temperature increase.

Detail 3-8. Relation of pulse energy and pulse duration at ultra-short laser pulses

The peak powers achievable with ultra-short pulses are typically in the regime of Megawatt (MW) to Terawatt (TW), depending on pulse duration and pulse energy. So, for example, a pulse with the duration τ_p = 1 ps and a pulse energy E_p = 300 μJ (1 μJ = 0.000001 Joule) has a peak power of about 300 MW. If pulses with this energy were used to heat up 0.25 l of water (the volume of a large coffee cup) from room temperature to boiling point, about 125 million pulses would be required. Focused on a spot of 100 μm, the intensity during one pulse is about 3.8 TW/cm^2, which is the same as about 1300 times the peak power of the power plant of Hoover Dam on the Colorado River, USA (P_{max} = 2.8 Gigawatt) focused on 1 cm^2.

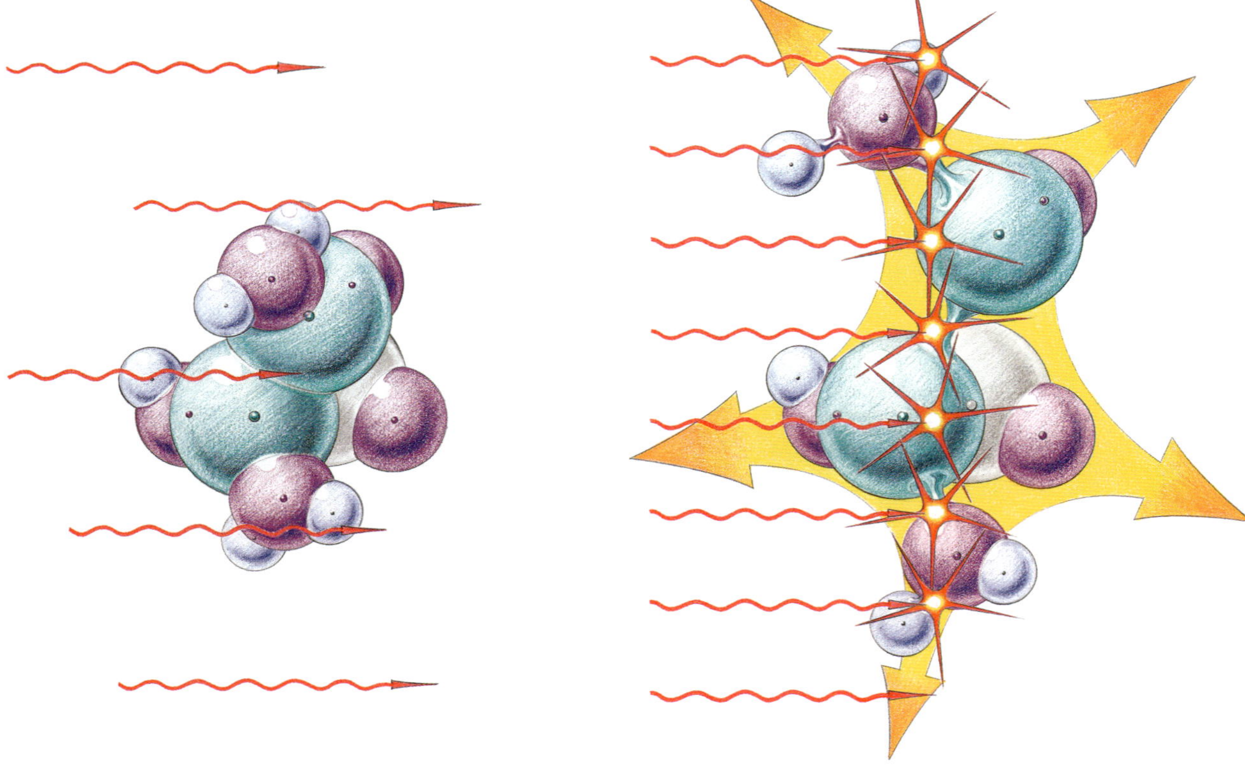

Fig 3-66 Graphical illustration of the plasma-induced ablation. The electrons can leave the atomic compound. Thus the atomic bindings to the material are cracked and electrons and free ions form a plasma.

Usually, ablation energies for dental enamel applied with pulses of ~1 ps duration are about 100 µJ. Conventional laser systems with pulse durations around 150 µs use pulse energies of 250 mJ, i.e., 2,500 times more.

Detail 3-9. Plasma formation and ablation of material

Mindermann et al.[78], being one of the first groups in this field, described in detail the mechanisms of plasma-mediated ablation as follows: "power densities $>10^{11}$ W/ cm^2 are obtainable with picosecond pulses with sufficient pulse energy and focusing conditions. Thus, an electric field of about 10^7 V/cm can be generated at the focus spot. A microplasma is induced with an absorption coefficient much higher than that of enamel. Consequently, the laser beam is absorbed totally by the plasma. The ablation itself is caused by the ionization of the enamel and the shock wave generated by this. Advantages of this interaction mechanism are the low thermal effects and the lack of crack formation in enamel". The validity of this model was proven by numerous publications and consequently elaborated for the regimes of femto-, sub-pico- and picosecond pulse durations.

The initiation of the plasma development is driven by multiphoton absorption (MPA): the irradiating intensity is so high that the valence electrons of the atoms in the affected matter can absorb not only one, but two or even more photons at once. Hence they gain enough energy to leave the atom, thus creating plasma.

The generated free electrons are further accelerated by absorption of the incident light. On their way through the plasma they collide with other

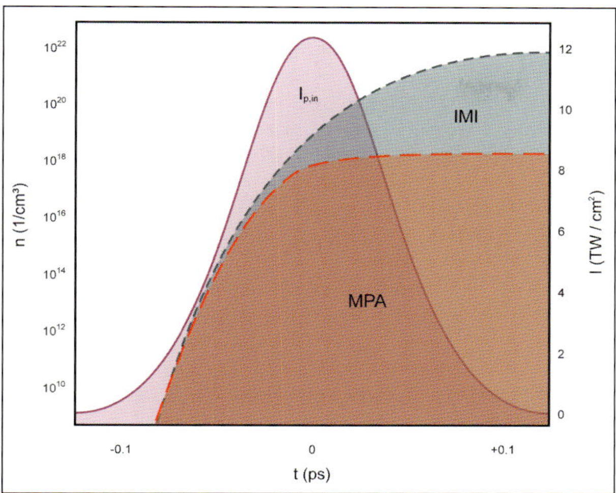

Fig 3-67 Development of the plasma during pulse duration: the electron density *n* in the plasma initially is created by multiphoton absorption (MPA). After the pulse peak it is mainly increased by impact ionization (IMI).

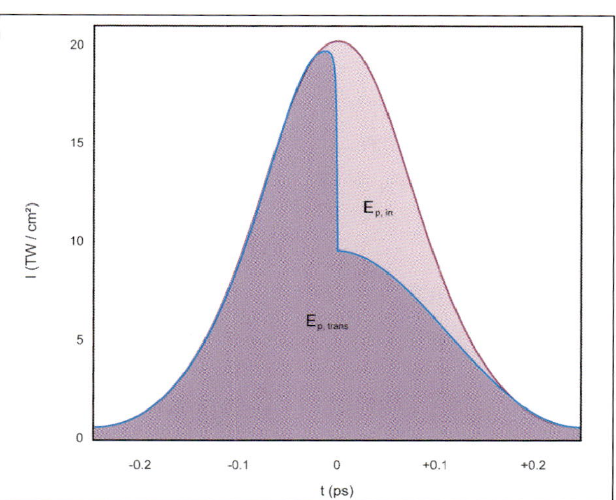

Fig 3-68 Plasma reflection: a part of the incident pulse energy $E_{p,\ in}$ is reflected on the plasma layer; this reduces the pulse energy $E_{p,\ trans}$ that can be transmitted into matter.

atoms and transfer a quantum of their energy to them. Hence additional free electrons are produced. This process is called impact ionization. As depicted in Fig 3-67, MPA is the dominant process during the leading edge of the incident light pulse. As soon as the light pulse has passed its maximum, MPA breaks down and further electrons are produced only via impact ionization.

As the free electrons absorb a significant part of the light pulse, the plasma is heated up rapidly. Moreover the plasma becomes highly reflective after it has reached a critical electron density. The heating of the plasma leads to its expansion due to thermodynamical laws. Thus it is blown out easily as the ions and free electrons have overcome the material bonds. This is the way matter is ablated.

The absorption and, further on, the reflectivity of the plasma yield very important benefits for the temperature development in the remaining material: Nearly all the energy during plasma-mediated ablation is absorbed in a layer of about 1 µm thickness. As the incident light is well absorbed by the generated plasma, the deposited energy stays spatially well confined in this layer and is removed again by its expulsion. Furthermore, as the plasma becomes reflective over a critical electron density (in Fig 3-68 this is reached at approximately the peak of the pulse), the rest of the energy contained in the trailing edge of the incident pulse (that is not needed any more for generation or heating of the plasma) is reflected and therefore is prevented from penetrating into the matter and heating it up.

As the plasma plume has a lifetime of about 100 ps, the reflection is very reliable even for longer pulse durations. This benefit is impossible for other ablation mechanisms such as the thermal ablation where no plasma is created.

3.4.5.4 Irradiated Area and Scanning of Ultra-Short Laser Pulses

It was discussed above that the initiation of plasma-mediated ablation depends on the pulse energy, the pulse duration and the irradiated area. These three parameters determine the power density applied on the target surface. The ablation threshold, of course, is a specific material parameter depending on the pulse duration, but generally the intensity has to reach some hundred GW/cm^2.

As the available pulse energy and pulse duration are limited by the laser system as well as by the threshold of destruction of the optical components, sharp focusing of the laser beam has to be achieved. Usually, spot diameters ranging from some tens of μm up to ~ 0.1 mm provide an energy density for reliable plasma generation. But these spot diameters are so small that they are only suitable for micro-preparation. For the treatment of larger areas the laser beam has to be moved over a certain area. This operation mode is called "scanning" of the beam, and it has to be performed by an automatic device that guarantees a constant energy distribution over the irradiated area, as depicted in figure 3-69. By applying different scanning algorithms it is possible to produce cavities of different shape, like those shown in Fig 3-70.

Detail 3-10. Development of Pulse Efficiency and Temperature Rise during Scanning

One goal for scanning the laser beam automatically over a certain area is to make handling for the dentist more efficient. Other even more important aspects are the advantages arising in terms of preparation quality and heat distribution in the irradiated tooth.

It has been shown that pulse efficiency drops rapidly if several pulses are delivered on the same spot (e.g., Kim et al.[79]). Additionally, the temper-

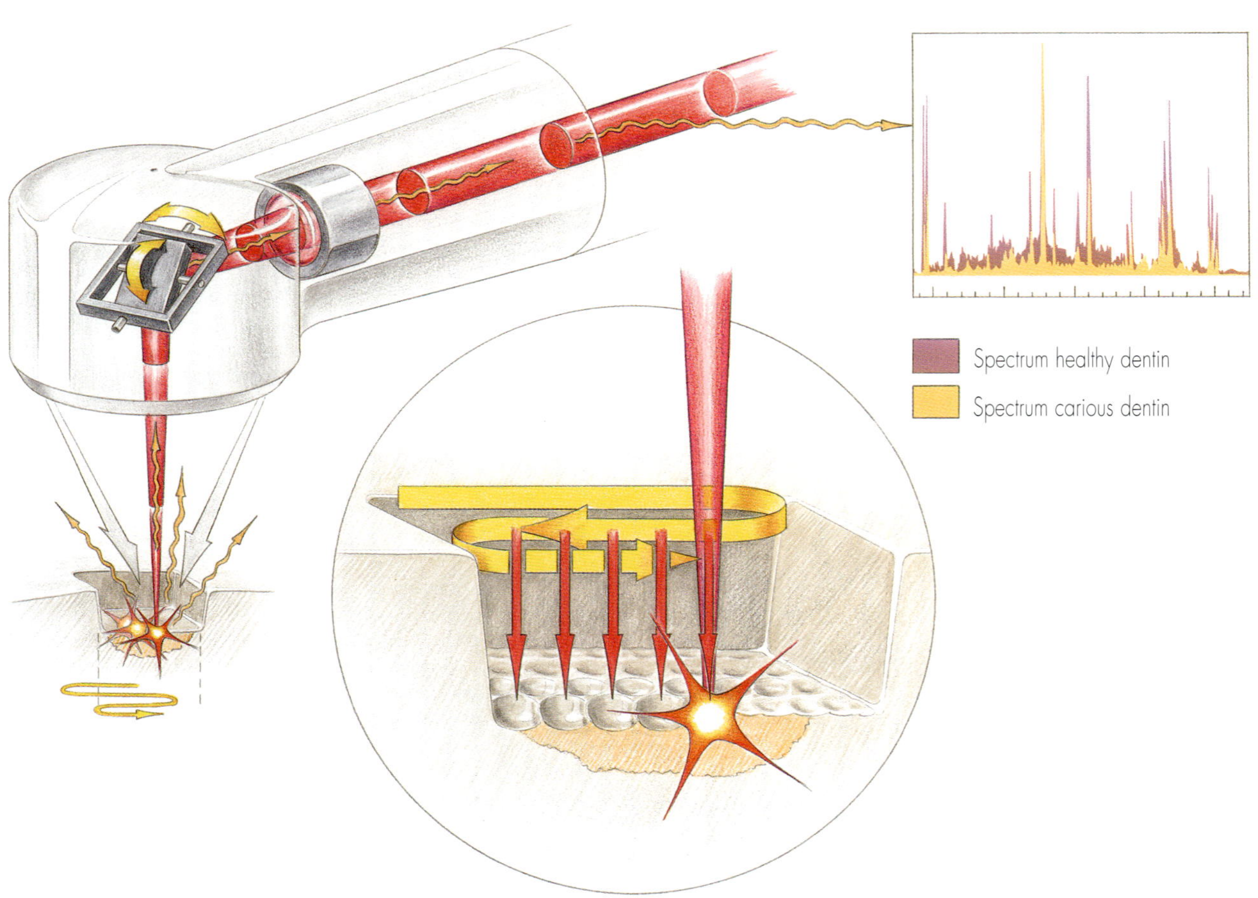

Fig 3-69 Depiction of a scanning hand piece.

ature increase in the tissue can be reduced significantly if fewer pulses hit the same spot. Both can be explained by a reduction of cumulative effects: if a longer train of subsequent pulses is delivered to the same spot, the drilled hole becomes deeper and is very narrow. Thus the lateral region of the incident beam touches the hole's walls. According to the grazing incidence the energy density on the cavity walls is very low and cannot cause ablation any more. Additionally, the grazing light is scattered and undergoes multiple reflections in the hole. At each reflection a certain amount of the light becomes absorbed. Thus a significant part of the pulse energy gets lost on its way to the bottom of the hole, where the next ablation should occur. The deeper the hole, the more light is scattered and absorbed, thereby reducing ablation efficiency and increasing the temperature in the tissue.

When the laser beam is scanned over a larger area, scattering can occur only at the rim of the scanning pattern and there only at one side of the beam (maximally on two sides if there is a sharp corner in the pattern). Thus, the pulse energy can be applied very efficiently even in very deep holes (see Figs 3-70).

The heat accumulation is further reduced during scanning because the amount of energy that is always transferred to the lattice (see Detail 1-9) can be removed very rapidly by conventional thermal convection until the scanned laser beam reaches the same spot again.

3.4.5.5 Benefits of Ultra-short Laser Pulses in Working with Biological Tissues

The very short interaction times of the laser pulses with the treated material, the nearly perfect confinement of the deposited energy in the irradiated volume, the expulsion of the deposited energy with the ablation products (i.e., the plasma), and the small ablated volume per pulse, make plasma-mediated ablation very suitable for surgical procedures where the highest degree of precision with a nearly complete absence of collateral damage has to be achieved. Also, for the treatment of lesions in dental hard tissue the application of this technology is very well suited. Here it is possible to generate cavities of a very precise shape with a well-defined inclination of the walls as depicted in Fig 3-70.

The bottom and the walls of the cavity produced show a micro-retentive pattern and opened dentinal tubules (Fig 3-71). The complete absence of a smear layer could allow a direct application of composite materials without etching.

Besides the possibility of producing cavities with geometrically well-defined walls, the laser generally has a certain selectivity in the ablation of healthy and carious tissue. It is based on the higher ablation rate of carious substances already known from thermomechanical ablation. In plasma-mediated ablation, it is amplified by the precision removal of material. Thus, not only precise cavities reaching deep into the healthy tissue, like those in standard preparations, can be generated.

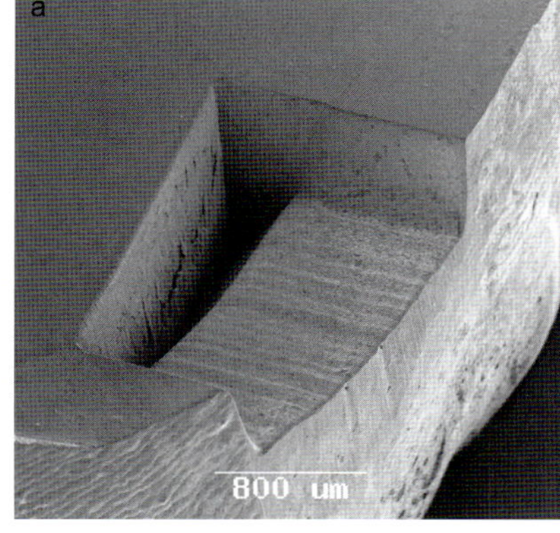

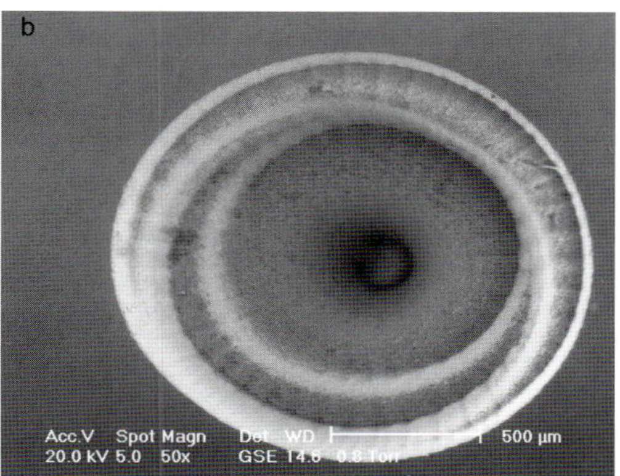

Fig 3-70 Examples of cavity shapes achieved by different, free programmed scanning algorithms a.) courtesy of A. Kasenbacher, Traunstein, Germany, and b.) courtesy of J. Serbin, Laser Zentrum Hannover, Germany.

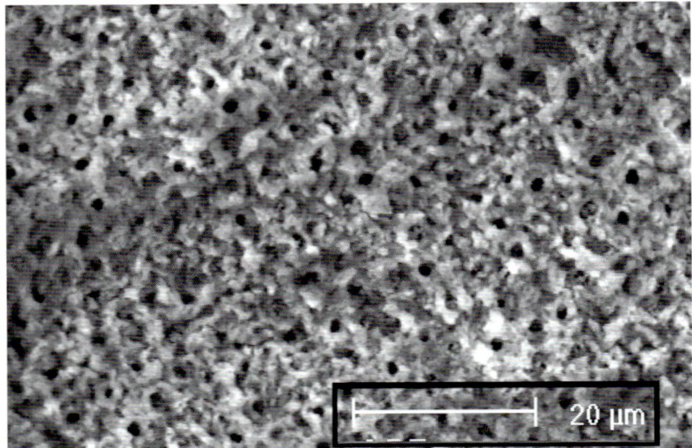

Fig 3-71 Open dentinal tubules and micro-retentive pattern after laser irradiation.

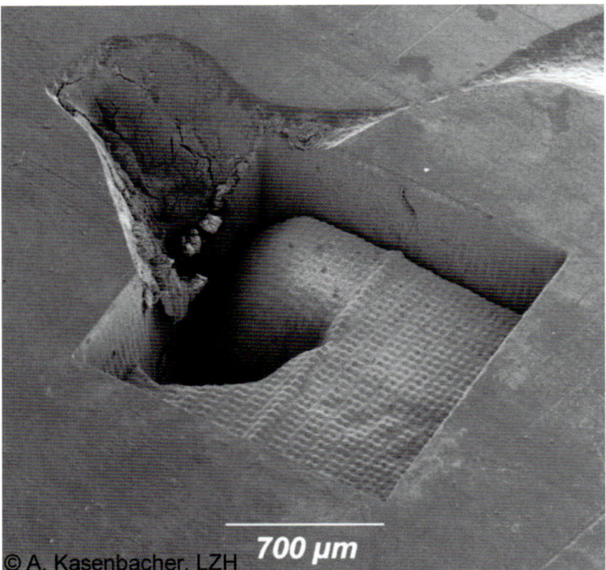

Fig 3-72 Selective ablation of healthy and carious tissue: for better illustration of selective ablation a rectangular cavity was laid over an irregularly shaped carious lesion (upper left quarter). The energy was held constant over the whole area (i.e., each spot in the base of the cavity was irradiated with the same ablation energy). The orthogonal faces of the cavity show the ablation in healthy dentin. The irregular shaped, steep falling surfaces show the significantly higher ablation in carious tissue (picture courtesy of A. Kasenbacher, Traunstein, Germany, and J. Serbin, Laser Zentrum Hannover, Germany).

It is also possible to produce really minimally invasive cavities in which virtually only the carious tissue is ablated (see Fig 3-72). This natural given selectivity can be further supported and controlled by spectral analysis of the generated plasma sparks.

Spectral analysis as a standardized measuring method allows a reliable diagnosis of the treated tissue.[80] Here, the different chemical composition of the tissues is used. Healthy enamel, healthy dentin, carious enamel, carious dentin and dentin near to the pulp each contain different elements causing characteristic spectroscopic lines in the generated plasma.

Since certain spectral regions stay nearly constant in healthy and carious tissue, they can be used as a reference for each analysis. Hence, the procedure is virtually independent of boundary conditions such as intensity of the plasma spark or brightness of the surroundings; it thereby achieves an accuracy superior to that of most methods used nowadays, and is suited for diagnosis before treatment as well as for online monitoring during ablation. Combined with the small ablation depth per pulse, a very accurate ablation of carious tissue can be achieved.

Hence, it also allows the precise diagnosis and treatment of the well known "white spots kept under observation" at an early stage.

From the mentioned facts it can be seen that during recent years there was a paradigm shift in ablation research: before, high pulse energies at low repetition rates were believed to be crucial for fast ablation suitable for practical applications. But since an ultra-short pulse has the energy to convert only a very thin layer into plasma, and the plasma shielding effect (see detail 3-9) additionally inhibits a deeper penetration of the laser energy into the matter very effectively, this aim was not realistic. Moreover, application of significantly more pulse energy than minimally necessary would eliminate the key advantage of conservative tissue preparation: the minimal energy deposition in the remaining tissue.

So it was found that applying minimal pulse energy at extremely high pulse repetition rates would be better for high ablation rates, being in good compliance with the proverb

"constant dripping wears away the stone".

The pulse repetition rates for an acceptable ablation rate of about 4.5–5.0 mm^3/min are situated around 45 kHz, and have already been realized. With a pulse energy of about 100 μJ at $\tau_p \sim$ 1 ps this yields an average power of 4.5 W, already comparable to the power of conventional Er-laser systems for dental hard-tissue treatment.

3.4.5.6 Actual Limitations of Ultra-Short Pulse Laser Systems

The main problems of the ultra-short pulse laser systems that have inhibited their broad application in practice until now were their size, their sensitivity to environmental changes and of course their very high price. But since basic research has produced many innovative concepts that improved the size and stability of these systems by several orders of magnitude, it should be not a question of decades but only of some years until the suitable laser systems will be available for clinical use. One of the best indications for this optimism is that some of the leading laser companies in the world have put considerable effort in resent years into bringing these concepts to a high degree of development. Some of the developments really do seem poised for a breakthrough for industrial use. One of them, for instance, is the thin-disk laser[79] which, together with other devices, has reduced the size and costs of such laser systems radically.

But even if the results of the in-vitro experiments with this technology look very promising, and we believe it to have a high potential for minimal invasive medical therapies, it still has to prove its suitability for clinical applications in the coming years.

3.5 Other Laser Types

As already mentioned at the beginning of this chapter, only the erbium-based laser systems were able to succeed in the removal of dental hard substances. But as many studies have been performed on this topic also with other wavelengths, it is time to take a look at them now.

3.5.1 The CO_2 Laser

The CO_2 laser was investigated very early for dental hard-tissue removal, as it was one of the first available laser systems with a sufficiently high output power.[3] Its first disappointing results were confirmed in new studies performed during the 1980s.[81,82] Even during recent years, studies on the usability of the CO_2-wavelength of $\lambda = 9.6$ µm have been performed. In most of them, different devices and methods for reducing the high thermal impact on the residual tissue were investigated.

In 2002, Mullejans et al.[83] investigated the microleakage of filled class V cavities in an in vitro study. As they reported no cracks or carbonization in the prepared cavity walls, they found the CO_2 laser to be usable. But still they found the cavity walls to be so smooth that microleakage could not be prevented without additional bonding.

In her PhD thesis, Glock[84] investigated the effect of lateral scanning of CO_2 pulses on local reduction of the thermal load. She stated that, even with this approach, no satisfactory results could be found, as even 10–20 s after the end of the treatment, a significant temperature rise in the pulp has to be expected, although she assumed a temperature rise of 6–10°C to be possible (and not 10°F as stated by Zach and Cohen[14]).

Taking into account that the wavelength of the CO_2 is absorbed much better in collagen than in water (see Fig 3-62), it seems to be evident that the interaction cannot avoid direct heating of the tissue. Thus, the usability of the CO_2 wavelengths in hard tissues will always be limited by the uncontrollable temperature rise induced.

3.5.2 The Nd:YAG Laser

Nd:YAG radiation is much less absorbed in dental hard tissue, thus having a high penetration depth. Hence, heat can be transported easily to deeper layers, inducing a profound heating of large volumes.

But as laser radiation is much better absorbed by carious than by sound enamel, Harris et al. tried a selective caries removal in enamel lesions.[85] They reported an efficient removal of carious tissue with simultaneous conservation of the underlying healthy regions. During the subsequent clinical and histological examinations of the pulp vitality, no abnormalities were found. Regarding Inoue et al.[23], who were able to detect cell damage only under the electron microscope, these results would have to be examined critically once more.

Nevertheless, as in endodontics a bactericidal effect in dentin was proven for the Nd:YAG laser down into a depth of 1 mm (explosion of cells and formation of megalospheres), a strong interaction of this radiation with deep layers of the tissue has to be assumed. Thus, the Nd:YAG laser has to be classified as not suitable for caries removal, because it bears a high risk of pulpal damage due to the high penetration depth and the additional heat transport deeper into the tooth.

3.5.3 The Ho:YAG Laser

In the beginning, the Ho:YAG-laser was believed to be suitable for dental hard-substance removal. But in later studies, such significant collateral heat damage was found that this had to be revised.[6] Nowadays, holmium lasers are no longer produced on a large scale. But in spite of this, this laser wavelength is much appreciated for surgical applications by users who are equipped with such a system; it is well suited for this purpose owing to its low penetration depth.

3.6 Practical Procedure in Laser-assisted Cavity Preparation – Clinical Work

3.6.1 Application of the Rubber Dam

Laser-supported cavity preparation should be analogous to the conventional treatment criteria, always with the use of the rubber dam. This guarantees a good view and facilitates the use of other materials. Iatrogenic damage of the bordering approximal area can be avoided because of the low absorption by the rubber dam of the wavelengths used. Since one of the domains of the laser preparation is defect maintenance with composites, the drying of the cavity is of great importance. The specific laser retention pattern also has to be secured from saliva and from contact with the mucosa or the tongue, as in conventional acid-etching techniques. The adhesive systems used with composite fillings only guarantee a strong bondage between the dental hard tissue and the compound under optimized dry working conditions and can even be influenced by the humidity of the breath.

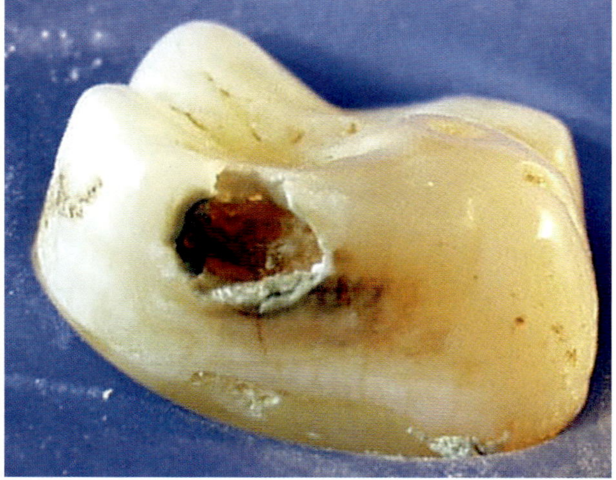

Fig 3-73 Display of the carious lesion after the application of a rubber dam.

3.6.2 Display of the Cavity

First of all, it is recommended to clean concrement and superficial detritus off the treated tooth with an ultrasound scaler or a polishing device, because these can influence the absorption of the laser. Before the first irradiation it should be checked whether all safety requirements are met (safety goggles, secured working area, a check of the laser parameters).

Analogous to the steps with rotating instruments, the carious lesion is prepared first. Therefore, the parameters recommended for enamel preparation by the producer are used. The laser beam should preferably be perpendicular and under water cooling, which in most systems is integrated in the hand piece. A strong enough water-spray is important under permanent suction cleaning because a too-thin or -thick water film can complicate the laser preparation. In this first working step, overhanging enamel areas are removed to allow access to the caries-damaged enamel and dentin.

Depending on the system used, one works contact-free with a visible laser spot or with contact supported through a stiff laser fiber. In any case, one should work in contact-free mode. Using free-beam handpieces (handpieces without a sapphire tip) a working distance has to be observed that assures the smallest possible diameter of the aiming laser beam (in most cases the same distance as from a conventional drilling handpiece to the instrument tip, see the manufacturer's instructions).

Handpieces with a sapphire tip have to be guided over the working area at a distance of 1 mm. Thus, the fiber won't get stuck on the surface, sufficient cooling is facilitated and a premature erosion of the fiber tip due to the annealing of adhered ablation particles can be avoided.

3.6.3 Caries Removal

It is recommended that the power of the laser be reduced while breaking through the enamel (see section 3.4.4). On the one hand, the thermal exposure of the pulp is reduced and, on the other hand, the removal of the carious dentin through lower energies is possible since the greater proportion of water in the damaged dentin causes a higher ablation rate, as was explained before (see section 3.4.2.2.5). With scanning of the carious area, a partly selective preparation is done under spray cooling and suction cleaning. If during the caries excavation the cavity is getting too close to the pulp, the energy of the system has to be reduced accordingly. During preparation close to the pulp, the work should be intermittent and the frequency reduced. (Note: in systems with an optimal pulse shape the reduction of the pulse frequency is not mandatory, since they allow for efficient ablation with much lower pulse energies compared to devices with higher settings, see section 3.4.2.2.) The total removal of the caries is controlled with the classic probe test or with the help of a caries indicator. On closer inspection, the laser-prepared areas are seen to have a matt surface that comes from the specific reflection-poor retention pattern.

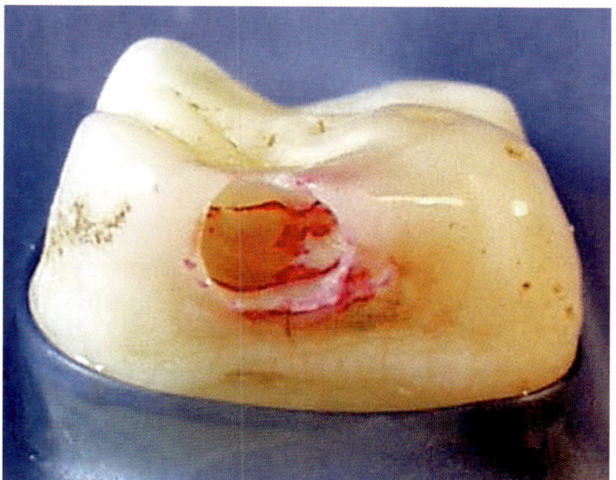

Fig 3-74 Primary caries removal, control with caries indicator.

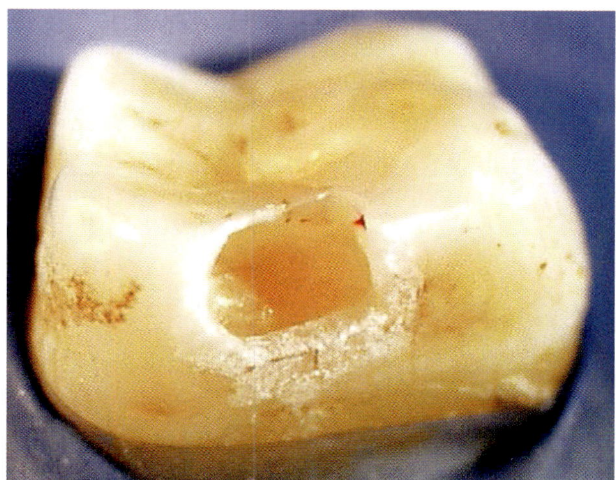

Fig 3-75 Completion of the cavity.

3.6.4 Completion of the Cavity

A possible finishing and beveling of the cavity mainly depends on the choice of the filling material. Using composites, some of the working steps necessary when rotating instruments are used can be left out. Finely tapered enamel lamelle are also removed with a carbide finishing bur or with an Arkansas stone. After a careful cleansing of the cavity with a water-spray and alcohol, the adhesive can be brought in and the composite filling can be finished as recommended by the manufacturer. As mentioned before, the treatment with preparation lasers leaves a micro-

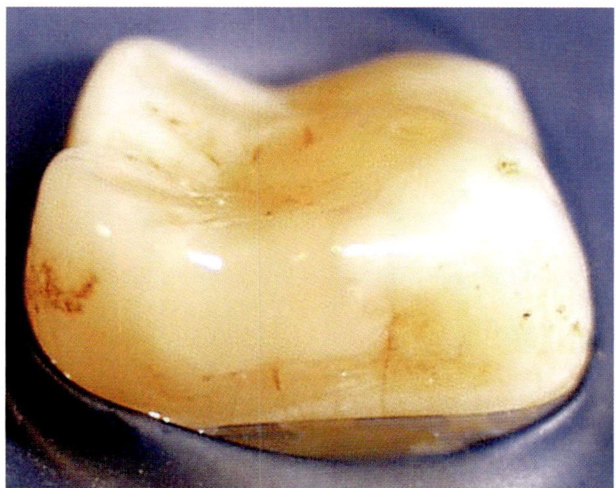

Fig 3-76 Definitive filling with composite.

roughness that is at least equal in adhesive power to the retentive pattern produced by etching with phosphoric acid. Therefore, acid etching is generally not necessary. If adhesive filling materials are not used, the same working steps as in conventional preparation of the cavity have to follow.

3.6.5 Choice of Parameters

The choice of the correct parameters is strongly dependent on the actual laser system applied. Therefore it is impossible to give general statements that are valid for all units. Depending on the manufacturer, a frequency range between 2 and 20 Hz and pulse energies from 50 to 1000 mJ are available. In addition, the ablation efficacy does not only depend on these two parameters, but also on many other factors (see section 3.4.2). Since nowadays an immense number of laser systems are available on the market, it would go beyond the scope of this book to expand on each individual laser and to give an objective recommendation. Each user is thus invited to scrutinize the manufacturer's guidelines for the individual laser and to work out the optimal parameters based on physical knowledge and his own clinical experience. In case of any doubt, the parameters have to be kept as low as possible in order to minimize the risk of collateral damage.

In general, it can be said that the highest pulse energies can be used for the ablation of enamel. When the preparation advances into the dentin, the output power can be reduced by one third; close to the pulp, it should be further decreased. The same holds true for the removal of resin or glass-ionomer fillings. If the surface should only be cleaned or roughened (e.g., when performing a fissure sealing or conditioning), the power can be reduced to one-half or one-third, even when working within enamel.

3.7 Clinical Cases

3.7.1 Cavity Preparation Class I, II and III

A 55-year-old patient with a class II in tooth 15, a class II in tooth 16 and additional occlusal cavities (class I) (see Figs 3-77a–c).

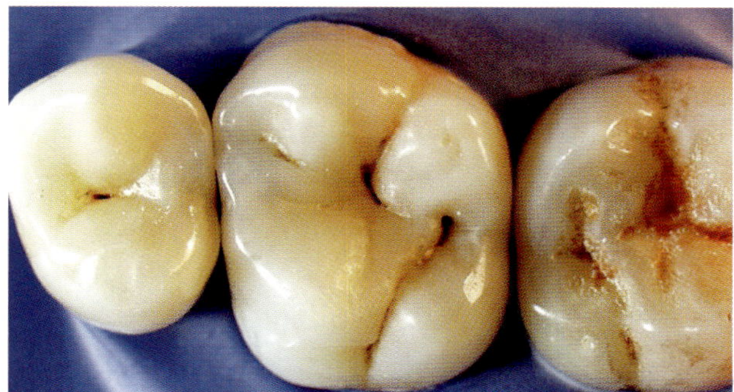

Fig 3-77a Occlusal display of discoloured fissures and interdental caries shimmering below the surface.

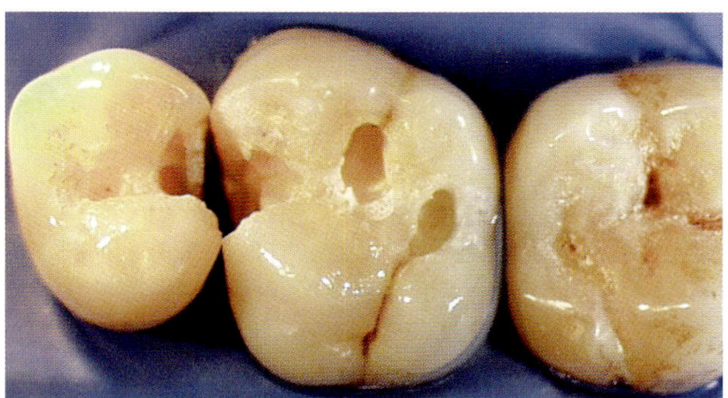

Fig 3-77b After preparation with the laser the full extension of the carious lesion is visible.

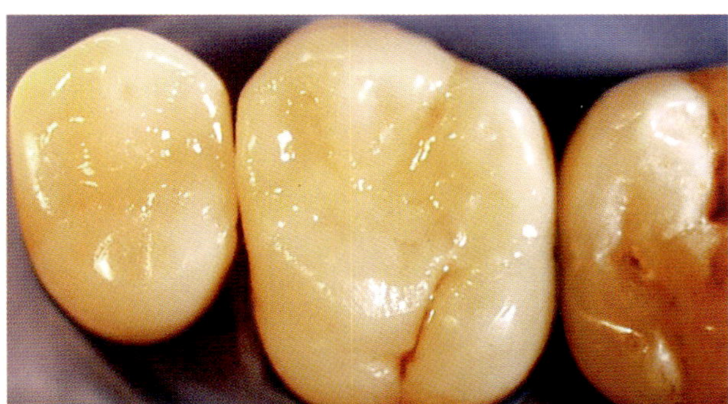

Fig 3-77c The completed composite fillings.

3.7.2 Fissure Sealing

Fissure sealing is one of the most popular indications for laser preparation, particularly in pediatric dentistry (see Figs 3-78a–c).

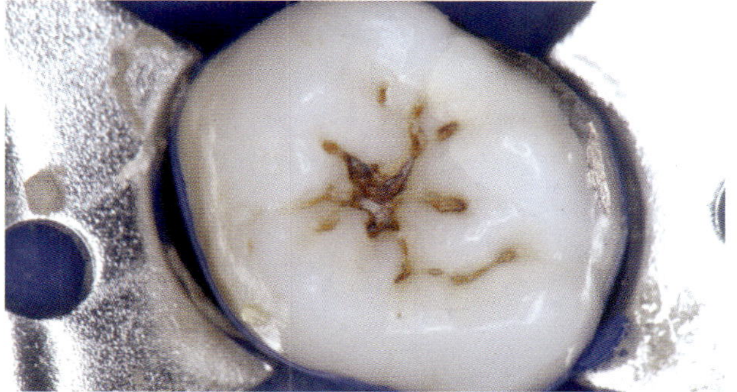

Fig 3-78a Discoloured fissures in an upper molar.

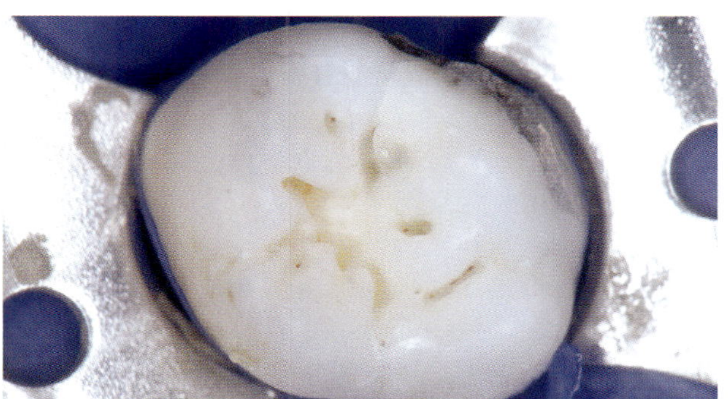

Fig 3-78b Situation after laser preparation.

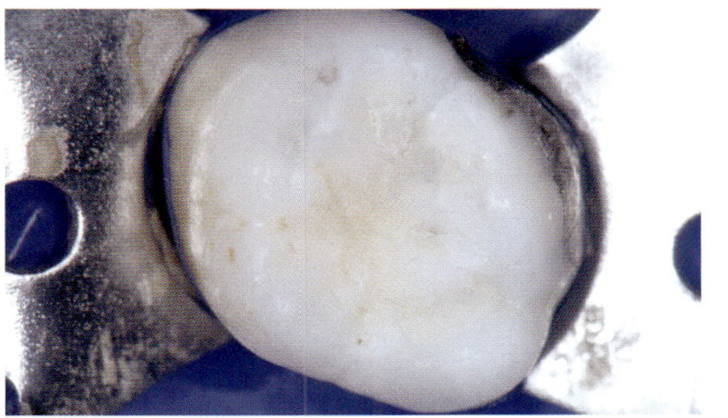

Fig 3-78c Completed fissure sealing.

3.7.3 Veneer

Treatment of a 40-year-old patient with a strongly discoloured, but vital tooth 12 (see Figs 3-77a–f).

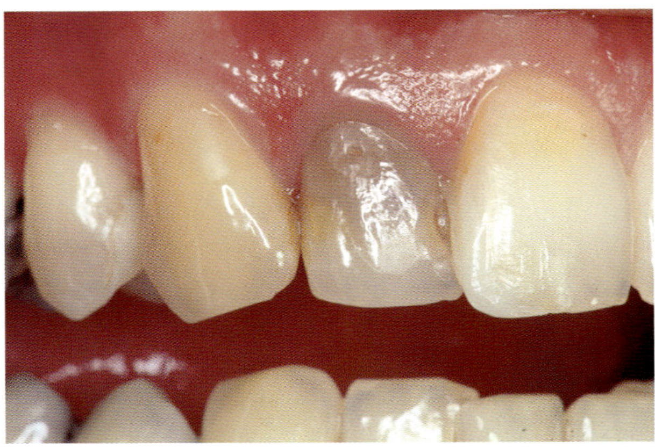

Fig 3-79a Shows the strongly discoloured tooth 12. Because of the intensity and the depth of the discoloration the tooth was scheduled to be restored with a veneer.

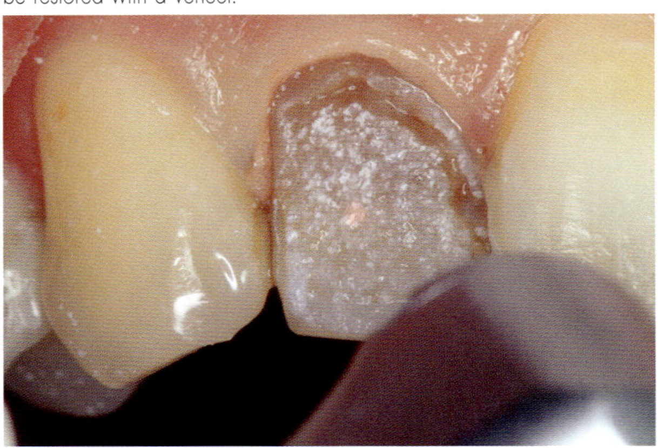

Fig 3-79b Illustrates the laser preparation, in this case with a non-contact hand piece.

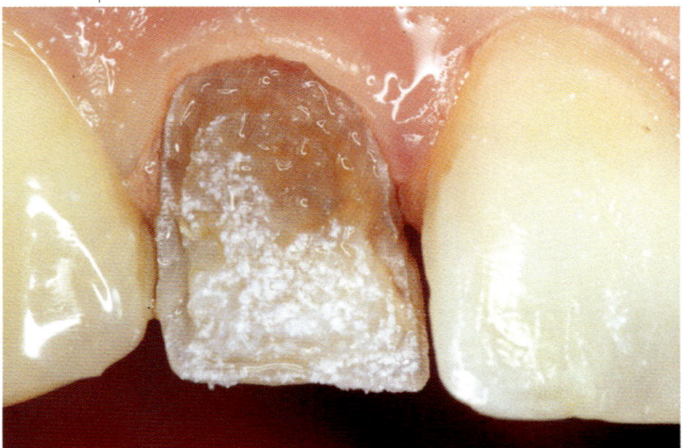

Fig 3-79c The highly retentive surface after laser preparation can be seen. No bleeding occurs on the gingival margin.

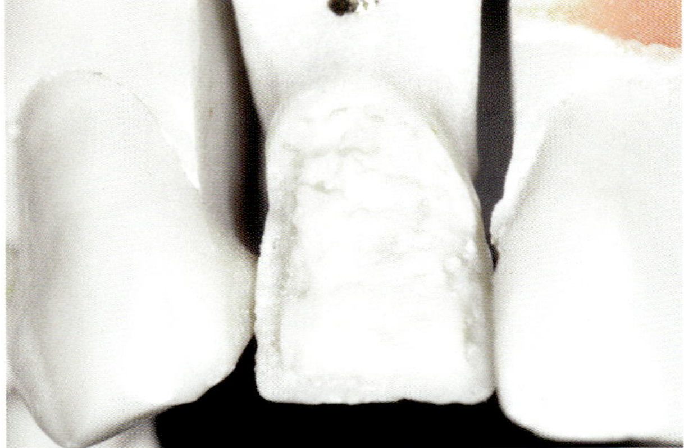

Fig 3-79d Also in the model cast the retentive surface is discernible.

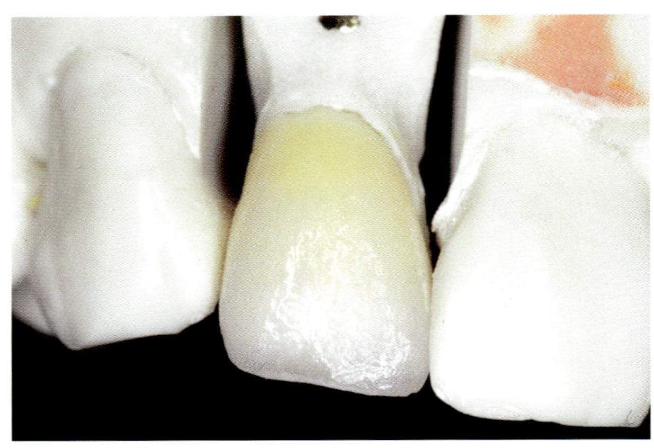

Fig 3-79e Shows the completed veneer on the model stump.

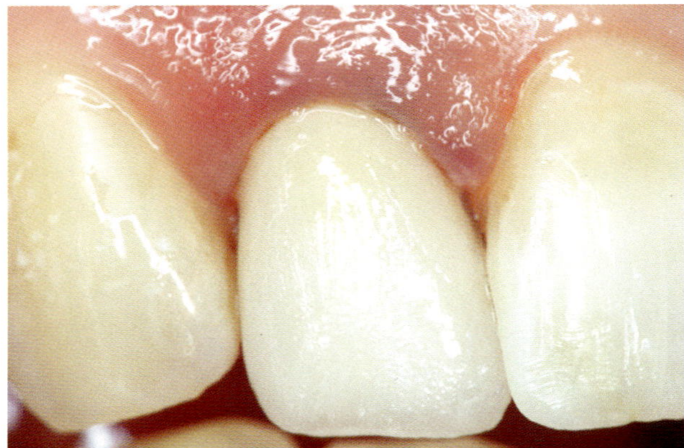

Fig 3-79f Finally shows the complete work in the mouth. For the cementage, no acid etching was necessary.

3.7.4 Gold Inlay

Treatment of a 20-year-old patient with hypersensitivity on the tooth 16. Because of the dimension of the cavity, a composite restoration was waived and a high-grade restoration with a cast gold filling was chosen (see Figs 3-80a–g).

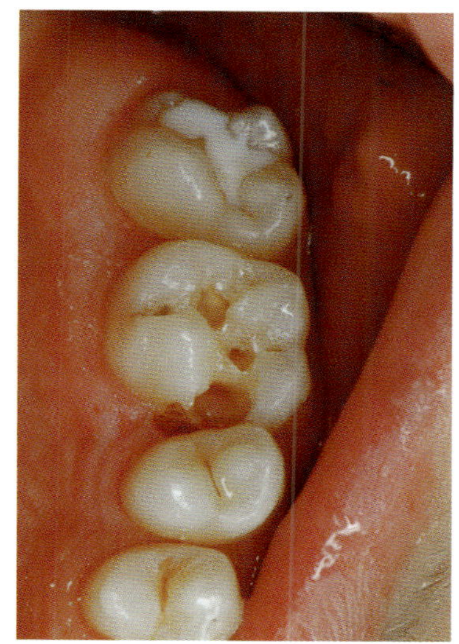

Fig 3-80c Shows the situation after the removal of the filling.

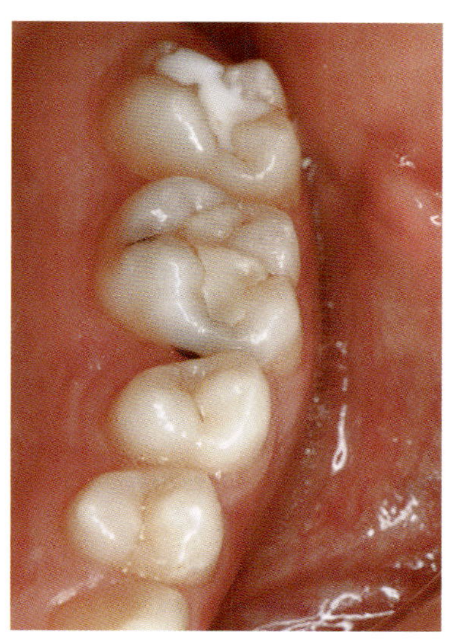

Fig 3-80a Shows the first quadrant with an insufficient resin filling on tooth 16.

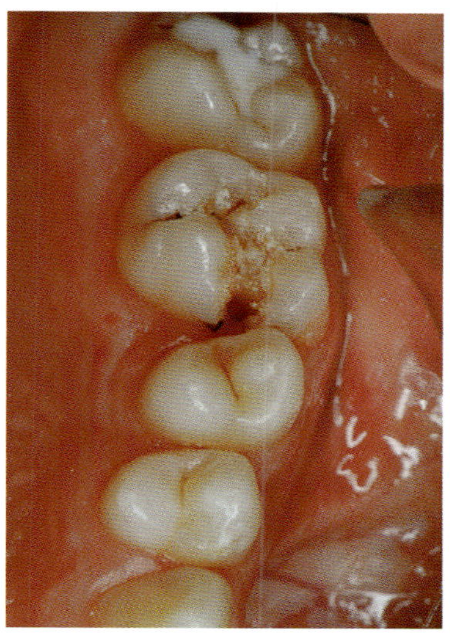

Fig 3-80d Illustrates the situation after the further extension of the preparation.

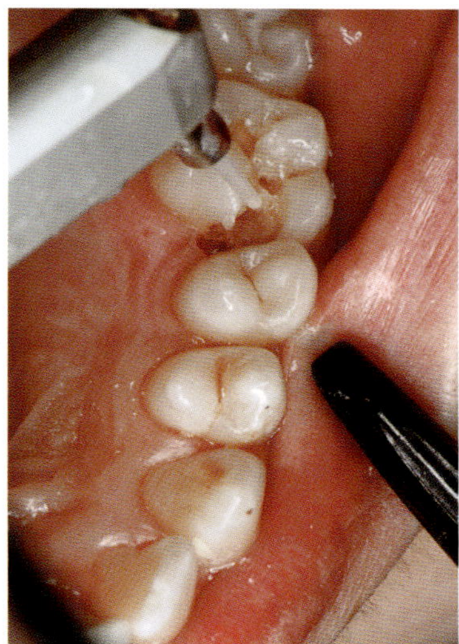

Fig 3-80b The resin filling is removed using an Er:YAG laser, in this case with fiber contact.

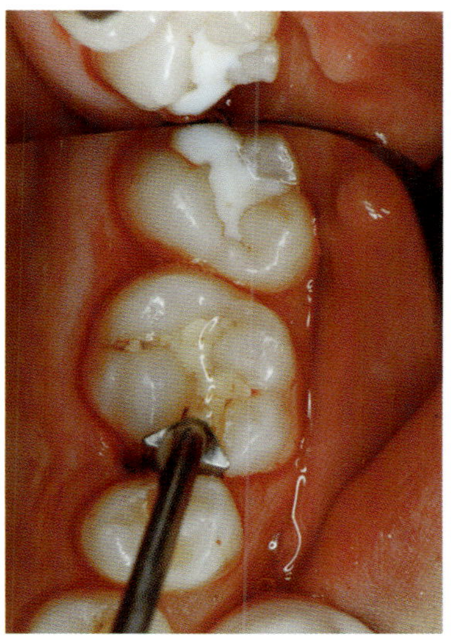

Fig 3-80e To achieve the desired smoothness of the preparation edges, a rework with an ultrasonic preparation system is necessary.

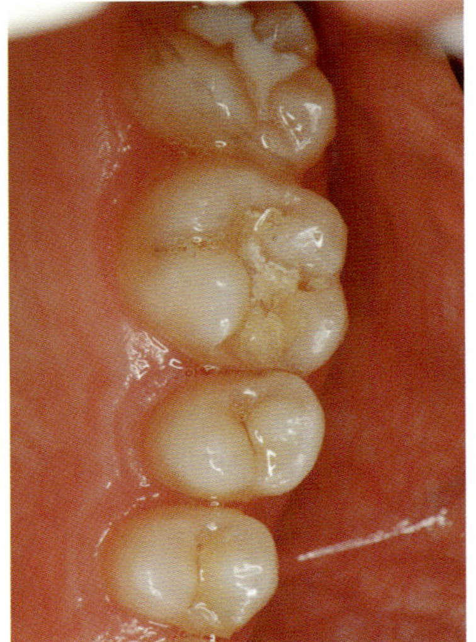

Fig 3-80f Preparation achieved as shown in Fig 3-80e.

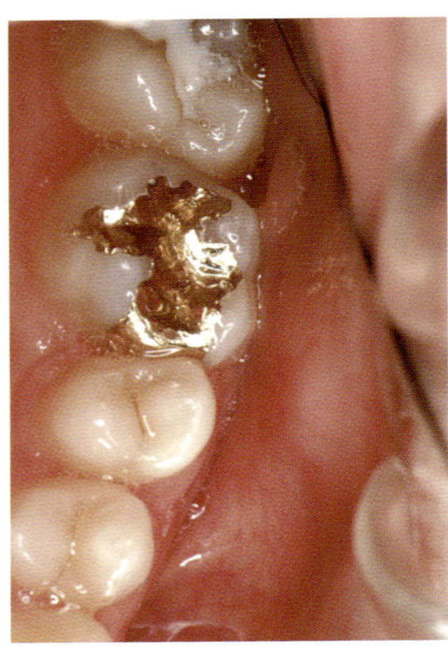

Fig 3-80g Finally shows the inserted gold inlay.

3.7.5 Ceramic Inlay

Treatment of a 19-year old patient with insufficient resin fillings in the molar region of the lower jaw. The patient insisted on a functional and esthetical high-grade restoration. Therefore, the indication was given for ceramic inlays (see Figs 3-81a–i).

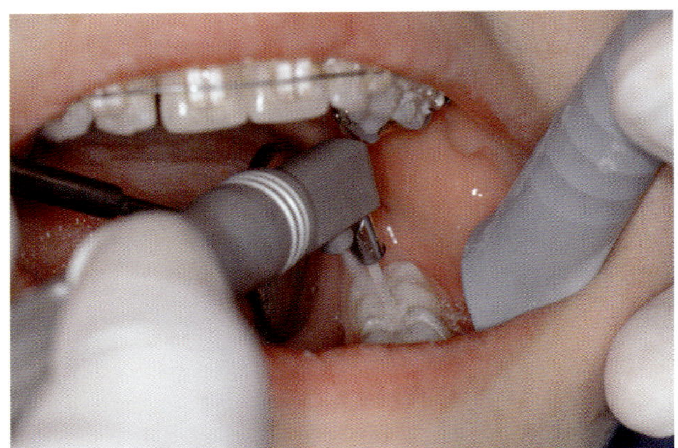

Fig 3-81b Illustrates the laser preparation under fiber contact. Note the cooling water spray.

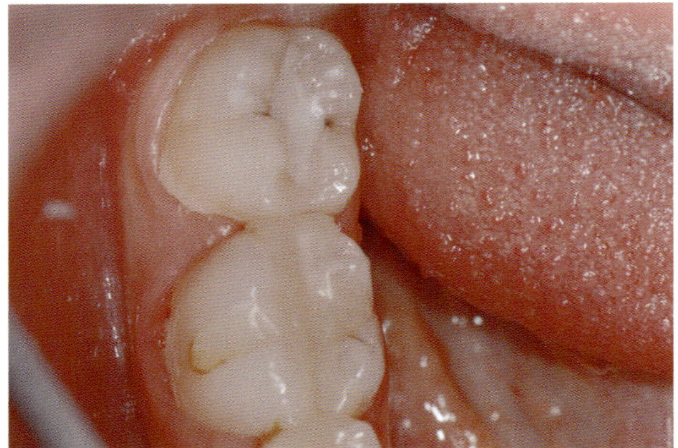

Fig 3-81a Shows insufficient resin fillings in teeth 36 and 37.

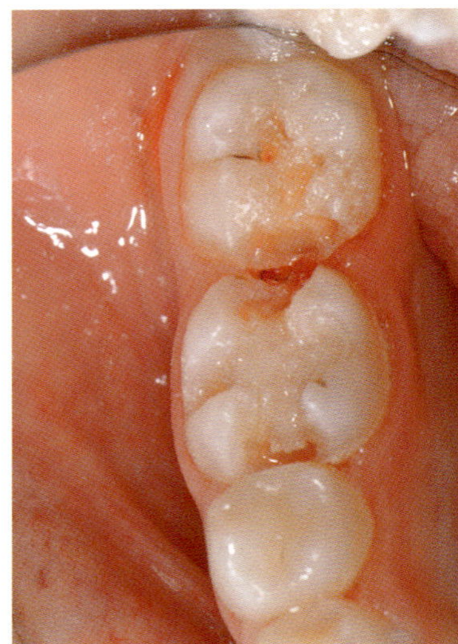

Fig 3-81c Shows the situation after laser preparation.

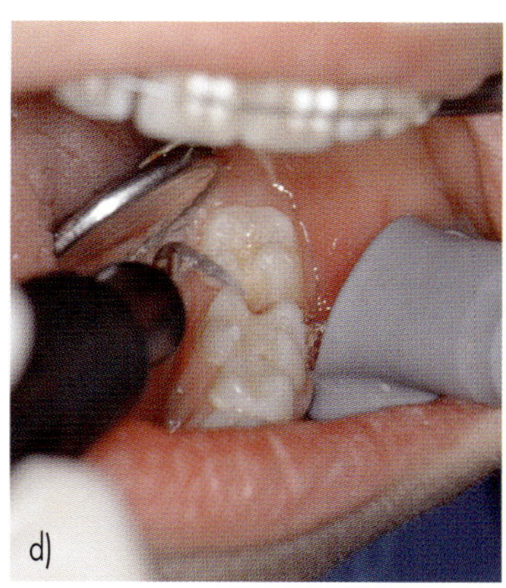

Fig 3-81d and e To achieve the desired smoothness of the preparation edges, a rework with an ultrasonic preparation system is necessary.

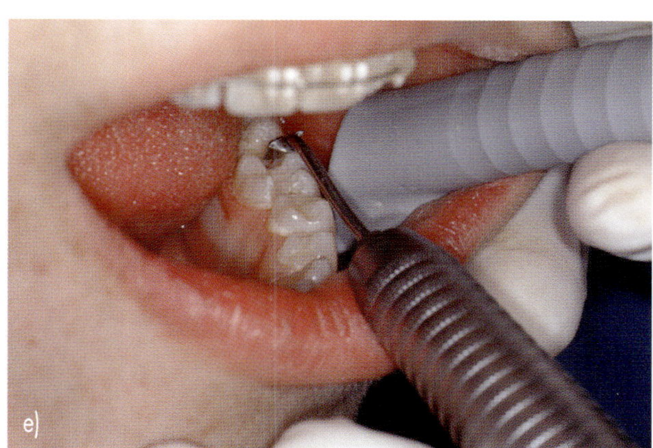

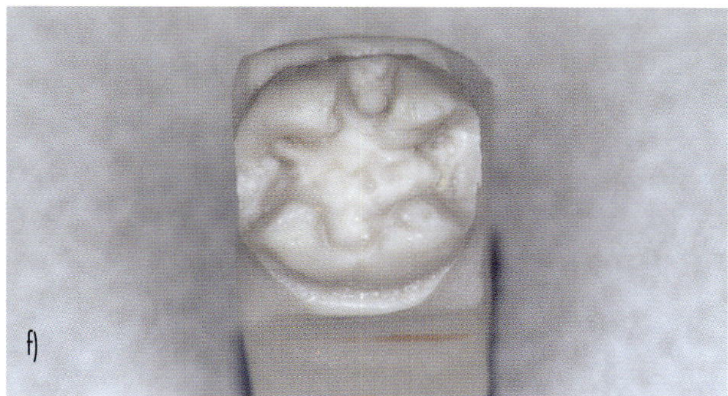

Fig 3-81f Tooth 36 in the cast model.

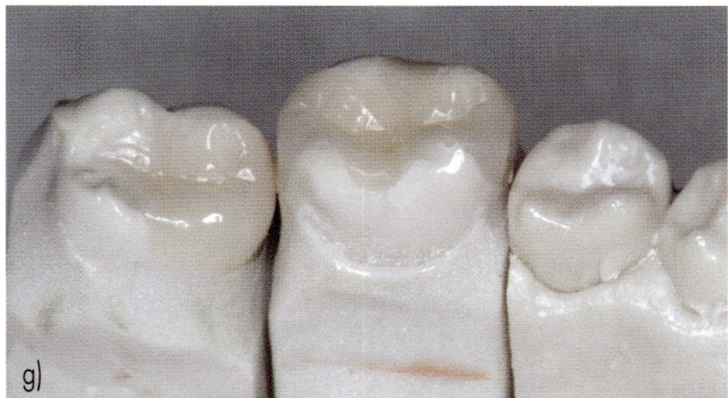

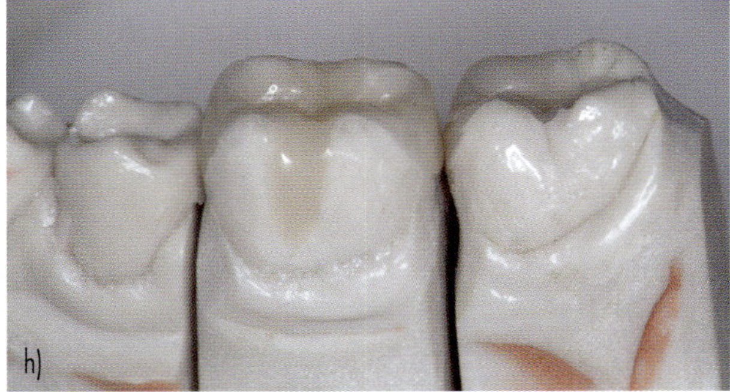

Fig 3-81g and h Completed ceramic inlays on the cast model.

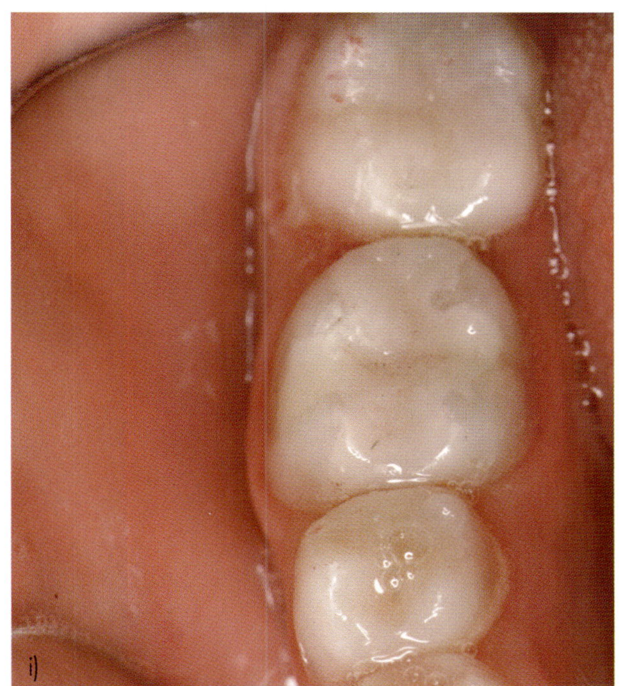

Fig 3-81i The cemented inlays in teeth 36 and 37.

3.7.6 Maryland Bridge

A 10-year-old boy lost teeth 11 and 21 through an accident. To straddle the time until an implant restoration, a Maryland bridge was customized (see Figs 3-82a–i).

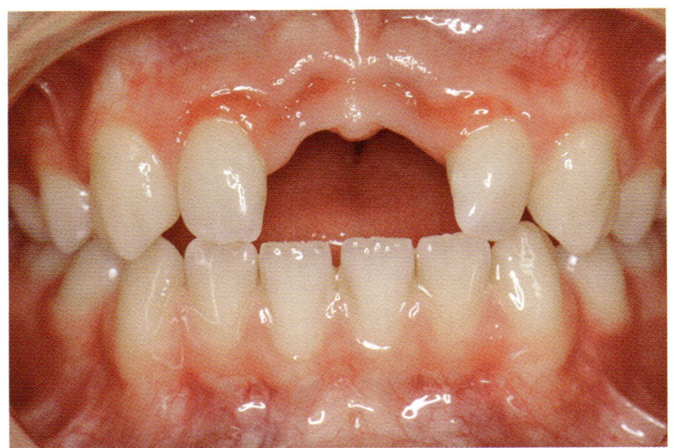

Fig 3-82a Gap in the region of teeth 11 and 21.

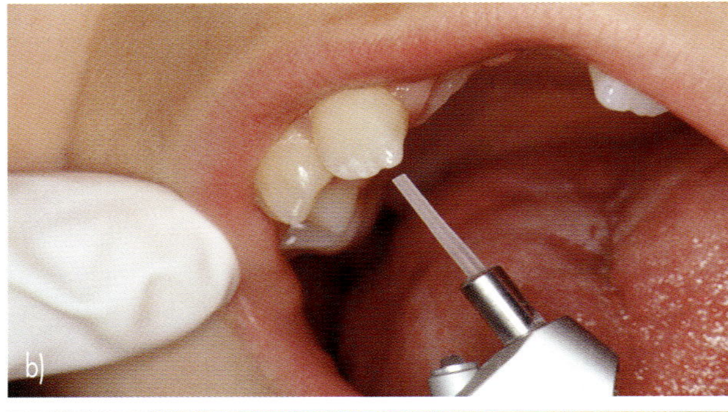

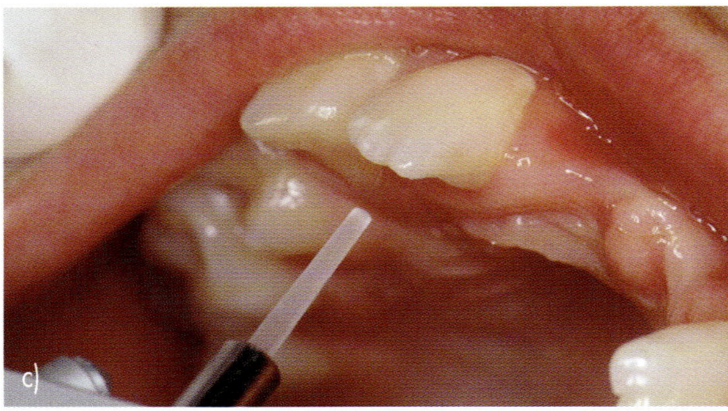

Fig 3-82b and c Preparation of the retentive palatinal facettes on teeth 12 and 22.

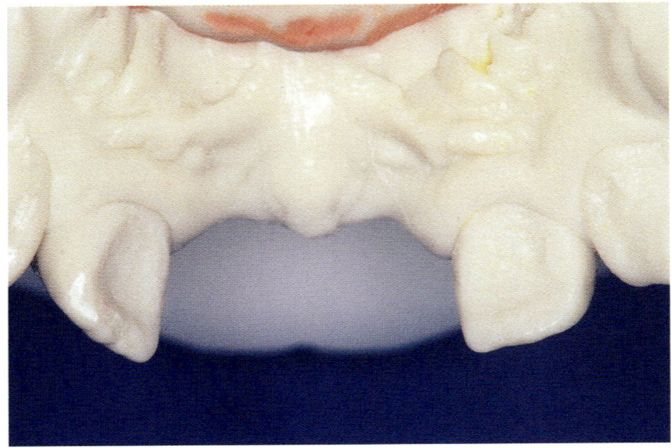

Fig 3-82d The situation in the model. The roughness of the retentive facettes is discernible.

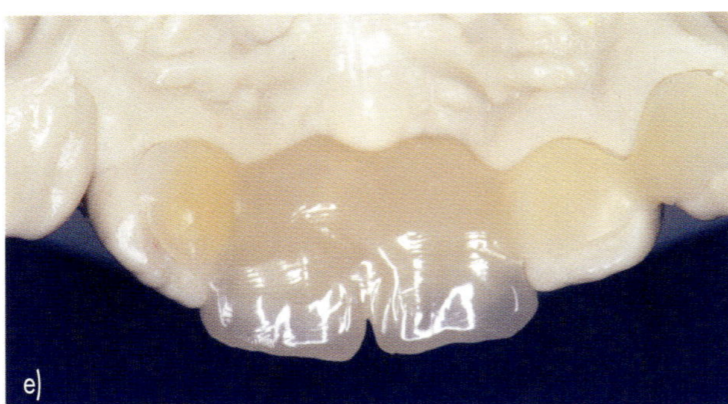

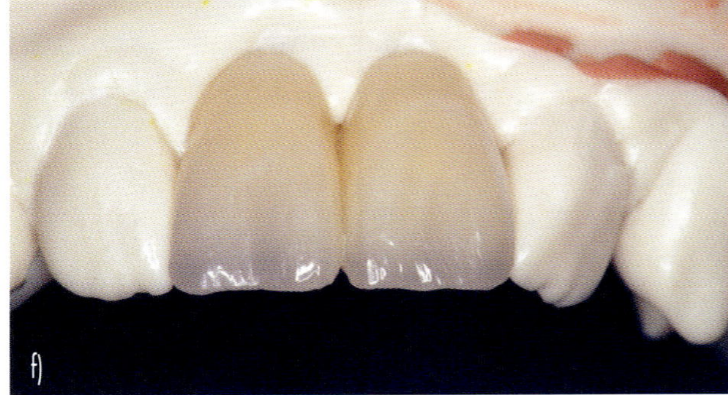

Fig 3-82e and f The completed Maryland bridge on the cast model.

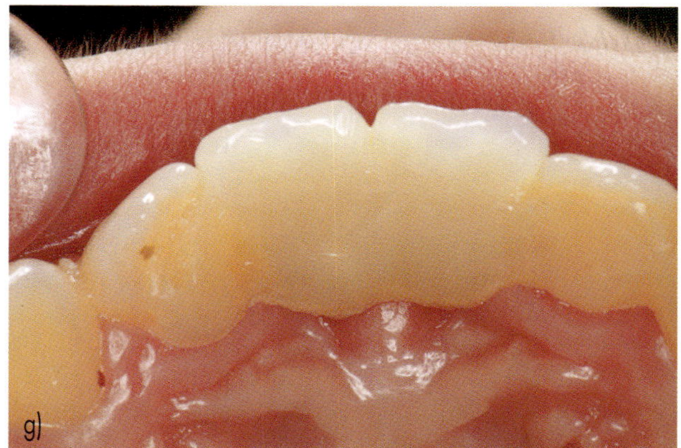

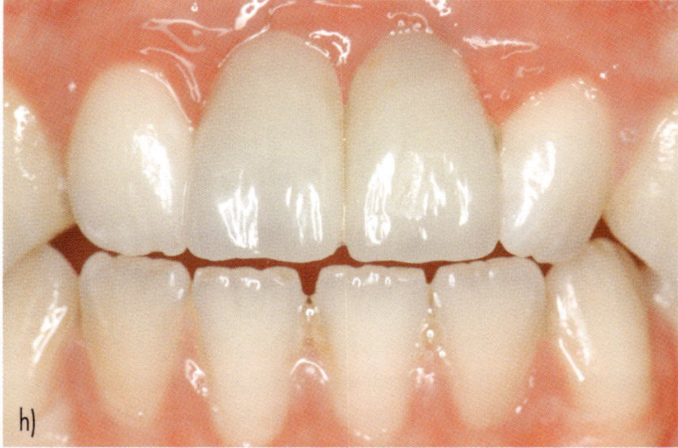

Fig 3-82g and h The completed restoration in the mouth.

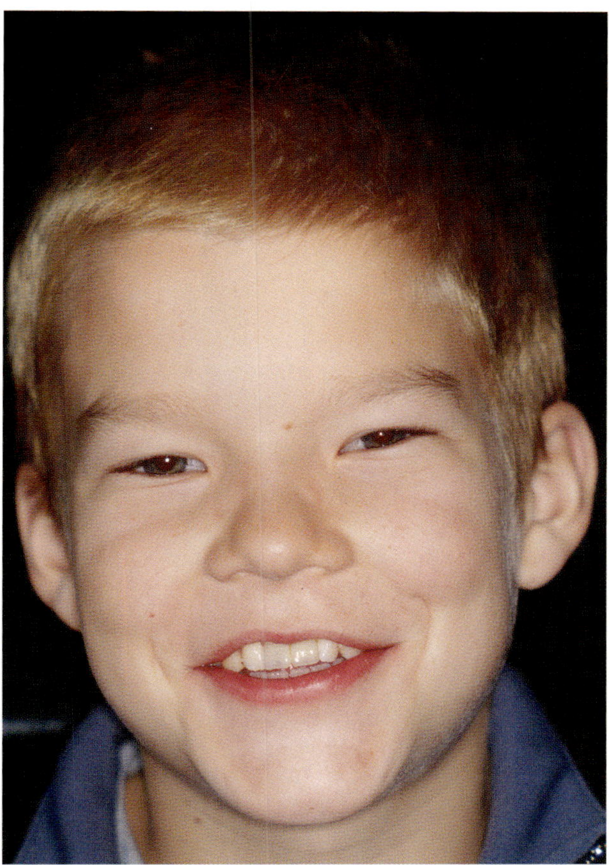

Fig 3-82i Shows the smile of the patient.

3.7.7 Esthetic Front Restoration

Treatment of a 20-year-old girl with 1-year-old resin fillings in the upper front, which partly showed large gaps and discolorations. An esthetic reconstruction was strongly requested (see Figs 3-83a–c).

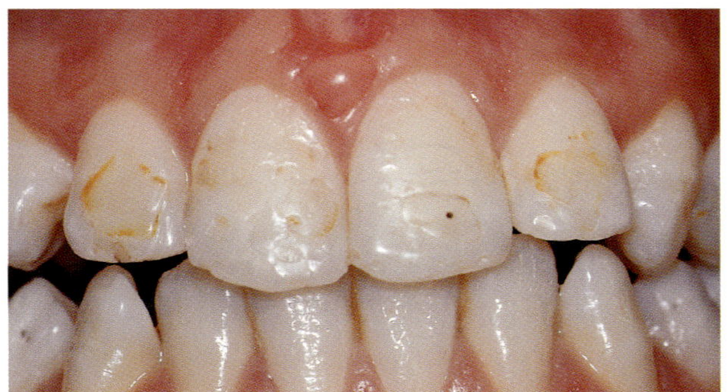

Fig 3-83a Shows the initial situation. Strong discolorations of the filling margins through gaps in the teeth 12–22.

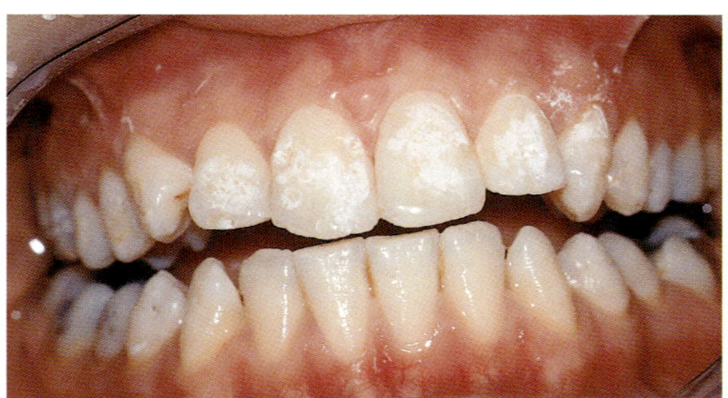

Fig 3-83b Situation after the treatment with an Er,Cr:YSGG laser. All the old fillings have been removed, with the same power settings as in enamel preparation.

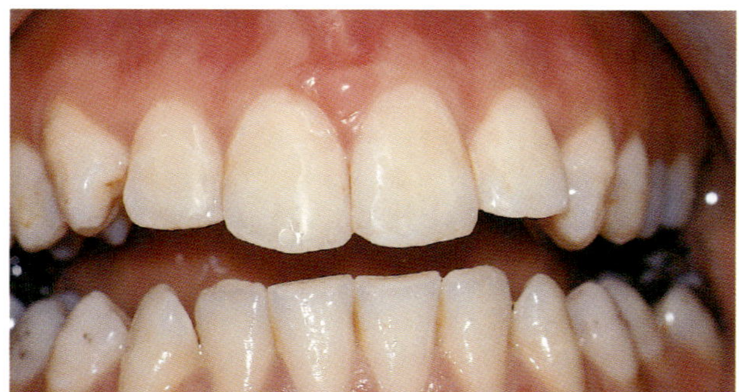

Fig 3-83c Shows the completed restoration after sandwich technique without acid etching.

3.7.8 Esthetic Reconstructions

A 32-year-old patient after an bicycle accident with fracture of teeth 21 and 22 (see Figs 3-84a–e).

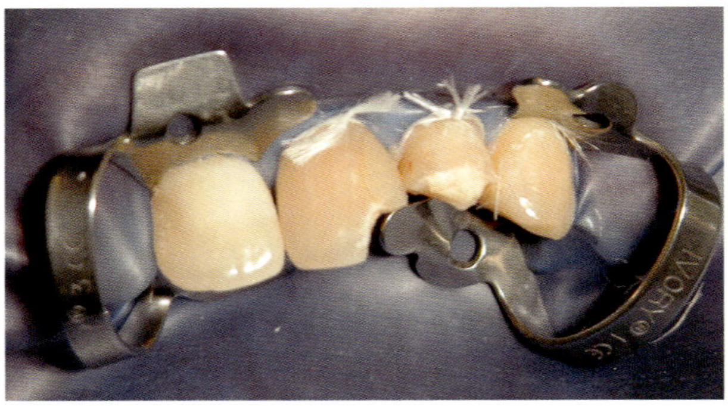

Fig 3-84a Shows the fractured front teeth immediately before the restoration.

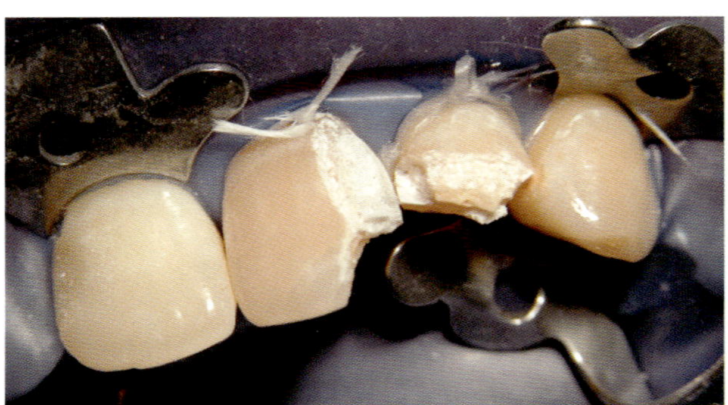

Fig 3-84b After preparation with an Er,Cr:YSGG laser.

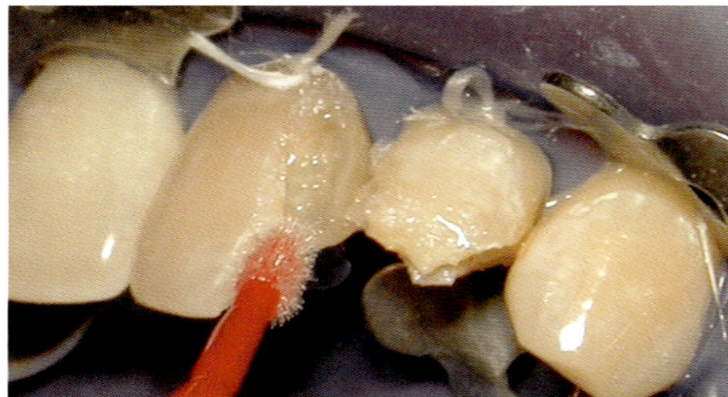

Fig 3-84c Application of the adhesive bonding.

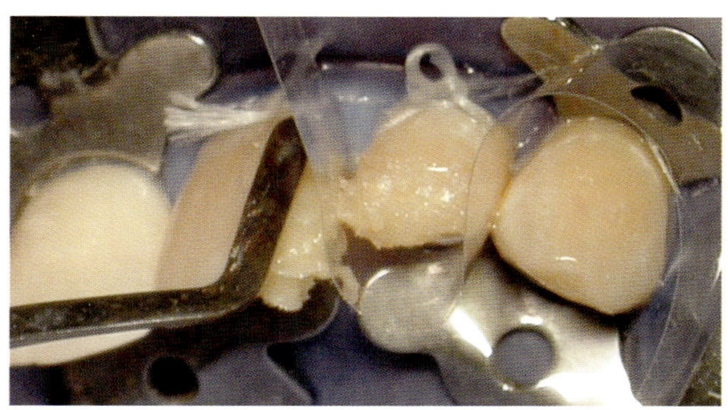

Fig 3-84d Sandwich technique (dentin and enamel shades).

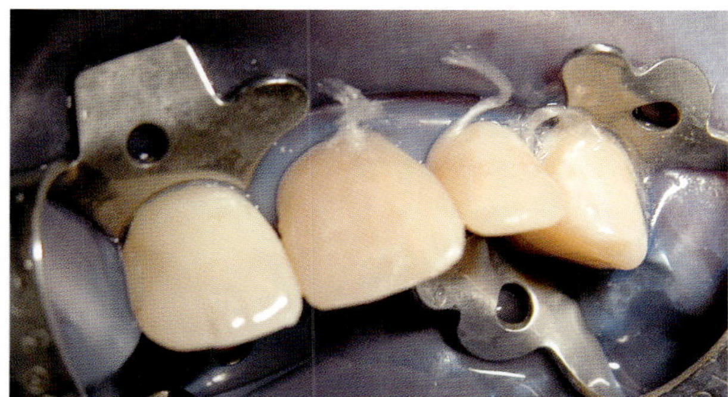

Fig 3-84e Completed restoration.

3.8 References

1. Stern R H, Sognnaes, R F: Laser beam effect on dental hard tissues. J Dent Res 43: 873, 1964
2. Gordon T: Single-surface cutting of normal tooth with ruby laser. J Am Dent Assoc 74: 398, 1967
3. Schulte W, Klaus H, Flach A, Geisbett: Lasereffekte an Zahnhartsubstanzen – Mikroskopische Untersuchungen. Dtsch Zahnärztl Z 20: 289, 1965
4. Melcer J, Chaumette M T, Melcer F, Dejardin J, Hasson R, Merard R, Pinaudeau Y, Weill R: Treatment of dental decay by CO_2 laser beam: preliminary results. Lasers Surg Med 4(4): 311–321, 1984
5. Melcer J: Latest treatment in dentistry by means of the CO_2 laser beam. Lasers Surg Med 6(4): 396–398, 1986
6. Niemz M H, Eisenmann L, Pioch T: Vergleich von drei Lasersystemen zur Abtragung von Zahnschmelz. Schweiz Monatsschr Zahnmed 103(10): 1252, 1993
7. Frentzen M, Koort H J, Kermani O, Dardenne M U: Preparation of hard tooth structure with Excimer lasers. In vitro study. Dtsch Zahnärztl Z 44(6): 431–435, 1989
8. Liesenhoff T, Bende T, Lenz H, Seiler T: Removal of hard tooth substance with Excimer lasers. Dtsch Zahnärztl Z 44(6): 426–430, 1989
9. Keller U, Hibst R: Experimental studies of the application of the Er:YAG laser on dental hard substances: II. Light microscopic and SEM investigations. Lasers Surg Med 9(4): 345–351, 1989
10. Hibst R, Keller U: Experimental studies of the application of the Er:YAG laser on dental hard substances: I. Measurement of the ablation rate. Lasers Surg Med 9(4): 338–344, 1989
11. Niemz M H, Eisenmann L, Pioch T: A comparison of 3 laser systems for dental enamel ablation. Schweiz Monatsschr Zahnmed 103(10):1252–1256, 1993
12. Niemz M H: Cavity preparation with the Nd:YLF picosecond laser. J Dent Res 74(5): 1194–1199, 1995
13. Kohns P, Zhou P, Stormann R: Effective laser ablation of enamel and dentine without thermal side effects. J Laser Appl 9(3): 171–174, 1997
14. Zach L, Cohen G: Pulp response to externally applied heat. Endotontics. Oral Surg Oral Med Oral Pathol 19(4): 515–530, 1965
15. Kerschbaum T, Voss R: The risk of crowns. Dtsch Zahnärztl Z 34(10): 740–743, 1979
16. Kerschbaum T, Voss R: Practical efficacy of crowns and inlays. Dtsch Zahnärztl Z 36(4): 243–249, 1981
17. Lussi A, Gygax M: Iatrogenic damage to adjacent teeth during classical approximal box preparation. J Dent 26(5–6): 435–441, 1998
18. Lussi A, Kronenberg O, Megert B: The effect of magnification on the iatrogenic damage to adjacent tooth surfaces during class II preparation. J Dent 31(4): 291–296, 2003
19. Moritz A, Schoop U, Goharkhay K, Szakacs S, Sperr W, Schweidler E, Wernisch J, Gutknecht N: Procedures for enamel and dentin conditioning: a comparison of conventional and innovative methods. J Esthet Dent 10(2): 84–93, 1998
20. Matson J R, Matson E, Navarro R S, Bocangel J S, Jaeger R G, Eduardo C P: Er:YAG laser effects on enamel occlusal fissures: an in vitro study. J Clin Laser Med Surg 20(1): 27–35, 2002
21. Pioch T, Matthias J: Mercury vapor release from dental amalgam after laser treatment. Eur J Oral Sci 106(1): 600–602, 1998
22. Frentzen M, Hamrol D: Kavitätenpräparation mit dem Er:YAG-Laser – eine histologische Studie. Dtsch Zahnärztl Z 55(2): 114–117, 2000
23. Inoue H, Izumi T, Ishikawa H, Watanabe K: Short-term histomorphological effects on Er:YAG laser irradiation to rat coronal dentin-pulp complex. Oral Surg Oral Med Oral Pathol Oral Radiol Endod 97: 246–250, 2004
24. Kato J, Moriya K, Jayawardena J A, Wijeyeweera R L: Clinical application of Er:YAG laser for cavity preparation in children. J Clin Laser Med Surg 21(3): 151–155, 2003
25. Cavalcanti B N, Lage-Marques J L, Rode S M: Pulpal temperature increases with Er:YAG laser and high-speed handpieces. J Prosthet Dent 90(5): 447–451, 2003
26. Oelgiesser D, Blasbalg J, Ben-Amar A: Cavity preparation by Er-YAG laser on pulpal temperature rise. Am J Dent 16(2): 6–98, 2003
27. Louw N P, Pameijer C H, Ackermann W D, Ertl T, Cappius H J, Norval G: Pulp histology after Er:YAG laser cavity preparation in subhuman primates – a pilot study. SADJ 57(8): 13–317, 2002
28. Tanabe K, Yoshiba K, Yoshiba N, Iwaku M, Ozawa H: Immunohistochemical study on pulpal response in rat molars after cavity preparation by Er:YAG laser. Eur J Oral Sci 110: 237–245, 2002
29. Takamori K: A histopathological and immunohistochemical study of dental pulp and pulpal nerve fibers in rats after the cavity preparation using Er:YAG laser. J Endod 26(2): 95–99, 2000
30. Jayawardena J A, Kato J, Moriya K, Takagi Y: Pulpal response to exposure with Er:YAG laser. Oral Surg Oral Med Oral Pathol Oral Radiol Endod 91(2): 222–229, 2001
31. Moritz A, Gutknecht N, Schoop U, Goharkhay K, Wernisch J, Sperr W: Alternatives in enamel conditioning: a comparison of conventional and innovative methods. J Clin Laser Med Surg 14(3): 133–136, 1996
32. Usumez S, Orhan M, Usumez A: Laser etching of enamel for direct bonding with an Er,Cr,:YSGG hydrokinetic laser system. Am J Orthod Dentofacial Orthop 122(6): 649–656, 2002
33. De Munck J, Van Meerbeek B, Yudhira R, Lambrechts P, Vanherle G: Micro-tensile bond strength of two adhesives to Erbium:YAG-lased vs. bur-cut enamel and dentin. Eur J Oral Sci 110(4): 322–329, 2002
34. Ceballo L, Toledano M, Osorio R, Tay F R, Marshall G W: Bonding to Er:YAG-laser treated dentin. J Dent Res 81(2):119–122, 2002
35. Zakariasen K L, MacDonald R, Boran T: Spotlight on lasers. A look at potential benefits. J Am Dent Assoc 122: 58, 1991

36. Arcoria C J, Lippas M G, Vitasek B A: Enamel surface roughness analysis after laser ablation and acid-etching. J Oral Rehabil 20: 213, 1993
37. Walsh L J, Abood D, Brockhurst P J: Bonding of resin composite to carbon dioxide laser – modified human enamel. Dent Mater 10: 162, 1994
38. Cooper L F, Mayers M L, Nelson D G A, Mowery A S: Shear strength of composite bonded to laser – pretreated dentin. J Prosthet Dent 60: 45, 1988
39. Keller U, Hibst R: Experimental studies of the application of the Er:YAG laser on dental hard substances. I. Measurement of the ablation rate. Lasers Surg Med 9: 338, 1989
40. Miller M, Truhe T: Lasers in dentistry: an overview. J Am Dent Assoc 124: 32, 1993
41. Visuri S R, Gilbert J L, Wright D D, Wigdor H A, Walsh J T: Shear strength of composite bonded to Er:YAG laser-prepared dentin. J Dent Res 75: 599, 1996
42. Burnett L H Jr, Conceicao E N, Pelinos J E, Eduardo C D: Comparative study of influence on tensile bond strength of a composite to dentin using Er:YAG laser, air abrasion, or air turbine for preparation of cavities. J Clin Laser Med Surg 19(4): 199–202, 2001
43. Martinez-Insua A, Da Silva Dominguez L, Rivera F G, Santana-Penin U A: Differences in bonding to acid-etched or Er:YAG-lased-treated enamel and dentin surfaces. J Prosthet Dent 84: 280, 2000
44. Staninec M, Xie J, Le C Q, Fried D: Influence of an optically thick water layer on the bond-strength of composite resin to dental enamel after IR laser ablation. Lasers Surg Med 33(4): 264–269, 2003
45. Hossain M, Nakamura Y, Tamaki Y, Yamada Y, Murakami Y, Matsumoto K: Atomic analysis and knoop hardness measurement of the cavity floor prepared by Er,Cr:YSGG laser irradiation in vitro. J Oral Rehabil 30(5): 515–521, 2003
46. Nair P N, Baltensperger M M, Luder H U, Eyrich G K: Pulpal response to Er:YAG laser drilling of dentine in healthy human third molars. Lasers Surg Med 32(3): 203–209, 2003
47. Shigetani Y, Okamoto A, Abu-Bakr N, Iwaku M: A study of cavity preparation by Er:YAG laser-observation of hard tooth structures by laser scanning microscope and examination of the time necessary to remove caries. Dent Mater J. 2002 Mar;21(1):20–31
48. Shigetani Y, Tate Y, Okamoto A, Iwaku M, Abu-Bakr N: A study of cavity preparation by Er:YAG laser. Effects on the marginal leakage of composite resin restoration. Dent Mater 21(3): 238–249, 2002
49. Gonzalez Bahillo J, Ruiz Pinon M, Rodriguez Nogueira J, Martin Biedma B, Varela Patino P, Magan Munoz F, Bahillo Varela M, Barciela Castro N: A comparative study of microleakage through enamel and cementum after laser Er:YAG instrumentation in class V cavity obturations, using scanning electron microscopy. J Clin Laser Med Surg 20(4): 197–201, 2002
50. Matsumoto K, Hossain M, Hossain MM, Kawano H, Kimura Y: Clinical assessment of Er,Cr:YSGG laser application for cavity preparation. J Clin Laser Med Surg 20(1): 17–21, 2002
51. Armengol V, Jean A, Enkel B, Assoumou M, Hamel H: Microleakage of class V composite restorations following Er:YAG and Nd:YAP laser irradiation compared to acid-etch: an In vitro study. Lasers Med Sci 17(2): 93–100, 2002
52. Ishizaka Y, Eguro T, Maeda T, Tanaka H: Effects of Er:YAG laser irradiation on human dentin: polarizing microscopic, light microscopic and microradiographic observations, and FT-IR analysis. Lasers Surg Med 31(3): 171–176, 2002
53. Corona S A, Borsatto M C, Pecora J D, Rocha de Sá R A, Ramos T S, Palma-Dibb R G: Assessing microleakage of different class V restorations after Er:YAG laser and bur preparation. J Oral Rehabil 30(10): 1008–1014, 2003
54. Wright G Z, McConnell R J, Keller U: Microleakage of class V composite restorations prepared conventionally with those prepared with ER:YAG laser: a pilot study. Pediatric Dent 15, 425
55. Setien V J, Cobb D S, Denehy G E, Vargas M A: Cavity preparation devices: effect on microleakage of Class V resin-based composite restorations. Am J Dent 14:157, 2001
56. Ceballo L, Osorio R, Toledano M, Marshall G W: Microleakage of composite restorations after acid or Er:YAG laser cavity treatments. Dent Mater 17(4): 340–346, 2001
57. Gutknecht N, Apel C, Schafer C, Lampert F: Related Articles, Microleakage of composite fillings in Er,Cr:YSGG laser-prepared class II cavities. Lasers Surg Med 28(4): 371–374, 2001
58. Rocca JP: ABSTRACT Alpe Adria Congress, Bled, May 7–8, 2004
59. Bertrand M F, Hessleyer D, Muller-Bolla M, Nammour S, Rocca J P: Scanning electron microscopic evaluation of resin-dentin interface after Er:YAG laser preparation. Lasers Surg Med 35(1):51–57, 2004
60. Kohara E K, Hossain M, Kimura Y, Matsumoto K, Inoue M, Sasa R: Morphological and microleakage studies of the cavities prepared by Er:YAG laser irradiation in primary teeth. J Clin Laser Med Surg 20(3): 141–147, 2002
61. Khan M F, Yonaga K, Kimura Y, Funato A, Matsumoto K: Study of microleakage at Class I cavities prepared by Er:YAG laser using three types of restorative materials. J Clin Laser Med Surg 16(6): 305–308, 1998
62. Niu W, Eto J N, Kimura Y, Takeda F H, Matsumoto K: A study on microleakage after resin filling of Class V cavities prepared by Er:YAG laser. J Clin Laser Med Surg 16(4): 227–231, 1998
63. Roebuck E M, Whitters C J, Saunders W P: The influence of three Erbium:YAG laser energies on the in vitro microleakage of Class V compomer resin restorations. Int J Paediatr Dent 11(1): 49–56, 2001
64. Quo B C, Drummond J L, Koerber A, Fadavi S, Punwani I: Glass Ionomer microleakage from preparations by an Er:YAG laser or high-speed handpiece. J Dent 30(4): 141–146, 2002
65. Dostalova T, Jelinkova H, Kucerova H, Krejsa O, Hamal K, Kubelka J, Prochazka S: Noncontact Er:YAG laser ablation: clinical evaluation. J Clin Laser Med Surg 16(5): 273–282, 1998
66. Apel C, Schäfer C, Gutknecht N: Demineralization of Er:YAG and Er,Cr:YSGG Laser-Prepared Enamel Cavities in vitro. Caries Research 37: 34–37, 2003

67. Vogel A, Venugopalan V: Mechanisms of Pulsed Laser Ablation of Biological Tissues. Chem Rev 103: 577–644, 2003
68. Bondarenko G V, Gorbatay Yu E, Kalinichev A G, Okhukov A V, Popov V K: A Comprehensive Study of NaCl Aqueous Solution at a Constant Pressure of 1000 bar in the Temperature Range 20–500 °C. Webpaper of the 4th International Symposium on High Pressure Process Technology and Chemical Engineering, September 22–25, 2002 Venice/Italy
69. Hibst R, Keller U: Effects of water spray and repetition rate on the temperature evaluation during Er:YAG laser ablation of dentine. SPIE 2623: 139–144, 1996
70. Hibst R: Technik, Wirkungsweise und medizinische Anwendung von Holmium- und Erbium-Lasern. Habilitationsschrift. Ecomed Verlag, Landsberg 1996
71. Seka W, Featherstone J D B, Fried D, Visuri S R, Walsh J T: Laser ablation of dental hard tissue: from explosive ablation to plasma-mediated ablation. SPIE 2672: 144–158, 1996
72. Mitra T: Ablation biologischen Hartgewebes mit gepulsten IR-Lasern. Dissertation. Heinrich-Heine-Universität, Düsseldorf 2002
73. Meister J, Apel C, Franzen R, Gutknecht N: Influence of the spatial beam profile on hard tissue ablation Part I: multimode emitting Er:YAG lasers. Lasers Med Sci 18: 112–118, 2003
74. Keller, U: Laser zur Zahnhartsubstanzbearbeitung – Vor- und Nachteile. Dtsch Zahnärztl Z 55: 85–91, 2000
75. Lukač M, Marincek M, Grad L: Super VSP Er:YAG Pulses for Fast and Precise Cavity Preparation. JOLA 4(3):171–174,2004
76. Stuart B C, Feit M D, Rubenchik A M, Shore B W, Perry M D: Laser-induced Damage in Dielectrics with nanosecond to subpicosecond Pulses. Phys Rev Lett 74(12): 2248–2251, 1996
77. Feit M D, Rubenchik A M, Shore B W: Unique Aspects of Laser Energy Deposition in the fs Pulse Regime. SPIE 2672: 243–249, 1996
78. Mindermann A, Niemz M H, Eisenmann L, Loesel F H, Bille J F: Comparison of three different laser systems for application in dentistry. SPIE 2080: 68–76, 1993
79. Kim B M, Feit M D, Rubenchik A M, Joslin E J, Celliers P M, Eichler J, Da Silva L B: Influence of pulse duration on ultrashort laser pulse ablation of biological tissue. J Biomed Opt 6(3): 332–338, 2001
80. Niemz M H: Laser-Tissue Interactions. Fundamentals and Applications. Springer, Berlin 1996
81. Melcer J, Chaumette M T, Melcer F, Dejardin J, Hasson R, Merard R, Pinaudeau Y, Weill R: Treatment of dental decay by CO_2 laser beam: preliminary results. Lasers Surg Med 4(4): 311–321, 1984
82. Melcer J: Latest treatment in dentistry by means of the CO_2 laser beam. Lasers Surg Med 6(4): 396–398, 1986
83. Mullejans R, Eyrich G, Raab W H, Frentzen M: Cavity preparation using a superpulsed 9.6-micron CO_2 laser-a histological investigation. Lasers Surg Med 30(5): 331–336, 2002
84. Glock K: Bearbeitung von Zahnhartsubstanzen mit dem CO_2-Swiftlase®-Lasersystem – eine In-vitro-Studie. Dissertation. Technische Universität München 2000
85. Harris D M, White J M, Goodis H, Arcoria C J, Simon J, Carpenter W M, Fried D, Burkart J, Yessik M, Myers T: Selective ablation of surface enamel caries with a pulsed Nd:YAG dental laser. Lasers Surg Med 30(5): 342–350, 2002

4

Photopolymerization

P. Verheyen, A. Moritz. L. J. Walsh

with contributions from R. Blum

4.1 Introduction

The treatment of carious lesions has always been accompanied by the search for the ideal filling material. At the end of the 19th century, amalgam began to be accepted worldwide as the material of choice. This occurred after a lengthy debate between the "Gold-group", those who stated that only gold fillings and gold restorations were acceptable, and the "Silver-group", the defenders of the early silver-mercury alloys. In the 1950s, the introduction to dentistry of the "Bowen-resin" and Buonocore's trials in dental-resin adhesion saw the start of what would become a complete change in handling dental defects and caries. It was the beginning not only of restoring function but esthetics as well, and of dental treatments with more consideration given to hard tooth structures.

Due to this set of developments, G.V. Black's statement, "Extension for Prevention", was questioned for the first time. And nowadays, prevention and minimally invasive dentistry go hand in hand. Modern dentistry approaches a dental lesion as conservatively as possible. That is, removing only the sick and infected part of the tooth and conserving the maximum amount of sound tooth structure. These minimally invasive techniques are the result of decades of developing new materials and products for tooth restoration, and improved techniques and products which increase the quality of adhesion.

Chemically-cured materials were replaced by UV curing in the late 1970s, and succeeded afterwards by visible-light-curing materials. Initially, it was only possible to adhere to enamel. But the 1990s saw the vast improvement of dentin adhesion, the evolution of effective caries-prevention techniques and a range of new technologies to treat dental defects and lesions. These include air-abrasion, the chemical dissolving of caries, and laser techniques such as PAD (Photo Activated Disinfection, see chapter 12), caries diagnosis by laser fluorescence, caries prevention by laser irradiation (see chapter 5) and laser cavity preparations (see chapter 3).

Towards the end of the 20th century caries prevalence had dropped. Not only the number of lesions declined but also their extent. Smaller lesions are ideally treated with adhesive filling materials, saving tooth structure and enhancing longevity. Minimal invasive interventions should be chosen whenever possible.

However, despite new preparation techniques, high quality restorative materials and sufficient bond strengths to enamel and dentin, many restorations still fail. The question to be answered then is whether clinical results can be improved by a different approach to handling light-cured restorative materials.

4.2 In General

Restorations in the frontal teeth region and small occlusal fillings or fissure sealings represent the ideal indication for light-cured composite materials. As was the case a century ago, researchers are still debating which material should be the restorative material of choice, particularly for the premolar and molar region. Nevertheless, there is an ongoing tendency to use direct light-cured materials. These direct light-cured restorative materials offer many benefits when compared to silver alloys and indirect restorations. Preserving tooth structure, which can then be bonded to the restorative material with a tight seal, is the most important benefit. Additional benefits include excellent esthetics and the extensive field of applications (Table 4-1)[1].

A decreased stability against masticatory pressure compared to silver alloys only has to be taken into account when dealing with large fillings in the molar region. At the same time, the durability of light-cured fillings can be remarkably improved by the use of innovative curing techniques (also see section 4.4).

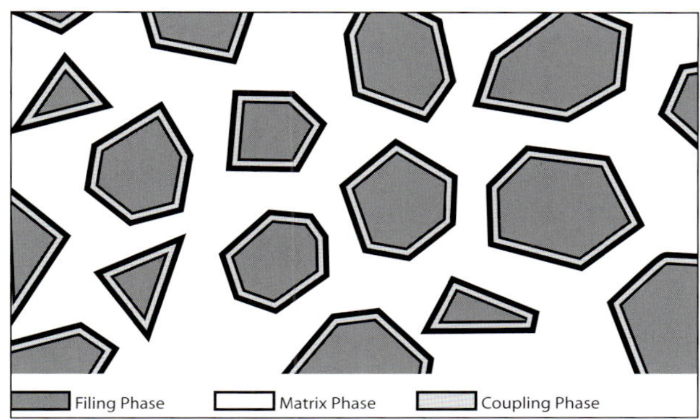

Fig 4-1 Components of composite materials (According to Roeters, De Kloet[2]).

Table 4-1 Restorative materials and pertinent indications for use (According to Lutz and Krejci[1]).
= under development, = indication, = experimental

MATERIAL CLASS AND MATERIAL	AMALGAM	AMALGAM SUBSTITUTE	AMALGAM ALTERNATIVES			
Restorative/Reconstructive work	Non-gamma-2	Compomer	Composite	Ceramic	Metal-Ceramic	Gold Metal
Fissure Sealing						
Preventive Resin restoration			indication			
Adhesive Filling			indication			
Adhesive Class V Filling		experimental	indication			
Conventional Class V Filling	indication	experimental	indication			
Bull-shaped Class I/II Filling	indication	experimental	indication			
Box-shaped Class I/II Filling	indication	experimental	indication			
Cuspal Coverage	indication		indication			
Inlay			indication	indication	indication	experimental
Onlay			indication	indication	indication	experimental
Partial Crown			indication	indication	indication	experimental
Full Crown			experimental	indication	indication	experimental
Bridge			experimental	experimental	indication	experimental

As there is a wide range of light-cured filling materials, it is important to have a basic knowledge of their composition. They consist of three basic substances: an inorganic or filler phase, an organic or matrix phase and a coupling or binding phase[2](Fig 4-1).

Components of the filler phase are either crystalline quartz (SiO_2) or heavy metal glasses (lithium-aluminum-silicate, borosilicate) to make the filling material radiopaque. They are commonly designated as macrofillers made by a crushing and milling action. In contrast, the microfillers are made by a chemical reaction. Nowadays, modern filler technology combines mechanical and chemical methods for the production of different fillers. Therefore, the filler is usually more rounded, less sharp (see Fig 4-5b). Particle size ranges from one micron to several microns. The latest nano-technology-created materials have a particle size smaller than 1 micron. Classifications are based upon the particle size and mode of distribution. Particles can be chemically altered by the manufacturer to create splintered, sintered or spherical prepolymerates or sintered agglomerates, and fibers can be added to reinforce the composite[3](Fig 4-2).

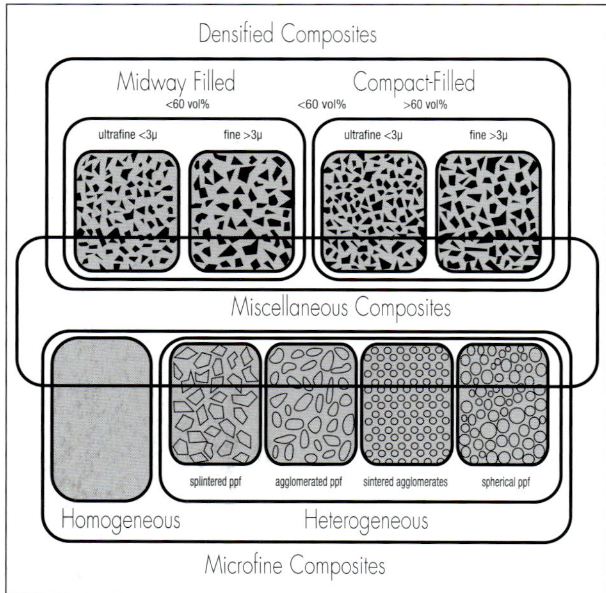

Fig 4-2 Categorization of composites. (With the permission of Dental Materials, according to Willems et al.[3]).

The matrix phase contains three different groups of components. First the building blocks of the polymer network (oligomers, monomers), second the components that control the setting reaction and third a group of esthetic enhancing substances.

Oligomers such as bisphenol A-glycidyl-methacrylate (BIS-GMA) or Bowen-resin are the most commonly used; also included are urethane dimethacrylate (UDMA), tricyclodecane dimethacrylate (TCDDMA) and more. They can be chemically altered like the latest Ceromers (Ceramic Optimised Polymers), OCMs (Organically Modified Composites) or ACTs (Advanced Composite Technology).

Monomers like triethylene glycol dimethacrylate (TEGDMA) or bisphenol A-dimethacrylate (BIS-DMA) are added mainly to regulate viscosity. They absorb less water than the oligomers and have better color stability. But they increase polymerization shrinkage.

Photo-initiators are mostly camphoroquinone, followed by benzoylperoxides or benzoylalkylethers. An aliphatic amine such as N,N-dimethyl-paratoluidine, N,N-dimethylaminoethyl methacrylate or N,N-diethanol-p-toluidine acts as a photo-accelerator.

Photo-inhibitors, a hydroquinone monomethylether or butylhydroxytoluene, are used to prevent polymerization during storage. Finally, several components are added to enhance the esthetic and tooth-like appearance of the filling material. These are color pigments and stabilizers, UV absorbers and modulators of fluorescence.

The bonding phase consists of an organosilane, which surrounds the filling particles and creates a bonding to the matrix phase. It constitutes 1–6% of the weight of the filling particles.

Selecting the proper material in a given clinical situation is important. This is not easy as there is an increasingly wide variety of available products. Classification by Willems et al.[3] of the then current materials shows the importance and difficulty of selecting the right product (Tables 4-2 to 4-6) (Figs 4-3 to 4-9).

Table 4-2 Densified composites: midway-filled (According to Willems et al.[3]).

Densified Composites: Midway-Filled									
Products	MPS	Mo	Ra	Y-Mod	Vol% A	Vol% B	CS	HV	RO
Ultrafine Midway-Filled Composites									
Command Ultrafine*	1.1	0.9	0.21	14.803	52.5	49.9	344	87	–
Herculite conden-Sable	0.9	0.8	0.12	14.871	52.6	58.0	414	65	–
Herculite XR	1.0	0.8	0.12	16.042	55.2	57.0	397	74	227
Charisma	0.7	–	–	14,060	50.7	59.4	417	81	–
Conquest DFC	0.8	–	–	17.511	58.1	68.5	483	95	–
Biogloss	3.4	3.9	0.34	15.190	53.3	51.9	350	73	–
Brilliant	2.8	3.1	–	16.586	56.3	53.9	328	–	–
Brilliant Direct Inlay	2.2	2.0	0.20	17.176	57.5	56.5	342	85	223
Brilliant Lux	2.1	1.8	0,19	14.451	51.7	49.8	330	70	232
Brilliant Dentin	3.6	10.0	0.11	15.821	54.7	55.2	377	84	231
Lumifor	2.0	1.8	0.21	13.208	48.6	54.8	–	84	217
Pekafill	1.7	1.2	–	15.514	54.0	55.2	–	84	173
Post Comp II LC	2.7	2.8	–	16.079	55.3	70.0	345	97	231
Prisma APH	3.1	3.5	0.29	13.644	49.7	–	383	77	269
Fine Midway-Filled Composites									
Ful-Fil compules	6.0	8.1	0.39	13.812	50.2	52.3	372	87	255
Ful-Fil*	6.0	8.1	0.50	14.465	51.7	52.8	–	97	–
Pertac Hybrid	4.2	8.1	–	15.062	53.1	61.0	450	126	–
Gem,CCI	7.6	11.2	0.94	18.487	59.9	61.8	–	117	–
Gem-Lite I	9.3	12.4	0.46	–	–	64.4	–	144	–
Prisma-Fil Compules	8.4	12.4	0.68	13.362	49.0	51.0	353	79	253
Prisma-Fil	7.3	10.0	0.60	14.251	51.2	52.0	–	83	272
Superlux Molar	5.5	4.3	–	13.984	50.6	60.0	343	90	–

MPS: Mean particle size (µm); **Mo:** mode of the particle size distribution (µm); **Ra:** Intrinsic surface roughness (µm); **Y-Mod:** Young's Modulus of elasticity (MPa); **Vol%A:** inorganic filler volume percentage as calculated according to Braem (1985); **Vol%B:** inorganic filler volume percentage as obtained from the manufacturers; **CS:** compressive strength (MPa); **HV:** Vickers Hardness (k/mm^2); *****: Young's modulus data taken from Braem (1985); **RO:** Radiographic Opacity taken from Willems et al. (1991b).

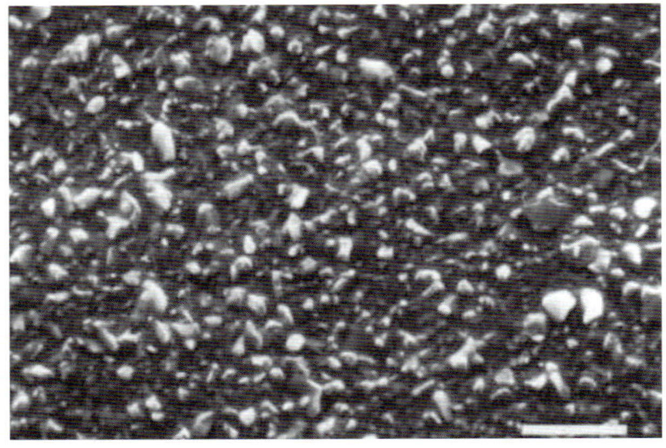

Fig 4-3 Command Ultrafine, an ultrafine midway-filled, is composed of very fine barium-glass particles with an average particle size of 1.1 µm. This type of composite yields good esthetics and is strong enough to withstand masticatory stresses in anterior restorations (bar = 10 µm). (With the permission of Dental Materials, according to Willems et al.[3]).

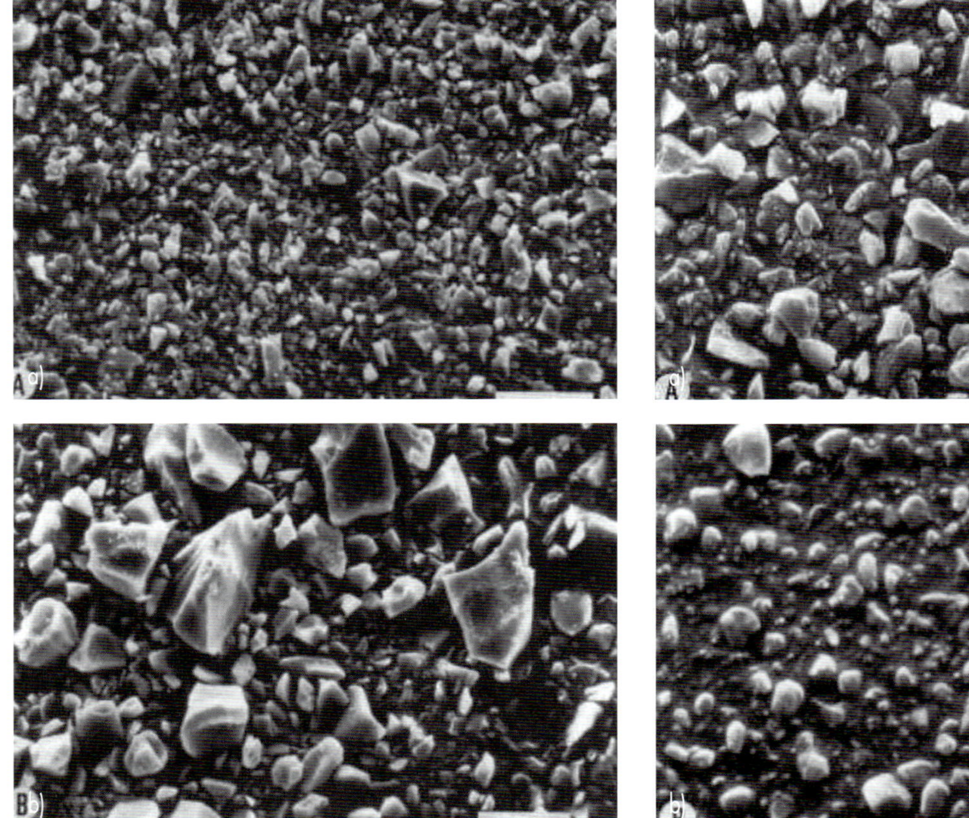

Fig 4-4a and b Full-Fil Compules (a) is a fine midway-filled composite. Due to its fairly large particles, it is less esthetically pleasing than the ultrafine midway-filled composites. Graft LC (b) is a fine compact-filled composite. Its big filler particles are expected to increase the occlusal wear rate of the material. These resin composites are therefore less suitable for posterior use (bar = 20 µm). (With the permission of Dental Materials, according to Willems et al.[3]).

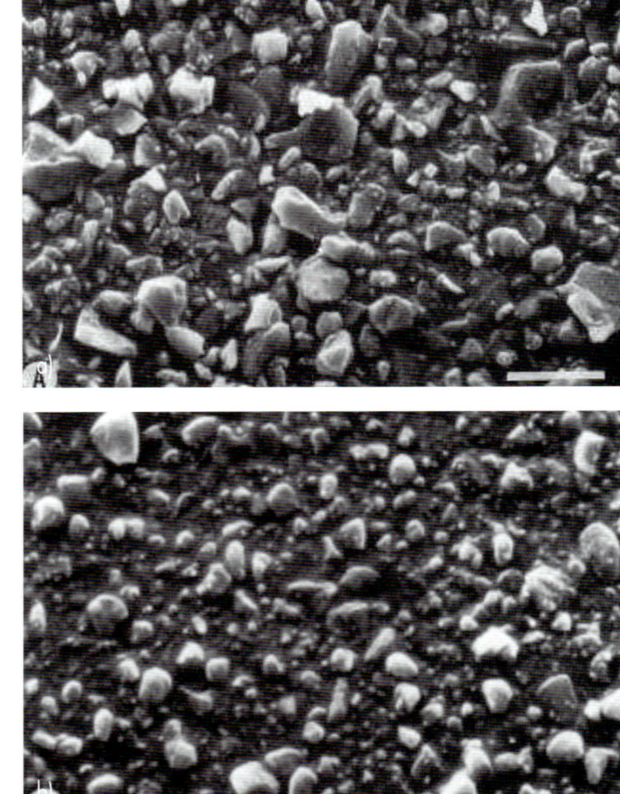

Fig 4-5a and b Both ultrafine compact-filled composites Adaptic II (a) and P-50 5APC (b) are heavy materials filled with rather small inorganic particles. Adaptic II displays more angular-shaped inorganic filler particles with an overall mean diameter of 3.2 µm, whereas P-50 APC is made up of particles that have a more rounded shape. At present, both these materials are the resin composites of choice for restoring posterior cavities (bar = 10 µm). (With the permission of Dental Materials, according to Willems et al.[3]).

Table 4-3 Densified composites: compact-filled (According to Willems et al.[3]).

Densified Composites: Compact-Filled									
Products	MPS	Mo	Ra	Y-Mod	Vol% A	Vol% B	CS	HV	RO
Ultrafine Compact-Filled Composites									
Adnplic II	3.2	3.9	0.48	21.875	65.6	66.5	380	106	238
P-30	2.8	7.3	0.67	23.385	67.8	69.0	340	107	228
P-30 APC	3.0	2.5	0.71	23.155	67.5	69.0	394	157	217
P-50 APC	2.1	1.2	0.48	25.007	70.1	77.0	395	159	277
Pallique Lite Posterior	3.6	5.9	–	26.293	71.8	73.0	421	143	–
Valux	2.4	2.3	0.27	19.728	52.1	–	430	107	240
Z-100	1.0	0.8	0.27	21.030	64.3	71.0	416	120	–
Fine Compact-Filled Composites									
Bis-Fil	6.2	10.0	0.80	19.991	62.6	74.0	345	102	195
Bis-Fi1 P	–	–	–	20.219	63.0	74.0	339	114	195
Clearfil Photo Posterior	7.5	10.0	0.53	25.343	70.5	71.0	408	159	189
Clearfil Ray	8.0	10.0	1.18	27.384	73.1	69.0	350	–	–
Clearfill Ray Posterior	8.2	12.4	0.65	26.435	72.0	71.0	408	174	174
Estilux Hybrid VS	8.8	12.4	0.90	22.594	66.7	68.4	345	130	133
Estilux Posterior CVS	9.6	12.4	1.48	24.508	69.4	68.4	345	133	126
Graft	6.7	8.1	1.26	21.719	65.4	–	332	128	164
Marathon	7.9	10.0	1.07	20.343	63.2	68.0	299	100	245
Occlusin	8.6	12.4	0.99	23.774	68.4	69.0	348	125	322
Opalux	8.9	12.4	0.79	22.336	66.3	–	277	111	153
P-10 (Pasta A-B)*	5.1-3.6	10.0-3.9	1.02	25.117	70.2	69.1	390	174	–
Photo Clearfil	7.9	10.0	1.17	25.225	70.4	69.0	350	166	65
Visio-Molar Radiopaque	7.5	10.0	1.08	26.754	72.4	68.4	400	188	220

MPS: Mean particle size (μm); **Mo:** mode of the particle size distribution (μm); **Ra:** Intrinsic surface roughness (μm); **Y-Mod:**Young's Modulus of elasticity (MPa); **Vol%A:** inorganic filler volume percentage as calculated according to Braem (1985); **Vol%B:** inorganic filler volume percentage as obtained from the manufacturers; **CS:** compressive strength (MPa); **HV:** Vickers Hardness (kg/mm^2); *: Young's modulus data taken from Braem (1985) **RO:** Radiographic Opacity taken from Willems et al. (1991b).

Table 4-4 Microfine composites (According to Willems et al.[3]).

Microfine Composites										
Products	MPS	PPF	Mo	Ra	Y-Mod	Vol% A	Vol% B	CS	HV	RO
HMC with splintered prepolymerized fillers										
Certain	0.04	14.2	15.3	0.08	8.770	34.9	31.4	365	43	44
Durafill*	0.04	17.0	18.9	0.11	6.085	22.6	37.5	463	48	–
Durafill VS	0.04	15.5	25.9	0.16	6.154	23.0	37.5	474	45	< 40
Estetic Microfill*	0.04	11.7	15.3	–	6.473	24.7	36.1	415	–	–
Helio Progress	0.04	17.9	18.9	0.12	9.098	36.1	43.0	330	50	< 40
Heliosit*	0.04	13.6	15.3	0.07	6.401	24.3	24.3	400	36	48
Isomolar*	0.04	16.5	25.9	–	9.619	38.0	45.3	390	–	–
Isopast (Base-Cat)*	0.04	20.8-12.8	39.5-15.3	0.13	5.436	18.8	23.2	359	–	–
Microrest AP	0.04	17.0	32.0	–	8.679	34.5	17.1	304	–	–
Multifill VS	0.04	16.6	39.5	–	7.833	31.1	–	–	55	63
Perfection 0.04	–	–	–	5.620	20.0	–	–	25	< 40	–
Prisma-Microfine Comp 0.04	25.5	48.8	0.22	6.612	25.4	–	–	42	–	–
Prisma-Microfine	0.04	29.8	54.2	0.19	5.700	20.4	–	262	39	48
Silar Paste (A-B)*	0.04	20.8-21.3	18.9-48.8	0.13	9.075	36.0	35.4	283	–	–
Silux*	0.04	20.0	39.5	0.10	9.372	37.1	36.3	344	46	< 40
Silux Plus	0.04	22.0	39.5	0.13	9.466	37.5	–	–	59	47
Superlux Solar	0.04	16.0	31.9	–	7.905	31.4	41.0	324	55	–
HMC with agglomerated prepolymerized fillers										
Adaptic LCM	0.04	13.0	18.9	0.21	9.692	38.3	–	498	55	< 40
Answer (Uni-Cat)*	0.04	13.3-20.7	12.4-32.0	0.16	9.932	39.1	39.7	303	63	–
Heliomolar*	0.04	12.4	18.9	0.09	10.612	41.3	49.1	325	61	–
Nimetic Dispers*	0.04	13.8	13.9	–	10.147	39.8	40.5	455	–	–
HMC with sintered agglomerates										
Amalux *	0.04	12.4	32.0	0.22	13.372	49.0	39.0	304	47	–
Amalux Sintergel NC	0.04	5.2	5.3	0.25	11.918	45.2	39.0	–	70	61
Sinterlux 2*	0.04	8.0	5.9	0.33	9.384	37.2	–	–	55	–
HMC with spherical prepolymerized fillers										

HMG: heterogeneous microfine composites; **MPS:** mean particle size (μm); **PPF:** mean particle size of prepolymerized fillers and sintered agglomerates; **MO:** mode of the particle size distribution (μm); **Ra:** Intrinsic surface roughness (m); **Y-Mod:** Young's Modulus of elasticity (MPa); **Vol%A:** inorganic filler volume percentage as calculated according to Braem (1985); **Vol%B:** inorganic filler volume percentage as obtained from the manufacturers; **CS:** compressive strength (MPa): HV: Vickers Hardness (kg/mm^2); *: Young's modulus data taken from Braem (1985) **RO:** Radiographic Opacity taken from Willems et al (1991b).

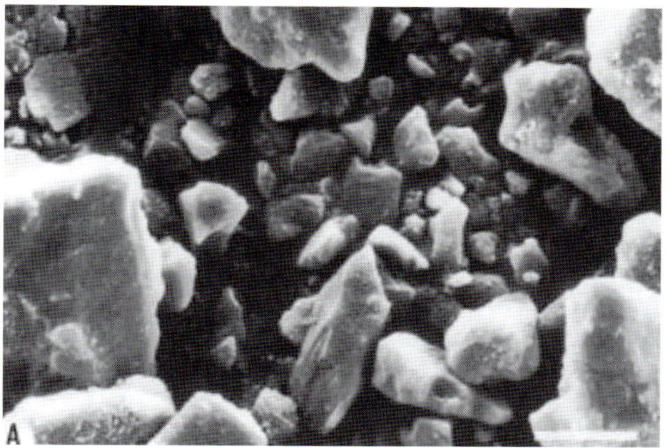

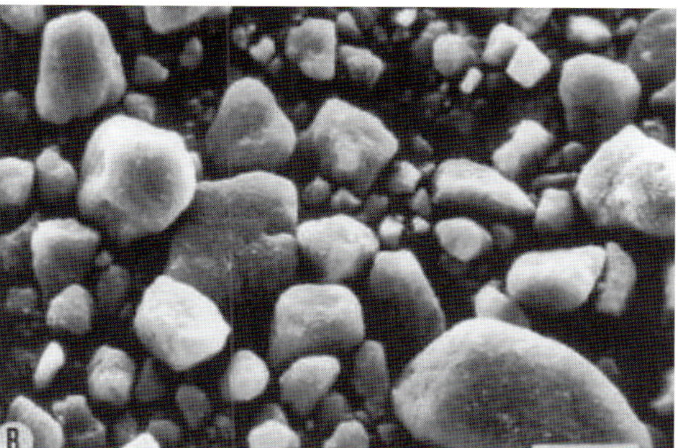

Fig 4-6a and b Silux Plus (A) is a light-cured heterogeneous microfine composite with splintered prepolymerized fillers. Answer (B) is a chemically-cured heterogeneous microfine composite with agglomerated prepolymerized fillers. Both materials have approximately the same properties. They differ mainly in the manufacturing process of their polymerized filler particles. Silux Plus contains fillers of a more angular shape whereas the filler particles of Answer are more round (bar = 20 µm). (With the permission of Dental Materials, according to Willems et al.[3]).

Table 4-5 Traditional composites (According to Willems et al.[3]).

Traditional Composites									
Products	MPS	Mo	Ra	Y-Mod	Vol% A	Vol% B	CS	HV	RO
Adaptic (80'S)*	15.4	18.8	1.26	21.412	64.9	56.3	234	–	–
Adaptic Radiopaque (Uni-Cat)*	13.5-8.1	18.8-12.4	1.08	19.616	61.9	55.0	240	121	–
Aurafill*	8.6	12.4	0.85	17.935	58.9	62.0	345	105	119
Clearfill*	9.7	12.4	0.83	20.373	63.2	58.1	252	93	–
Concise*	–	–	1.44	22.531	66.6	56.8	241	–	–
Epolite 100*	10.1	12.4	1.46	18.206	59.4	53.0	253	107	79
Estilux Posterior*	9.5	12.4	0.88	17.408	57.9	58.1	294	96	137
Estilux Posterior XR1*	5.1	11.1	–	21.805	65.5	66.2	–	–	232
Estilux Posterior XR2*	8.8	12.4	–	–	–	–	346	–	230
Miradapt*	7.8	10.0	1.01	20.320	63.1	60.1	310	112	–
Nimetics(Uni-Cat)*	14.4-12.4	32.0-25.9	0.91	20.908	64.1	58.9	330	149	–
Visio Fil	7.5	8.1	1.23	21.723	65.4	64.4	350	160	71
Fiber-Reinforced Composites									
Products	MPS	Mo	Ra	Y-Mod	Vol% A	Vol% B	CS	HV	RO
Restolux SP-4	11.2	15.3	1.19	23,839	68.5	–	–	125	163

MPS: Mean particle size (µm); Mo: mode of the particle size distribution (µm); Ra: Intrinsic surface roughness (µm); Y-Mod: Young's Modulus of elasticity (MPa); Vol%A: inorganic filler volume percentage as calculated according to Braem (1985); Vol%B: inorganic filler volume percentage as obtained from the manufacturers; CS: compressive strength (MPa); HV: Vickers Hardness (kg/mm^2); *: Young's modulus data taken from Braem (1985); RO: Radiographic Opacity taken from Willems et al. (1991b).

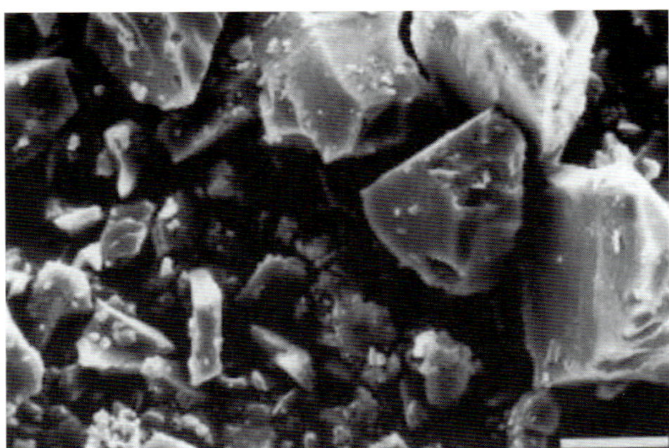

Fig 4-7 Adaptic is a traditional composite. These composites are older materials and are now rarely used (bar = 20 µm). (With the permission of Dental Materials, according to Willems et al.[3]).

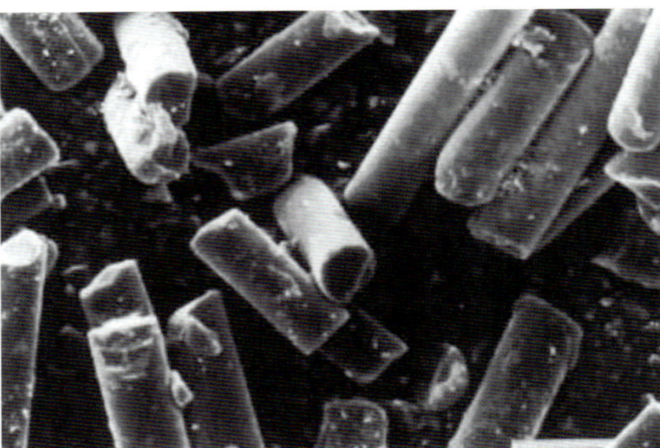

Fig 4-8 The fiber-reinforced composite Restolux SP-4 contains glass ceramic fibers with a maximum length of 300 µm, which are embedded in resin matrix (bar = 20 µm). (With the permission of Dental Materials, according to Willems et al.[3]).

Table 4-6 Miscellaneous composites (According to Willems et al.[3]).

Miscellaneous Composites									
Products	MPS	Mo	Ra	Y-Mod	Vol% A	Vol% B	CS	HV	RO
with splintered prepolymerized fillers									
Bell firm (Uni-Cat)	2.0-7.4	0.8-10.0	0.96	–	–	–	324	–	–
Bis-Fil M	10.4	12.3	0.58	12.882	47.8	59.0	301	63	87
Clearfil Lustre	12.9	12.4	0.74	11.511	44.0	–	387	100	< 40
Palfique Estelite	13.4	15.3	–	12.132	45.8	56.0	373	63	–
Palfique Lite	15.1	15.3	–	12.118	45.8	56.0	373	70	–
with agglomerated prepolymerized fillers									
Visio Dispers*	15.0	15.3	0.26	10.786	41.8	47.6	455	63	232
Heliomolar.Radiopaque	13.1	15.3	0.13	9.755	38.5	48.0	340	56	230
with sintered agglomerates									
Amalux 2	6.4	4.7	0.44	14.166	51.0	–	343	89	118
with spherical prepolymerized fillers									
Pekalux	16.1	15.3	0.18	5.973	22.0	54.7	275	27	< 40

MPS: Mean particle size (µm); Mo: mode of the particle size distribution (µm); Ra: Intrinsic surface roughness (µm); Y-Mod: Young's Modulus of elasticity (MPa); Vol%A: inorganic filler volume percentage as calculated according to Braem (1985); Vol%B: inorganic filler volume percentage as obtained from the manufacturers; CS: compressive strength (MPa); HV: Vickers Hardness (kg/mm^2); *: Young's modulus data taken from Braem (1985) RO: Radiographic Opacity taken from Willems et al. (1991b).

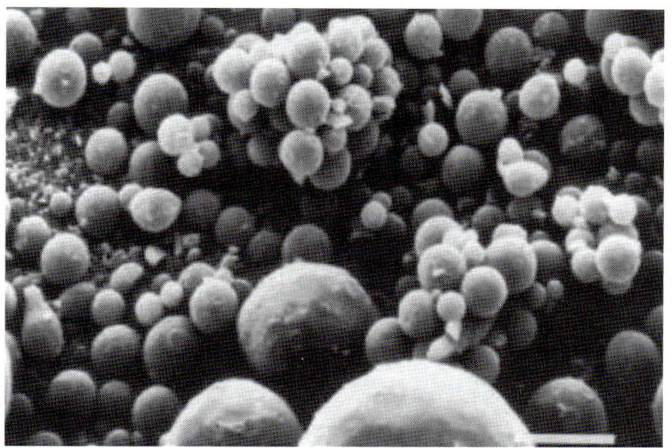

Fig 4-9 The spherical prepolymerized filler particles of Pekalux, a miscellaneous composite, are clearly apparent (bar = 20 µm). (With the permission of Dental Materials, according to Willems et al.[3]).

Table 4-7 Evaluation of the radiation intensity of polymerization lamps in dental practices (according to Barghi et al.[19]).

GROUP RATING	NUMBER OF UNITS	PERCENT OF TOTAL
A. Adequate	114	54.59%
B. Adequate with increased time	33	15.80%
C. Inadequate	62	29.70%

Clinically handling these light-cured materials is a more laborious task than the traditional restorative techniques, and the clinical behavior of a composite filling largely depends upon the polymerization reaction inside the material[4]. Poor polymerization leads to an insufficient conversion rate. As a result, restorations have weaker physical properties, less wear resistance, and increased moisture absorption and discoloration. There is less adhesion to enamel and dentin with increased micro-gap formation and micro-leakage leading to bacterial invasion, pulp irritation and secondary decay. Finally, more untreated monomers will be leached out of a poorly polymerized filling. Side effects at the pulp again are possible[5–18].

So proper polymerization is one of the basic requisites in tooth restoration with light-cured materials. Studies carried out in the Netherlands and the USA show astonishing results (Table 4-7)[19].

The quality of halogen lamps was tested in dental practices on a random basis. Only about 55% of the lamps could provide adequate polymerization; 16% only with increased exposure time. And nearly 30%, or 1 out of 3, did not allow suitable polymerization to take place.

Effective polymerization requires, in a decreasing order of importance: quality and quantity of the energy delivered by the light source, an incremental filling technique, correct light exposure time and the correct distance from the light source to the material[4].

4.3 Photopolymerization Reaction

Polymerization is always initiated by free radicals. Fig 4-10 shows a schematic representation of the formation of free radicals by the different types of initiator systems[20].

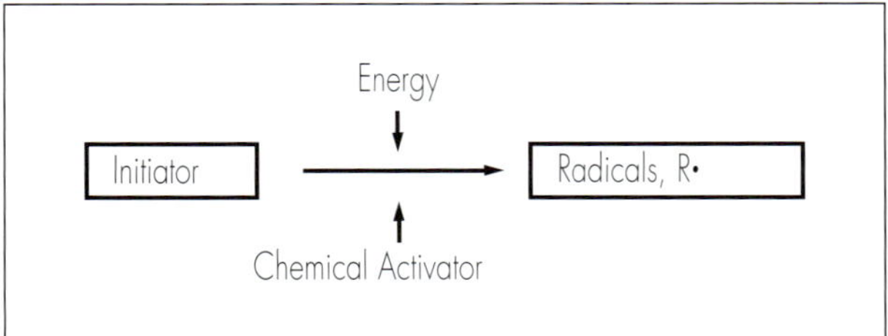

Fig 4-10 Polymerization is initiated by free radicals. Schematic representation of the formation of radicals by different types of initiator systems (According to Ruyter[20]).

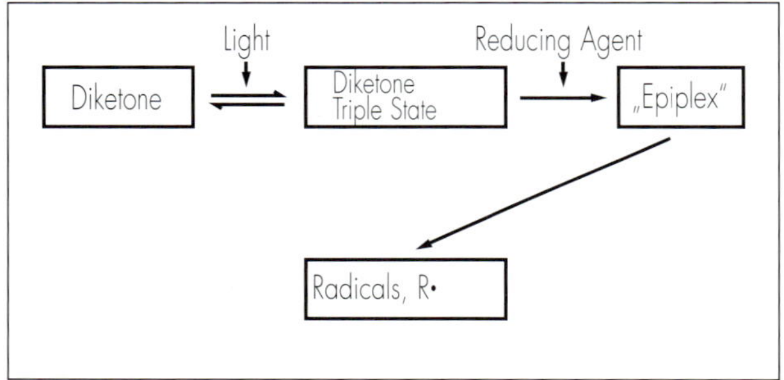

Fig 4-11 Free radicals formed from a diketone and a reducing agent during light exposure (According to Ruyter[20]).

Chemical polymerization and polymerization by UV light are no longer used because of several disadvantages compared to visible light curing. Photopolymerization or visible light curing occurs when free radicals are formed from a diketone and a reducing agent during light exposure (Fig 4-11)[20].

The most commonly used photo-initiator or diketone is camphoroquinone. It absorbs the radiation energy and is transferred to excited states. At the appropriate excited state (triplet state), it combines with the photo-accelerator or reducing agent, e.g., N,N-dimethylaminoethyl methacrylate, to form a complex in an excited state (epiplex) which breaks down to give reactive free radicals. These free radicals trigger the polymerization reaction. But first they react with the oxygen on the surface layer and the added photo-inhibitor, e.g., p-hydroquinone. Then they affect the oligomers and monomers present in the material, to form chains of polymers and cross-linking. A free radical (RAD®) stabilizes by giving its superfluous energy to a target molecule which has at each of its ends a double C binding (C=C). As a result, an electron out of the p-orbital of those double bindings is released, with the creation of a new free radical, affecting another oligomer or

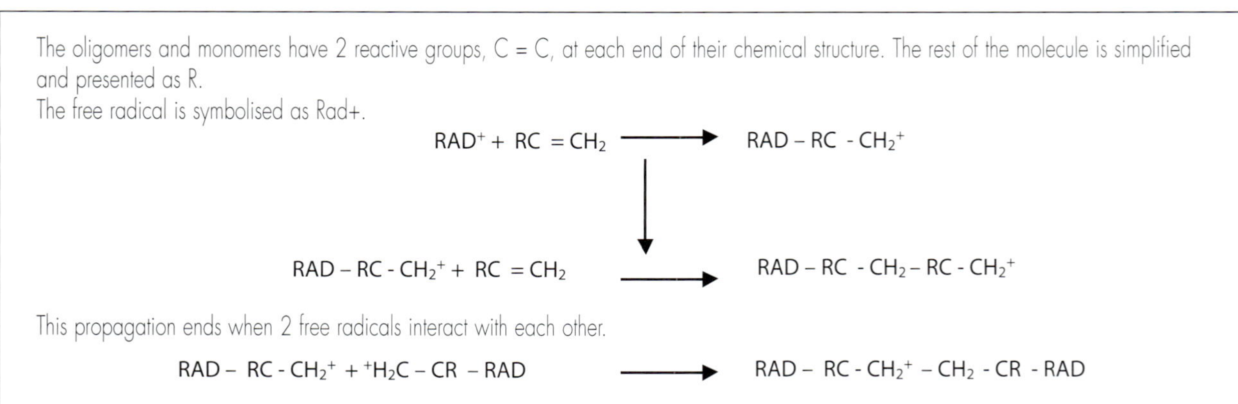

Fig 4-12 Schematic representation of the chemical proceedings in a polymerization reaction.

monomer and thus creating chains of polymers (Fig 4-12).

The formation of long polymer-chains, and a high degree of cross-linking is ideal. Figure 4-13 shows an idealized representation of a BIS-GMA-TEGDMA-system[20].

The factors that influence reaching this point are as follows: light propagation through the material depending on the type and concentration of the color and color pigments; the type and concentration of the filler-phase, of the oligomers, of the monomers and of the chemical additives; the type and concentration of the free radicals; the available wavelengths of the light source and its exposed energy level; exposure time, and the temperature of the material and its inherent speed-reaction time or T rate, which depends upon the concentration of free radicals [RAD®], and Kd, a constant, comprising several parameters such as the molecular concentration of the monomer and the diffusion speed in the solvent[21,22].

$$\text{T rate} = ([\text{RAD}^{®}]^{2})\,(\text{Kd})$$

Polymerization reactions, in general, start with an inhibition period (A), followed by a period with a constant reaction rate and formation of low-molecular polymers (B), and ending in the gel stage with auto-acceleration and the formation of polymer molecules with a high degree of polymerization and with cross-linking (C) and at a certain degree of conversion as shown in Figure 4-14[20].

The aim is to produce a high conversion rate, and this is dependent on the quality and quantity of available light energy.

In conclusion, photo-polymerization of light-activated materials is a difficult and complicated process with several variables, some of which the clinician can control and others the clinician cannot. The chemical constitution of the material used is out of the control of the dentist. But the right product, in any given clinical situation, can be chosen from the wide variety of commercially available materials.

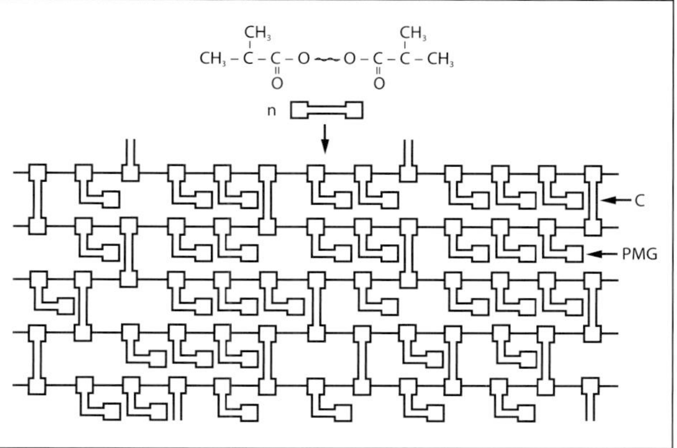

Fig 4-13 Simplified and idealized representation of the three-dimensional structure of copolymers of dimethacrylate monomers with cross-linking (C) and pendant methacrylate groups (PMG) (According to Ruyter[20]).

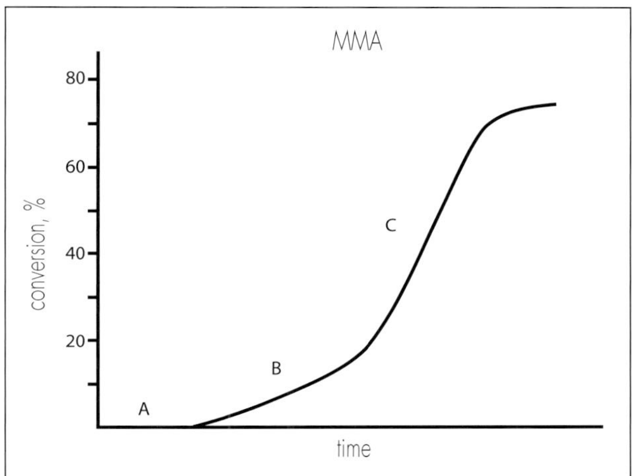

Fig 4-14 Bulk polymerization of methyl methacrylate (MMA). Plots of MMA conversion vs. time: A, an inhibition period; B, a period with constant reaction rate and formation of low-molecular polymers; C, the gel stage with auto-acceleration and the formation of polymer molecules with a high degree of polymerization (According to Ruyter[20]).

Proper material handling and effective clinical techniques are essential, and these factors are fully under the dentist's control.

In addition, the dentist can control the quality of the light source, the quality and quantity of the light energy delivered and the wavelengths applied, all of which influence the clinical results.

Albers et al.[15] formulated a very practical nomenclature to allow precise determination and specification of all the parameters involved in the complicated process of photopolymerization (Fig 4-15)[15].

1. Wavelength Requirements of the Composite.
SR = Spectral Requirements for Photopolymerization.
The bandwidth of wavelengths necessary to activate the photoinitiator(s) in a specific composite; the bandwidths that absorb light energy and form the free radicals necessary for polymerization.

2. Wavelength Generated by the Curing Unit.
SE = Spectral Emission for Photopolymerization.
The effective bandwidth of wavelengths emitted by a curing unit for photopolymerization.
The SE bandwidth should overlap or be congruent with the absorption range(s) of the photoinitiator(s) in the resin composite.

3. Intensity of Wavelength the Curing Unit Emits.
PD = Power Density.
The total power (mW or W) emitted by a curing unit within the stated effective bandwidth or SE, divided by the spot size of the curing tip (cm^2).

4. How Much Total Energy is Applied.
ED = Energy Density.
The power density (PD) multiplied by the exposure time(s).

5. The Energy the Composite Needs.
EOP@D = Energy Density for Optimal Polymerization at a Specified Depth.
For example: 16 indicates that optimal polymerization can be achieved for a 2-mm increment with an ED of 16 J/cm^2, specified by the composite manufacturer.

6. How the Energy is Applied.
EAS = Energy Application Sequence.
The way or sequence in which a clinician uses the curing unit to polymerize a composite. Since ED is the product of PD and exposure duration, the clinician will typically choose the highest power density and shortest exposure time necessary to reach the ED equal toth specified EOP@D. The decrease or savings in exposure time is not inversely proportional to increases in PD; therefore, EOP@D may have differing values depending on the PD utilized.

Fig 4-15 Dental terms for polymerization of resins: a nomenclature. (According to Albers et al.[15]).

4.4 Laser Photopolymerization versus Traditional Methods

Photopolymerization starts when radiation energy is absorbed by a photo-initiator or diketone. Camphoroquinone is most commonly used[6]. It has an absorption spectrum between 460 and 492 nm with a peak at 468: $\lambda_{max} = 468$ nm (Fig 4-16)[23].

De Gee et al.[24] analyzed the spectral emission and relative intensity output of the available light sources[24]. Halogen lamps show the broadest spectral emission, from 300 to 1300 nm (Fig 4-17). Wavelengths beneath 400 nm and above 500 nm have to be filtered out, because only wavelengths between 400 and 500 nm produce useful energy for photo-polymerization. Beneath 400 nm there is the possibility of potentially dangerous UV light, and above 500 nm there is possible heating and pulp-damaging infrared light. Intensity outputs range between 400 and 600 mW/cm^2. Latest devices can generate up to 1000 mW/cm^2.

Plasma arc devices have the same spectral emission, but different relative intensities at the different wavelengths (Fig 4-18). Argon gas or xenon gas are used to generate the light energy. The argon device filters out wavelengths beneath 445 nm and above 505 nm. The xenon type filters out wavelengths beneath 430 nm and above 500 nm. Energy densities range from 1600 to 2000 mW/cm^2.

LEDs, or indium-gallium-nitride light emitting diodes, generate a smaller emission spectrum with a peak around 470 nm (Fig 4-19). Yet the energy densities that they can generate are modest. Future developments look very promising.

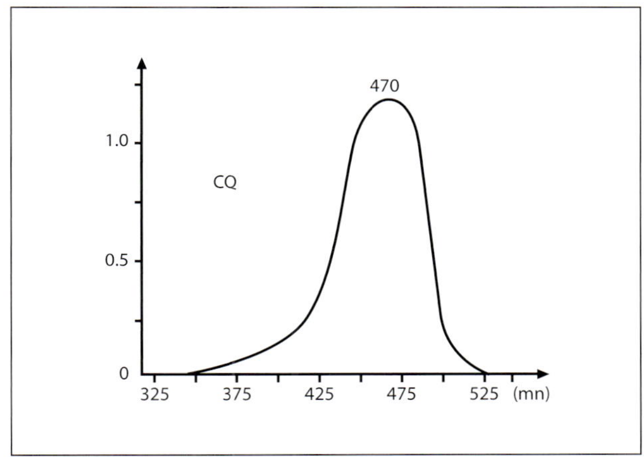

Fig 4-16 Camphoroquinone absorption coefficient curve (According to Cipolla[23]).

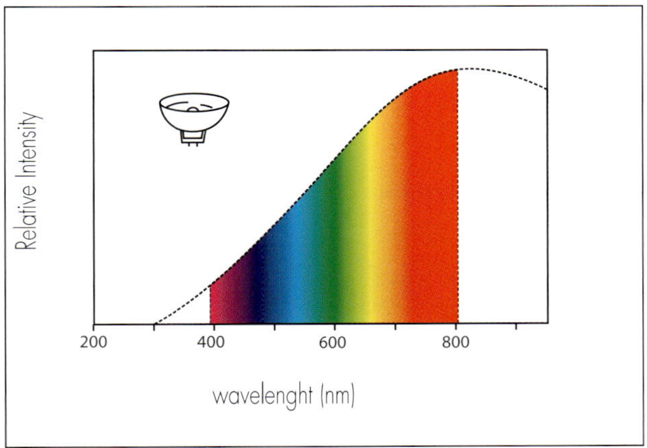

Fig 4-17 Spectral emission of a halogen lamp. Emission in the visible range is colored (According to De Gee[24]).

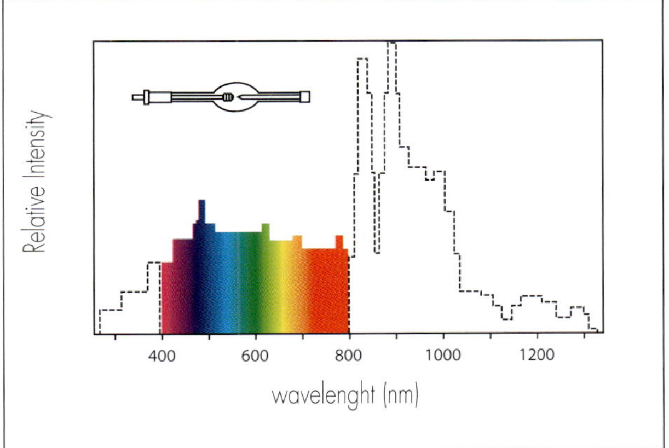

Fig 4-18 Spectral emission of plasma arc devices. Emission in the visible range is colored (According to De Gee[24]).

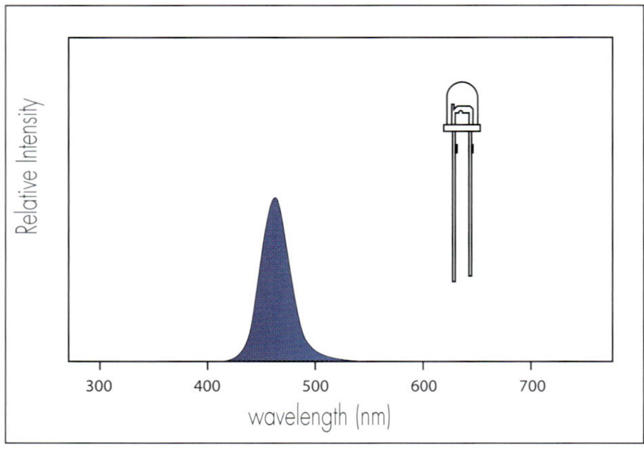

Fig 4-19 Spectral emission of an LED. Emission in the visible range is colored (According to De Gee[24]).

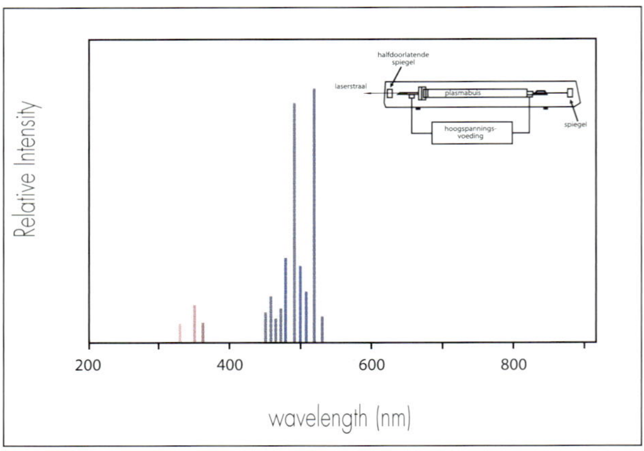

Fig 4-20 Spectral emission of an argon laser. (According to De Gee[24]).

Argon lasers produce a limited number of very specific wavelengths (λ) of light energy, with 476 nm, 488 nm and 514.5 nm the most important (Fig 4-20). The green 514.5 nm can be filtered out, but has no influence on the polymerization reaction, tooth structures or the oral environment. Argon lasers can produce extremely high energy densities.

Furthermore, laser light has unique properties (see chapter 1). It is monochromatic, which means it consists of only one single wavelength. It is coherent, i.e., all waves are travelling in phase. And it is collimated, so it travels in just one direction. These features add benefits to argon laser photopolymerization. The unique wavelength of 488 nm provides important energy because it is in the maximum absorption range of the camphoroquinone (Fig 4-16). It has a high penetration depth and an excellent diffusion throughout the composite layer. The thin delivery fiber of 300 µm gives easy access to every region in the mouth. Energy densities do not decrease with increased distance from the target material. Power output and energy densities are adjustable and controllable. Features to be noted and discussed when light curing with an argon laser are: the reduction in polymerization time and the quality of the polymerization reaction, the pulpal response, the physical properties of the cured materials, the management of the inherent polymerization shrinkage and the caries preventive action.

Blankenau et al.[25] measured the wavelength range and the peak average wavelength of different VLC (Visible Light Curing) units. They showed a wide range of spectral emissions, even after filtering. Camphoroquinone has a maximum absorption of light energy between 460 and 492 nm. Therefore, only 1/3 of the power output provided by conventional light sources is really influencing and activating the photo-initiating system of light-cured materials using camphoroquinone as a photo-initiator (Fig 4-21)[26]. The light they emit is incoherent and is therefore out of phase, with different waves overlapping each other, thus reducing each other's photon energy or even neutralizing each other. However, laser light is coherent and monochromatic. The photons travelling in phase do not interact with each other, and all of the energy produced by the 488 nm wavelength is capable of interacting with the camphoroquinone molecules present in the target material. The efficient initiating process induces an equal chemical response leading to a reduction in exposure time[27].

Curing Times™ [28] listed a table with the optimal parameters for curing of all of the commonly used light-cured materials. With a few exceptions, they all use camphoroquinone as a photo-initiator

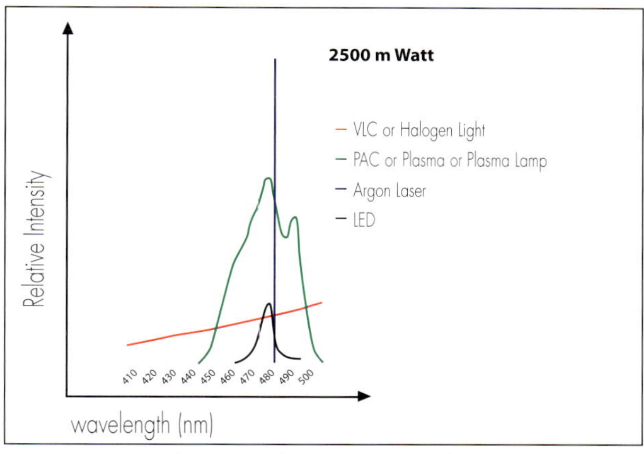

Fig 4-21 Spectral emission of VLC, PAC, argon laser and LED.

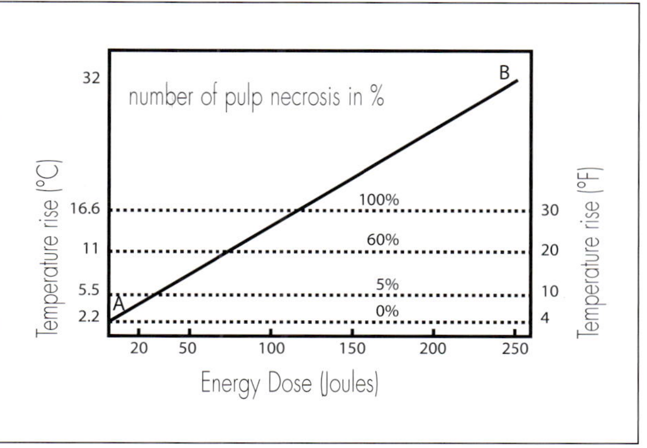

Fig 4-22 Relationship of pulp temperature elevation to pulp necrosis. (From J Endodent 1989;15:302-305. Reprinted with permission).

and are thus capable of being light-cured by the single wavelength energy of a laser. Their findings correspond with those of Kelsey et al.: to achieve optimal polymerization, specific time and power settings are required[27].

The energy flux, or the amount of energy delivered, depends on the average power output, the time of interaction and the area of exposure.

$$E = \frac{W \times S}{\mathrm{cm}^2}$$

E = energy flux
W = watt
S = second

The different chemical constitutions of the light-cured materials makes them respond differently to a given energy flux, and within it, to variations in time and power setting[27].

Laser devices permit these precise and controllable settings and provide optimal polymerization for the material to be handled. The general consensus is that laser exposure times should be 25% of the recommended time for VLC devices, and with average power settings of 350 mW[6]. There is a direct correlation between power settings and reaction speed. The higher the laser power output, the faster polymerization takes place. But above a certain threshold, there is an equal decrease in the quality of the polymerization[27].

Besides an increased reaction speed with decreased exposure time, polymerization is accomplished more efficiently, resulting in a higher conversion rate[7,8,29]. Measurements by high-performance liquid chromatography show for the polymerization of micro-fine composites a reduction in unpolymerized TEGDMA of 31%, and for BIS-GMA of 40%, when laser cured compared to VLC curing. This occurs with reduced exposure times[8]. Visible light curing provides lower conversion rates compared to laser curing, achieving cured materials with fewer residues. These residues may be potentially dangerous when leaking to the pulp or to the oral environment.

Another concern for the vital pulp is an increase in temperature whilst curing. The critical threshold is 5.6°C, with temperature increases above this causing irreversible damage to the pulp[30]. There is a direct correlation between pulpal temperature rise and percentage of pulpal necrosis (Fig 4-22).

Launay et al.[31] measured the temperature change in the pulp chamber with different settings, beam sizes and exposure times. Powell et al. concluded that the energy densities generated during laser curing did not affect the pulp or the surrounding enamel[32,33]. Anic et al.[34] measured a temperature increase of only 2.5°C while laser curing

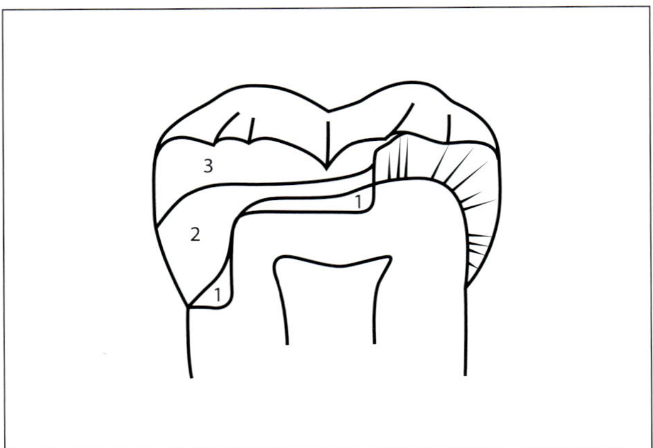

Fig 4-23 Composite restorations made in several independently cured layers in order to promote preservations of an adaptation to the cavity wall. (According to Davidson[39]).

class I restorations in vitro. The highest surface temperature of the cured resins was 13.8°C, which was due to the exothermic polymerization reaction and the light energy. This is one-third that shown by Lloyd[35] in studies with conventional light sources.

Puckett et al.[36] measured the degree of polymerization, comparing argon laser to VLC. They noted a significant difference in Brinell hardness in favor of argon curing, and this is with 1/3 of the exposure time: argon 10 s vs. VLC 30 s. The argon laser also has a higher penetration depth in the cured resin layer and produces better physical properties.

Severin et al.[37] showed that the higher energy density, combined with the ideal wavelength produced by an argon laser, improves the hardness of the cured resins, increases the polymerization rate with improved compressive and tensile strengths, and reduces the shrinkage stress at the interface. Blankenau et al.[38] indicated that the adhesion to dentin and enamel is proportional to the energy flux applied.

In clinical terms, these features show less pulp irritation and less post-operative sensitivity. And the energy flow needed is higher when using VLC. Curing three layers of composite material (Fig 4-23) for 40 s with a halogen light and with an energy density of 400 mW/cm^2 produces a total energy flux of 48 J/cm^2. Using an argon laser at 1000 mW/cm^2 for three passes of 10 s generates a total energy flux of only 30 J/cm^2.

A study of the physical and mechanical properties of filling materials is useful in predicting the clinical behavior of a restoration[4]. Blankenau et al.[9], Kelsey et al.[10], and Waknine and Cipolla[40] showed an enhancement of the physical properties of resin restorative materials by laser polymerization.

Compressive strength values give an indication of the resistance to fractures when the filling material is subject to compression forces whilst chewing. They give an idea of how the material functions over time.

For two different kinds of composite materials, Silux (MP) (a microfine composite) and P50 (a densified compact filled composite), compressive strength measurements show higher values after laser polymerization than VLC, and with reduced exposure times.

Mean values for diametrical tensile strength are significantly higher after laser polymerization and with a total exposure time of 1/4, compared to VLC. They indicate a higher resistance to lateral tensile forces during function.

Transversal flexural strength values are in direct correlation with the resistance to distortion of the material when loaded. They give an indirect indication of the resistance to fatigue wear.

The flexural modulus indicates the stiffness or rigidity of the cured filling material. It is ideal to have the same values for enamel, dentin and the cured composite, so that distortion will be uniform when loaded. If the filling material shows a lower flexural modulus, it will be compressed more than the surrounding tooth structures during chewing. This causes high tensile forces and shear stresses to the tooth-filling interface, with fractures in the marginal seal, micro-leakage and secondary decay formation. Laser polymerization increases the values of the flexural modulus.

A study by Powell et al.[41] investigated the diametrical tensile strength values of a later generation of composite materials. They looked at the influence of different power settings of the argon laser and at different exposure times of the VLC units. They compared 10-s argon curing to 40-s visible light curing. Previous results could be confirmed.

Blankenau et al.[42] showed improved diametrical tensile strength values for laser-cured pit and fissure sealants. They demonstrated equal or improved physical properties for light-cured liners and glass-ionomer materials[11].

The higher degree of conversion rate with a more profound polymerization and the decrease of the remaining unpolymerized monomer produces enhanced physical properties after laser curing[8,10]. And the conversion rate will undoubtedly affect chemical stability as well as fatigue wear in light-cured materials[43]. Wear rate, and resistance to wear, are important features in predicting the clinical behavior of composite resin restorations[43].

- Abrasive wear occurs when a hard surface slides against a softer one and is related to the friction between two sliding bodies, called two-body abrasive wear.
- Erosive wear occurs when a medium containing hard abrasive particles lies between the sliding surfaces and causes three-body abrasive wear or erosive wear.
- Corrosive wear is the result of a chemical reaction. In composites, moisture absorption leads to corrosive wear.
- Fatigue wear results from repeatedly overloading the surface beyond its elastic limit. With brittle materials, particularly, this can lead to crack formation, as the material just below the surface is usually strained to a higher extent than the surface itself (Fig 4-24)[43].

Glasspoole et al.[44], however, found no statistically significant difference in wear rate in vitro between laser polymerization and VLC.

Measurements of post-polymerization strength showed that laser curing yielded initially higher values compared to VLC. This difference decreased

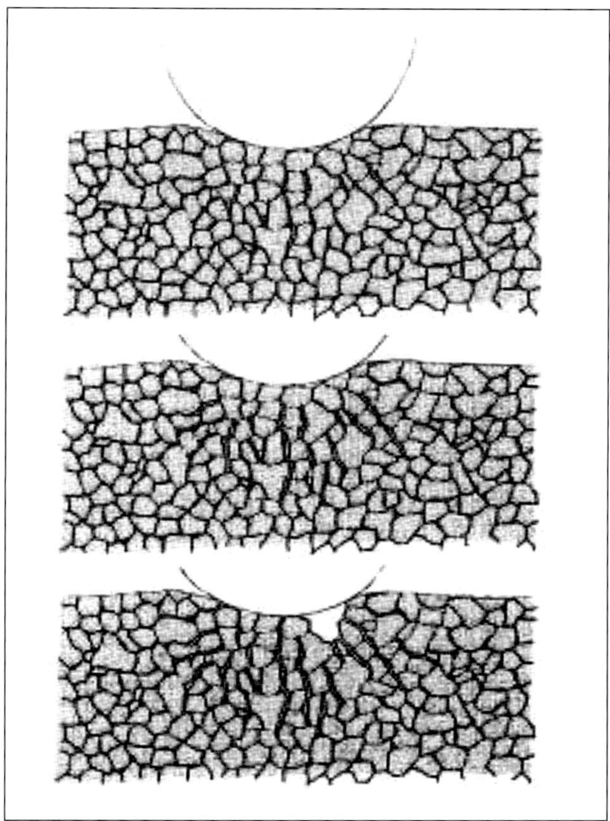

Fig 4-24 Schematic representation of the various successive stages of damage in a composite after static loading at direct contact (According to Davidson[39]).

time[9]. Nevertheless, these initial higher values may be clinically important when finishing and polishing the restoration after curing, and with the direct loading during chewing.

Frentzen and Koort[45] concluded that the homogeneous penetration of the laser light induces an improved marginal seal due to a reduction of the shrinkage stresses toward the light source. Shanthala and Munshi[46] stated that the superior polymerization induced by the energy of a laser improves bond strengths to enamel in primary teeth as well as in permanent teeth.

Powell et al.[47], Sedivy et al.[48] and Hinoura et al.[49] showed the same results.

Bond strength to dentin is highly dependent on the energy density generated by the light source and the wavelength, which should ideally be as close to the λ_{max} of camphoroquinone as possible[37].

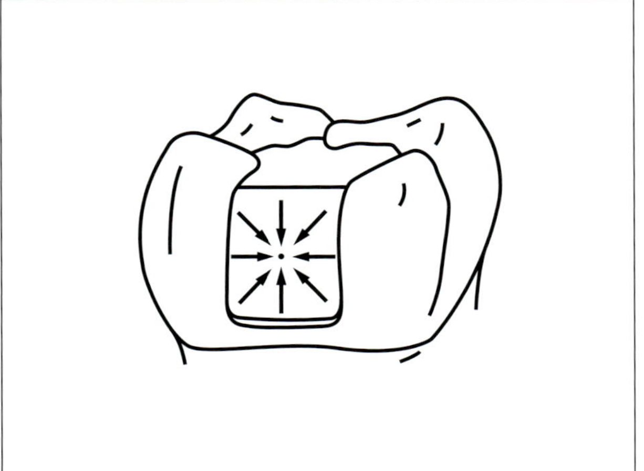

Fig 4-25 Chemically-cured composite resins shrink toward the geometric center of the mass. This leaves a small contraction gap at the gingival margin. The composite resin is strongly bonded to enamel on both the lingual and buccal walls preventing gaps at these walls; however, there may be stresses set up in both the tooth and the composite resin (According to Pollack[53]).

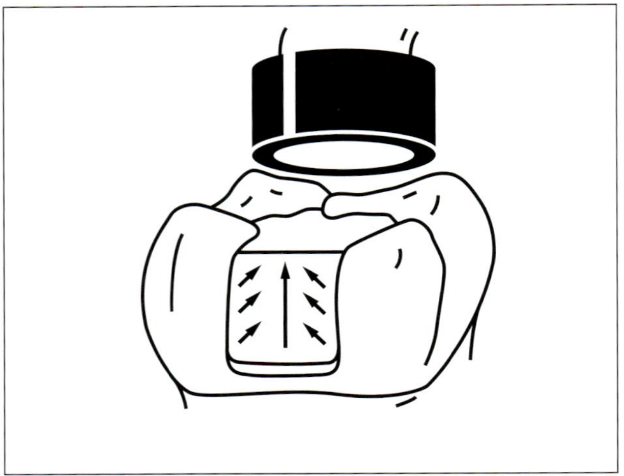

Fig 4-26 Photocured composite resin shrinks toward the light source because the composite resin closest to the light hardens first. This, in turn, pulls the softer composite resin from the gingival areas, creating a gap. The mass of composite resin being pulled to the occlusal area is twice that found in chemically-cured resins, hence the gingival contraction gap is twice as large (According to Pollack[53]).

Blankenau et al.[12] reported an increase of bond strengths to dentin of 21–24% after laser polymerization.

An interesting finding in the research of Hinoura et al.[49] is that there is little to no effect evident in changing the distance from the fiber tip to the resin surface while laser curing. This is contrasted with LC, which shows a significant decrease in bond strength from increasing the distance from the light tip to the resin surface. This was confirmed by Blankenau et al.[50] and Powell and Blankenau.[51]

Frentzen and Koort[45] reported a reduction of the polymerization stresses toward the light source when using an argon laser for photopolymerization. Polymerization shrinkage is inherent in all light-cured filling materials and is dependent on the organic phase-inorganic phase ratio. A higher degree of the organic matrix increases the shrinkage. Increased filler phase decreases shrinkage.

VLC and laser curing cause the same amount of polymerization shrinkage at any given rate of conversion[52]. The higher the conversion rate, the more monomers and oligomers have interacted with equally increased shrinkage[51], but with improved physical properties[9] and reduced cytotoxicity[52]. Laser curing shows a higher conversion rate[52].

In chemically-cured materials, polymerization shrinkage is directed towards the center (Fig 4-25)[53]. VLC causes polymerization shrinkage towards the light source (Figs 4-26 and 4-27)[53].

Kelsey et al. stated that the homogeneous penetration of the resin by the laser beam should result in improved marginal integrity by reducing the amount of polymerization shrinkage toward the curing light[7] (Fig 4-28).

Laser curing gives a uniform and immediate penetration of the light energy into the composite mass as a whole. Polymerization starts at the same time in every portion of the composite layer, on the surface as well as on the bottom. Thus, the shrinkage is directed to the adhesive layer on the cavity wall and on the bottom, resulting in an improved integrity at the interface and an

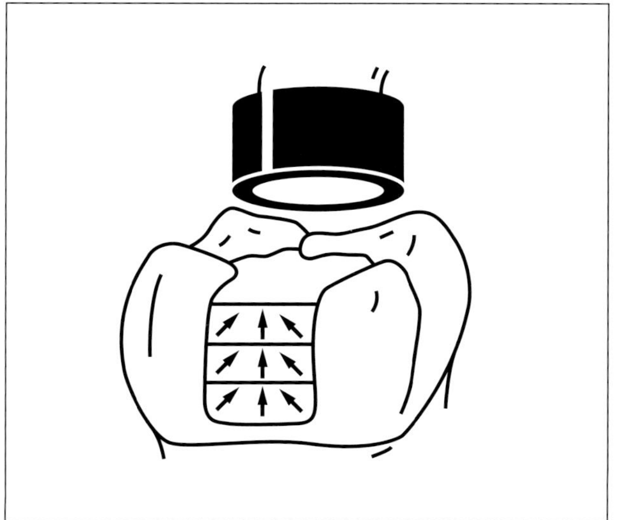

Fig 4-27 Incremental curing reduces, but does not completely eliminate, the gingival contraction gap (According to Pollack[53]).

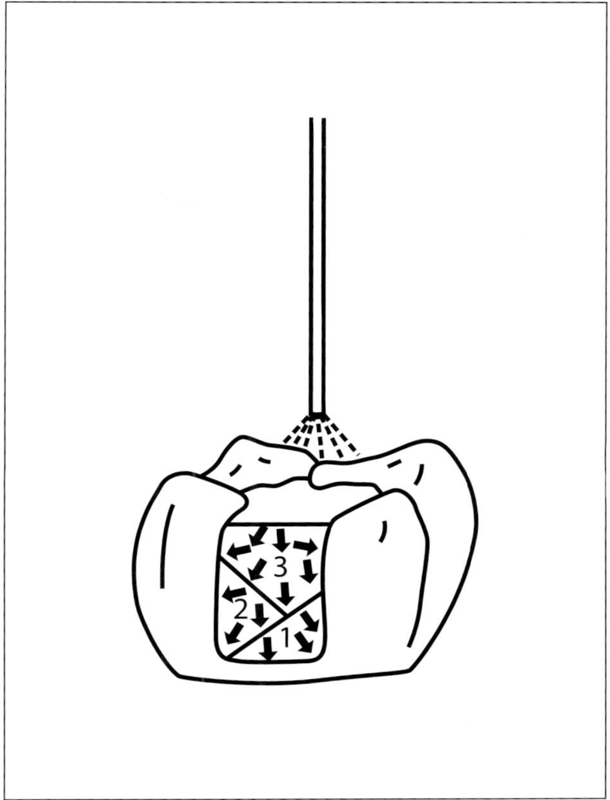

Fig 4-28 Direction of the polymerization shrinkage during incremental laser curing.

improved marginal seal. De Gee[24] concluded that the higher the energy density of the light source, the less polymerization shrinkage stress occurs. He postulates a difference in the chemical progress of photopolymerization with increased energy densities.

Through the generation of a higher concentration of reactive camphoroquinone radicals, the start of the polymerization reaction yields more and shorter polymer chains, with increased flow and elasticity in the material during the initial polymerization process.

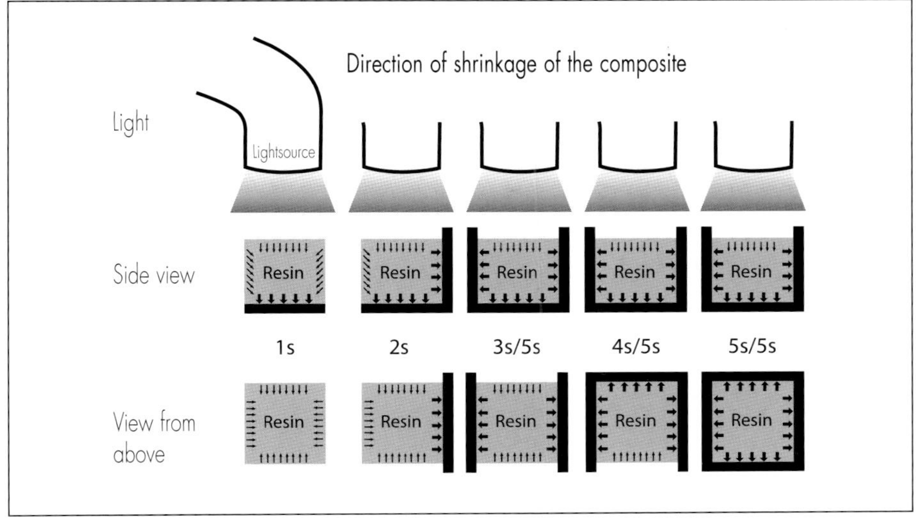

Fig 4-29 The configuration factor (C-factor) is the following relationship: the number of surfaces bonded, divided by the number of surfaces unbonded. As the configuration factor rices, the effects of polymerization stress and strain become more significant in maintaining marginal seal. (Adapted from Feilzer, AJ, De Gee, AJ, and Davidson CL. "Setting stresses in composite resin in relation to the configuration of the restoration". Dent Res 1990,6: 167-171) (According to Albers[54]).

Cavity design is another factor of influence (Fig 4-29)[39,54]. Controversially, Versluis et al.[55] stated that incremental filling yields greater polymerization shrinkage effects and, perhaps more significantly, higher tensile stress concentrations at the restoration-enamel interface than does bulk filling of a cavity. There are many factors involved during the polymerization process that may affect the resulting shrinkage stresses and their impact upon the integrity of the tooth-restoration complexes. Versluis et al.[55] concluded that there are other factors that favor incremental filling over bulk placement (e.g., densification, adaptation, thoroughness of cure and bond formation). However, their studies conclude that it is very difficult to prove that effective reduction in overall shrinkage stress, and hence in deformation of the remaining hard tissue walls, are sufficient reason to prefer incremental filling over single bulk filling.

Laser curing used with their suggested technique of single bulk filling may improve the thoroughness of cure and bond formation.

4.5 Improved Clinical Performance of Laser Cured Materials

Laser light is proven to be able to change the morphology of enamel, dentin and cementum, giving increased resistance to acid solubility[56–65] (see chapter 5). The light energy of an argon laser is highly efficient for this purpose, with the additional benefit of being pulp friendly[31,34,66]. Westerman et al.[13,14] showed that very low energy densities (10–15 J/cm^2) are sufficient to achieve an increased acid resistance. These densities are below the threshold energy density for photopolymerization. A caries-preventive effect occurs during laser curing. Hicks et al.[15] showed that the threshold pH for enamel dissolution in acid can be increased from 5.5 to 4.78 by argon laser irradiation. This means that an acid concentration of five times higher is needed to induce enamel demineralization. Hicks et al.[16] came to this conclusion after a study on caries progression in sealants after argon laser polymerization. They performed additional research, which confirmed their previous results[17]. Laser energy induces a decrease in the organic, carbon and water content of enamel. This leads to a contraction of the A-axes of the enamel prisms with a decreased acid solubility.

Anic et al.[34] showed surface melting and superficial sealing of the enamel surface with a maximum increase in pulpal temperature of 4°C. Oho and Morioka[18] reported the formation of microspaces and birefringence, capable of capting the dissoluted ions during demineralization, and capable of their reprecipitation during the process of remineralization. There is also an increased affinity to calcium, fluoride and phosphate ions. Furthermore, the conditioning of the enamel surface during argon laser irradiation facilitates the uptake of fluoride, producing an improved reduction in demineralization after an acid attack[15,17,65,66]. Curing sealants with argon laser energy produces the beneficial effects of reduced solubility of the surrounding enamel[17] and decreased micro-leakage[12,42,67,68]. It significantly reduces the depth of the lesions in models of caries initiating and progress in vitro[13,16]. It improves diametric tensile strength[42] and helps achieve a dry operation field[69]. Hicks et al.[16] studied the formation of caries-like lesions around argon laser-cured and visible light-cured sealants. Visible light curing showed an increase of 81 μm in depth of lesion over time, compared to only 32 μm with argon laser curing.

Westerman et al.[70] investigated artificial caries formation on the surface of a root. They came to the same conclusion of reduced caries progression after laser polymerization. They found an overall increase of 114 μm in lesion depth with VLC, compared to only 65 μm with laser curing. These results show a significant increase in the resistance to demineralization and caries formation in cementum and dentin due to argon laser irradiation.

The same results were demonstrated by Hicks et al.[17] in sound enamel. They found an overall depth increase of 66 μm in the lased lesions compared to 104 μm in the control lesions.

An additional feature of the light of an argon laser is early interproximal caries detection[71,72]. It has been demonstrated that when the blue-green light of an argon laser passes through a carious lesion, a wavelength shift to the orange-red ($\lambda > 540$ nm) occurs. Decalcified areas appear as dull, opaque, orange-colored zones. Even the appearance of enamel fractures can be detected[73].

4.6 Caries Prevention by Laser and with Laser Activated Fluoride

Human dental enamel comprises approximately 94 to 96% by weight of hydroxyapatite (HAP), with a nominal chemical formula of $Ca_{10}(PO_4)_6(OH)_2)$[74]. Because of the presence of carbonate (CO_3^{2-}), the enamel mineral is more properly termed a carbonated hydroxyapatite.

Numerous studies have shown that irradiation of human dental enamel with laser energy at particular wavelengths in the visible and infra-red regions results in greater resistance to acid and cariogenic attacks (see chapter 5). The effect was first documented in the early 1970s, but was not subjected to intense investigation until the mid 1980s[59,75,76].

Laser-activated fluoride forms an important part of the modern armamentarium for caries prevention. The value of laser treatment for caries prevention is now becoming recognised even by those outside the field of laser dentistry. For example, a recent review of emerging caries prevention strategies included an overview of some key studies in laser caries prevention[77]. The authors commented that the accumulated data from laboratory studies on lased enamel and dentin was very positive regarding the ability of laser treatment to increase the resistance of tooth structure to caries and acid attacks.

A common theme in studies of laser caries prevention is that the mechanism of action is complex, and involves both chemical and physical effects. The published literature suggests that slightly better results are obtained for visible lasers when the enamel or root surface site is first treated with fluoride (either neutral sodium fluoride, or acidulated phosphate fluoride) and then lased, compared with the reverse sequence.

For infrared lasers (CO_2 and Nd:YAG), the optimal sequence is the reverse. However, the therapeutic difference is so small as not to be clinically significant (typically 6-10 %), should the sequence be reversed[78–80].

The resistance conferred by laser irradiation alone, or laser irradiation combined with fluoride, is of considerable clinical importance. Using these therapies, the practicing dentist can alter the likelihood of caries initiation and caries progression in a patient with high caries risk. Even if caries does develop and progress, the depth of the lesion at a lased enamel or root surface site will be reduced by as much as one half compared with an unlased site.

In other words, laser preventive therapy can be applied to prevent caries developing, or to reduce the progression rate of existing lesions on the enamel and root surfaces of teeth[78,79,81].

4.6.1. Laser Preventive and Laser-Fluoride Effects on Enamel with the Argon Laser

Numerous studies have reported the beneficial effects of low fluence argon laser treatment on enamel in terms of increased caries resistance (Table 4-8). In a recent and typical in vitro study, irradiation with the argon laser (231 mW, 11.5 J/cm^2,10 seconds) reduced lesion depth by 15%, while there was a 33–46% decrease in lesion progression when using an artificial caries model to study caries initiation and progression[82].

Other studies have reported reductions of between 31and 50 % in caries initiation and progression, using similar laser parameters[70,78,79]. Taken together, the published in vitro studies have shown reductions in lesion depth, with only a few percentage points of difference between

Table 4-8 Laboratory studies of caries prevention using the argon laser.

Study	Power (mW)	Fluence (J/cm^2)	Spot size (mm)	Time (s)	ToothSurface
Hicks et al. 1993	250	12	–	10	Enamel
Westerman et al. 1994	231	11.5	5	10	Root
Hicks et al. 1995	2000	100	5	10	Root
Hicks et al. 1995	250	12	5	10	Enamel
Westerman et al. 1996	231	11.5	5	10	Enamel
	2000	100	5	10	Enamel
Hicks et al. 1997	250	12	–	10	Root
Westerman et al. 1999	230	11.5	5	10	Root
Blankenau et al. 1999	250	12	5	10	Enamel
Anderson et al. 2000	230	11.5	5	10	Enamel
Westerman et al. 2002	231	11.5	5	10	Enamel
	270	13.5	5	10	Enamel

low and moderate argon laser fluences (e.g. 10 vs. 100 J/cm^2).[70,78,79] Importantly, irradiation of tooth surfaces with low-fluence argon laser radiation (250 mW, 12 J/cm^2, 10 seconds) has been shown to reduce demineralisation of tooth structure under clinical conditions.[83]

In the most recent laboratory study of the argon laser preventive effect, Westerman et al.[82] exposed buccal windows of sound enamel on 20 molar teeth to low-fluence argon laser irradiation, while the lingual windows of enamel served as matched controls. Caries-like lesions in the enamel were then created using an acidified gel. Longitudinal sections were evaluated by polarized light microscopy to assess the depth of the body of the lesion after lesion initiation (8 weeks) and lesion progression (12 weeks): Depths for lesion initiation and progression were reduced by 61-78 % at 8 weeks, and 50-69 % at 12 weeks. Thus, argon laser irradiation may be particularly useful for reducing the caries susceptibility of sound enamel in at-risk patients, and may also have value for treating white spot lesions.

At first, it was thought that the preventive effect was due to the λ = 488 nm (blue) rather than the λ = 514.5 nm (green) wavelength of the argon laser. Nevertheless, all but one laboratory study of the caries preventive effects of the argon laser have used just the blue wavelength[70], and thus could not validly compare the two.

More recent work in our laboratory using a range of visible-light laser wavelengths has shown that preventive effects do in fact occur with visible green wavelengths, including that from the KTP laser (λ = 532 nm).

The combination of low-fluence argon laser radiation (10-12 J/cm^2, 10 seconds) with fluoride preparations results in even greater reduction in lesion depth than when either modality is used alone. Fox et al.[65] demonstrated that the combination of laser irradiation and fluoride greatly decreased mineral loss after a strong acid challenge, relative to unlased enamel. Lesion depth reductions with argon laser combined with 1.23% acidulated phosphate fluoride (APF) have been reported as 25%[85], >50%[78], and 51-55%[84].

Because these findings are similar to the results obtained with moderate fluence levels (100 J/cm^2), clinically one only needs to employ lower fluence levels in order to achieve a useful result. When argon lasers are used for resin polymerization[8,10,47] or for photochemical whitening (Smartbleach®), the opportunity presents at the same appointment to treat the teeth with laser-fluoride combination therapy, with the aim of reducing the risk of further caries.

Moreover, there are data indicating that the fluoride preparation does not have to be acidulated in order to obtain a laser-fluoride effect. In a recent laboratory study, Anderson et al.[85] reported that the combination of the argon laser and 2% neutral sodium fluoride gave a reduction in lesion progression of 29%.

4.6.2 Mechanisms of Action: Enamel

A variety of mechanisms involving chemical or physico-chemical changes have been postulated to explain laser preventive and LAF (Laser activated fluorides) effects. A decrease in the permeability or solubility of enamel (or a combination of both) is a common explanation for the effect of laser radiation on enamel.[86–88]

Studies of the effect of laser irradiation on human dental enamel have reported changes in the crystal structure of hydroxyapatite, together with a reduction in the extent of dissolution following acid challenge[76,89,90]. Scanning electron microscope studies of the effect of CO_2 laser on enamel reveal that the type of structural change induced in enamel by lasing is influenced by both the wavelength and the fluence of the laser radiation[57].

Fowler and Kuroda[86,87] have suggested that irradiation with high-intensity infrared laser radiation ultimately leads to the formation of pyrophosphate, which is responsible for decreased enamel solubility in acidic conditions. According to their predictions, the temperature at the laser-irradiated enamel surface increases from the ambient temperature to reach approximately 1400°C. Based upon this temperature range, they predicted that several phase changes would occur with lasing, one of which was the conversion of hydroxyapatite to beta-TCP (beta-$Ca_3(PO_4)_2$).

Fox et al.[65] have demonstrated that enamel lased with the CO_2 laser (continuous wave, 65 J/cm^2 for 2 seconds) has a reduced dissolution rate. Furthermore, in a separate study, the same group demonstrated that laser irradiation of enamel reduces the critical pH at which enamel dissolution occurs, from 5.5 to 4.8.

This critical pH is further reduced in the presence of fluoride, even at concentrations as low as 0.01 ppm, to 4.3[65,91]. This reduced critical pH means that the quantity of acetic acid necessary to reach the new threshold level is increased by six-fold. Comparison of the lased and unlased enamel that had been exposed to CO_2 laser radiation at the above parameters has confirmed reduced solubility by a factor of 6[65]. The same study also noted that enamel irradiated with the CO_2 laser had a greater affinity for calcium, fluoride and phosphate ions, a feature also noted after treatment of enamel with the argon laser[92].

Oho and Morioka[18] have reported that continuous-wave argon laser irradiation of tooth enamel (67 J/cm^2) leads to a reduction in water, carbonate and organic substances, resulting in the creation of 'microspaces'. The presence of these microspaces accounts for the observed increased uptake of fluoride in lased enamel. While the presence of microspaces could potentially be interpreted as areas of weakness, it must be recalled that during demineralization, a variety of ions are released from the enamel matrix and are leached out. Instead of diffusing into the surrounding environment, these ions become trapped in the microspaces. This effect may be due to the altered charge or surface reactivity of the molecules lining these spaces.

In terms of direct chemical changes, the creation of new products by laser radiation has been reported. Direct evidence for conversion of human enamel to α-tri-calcium phosphate and/or tetra-calcium phosphate, using Raman spectroscopy, has been presented.[93] In this study, enamel was exposed to CO_2 laser radiation, using irradiation conditions shown previously to give surface fusion (single pulse, spot size 0.8 mm, pulse duration 200 milliseconds, power 10 W, energy density 67 J/cm^2, power density 1700 W/cm^2)[93,94].

For comparative purposes, samples of enamel, tri-calcium phosphate (TCP) and pure hydroxyapatite were heated in air in a temperature-controlled furnace to 1200°C, and maintained at that temperature for one hour. The Raman spectra were recorded using both dispersive and Fourier-transformed (FT) Raman spectroscopy. When the spectra of laser-treated enamel were compared to heat-treated specimens of hydroxyapatite and enamel, it became clear that laser irradiation induced chemical changes which differed from those induced by heat treatment. Comparing the Raman spectra of lased enamel to hydroxyapatite and TCP, it was evident that high-fluence CO_2 laser irradiation of enamel caused the partial conversion of hydroxyapatite to TCP. These phases are only seen after treatment with the CO_2 laser at high energy densities, which causes dramatic elevations of the surface temperature. This effect is in contrast to the low energy densities used with the argon laser[18], which did no elicit such thermal changes.

In the study of Aminzadeh et al.[95], the effect of high-fluence CO_2 laser radiation was not merely a simple local heating effect as previously thought, since simple heating of enamel led to the formation of both TCP and $Ca(OH)_2$, while laser treatment of enamel resulted in the formation of TCP, but not $Ca(OH)_2$. These findings are consistent with the conclusions of other workers[96], which were based on infrared spectroscopy.

Thus, at a temperature of 1200°C, enamel partly converts to TCP and $Ca(OH)_2$. As suggested by Aminzadeh et al.[95], this can also be expressed chemically using an alternative chemical formula for hydroxyapatite: 3 molecules of TCP and one of $Ca(OH)_2$, that is $3Ca_3(PO_4)_2 \cdot Ca(OH)_2$, as opposed to the more common presentation of the formula, $Ca_{10}(PO_4)_6(OH)_2$.

Further mechanisms for LAF that have been proposed include:

1. The creation of surface coating, on lased tooth structure, which increases the affinity for fluoride, calcium and phosphate ions from endogenous and exogenous sources;
2. Swelling and denaturation of proteins on the enamel surface, with subsequent sealing of the surface pores;
3. Alterations of micro-organisms in plaque that may be irradiated; and
4. Stabilization and decreased solubility of hydroxyapatite[17,18,70,78–80].

Scanning electron microscopic (SEM) examination of enamel laser with the argon laser shows that modifications of proteins or minerals on or in the surface can occur. Westerman et al.[92] have shown that argon laser irradiated enamel has a slightly roughened surface, with sporadic globular deposits, and some micro-porosities (< 1 micron in diameter).

These features are exhibited after either high or low fluence argon laser irradiation. The surface area is increased in the former, while reduced surface micro-porosites are seen in the latter. The lased surface is rich in calcium, phosphate and fluoride ions, which optimises its resistance to a cariogenic attack.

4.6.3 Mechanisms of Action: Root Surfaces

Unlike enamel, the root surface of a tooth is more susceptible to acid dissolution and caries, a property attributed to its lower solubility product and higher critical pH.[97] Both dentin and cementum have a much lower mineral content and a correspondingly greater organic matrix content than enamel. Thus, during a cariogenic attack, the collagen-based organic component of the matrix can be degraded by bacterial enzymes while the lesser mineral phases are quickly solubilized by organic acids. Nevertheless, root surfaces exhibit a much greater ability to uptake fluoride than enamel, and demonstrate increased fluoride levels with advancing age.

Although irradiation of the root surface has been shown to be very effective at reducing caries susceptibility, the combination of fluoride with the argon laser is even more potent. Hicks et al.[78] reported a 54% reduction in lesion depth for teeth that had been treated with the argon laser (200 mW, 100 J/cm^2, 10 seconds) and acidulated phosphate fluoride (1.23 %) together. The combination resulted in a synergistic effect, gaining a greater reduction in lesion depth than either laser or fluoride alone.

Hicks et al.[78] have proposed that laser radiation may create a micro-sieve network in the root surface in the same way that micro-spaces are created in enamel. As in enamel, these micro-sieves may trap some of the more soluble mineral phases, effectively limiting the formation of a carious lesion.

Several studies have compared the surface morphology created by laser irradiation alone, fluoride alone, or the two in combination when used in a root surface. Scanning electron microscopic examination of a sound root surface shows a relatively smooth, undulating appearance, with no cavitations or exposure of dentinal tubules[97,98]. Root surfaces that have been exposed to acidulated phosphate fluoride alone show a homogeneous surface coating, with sporadic granular deposits (< 1 micron in diameter).[97] Irradiation of the root surface with low-fluence argon laser radiation alone (231 mW, 11.5 J/cm^2, 10 seconds) creates an irregular, roughened surface with frequent granular and globular deposits (1–3 microns in dimension) and micro-porosities (< 1 micron in diameter).[98] These microporosities are believed to aid in the uptake of fluoride, enhancing resistance to caries attack.

A similar morphological appearance is attained when the treatment is undertaken with the argon laser at a high fluence (100 J/cm^2); however the particle size is slightly greater (> 2 microns), and there are more pores and surface depressions (2–3 microns). The combination of the argon laser and fluoride results in a root surface with a homogenous appearance, and more prominent and frequent, globular, adherent precipitates (1–2 microns). The morphology of these deposits resembles calcium fluoride (CaF_2).[97] From this, it appears that argon laser irradiation of the fluoride treated root surface unveils the dense coating created by the fluoride, exposing the underlying globular and spherical deposits (presumably CaF_2).

There is no damage to the root surface at either low or high fluence levels with the argon laser, and no evidence of cavitation, crazing or cratering.[92,97] The cementum shows no voids, and there is no exposure of the dentinal tubules. This is in sharp contrast to the thermal effects which can occur when infrared lasers are used at high fluence on the root surface.

4.7 General Considerations

Argon laser curing of light-activated materials adds substantial benefits to the clinical behavior of tooth restorations in time and allows the practitioner a more relaxed, but secure and safe way of operation. Nevertheless, one has to take into consideration the narrow bandwidth or spectral emission of an argon laser, and the ever extending list of new and improved devices for photopolymerization.

A concern while using an argon laser as a curing device is its limited spectral emission (Fig 4-30)[99].

Besides camphoroquinone (CQ), other photoinitiators can be used to induce photopolymerization. Due to the slightly yellow color of camphoroquinone, phenyl-propanedione (PPD) or Lucerin TPO (L TPO) may be used, especially when dealing with very light colors of composite materials such as the special "bleaching colors". These photo-initiators have a different SR or spectral requirement[5] than CQ has[99], given that the SE or spectral emission[5] of an argon laser overlaps the absorption range of PPD only in a limited way, but does not overlap at all nor is congruent with the absorption range of L TPO (Fig 4-31)[99].

Before using an argon laser as a curing device, the manufacturer's instructions for use have to be consulted to be sure the product's spectral emission for photopolymerization (SE) and the (EOP and D) energy density for optimal polymerization at a specified depth are congruent with the features of the laser device used.

Furthermore, the "conventional VLC" devices are being replaced by "improved" ones with increased power- and energy densities. Obviously, there was a strong need for this as the minimum energy density for proper polymerization should be 400 mW/cm^2 [5] and this was rarely obtained with the conventional halogen lamps[99].

But as with all halogen-light-based curing devices, energy output decreases with time, even with the improved devices[99], and a proper radiant exitance meter has to be used regularly to measure the real irradiance (W/cm^2).

Plasma lamps with a narrow bandwidth were followed by plasma lamps with broader bandwidths to overcome the problem of insufficient spectral emission. A problem with all plasma lamp devices is that they generate an improper polymerization at the curing times recommended by the manufacturer, resulting in a conversion rate far too low and an insufficient Vickers hardness at depth[99].

The first generation of LEDs had a limited spectral emission and the energy densities they

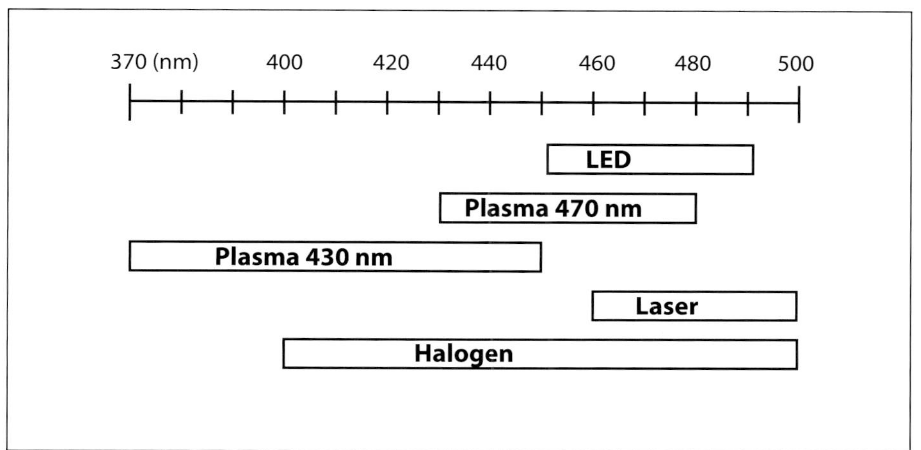

Fig 4-30 Emission spectra (According to Burtscher[99]).

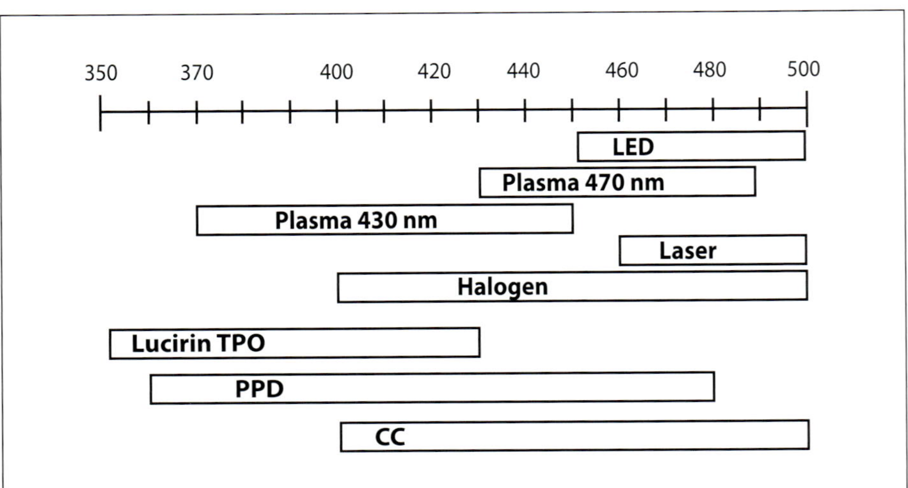

Fig 4-31 Initiators and light sources (According to Burtscher[99]).

could generate were too low. The next generation of "super LEDs" dealt with the problem of insufficient power output. And the latest generation of super LEDs with a broad bandwidth incorporate two types of diodes with different wavelength peaks, designed to activate separate photo-initiators and produce proper polymerization in depth[99]. The search for the ideal curing device is a difficult task, and the choice for it should be based upon a profound knowledge of the pros and contras of each device and upon the personal needs and demands of the operator.

4.8 Clinical Procedure of Photopolymerization by an Argon Laser

Photopolymerization of light-cured dental materials by means of an argon laser provides superior clinical results. Failures due to improper clinical handling or technical problems can be reduced. The technique offers a reduction of 75% in curing time. The distance to the light source is not as critical compared to VLC. The energy flow is controllable and adjustable. The physical properties of the light-cured material are improved, and reduced pulp irritation and lower post-operative sensitivity are demonstrated. It offers a better management of the inherent polymerization shrinkage with an improved adhesion and marginal seal. In addition to the decay-prevention properties of the argon laser, long-lasting clinical results may be predicted.

Good access to the material to be polymerized is a critical prerequisite when using VLC[5]. Albers et al.[5] demonstrated that while curing with visible light, not only the distance of the light source to the surface to be polymerized, but even the angle of the light source to the filling surface, are important[5] (Figs 4-32 to 4-34). And that due to a limited penetration depth of this multi-wavelength energy source, the conversion rate of the filling material decreases when depth increases[5] (Fig 4-35).

The thin delivery fiber of 200 or 300 mm, the small sterilizable hand piece and the disposable flexible tips of a laser device, allow easy access throughout the various regions of the mouth and may counteract these limitations of VLC devices, plasma lamps, PACs and LEDs. Furthermore, the easy access, together with the higher penetration depth of this single-wavelength energy source, enables polymerization through enamel and dentin layers (Figs. 4-36 to 4-41).

The tip diameter of conventional curing devices determines the number of curing cycles required for the full coverage of the surface of a composite layer[54] (Fig 4-42).

The spotsize of a laser device, however, is adjustable, making it possible to access the depth

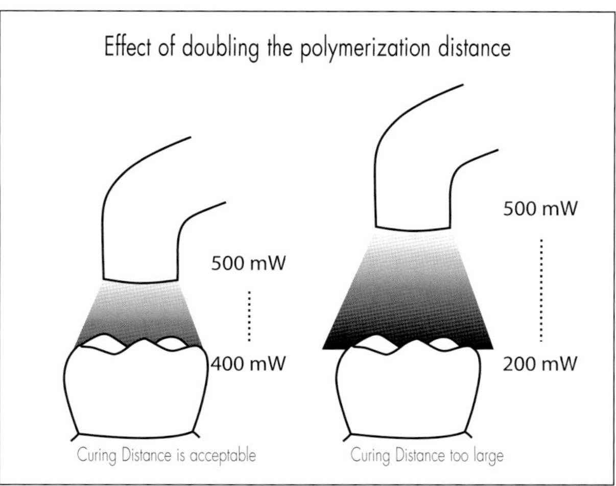

Fig 4-32 With deep restorations and those with poor access, the distance between the light guide and the composite can increase. This will generally reduce the power density at the surface by over 70% (According to Albers et al.[5]).

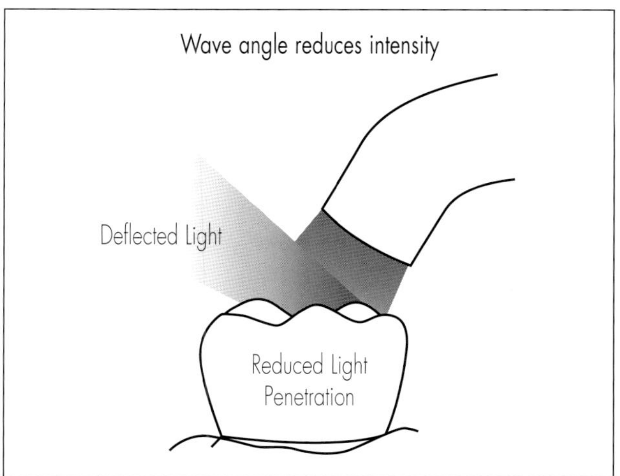

Fig 4-33 Light applied at an angle will reflect from a surface, which reduces its penetration into a composite (According to Albers et al.[5]).

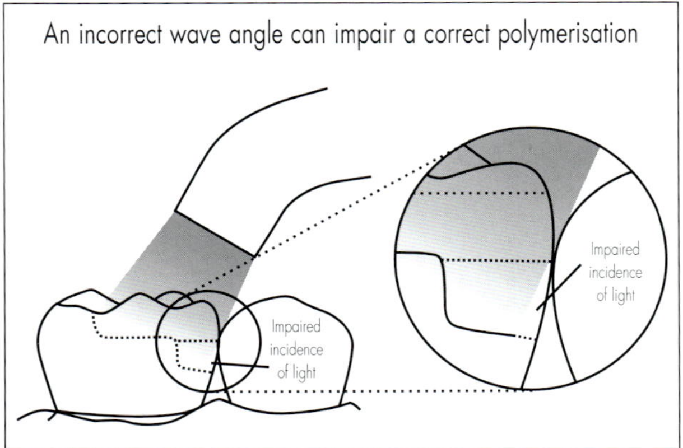

Fig 4-34 With deep restorations, particularly those far back in the arch, a direct path of light to the entire restoration can be blocked. The critical area of the gingival margin is most commonly affected (According to Albers et al.[5]).

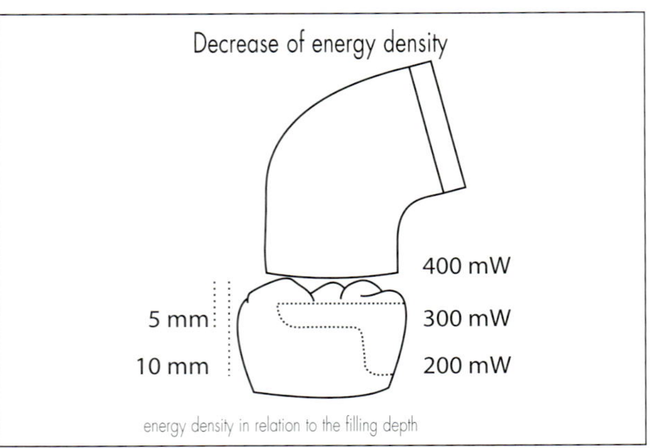

Fig 4-35 This illustration shows a 50% decrease in light intensity to deeper areas of the preparation (According to Albers et al.[5]).

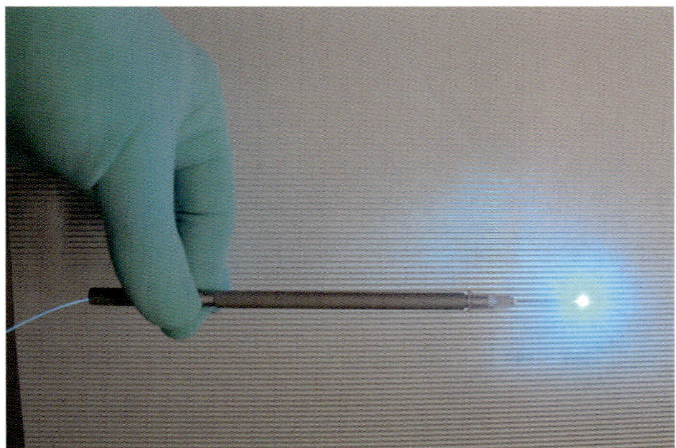

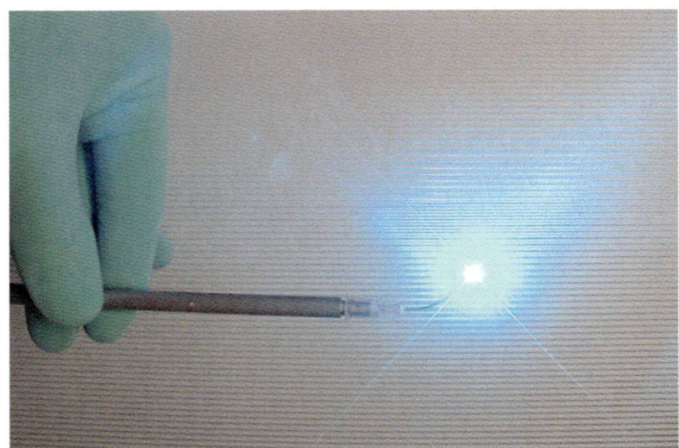

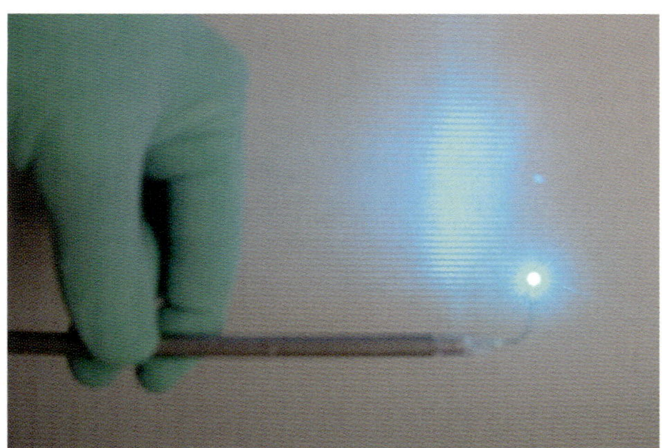

Fig 4-36–4-38 Thin delivery fiber. Small, sterilizable handpiece with flexible disposable tips.

of a distal interproximal cavity (Figs 4-39 and 4-40) as well as the full labial surface of the upper front teeth (Fig 4-41), eliminating the need for multiple curing cycles, and eliminating the need for an extended number of light guides[54] (Fig 4-43).

Bracket bonding can be achieved by a lateral exposure, with an immediate and superior bond and a decrease in acid solubility of the surrounding enamel, and an equal prevention of the appearance of white spot lesions[26] (Figs 4-44 and 4-45).

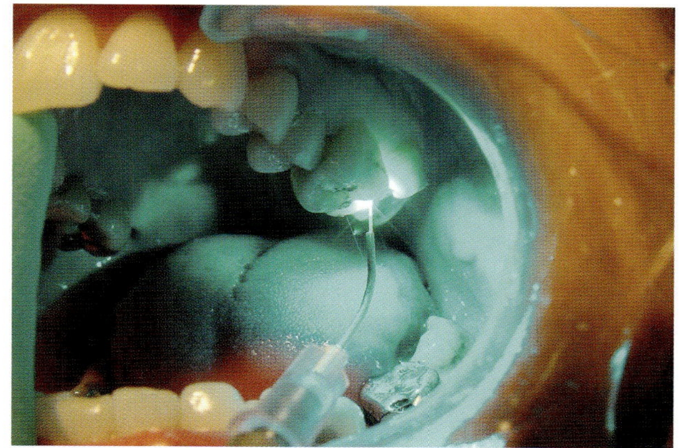

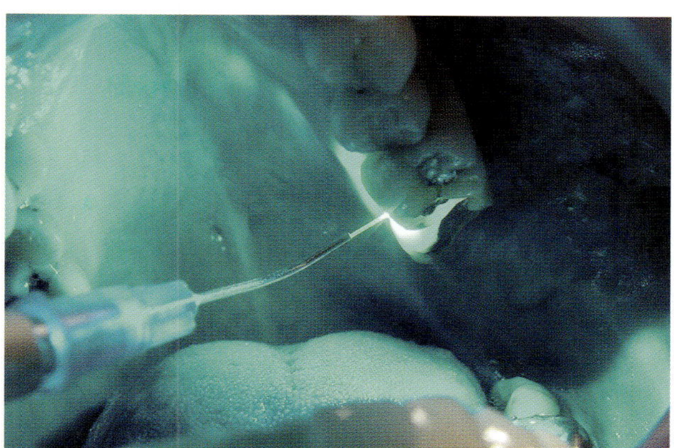

Fig 4-39 and 4-40 Easy accessibility to different areas of the oral cavity.

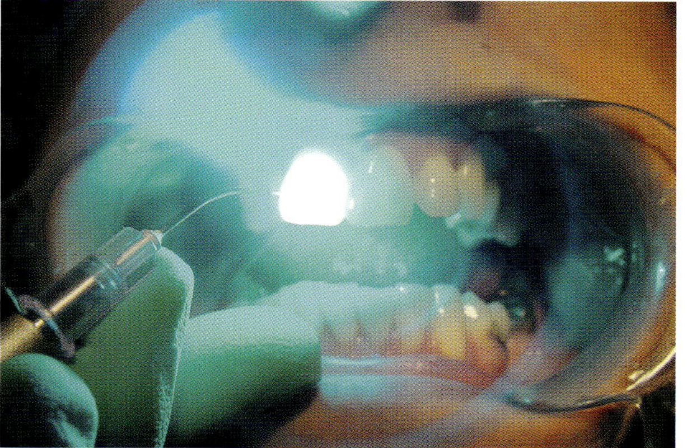

Fig 4-41 Adjustable spot size, covering an entire labial surface.

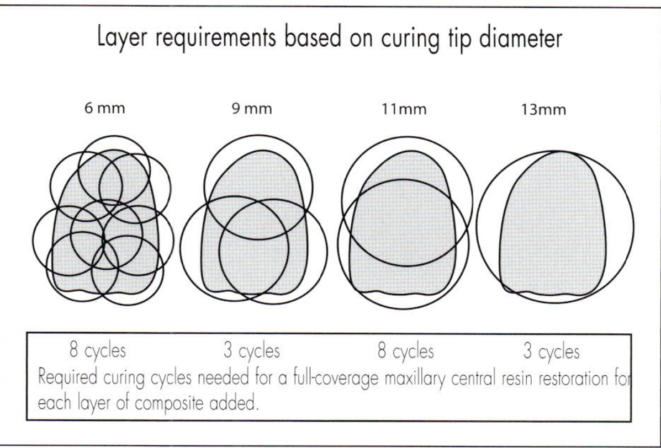

Fig 4-42 Layer requirements based on curing tip diameter (according to Albers[54]).

Fig 4-43 Typical light guides for a visible light curing system (according to Albers[54]).

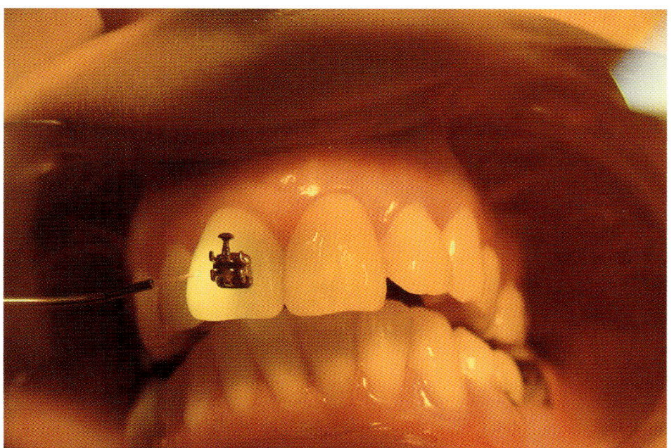

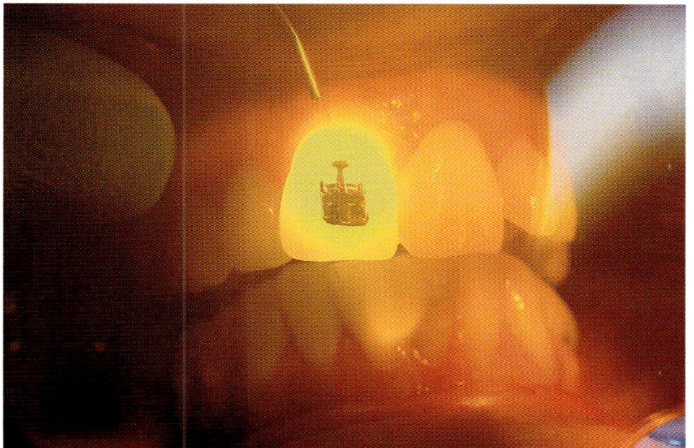

Fig 4-44 and 4-45 Bracket bonding technique together with caries prophylaxis

4.9 Clinical Cases

4.9.1 Introduction

In daily practice, the marked reduction of exposure time represents the greatest advantage of photopolymerization. Clinicians are than more likely to respect incremental filling techniques. Good access to all cavities, and the right quality and quantity of light energy, results in superior clinical performance of the cured filling materials[26].

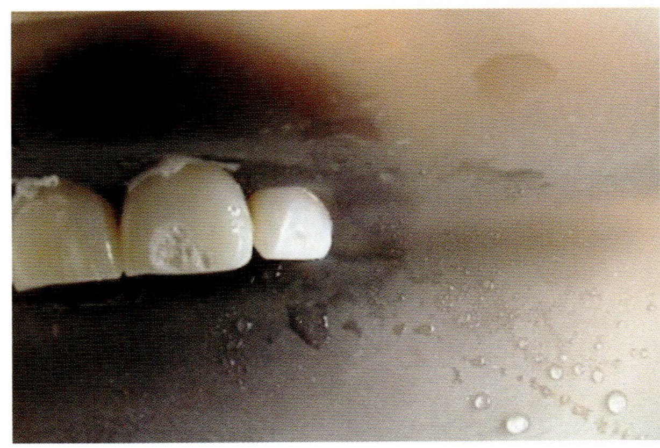

Fig 4-46b

Case 1

A 13-year-old girl with pronounced white-spot lesions on the central incisors (Fig 4-46a). Demineralized zones were carefully removed with an Er:YAG laser (Figs 4-46b,c), and bonding material was applied (Fig 4-46d) and photopolymerized. Final result after finishing and polishing shows fine esthetics (Fig 4-46e).

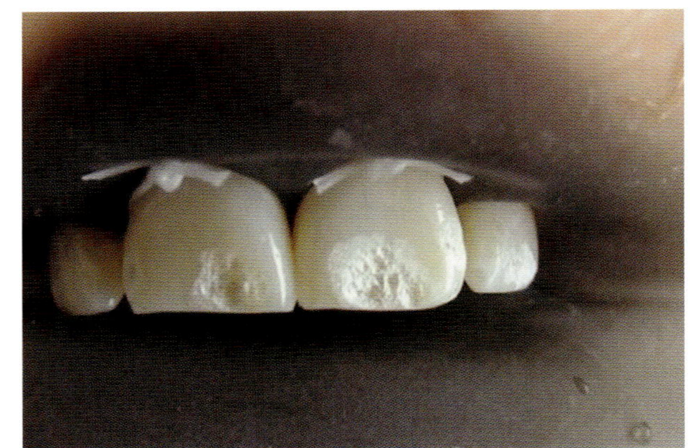

Fig 4-46c

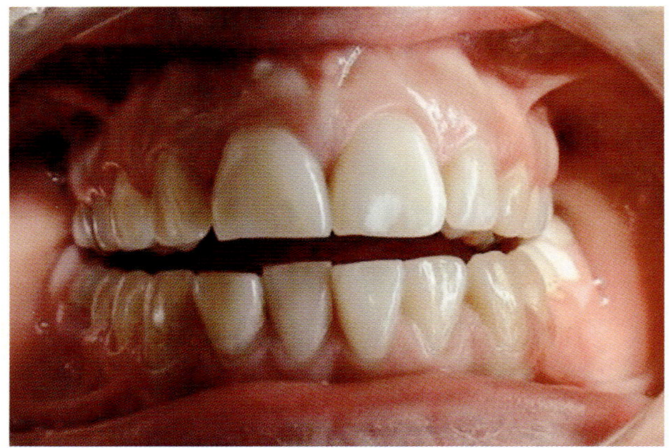

Fig 4-46a

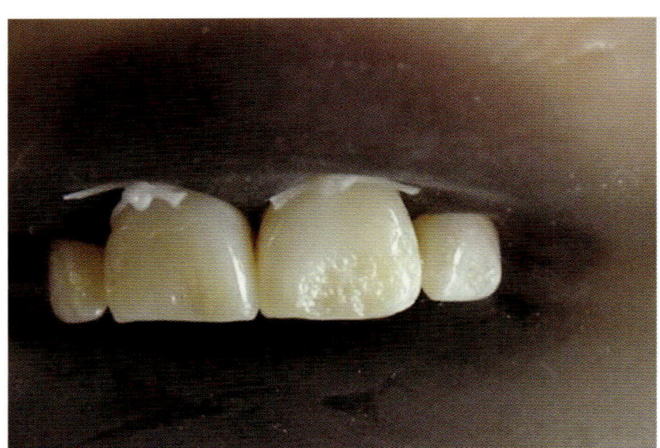

Fig 4-46d

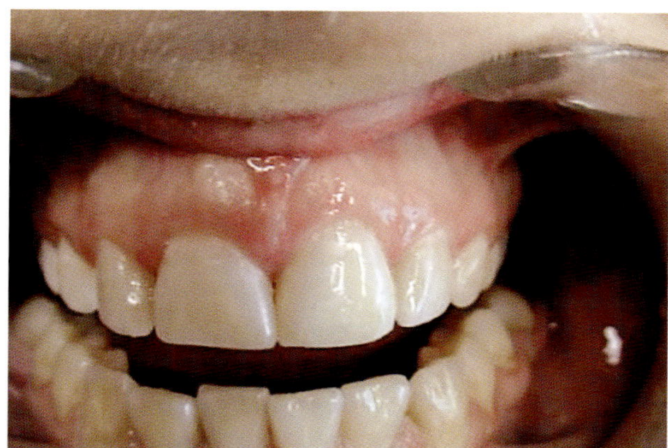

Fig 4-46e

These cases generally offer no problems: no difficult layer technique, and easy access to the composite to be cured. In function, there is less direct loading on these fillings, and less stress is generated..

The following examples demonstrate extreme cases of direct composite techniques, in which the use of laser photopolymerization offers additional benefits in achieving good clinical and long-lasting results.

The choice of direct composite techniques was to preserve as much sound tooth structure as possible. The financial situation of the patient to be treated is also a consideration. In some cases, extraction was the only other treatment option.

4.9.2 Esthetic Dentistry

Direct resin placement offers a technique with unlimited possibilities. It is more conservative and requires less preparation than veneers or crowns. The practitioner can control the clinical outcome. There is a superior bond to enamel and dentin, with less marginal gap formation.

Laser photopolymerization can reduce treatment time. The higher degree of polymerization, i.e., conversion rate, results in less shipping and an increased surface hardness with improved long-term esthetics. If proper polishing is performed, restorations maintain their condition, lustre and brightness. The unpolymerized surface layer has to be removed due to inhibited polymerization caused by the presence of oxygen. This removal should be performed with rubbers with water-cooling and pastes, rather than burs or slices. Ideally, the final composite layer should be shaped to its finished form before curing. This can be achieved by using porcelain brushes, as used by dental technicians. Thin aluminum foil can be inserted interproximally, and placed on to the adjacent teeth, instead of thick plastic strips that adhere to the composite material. Profin® (Dentatus, Sweden) offers superior gingival recontouring and finishing[26].

Case 2

A 29-year-old male patient wanted to improve esthetics in the upper front region. The existing composite fillings mesial on teeth 11 and 21 were renewed, other front teeth veneered (Figs 4-47a,b).

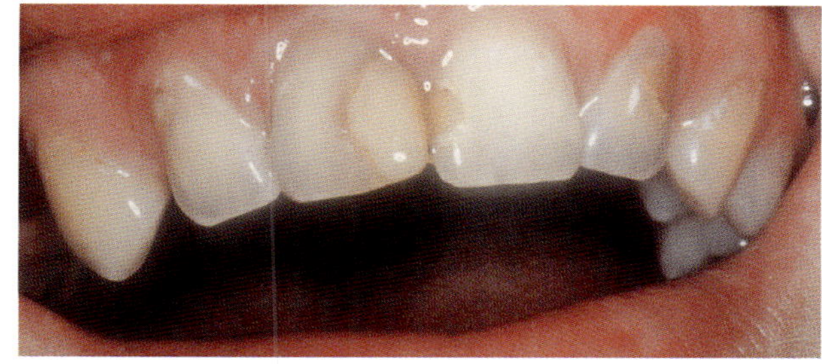

Fig 4-47a

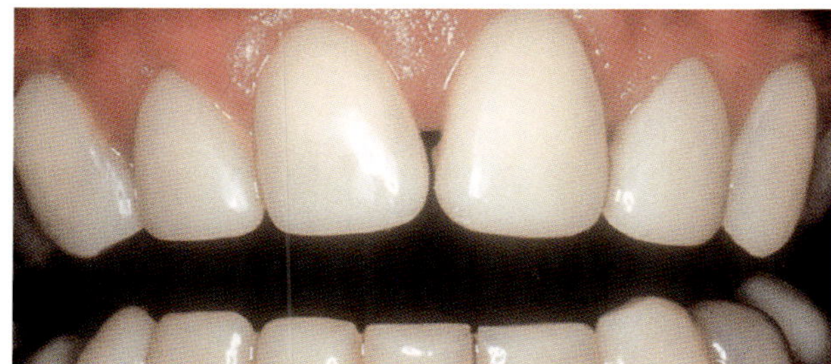

Fig 4-47b

Case 3

The same request from a 32-year-old female patient. Failing composite restorations were replaced (Figs 4-48a,b).

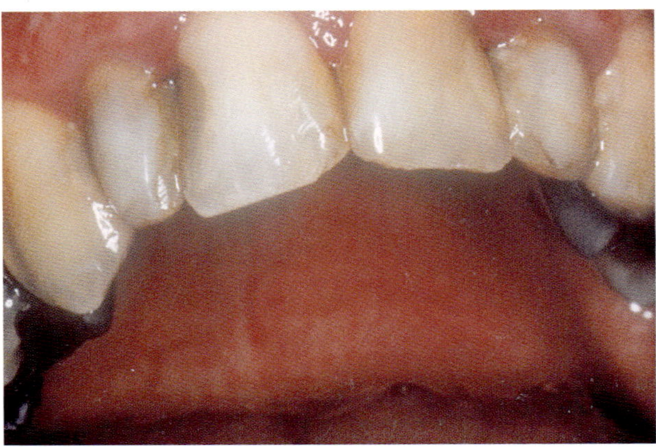
Fig 4-48a

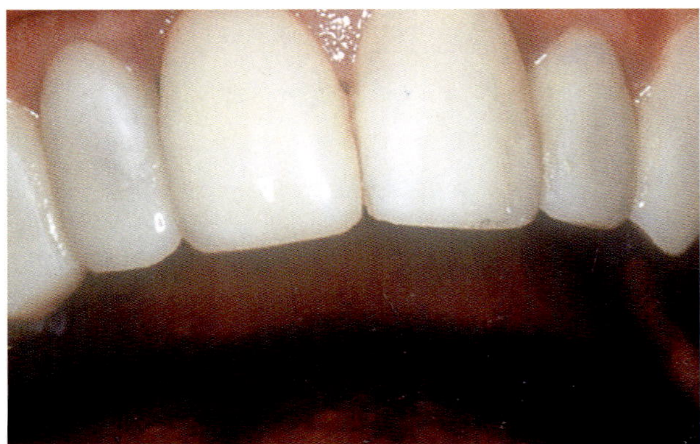
Fig 4-48b

Case 4

Full upper and lower treatment from second premolar to second premolar in a 38-year-old male patient. Apart from poor esthetics, there was a high degree of demineralization and loss of enamel due to working in the chemical industry (Figs 4-49a,b).

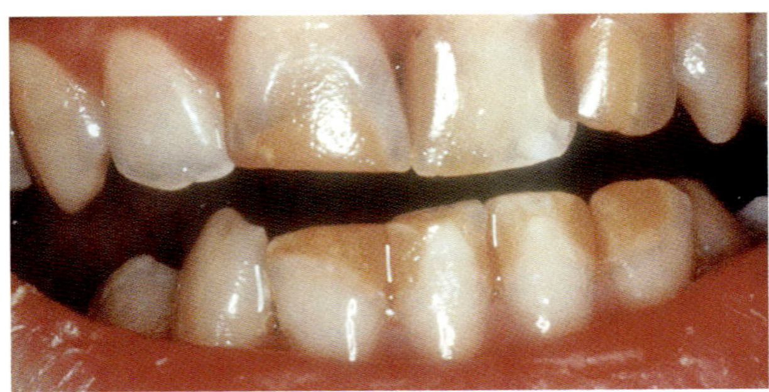
Fig 4-49a

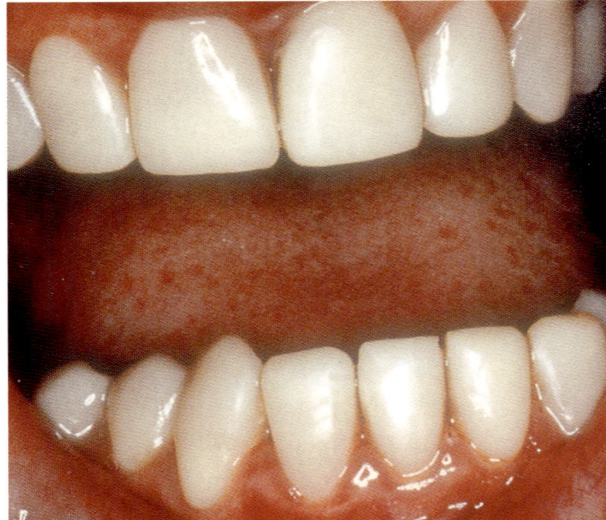
Fig 4-49b

Case 5

A 34-year-old male patient showing amelogenesis imperfecta with malformations, agenesis of the lateral upper incisors and very poor quality of enamel, also with esthetic problems (Figs 4-50a–c).

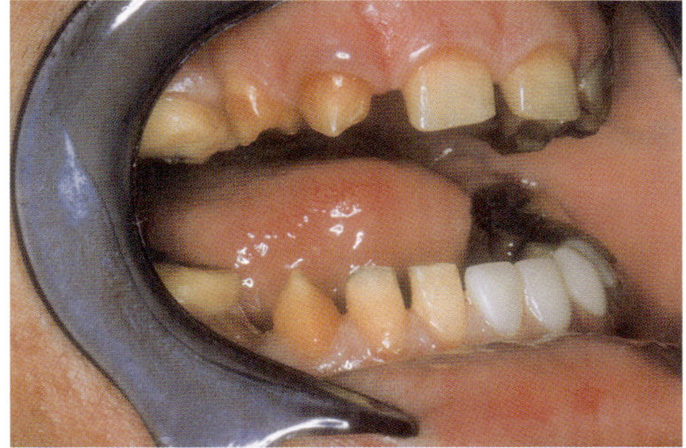

Fig 4-50a

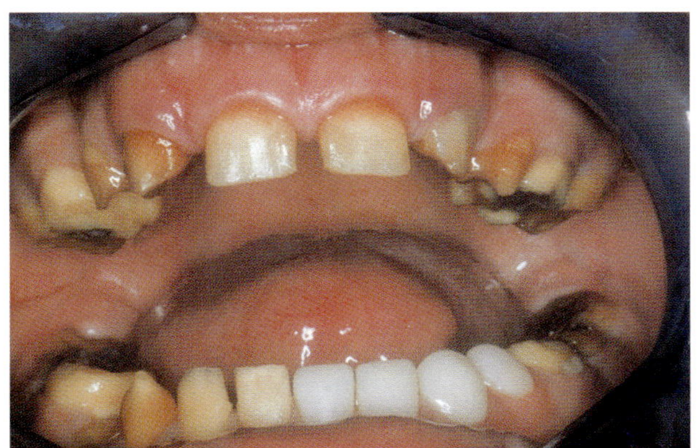

Fig 4-50b

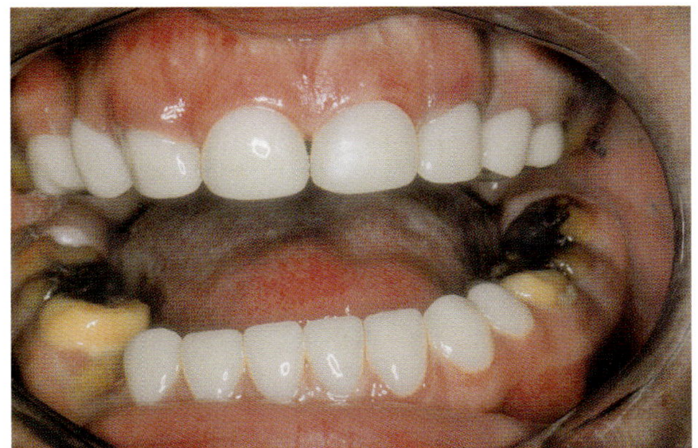

Fig 4-50c

Case 6

Poor esthetics with bad gingival adaptation of the six existing metal–resin crowns in the upper front. Improved esthetics and gingival conditions after removal of the resin and reshaping the metal of the crowns, followed by direct composite veneering in a 28-year-old male patient (Figs 4-51a,b).

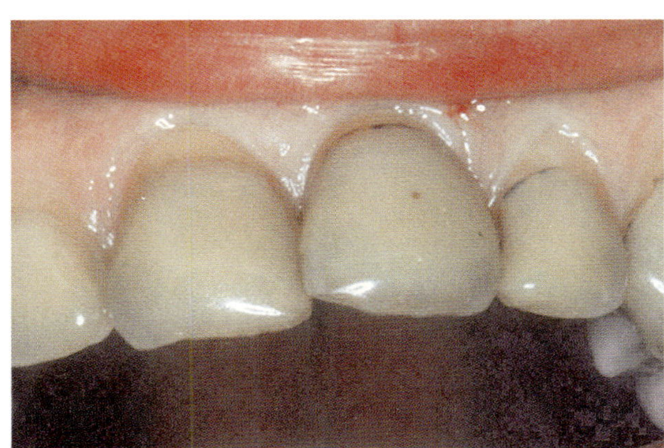

Fig 4-51a

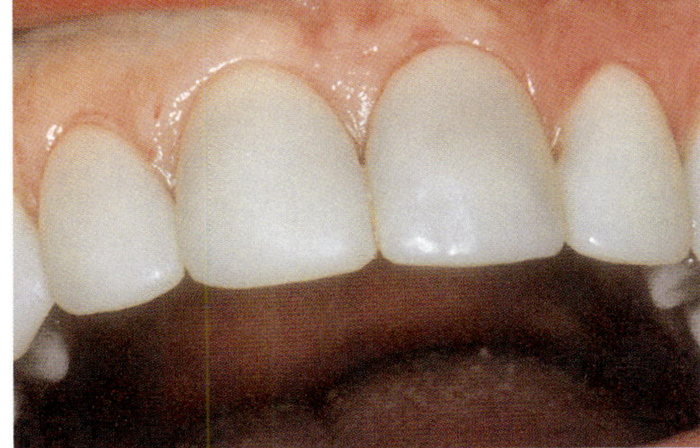

Fig 4-51b

Case 7

Same request from a 24-year-old female not happy with the outcome of metal–ceramic restorations on the central and lateral upper incisors. Conditioning of porcelain with very aggressive and toxic hydrogen fluoride (HF) can be replaced by air-abrasion techniques. In addition, with a proper ceramic-liner or silane agent, sufficient clinical bonding can be achieved with improved esthetics (Figs 4-52a,b).

Case 8

Severe tetracycline staining together with an unesthetic inclination of the central incisors in a 33-year-old male patient. Only the extended parts of the incisors were ground, retaining tooth vitality and achieving a good esthetic result (Figs 4-53a,b).

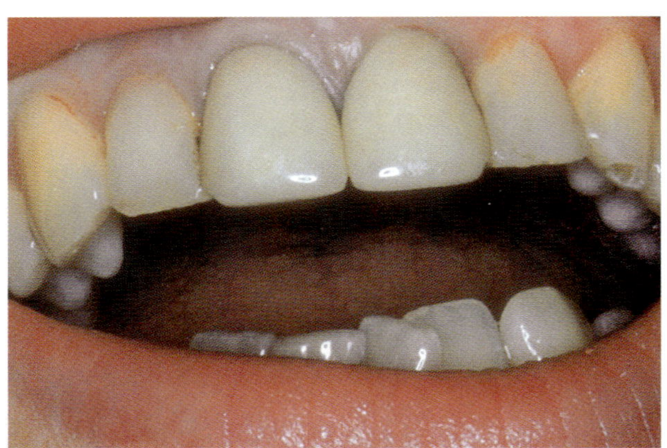

Fig 4-52a

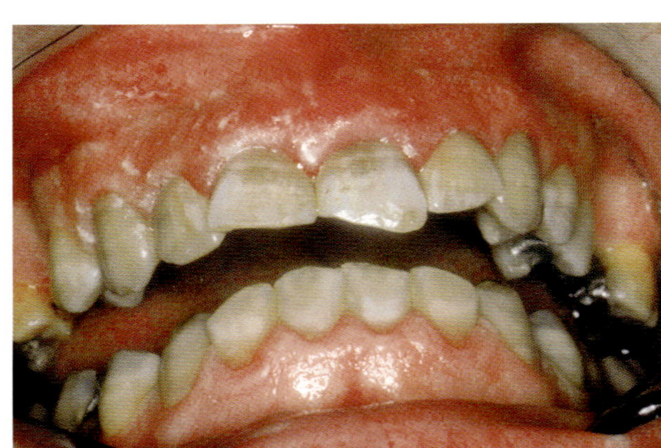

Fig 4-53a

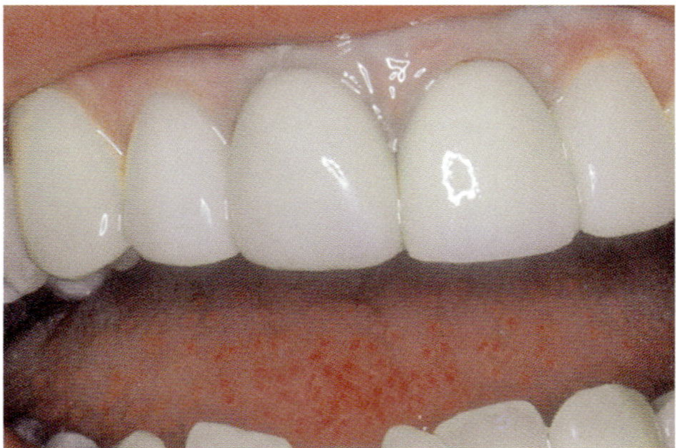

Fig 4-52b

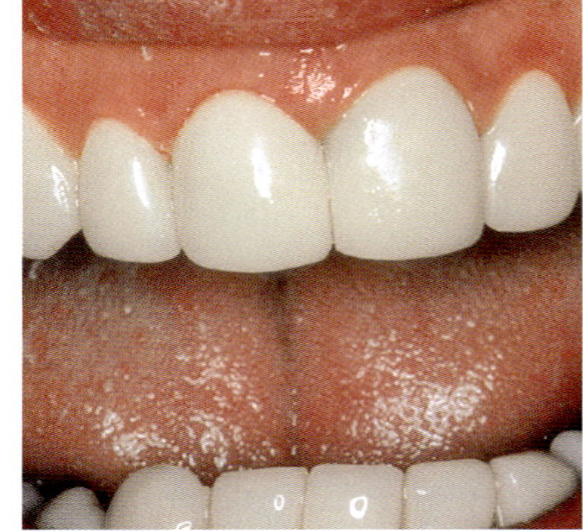

Fig 4-53b

Case 9

Several cases demonstrate the good clinical outcome over a period of time. Composite veneers in a 36-year-old female patient after 9 years in function (Fig 4-54a). In a 33-year-old female patient after 7 years (Fig 4-54b). After 8 years in a 38-year-old female patient (Fig 4-54c).

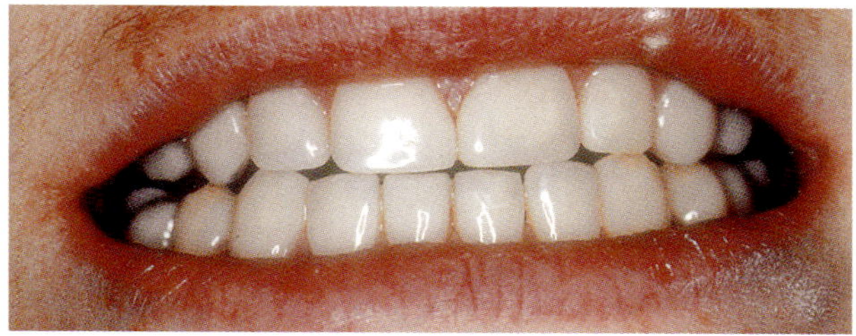
Fig 4-54a

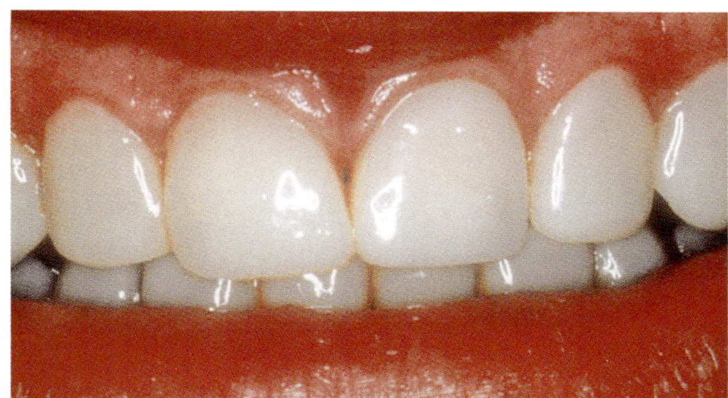
Fig 4-54b

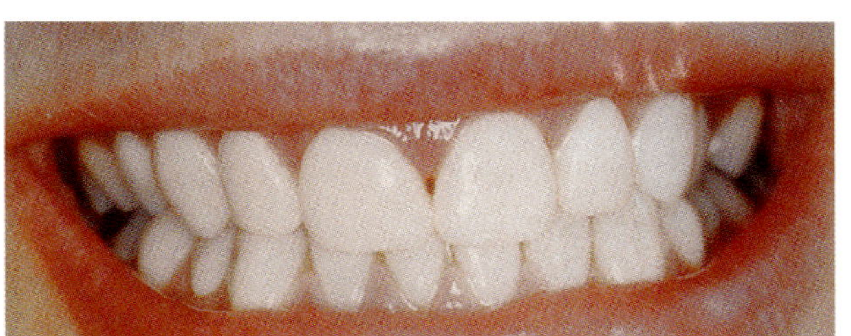
Fig 4-54c

Case 10

Proper reparation after failure of a veneer or after an accident can easily be achieved. A 40-year-old male patient showed an incisal fracture in the composite on tooth 12 after a car accident. The patient also presented a deep mesio-incisal fracture of tooth 21 and a complete loss of the crown of the right central incisor. Invisible restorations can be achieved. Once the oxygen-inhibited surface layer of the composite material is gone, it is not possible to achieve proper bonding. It is therefore important to condition the remaining composite and this can be done by air-abrasion or erbium-YAG laser. Special composite bonding agents should be used (Figs 4-55a,b).

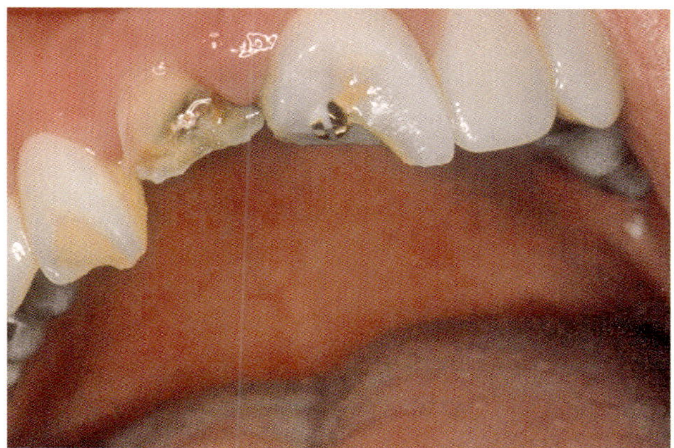
Fig 4-55a

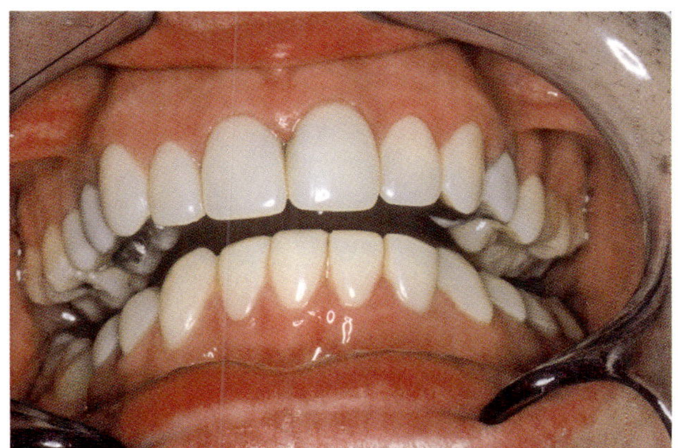
Fig 4-55b

4.9.3 High Caries Sensitivity

The higher acid resistance of enamel and dentin after argon laser irradiation during photopolymerization of the filling materials offers substantial benefits in these cases. Sensitivity to caries decreases. Furthermore, the decrease in polymerization shrinkage stresses improves bonding, and a good marginal seal with less gap formation can be achieved. Bacterial infiltration, and hence secondary decay, can be reduced. The lower build up of heat in the vital pulp reduces post-operative sensitivity, certainly in deep dentin lesions. Higher conversion rates with a smaller quantity of residual monomers means less toxicity for the pulp[26].

Case 11

A high caries incidence in a 47-year-old male patient produced poor esthetics and a neglected appearance (Fig 4-56b). As a salesman, he wished to improve his appearance. Previous restorations failed shortly after treatment, and consequently the patient did not visit a dentist for some time. Proper clinical techniques combined with argon laser photopolymerization offer substantially improved clinical performance of the restorations with equally satisfactory esthetics (Figs 4-56a–d).

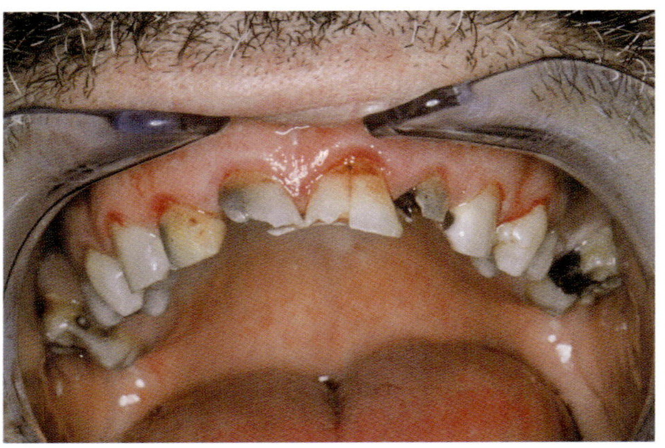

Fig 4-56a

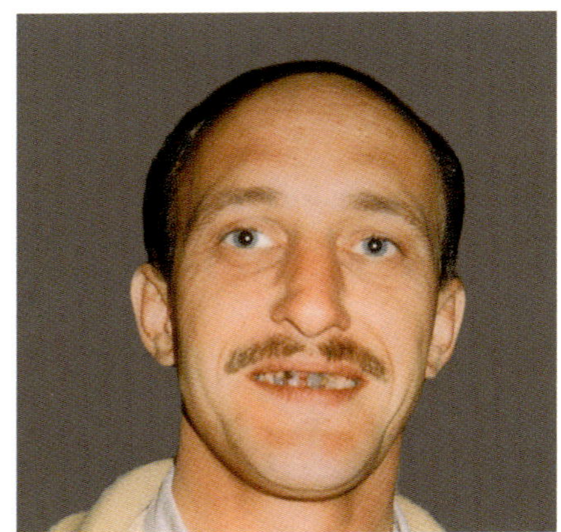

Fig 4-56b

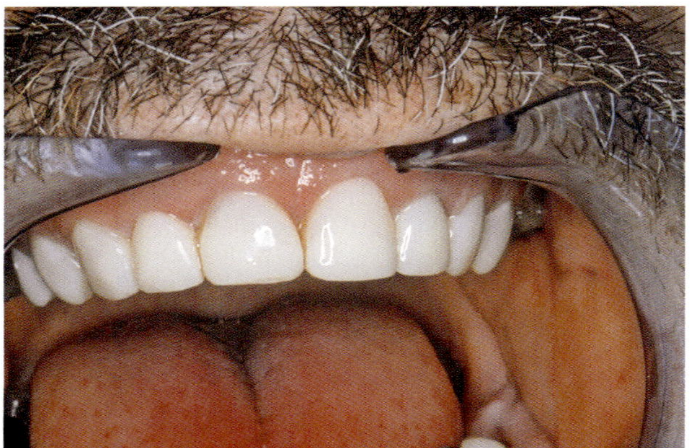

Fig 4-56c

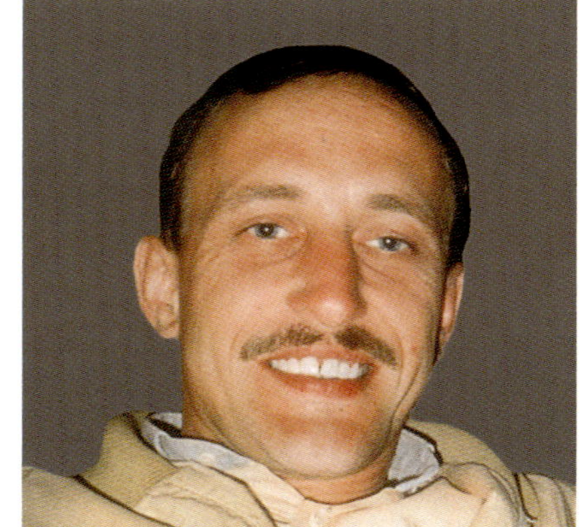

Fig 4-56d

Case 12

An 18-year-old male patient who was a refugee from Vietnam at the age of 3. The lack of basic nutrition during childhood and further continual regurgitation had led to deficient mineralization of the dentin and enamel with disastrous results. During treatment, preparations were performed as conservatively as possible, trying to maintain as much healthy tissue as possible. The front region and entire molar region had to be restored. After 8 years and a control visit every 6 months, the dental condition of this patient could be maintained without the need for additional restorations (Figs 4-57a–d).

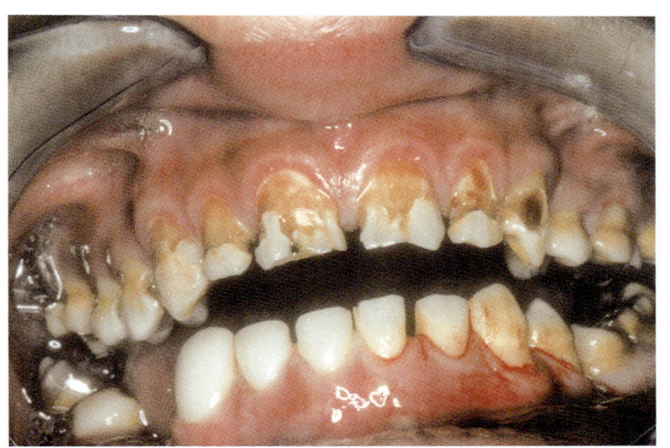

Fig 4-57a

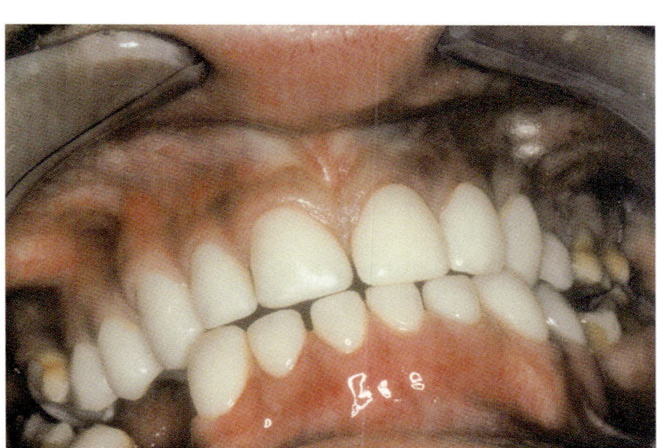

Fig 4-57b

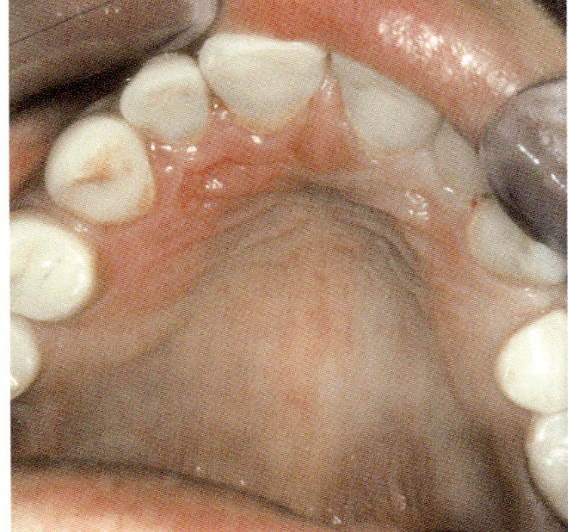

Fig 4-57c

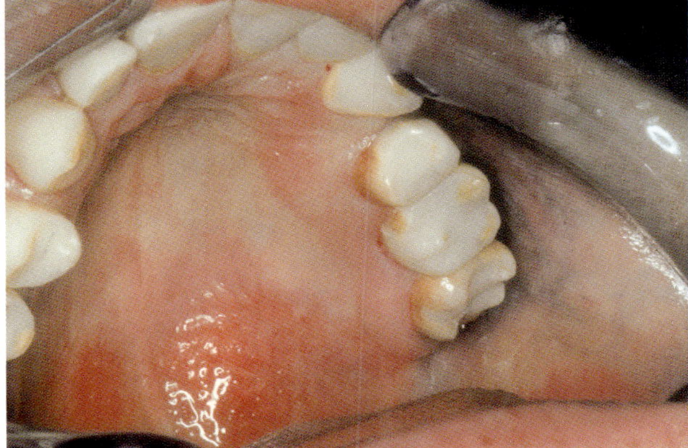

Fig 4-57d

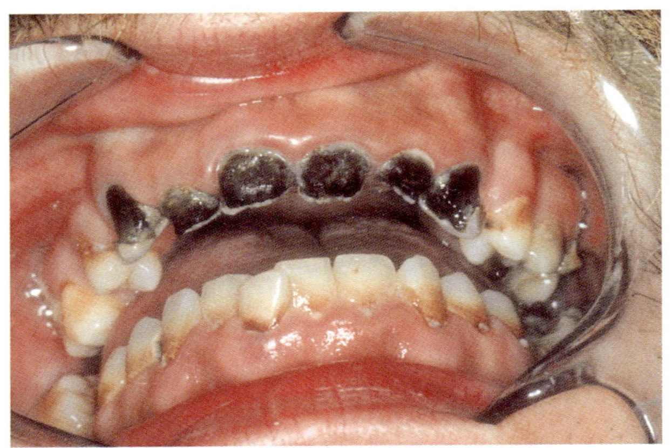

Fig 4-58a

Case 13

Appearance of rampant caries in the upper front region in a 26-year-old male patient. During restoration, no pins were used and every tooth could be restored without root canal treatment. After four and a half years, restorations are functional and with intact tooth vitality (Figs 4-58a,b).

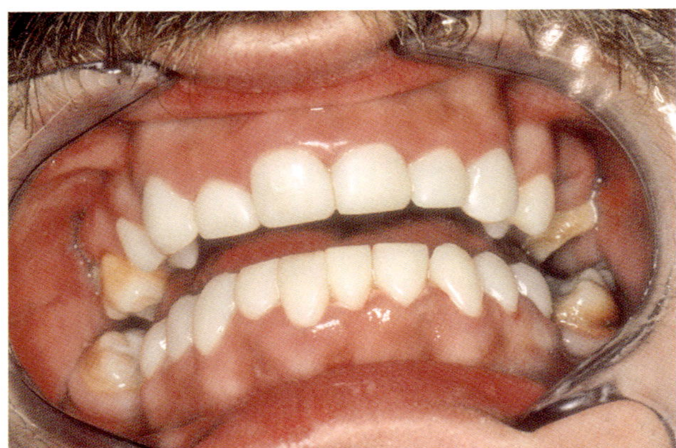

Fig 4-58b

4.9.4 Functional Problems

In cases where there is a high loss of tooth material due to abrasion, erosion, attrition, or loss of supporting teeth in the premolar–molar region, the argon laser combined with direct composite techniques can achieve improved physical properties. Due to the improvement in dentin bonding in the 1990s, restorations without pins or posts are now possible, even in the worst cases. In this way the living pulp can be preserved and even longer-lasting clinical results can be achieved[26].

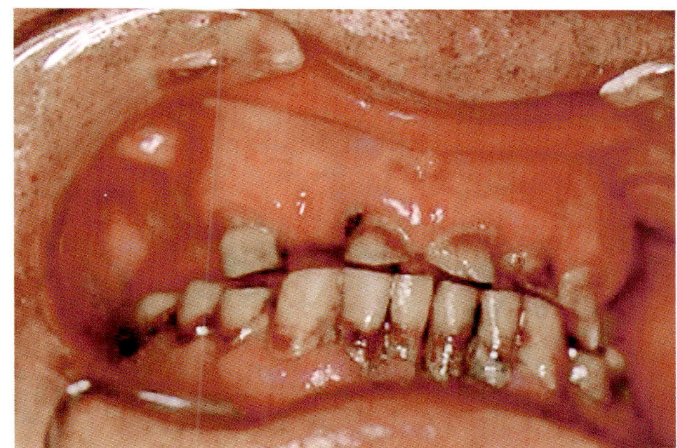

Fig 4-59a

Case 14

Due to the loss of all premolars and molars in the maxillary zone, dramatic attrition of the upper front teeth occurred. Very bad oral hygiene together with excessive force during use had led to the loss of periodontal tissue in the lower front region. This male patient was only 52 years old and had a history of prosthetic trials. He lost confidence in fixed dentures because they had led to the loss of his distal teeth. None of his six removable dentures satisfied him. Prolonged efforts to adapt to them failed. The situation improved with direct composite restorations and a directly resin-bonded bridge for replacement of tooth 12. Superior physical properties after argon laser polymerization guarantee a clinical life of the restorations of several years (Figs 4-59a,b).

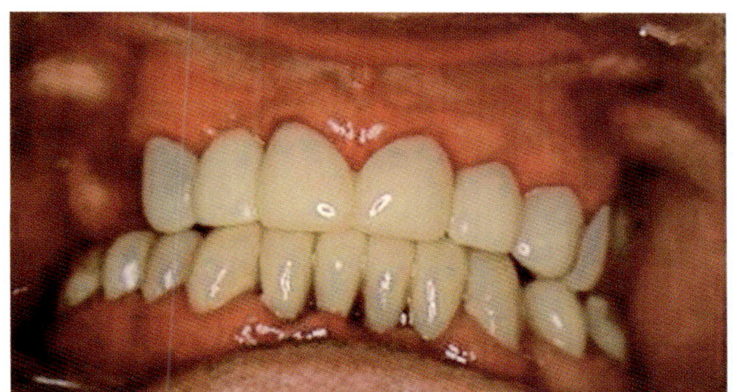

Fig 4-59b

4.9.5 Orthodontic Problems

"Move it or fake it". Move it, or orthodontic treatment, is always the first treatment of choice. "Fake it" can be done under a number of circumstances: classical treatment fails or is too risky in mostly elderly patients; or extended bone surgery is needed and the patient does not want it; or treatment is too time-consuming and the outcome unpredictable. A combination of the previously mentioned benefits of argon laser treatments allows spectacular improvements in esthetics as well as in function, with long lasting results and without irreversible damage to the teeth[26].

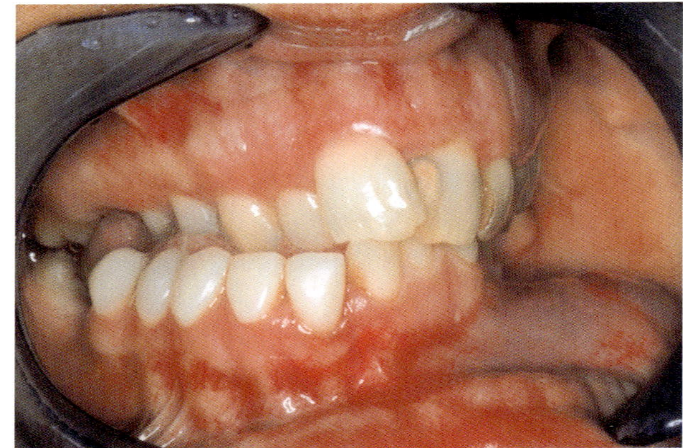

Fig 4-60a

Case 15

Dramatically failing occlusal situation in a 30-year-old female patient. Prior to orthodontic treatment, extensive bone surgery was needed which she refused. Besides esthetic complaints, she mostly suffered from poor functionality. The situation could be improved by direct composite resin application and argon laser treatment, and without the need for surgery (Figs 4-60a,b).

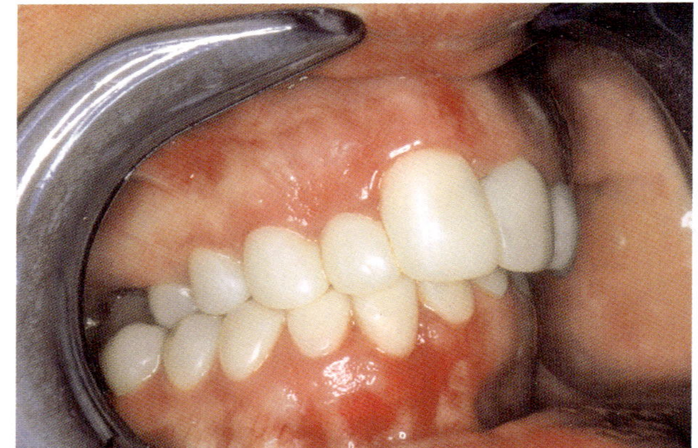

Fig 4-60b

4.9.6 Periodontal Problems

Severely periodontally compromised teeth can be preserved for several years by combining direct composite restorations, laser photopolymerization and a splint. Splints can be applied internally or externally. They may consist of a metal wire like Dentaflex® (Dentaurum, Germany) or of annealed stainless steel, such as Perfomat® (Dentaire SA, Switzerland). A whole series of non-metal splints can be used such as DVA Reinforcement Fibres® (DVA, USA), Splintmat® (Dentaire SA, Switzerland), Ribbond® (Ribbond, Inc., USA), or Connect® (Kerr, USA). In most cases, splinting has to be seen as a measure to postpone extractions[26].

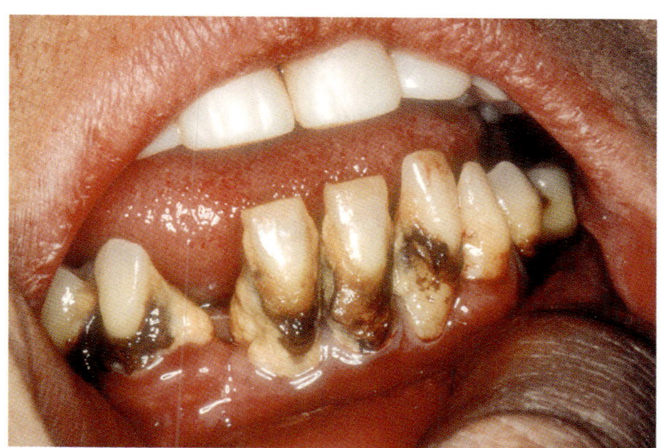

Fig 4-61a

Case 16

A 64-year-old female patient with full upper dentures and a dramatic periodontal situation in the lower arch. Continual problems in adapting to her dentures raised her request for preservation of her remaining dentition for as long as possible, but without removable dentures. A Connect® fiber splint was externally applied to the vestibular surface of the teeth. Together with direct composite veneers, a direct resin bonded bridge for replacement of tooth 42 was performed and argon laser polymerized. The argon laser was used for periodontal treatment as well. After more than 4 years, restorations and splint are still functional (Figs 4-61a,b).

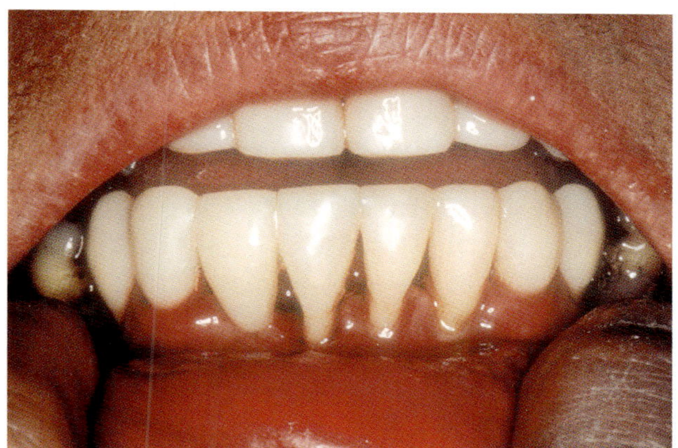

Fig 4-61b

4.9.7 Pediatric Dentistry

Reduced exposure times help to maintain a moisture-free operation field while treating young children. The biggest benefit, however, in using laser curing in children is increased caries resistance. Even if there are no cavities to be filled, the combination of argon laser irradiation and fluoridation is a powerful means of preventative dentistry. The best results are obtained by irradiation first, followed by the application of fluoride[26].

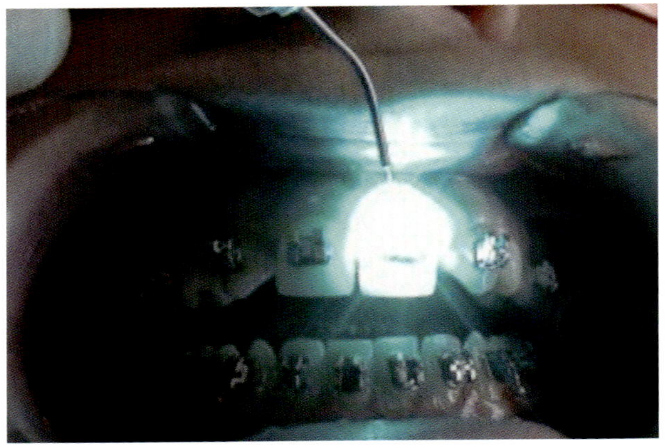

Fig 4-62a

Case 17

Laser photopolymerization for bracket bonding increases bond strength to the enamel in this 12-year-old female patient. There is a major reduction in treatment time, which assists in treating restless children. The fixed brackets could be loaded immediately and the laser irradiation will decrease possible demineralization and the appearance of white spot lesions during further orthodontic treatment (Figs 4-62a,b).

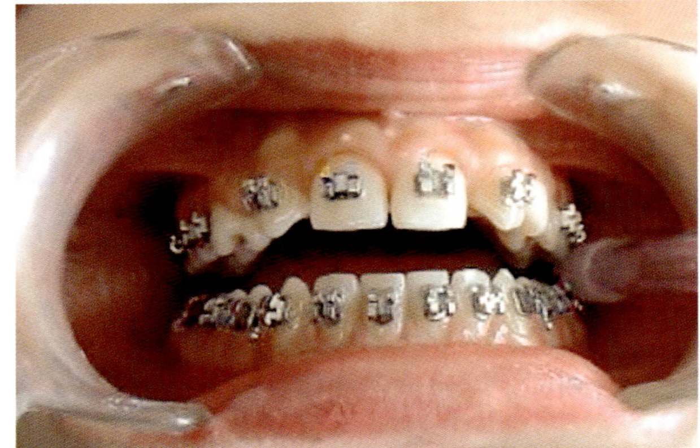

Fig 4-62b

4.9.8 Geriatric Dentistry

The combination of different treatment possibilities (perio, surgery, sterilization, hemostasis,...), and improved photopolymerization of resin restorations, together with increased decay resistance, makes the argon laser a preferred tool in geriatric dentistry. Exposed root surfaces caused by gingival recession are highly susceptible to decay. The loss of teeth with an increased loading on the remaining dentition causes high stresses at the crown–root interface with the appearance of abfraction lesions. Treating these root lesions in the neighborhood of the gingival tissues or beneath the gingival margin causes additional problems. Laser surgery provides easy access to the lesions, and hemostasis and inhibition of the sulcus fluid by laser irradiation facilitates a one-session treatment. High-quality restorations and excellent physical properties are obligatory if dentures have to be connected to the restored dentition[26].

Case 18

A 72-year-old male patient with few remaining teeth. Severe occlusal forces caused general abfraction lesions. These were treated together with an improvement of the occlusal situation by means of direct composite restorations and laser irradiation, creating a situation in which the new manufactured dentures could be fixed safely to the restored teeth (Figs 4-63a–f).

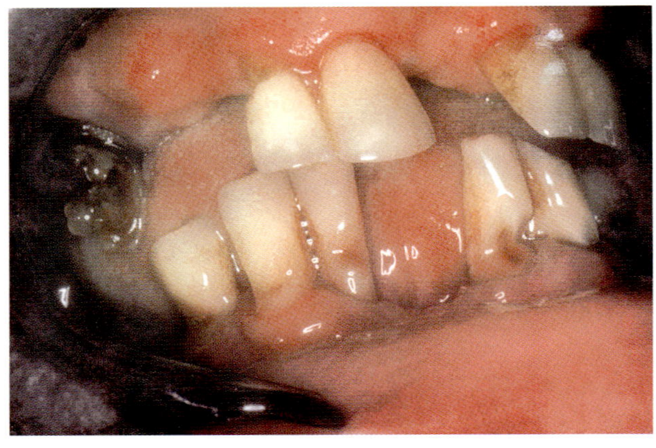

Fig 4-63a

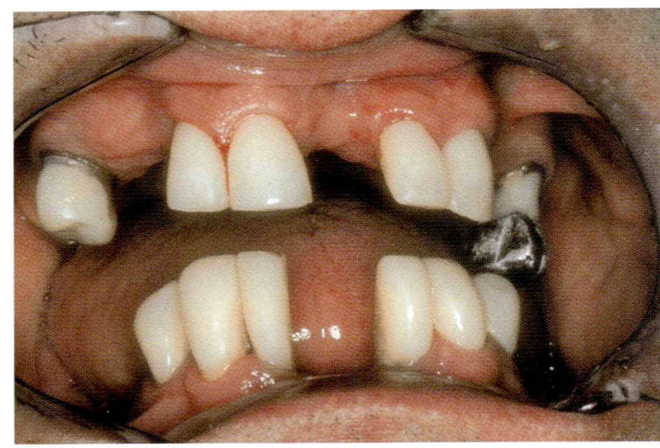

Fig 4-63b

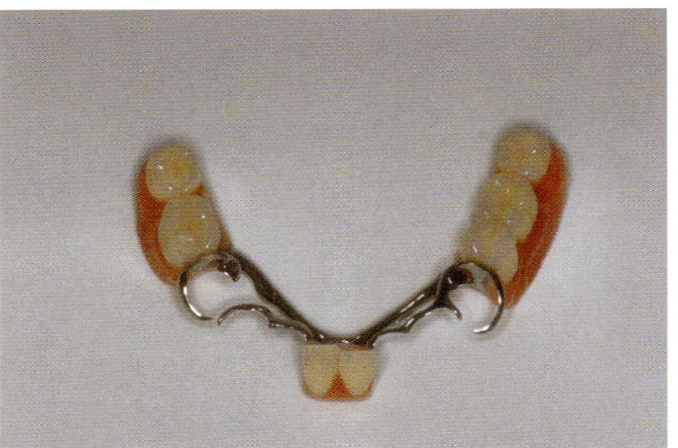

Fig 4-763c

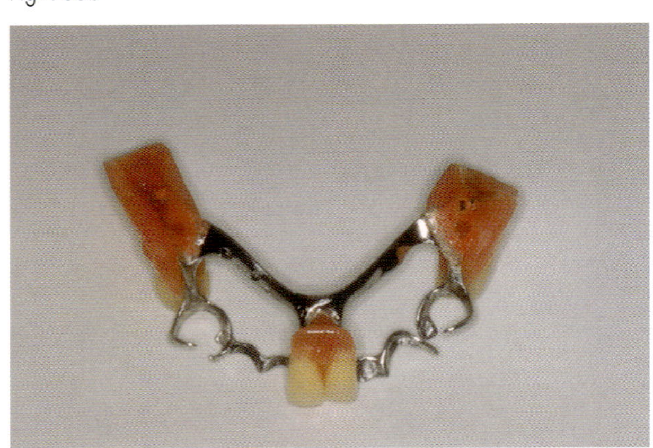

Fig 4-63d

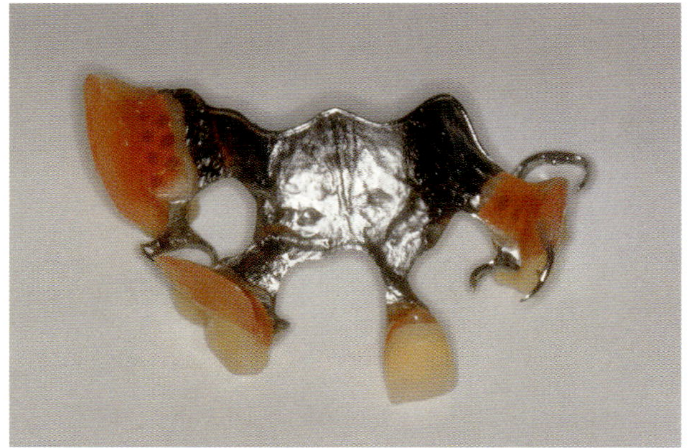

Fig 4-63e

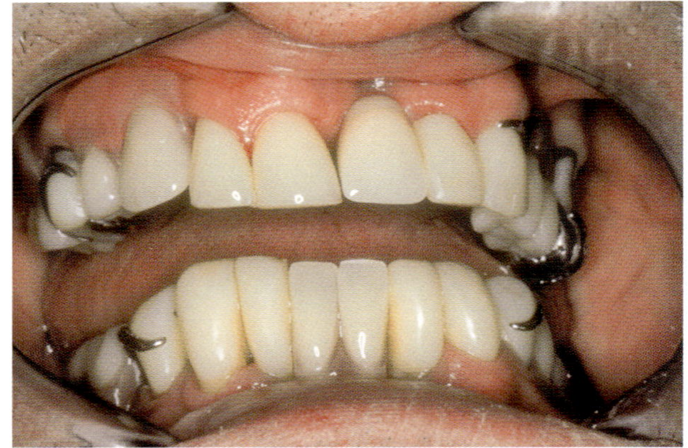

Fig 4-63f

4.9.9 Prosthetic Dentistry

Indirect veneers and full ceramic crowns and bridges are mostly fixed by means of either dual-cured or light-cured composite materials. Laser photopolymerization offers a substantial reduction in treatment time and an improved polymerization. Irradiation of the preparations prior to the placement of the restorations adds a substantial increase in functional life by preventing future secondary decay formation. The same goal is achieved at the most critical zone, the crown-tooth interface, during photopolymerization. Accidental bleeding and sulcus fluid can be controlled by laser irradiation[26].

Case 19

A 46-year-old male colleague required full ceramic crown restorations in the entire upper arch. All the benefits of argon laser applications were used to achieve the best possible result. Post-operative pictures were taken immediately after placement (Figs 4-64a–f).

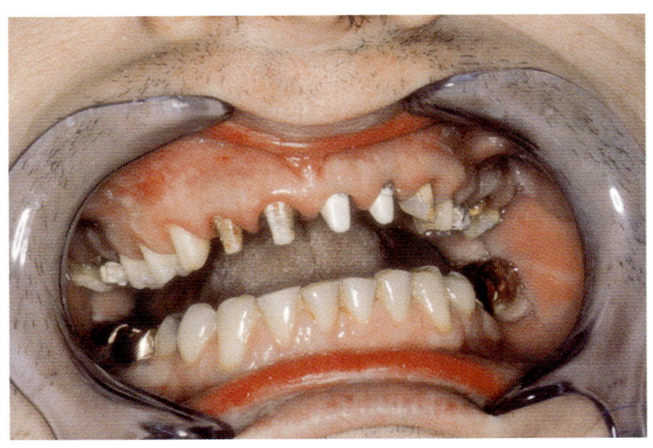
Fig 4-64a

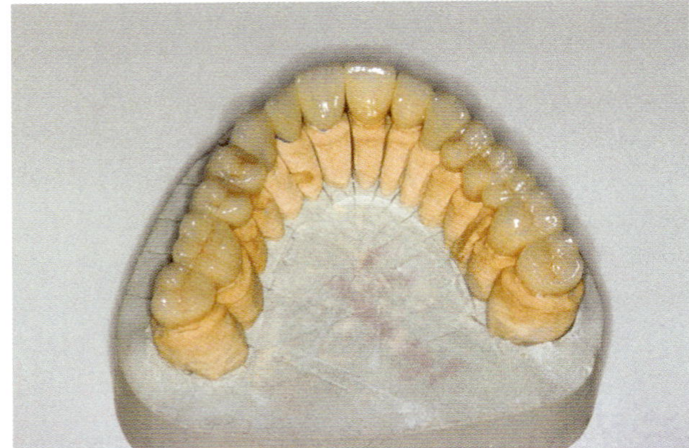
Fig 4-64b

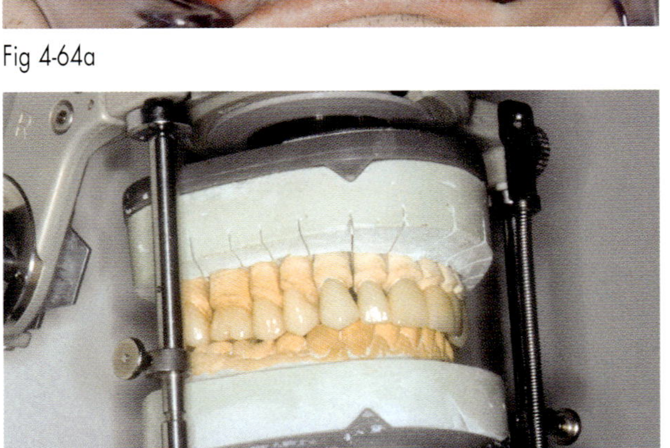
Fig 4-64c

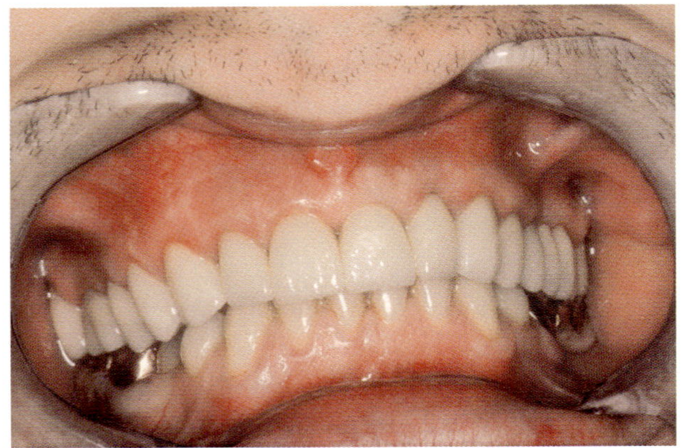
Fig 4-64d

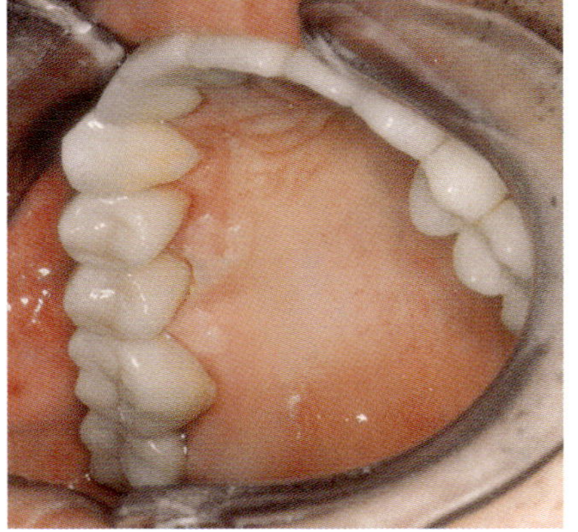
Fig 4-64e

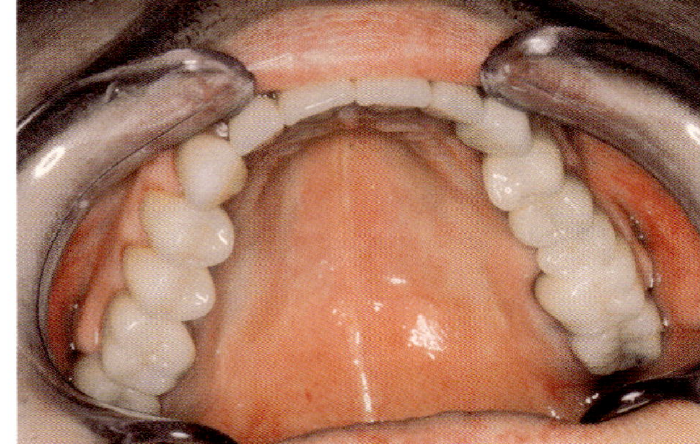
Fig 4-64f

4.10 References

1. Lutz F, Krejci I: Direct posterior filling materials. Vanherle G, Degrange M, Willems G. State of the Art on Direct Posterior Filling Materials and Dentin Bonding. Van der Poorten, Leuven 1993, 15–28
2. Roeters J, De Kloet H: Kosmetische Tandheelkunde met Composiet. Samson Stafleu, Alphen aan de Rijn, Brussel 1990
3. Willems G, Lambrechts P, Braem H, Vanherle G: Classification of composites. In: Vanherle G, Degrange M, Willems G: State of the Art on Direct Posterior Filling Materials and Dentin Bonding. Van der Poorten, Leuven 1993, 77–111
4. Vanherle G, Lambrechts P, Van Meerbeek B: Tandheelkundige Tijdingen 23: 84–85, 1995
5. Albers H F, Aso J, Foster D M: Resin Polymerization. Adept Report 6(3): 1–15, 2000
6. Blankenau R J, Kelsey W P, Kutsch V K: Clinical Applications of Argon Laser in Restorative Dentistry. In: Miserendino L J, Pick R M: Lasers in Dentistry. Quintessence Publ Co Inc 1995, 217–230
7. Kelsey W P, Blankenau R K, Powell G L: Application of the Argon Laser to Dentistry. Lasers Surg Med 11: 495–498, 1991
8. Blankenau R J, Kelsey W P, Powell G L, Shearer G O, Barkmeier W W, Cavel W T: Degree of composite resin polymerization with visible light and argon laser. Am J Dent 4: 40–42, 1991
9. Blankenau R J, Powell G L, Kelsey W P, Barkmeier W W: Post Polymerization Strength Values of an Argon Laser Cured Resin. Lasers Surg Med 11: 417–474, 1991
10. Kelsey W P, Blankenau R J, Powell G L, Barkmeier W W, Cavel W T, Whisenant B K: Enhancement of Physical Properties of Resin Restorative Materials by Laser Polymerization. Lasers Surg Med 9: 623–627, 1989
11. Blankenau R J, Kelsey W P, Anderson D M, Powell G L. Argon Laser Polymerization of G. I. Materials. J Dent Res 72(589): 177, 1993
12. Blankenau R J, Powell G L, Barkmeier W W, Kelsey W P: Argon Laser Effects on Dentin Adhesive Systems. J Dent Res 68: 32, 1989
13. Westerman G H, Hicks M J, Flaitz C M, Blankenau R J, Powell G L: Argon laser-cured sealants and reduced caries formation. J Dent Res 70: 493, 1991
14. Westerman G H, Hicks M J, Flaitz C M, Blankenau R J, Berg J, Powell G L: Argon laser irradiation in root surface caries. J Dent Res 71: 201, 1992
15. Hicks M J, Flaitz C M, Westerman G H, Blankenau R J, Powell G L, Berg J H: Enamel caries initiation and progression following low fluence energy argon laser and fluoride treatment. J Clin Ped Dent 20(1): 9–13, 1995
16. Hicks M J, Flaitz C M, Westerman G H, Blankenau R J, Powell G L, Berg J H: Caries-like lesion initiation and progression around laser-cured sealants. Am J Dent 6(4): 176–180, 1993
17. Hicks M J, Flaitz C M, Westerman G H, Blankenau R J, Powell G L, Berg J H: Caries-like lesion formation and progression in sound enamel following argon laser irradiation: an in vitro study. J Dent Child 60: 201–206, 1993
18. Oho T, Morioka T: A possible mechanism of acquired resistance of human dental enamel by laser irradiation. Caries Res 24: 86–92, 1990
19. Barghi N, Berry T, Hatton C: Evaluation of Intensity Output of Curing Lights in Private Dental Offices. J Am Dent Assoc 125: 992–996, 1994
20. Ruyter I E: Monomer systems and polymerization. Vanherle G, Smith DC. Posterior Composite Resin Dental Restorative Materials. Peter Szulc Publ Co, Utrecht 1985, 109–137
21. Harris J M: Analytical Chemistry 34, 1995
22. Harris J M: Journal of Physical Chemistry 97, 1993
23. Cipolla A J: Laser Curing of Photoactivated Restorative Materials. ILT Systems, Salt Lake City 1993
24. De Gee A J: Lampen in de lichtpolymerizatie. In: Van Steenberghe D, De Baat C, Braem M J A, Carels C E L, Roodenburg J L N, Snel L C, Van Welsenes W: Het Tandheelkundig Jaar 2002. Bohn Stafleu van Loghum, Houten 2001, 87–105
25. Blankenau R J, Kelsey W P, Cavel W T, Blankenau P: Wavelength and intensity of seven systems for visible light-curing composite resins: a comparision study. J Am Dent Assoc 106(4): 471–474, 1983
26. Verheyen P: Lasers in Dentistry and Maxillo-facial Surgery. European Laser Users and Research Association, Belgium 2000
27. Kelsey P W, Blankenau R K, Powell G L, Barkmeier W W, Stormberg E F: Power and Time Requirements of Use of the Argon Laser to Polymerize Composite resins. J Clin Laser Med Surg 10: 273–278, 1992
28. Curing Times™: Lasermed Inc 1996
29. Schuurs A H B, Moorer W R: Hormoonregelaars. Pseudo-oestrogeen in tandheelkundige composieten en sealants? Ned Tijdschr Tandheelkd 107: 490–494, 2000
30. Zach K, Cohen G: Pulp response to externally applied heat. Oral Surg Oral Med 19: 515–530, 1965
31. Launay Y, Mordan S, Cornil A, Brunetand J M, Moschetto Y: Thermal effects of lasers on dental tissues. Lasers Surg Med 7: 473–477, 1987
32. Powell G L, Morton T H, Whisenant B K: Argon laser oral safety parameters for teeth. Lasers Surg Med 13: 548–552, 1993
33. Duncan Y U, Powell G L, Higuchi W I, Fox J L: Comparison of three Lasers on Dental Pulp Chamber Temperature Change. J Clin Laser Med Surg 11: 119–122, 1993
34. Anic I, Pavelic B, Peric B, Matsumoto K: In vitro Pulp Chamber Temperature Rises Associated with the Argon Laser Polymerization of Composite Resin. Lasers Surg Med 19: 438–444, 1996
35. Lloyd C H: A differential thermal analysis for the heats of reaction and temperature rises produced during the setting of tooth colored restorative materials. J Oral Rehabil 11: 111–121, 1984
36. Puckett A, Bernett B, Drummond J, Holder R: Conventional light vs. laser photopolymerization. J Dent Res 72: 137, 1993

37. Severin C, Maquin M: Argon Ion Laser Beam as Composite Resin Light Curing Agent. In: Tamamoto H, Atsumi K, Kusakari H. Lasers in Dentistry. Elsevier Science Publ B V Biomedical Devision, Reims 1989, 241–246
38. Blankenau R J, Powell G L, Martinez, Ocanto R, Barkmeier W W. The argon laser and modified conventional light resin polymerization comparison. J Dent Res 73: 105, 1994
39. Davidson C L. Conflicting interests with posterior use of composite materials. In: Vanherle G, Smith D C: Posterior Composite Resin Detal Restorative Materials. Minnesota Mining, Utrecht 1985, 61–65
40. Waknine S, Cipolla A J: Lasers vs. Halogen Photopoly-meriztion-Characterization of VLC Composite Mechanical Properties. AADR, San Antonio Mar 12, 1995
41. Powell G L, Ellis R, Blankenau R J, Schouten R J: Evaluation of an Argon Laser and Conventional Light-Cured Composites. J Clin Laser Med Surg 13(5): 315–317, 1995
42. Blankenau R J, Powell G L, Cavel W T, Barkmeier W W, Anderson D: A Comparision of the Diameteral Tensile Strength Values of Pit and Fissure Sealants Polymerized with an Argon Laser and Conventional Light Source. Lasers Surg Med 12(2): 75–78, 1992
43. Davidson C L, Pallav P, De Gee A J: Wear Mechanisms of Dental Composites. In: Vanherle G, Degrange M, Willems G: State of the Art on Direct Posterior Filling Materials and Dentin Bonding. Van der Poorten, Leuven 1993, 119–129
44. Glasspoole E A, Blankenau R J, Barkmeier W W, Powell G L. Wear Rates of Argon Laser and Visible Light Polymerized Resins. J Dent Res 69: 126, 1990
45. Frentzen M, Koort M J: Lasers in dentistry: new possibilities with advancing laser technology. Int Dent J 40: 323–332, 1990
46. Shanthala B M, Munshi A K: Laser versus visible light cured composite resin: an in vitro shear bond study. J Clin Ped Dent 19(2): 121–125, 1995
47. Powell G L, Kelsey W P, Blankenau R J, Barkmeier W W: The Use of an Argon Laser for Polymerization of Composite Resin. J Esthet Dent 1: 34–37, 1989
48. Sedivy P, Ferguson D, Dhuze V, Kittleson R: Ortodontic resin adhesive cured with argon laser: tensile bond strength. J Dent Res 72: 176, 1993
49. Hinoura K O, Hiyazak M, Onore H: Influence of argon laser curing on resin bond strength. Am J Dent 6(2): 69–71, 1993
50. Blankenau R J, Powell G L, Martinez, Ocanto R, Barkmeier W W: The Argon Laser and Modified Conventional Light Resin Polymerization Comparison. J Dent Res 73(32): 105, 1994
51. Powell G L, Blankenau R J: The Effect of Beam Size on Composite Polymerization. J Dent Res 75: 146, 1996
52. Tare A W, Nicholls J L: Polymerization Shrinkage of Restorative Resins Using Laser and Visible Light Curing. J Clin Laser Med Surg 15: 137–141, 1997
53. Pollack B: Composite Resin. Fundamentals and direct technique restorations. Dale BG, Ascheim KW. Esthetic Dentistry. A clinical approach to techniques and materials. Lea & Febinger, Philadelphia, London 1993, 39–55
54. Albers H F: Tooth-Colored Restorations. Alto Books, Santa Rosa 1996
55. Versluis A, Douglas W H, Cross M, Sakaguchi R L: Does an Incremental Filling Technique Reduce Polymerization Shrinkage Stresses? J Dent Res 75(3): 871–878, 1996
56. Featherstone J D B, Nelson D G A: Laser effects on dental hard tissues. Adv Dent Res 1: 21–26, 1987
57. Mc Cormark S M, Fried D, Featherstone J D B, Glena R E, Seka W: Scanning electron microscope observations of CO_2 laser effects on dental enamel. J Dent Res 74: 1702–1708, 1995
58. Hsu J, Fox J L, Wang Z, Powell G L, Otsuka M, Higuchi W I: Combined Effects of Laser Irradiation/Solution Fluoride Ion on Enamel Denineralization. J Clin Laser Med Surg 16: 93–105, 1998
59. Nelson DGA, Shariati, Glena R, Shields CP, Featherstone JDB: Effect of pulsed low energy infrared laser irradiation on artificial carlies-like lesion formation. Caries Res 20: 289–299, 1987
60. Yamamoto S, Sato K: Prevention of dental caries by Nd:YAG laser irradiation. J Dent Res 59: 2171–2177, 1980
61. Boran T L, Peters J F M, Zakariasen K L: Effects of fluoride and CO_2 laser radiation on enamel demineralization. J Dent Res 71: 201, 1992
62. Yu D, Wong J, Otsuka P, Powell G L, Fok J L, Higuachi W I: Laser irradiated human enamel dissolution: influence of inhibitors. J Dent Res 69: 302, 1990
63. Peters J F M, Zakariasen K L, Boran T L, Borron J L: Effects of pulsed/nonpulsed CO_2 laser energy on enamel demineralization. J Dent Res 69: 302, 1990
64. Oho T, Morioka T: A possible mechanism of acquired resistance of human dental enamel by laser irradiation. Caries Res 24: 86–92, 1990
65. Fox J L, Yu D, Otsuka M, Higuchi W I, Wong J, Powell G: Combined effects of laser irradiation and chemical inhibitors on the dissolution of dental enamel. Caries Res 26: 333–339, 1992
66. Goodman B D, Kaufman H W: Effects of an argon laser on the crystalline properties and rate of dissolution in acid of tooth enamel in the presence of sodium fluoride. J Dent Res 56: 1201–1207, 1977
67. Blankenau R J, Taylor M H, Powell G L, Barkmeier W W: Microleakage of dental sealants cured with an argon laser. J Dent Res 69: 228, 1990
68. Blankenau R J, Powell G L, Barkmeier W W, Kelsey W P: Power requirements for laser polymerization of dental resin. Second World Congress ISLD, Paris May 1990
69. Blankenau R J, Powell G L, Cavel W T, Kelsey W P, Anderson D: Argon laser polymerized pit and fissure sealants. ISDL Third International Congress on Lasers in Dentistry 1992, 21
70. Westerman G H, Hicks M J, Flaitz C M, Blankenau R J, Powell G L, Berg J H: Argon laser irradiation in root surface caries: in vitro study examines laser's effects. J Am Dent Assoc 125(4): 401–407, 1994
71. Kutsch V K: Caries illumination with the argon laser: a clinical trial. ISLD. Third International Congress on Lasers in Dentistry 1992, 22
72. Alfano R R, Yao S S: Human teeth with and without dental caries studied by visible luminescence spectroscopy. J Dent Res 60: 120–122, 1981

73. Bjelkhagen H, Sunderstrom F, Angmar Mansson B: Early detection of enamel caries by luminescence ecxited by visible laser light. Swed Dent J 6(1): 1–7, 1982
74. Elliott J C: Structure, crystal chemistry and density of enamel apatites. Ciba Found Symp 205: 54–67, 1997
75. Stern R H, Sognnaes R F: Laser inhibition of dental caries suggested by first tests in vivo. J Am Dent Assoc 85: 1087–1090, 1972
76. Stern R H, Vahl J, Sognnaes R F: Lased enamel: ultra-structural observations of pulsed carbon dioxide laser effects. J Dent Res 51: 455–460, 1972
77. Clarkson B H, Rafter M E: Emerging methods used in the prevention and repair of carious tissues. J Dent Educ 65: 1114–1120, 2001
78. Hicks M J, Westerman G H, Flaitz C M, Blankenau R J, Powell G L, Berg J H: Effects of argon laser irradiation and acidulated phosphate fluoride on root caries. Am J Dent 8: 10–14, 1995
79. Hicks M J, Flaitz C M, Westerman G H, Blankenau R J, Powell G L: Root caries in vitro after low fluence argon laser and fluoride treatment. Compend Contin Educ Dent 18: 543–548, 1997
80. Tagomori S, Morioka T: Combined effects of laser and fluoride on acid resistance of human dental enamel. Caries Res 23: 225–231, 1989
81. Haider S M, White G E, Rich A: Combined effects of argon laser irradiation and fluoride treatments in prevention of caries-like lesion formation in enamel: an in vitro study. J Clin Pediat Dent 23: 247–257, 1999
82. Westerman G H, Flaitz C M, Powell G L, Hicks M J: Enamel caries initiation and progression after argon laser irradiation: in vitro argon laser systems comparison. J Clin Laser Med Surg 20: 257–262, 2002
83. Blankenau R J, Powell G, Ellis R W, Westerman G H: In vivo caries-like lesion prevention with argon laser: pilot study. J Clin Laser Med Surg 17: 241–243, 1999
84. Flaitz C M, Hicks M J, Westerman G H, Berg J H, Blankenau R J, Powell G L: Argon laser irradiation and acidulated phosphate fluoride treatment in caries-like lesion formation in enamel: an in vitro study. Pediat Dent 17: 31–35, 1995
85. Anderson J R, Ellis R W, Blankenau R J, Beiraghi S M, Westerman G H: Caries resistance in enamel by laser irradiation and topical fluoride treatment. J Clin Laser Med Surg 18: 33–36, 2000
86. Kuroda S, Fowler B O: Compositional, structural, and phase changes in in vitro laser-irradiated human tooth enamel. Calcif Tiss Int 36: 361–369, 1984
87. Fowler B O, Kuroda S: Changes in heated and in laser-irradiated human tooth enamel and their probable effects on solubility. Calcif Tiss Int 38: 197–208, 1986
88. Yamamoto H, Ooya K: Potential of yttrium-aluminum-garnet laser in caries prevention. J Oral Pathol 3: 7–15, 1974
89. Lenz P, Gilde H, Walz R: Enamel sealing studies with the CO_2 laser. Dtsch Zahnärztl Z 37: 469–478, 1982
90. Nelson D G A, Jongebloed W L, Featherstone J D B: Laser irradiation of human dental enamel and dentine. NZ Dent J 82: 74–77, 1986
91 Fox J L, Yu D, Otsuka M, Higuchi W I, Wong J, Powell G L: Initial dissolution rate studies on dental enamel after CO_2 laser irradiation. J Dent Res 71: 1389–1398, 1992
92. Westerman G H, Hicks M J, Flaitz C M, Powell G L, Blankenau R J: Surface morphology of sound enamel after argon laser irradiation: an in vitro scanning electron microscopic study. J Clin Pediat Dent 21: 55–59, 1996
93. Walsh L J, Perham S: Enamel fusion using a surgical carbon dioxide laser : a technique for sealing pits and fissures. Clin Prev Dent 13: 16–20, 1991
94. Walsh L J: Clinical evaluation of dental hard tissue applications of carbon dioxide lasers. J Clin Laser Med Surg 12: 11–15, 1994
95. Aminzadeh A, Shahabi S, Walsh L J: Raman spectroscopic studies of CO_2 laser-irradiated human dental enamel. Spectrochim Acta 55: 1303–1308, 1999
96. Wong J, Otsuka M, Higuchi W I, Powell G L, Fox J L: Effect of laser irradiation on the dissolution kinetics of hydroxyapatite preparations. J Pharm Sci 79: 510–515, 1990
97. Westerman G H, Hicks M J, Flaitz C M, Blankenau RJ, Powell G L: Combined effects of acidulated phosphate fluoride and argon laser on sound root surface morphology: an in vitro scanning electron microscopy study. J Clin Laser Med Surg 17: 63–68, 1999
98. Westerman G H, Hicks M J, Flaitz C M, Blankenau RJ, Powell GL: Argon laser irradiation effects on sound root surfaces: in vitro scanning electron microscopic observations. J Clin Laser Med Surg 16: 111–115, 1998
99. Burtscher P: Influence of Light Intensity on Essential Properties of Composites. Vivadent, München 2003

5

Caries Prevention

K. Goharkhay, A. Moritz

5.1 Introduction

The caries process is well understood[1]. Dental plaque on the surface of a tooth consists of a film of bacteria, some of which produce acids as by-products of their metabolism. These are the so-called acidogenic bacteria and, because they produce acids that can dissolve tooth mineral, they are also termed cariogenic[2]. The acids produced by the acidogenic bacteria when they metabolize fermentable carbohydrates are predominantly lactic, acetic, and propionic acids. Most importantly, lactic acid dissociates more readily than the other acids, producing hydrogen ions that lower the pH in the plaque rapidly[3]. As the pH is lowered, acids diffuse into the underlying enamel or dentin, dissolving the mineral. The two most important groups of bacteria that produce mostly lactic acid are *Streptococcus mutans* and lactobacilli[2]. Each group contains several species, each of which is cariogenic. *Streptococci* of the *Mutans* group include *S. mutans* and *S. sobrinus* species predominantly. *Lactobacillus* species are also prolific producers of lactic acid and appear in plaque before the observation of clinical caries[4,5]. These two groups of bacteria, separately or together, are primary causative agents of dental caries.

The mineral crystals of the teeth and bones are made of carbonated hydroxyapatite[6,7]. It is much more soluble than the hydroxyapatite that is commonly described as tooth mineral in the literature. Hydroxyapatite, in turn, is much more soluble than fluorapatite[8]. The carbonated apatite mineral contains about 3% carbonate in enamel and about 5% in dentin, substituting for phosphate in the crystal lattice and causing structural defects that make the mineral more acid-soluble.

Saliva plays a critical role in the prevention or reversal of the demineralization process, providing calcium in the plaque fluid, proteins and lipids that form a protective pellicle on the surface of the tooth, antibacterial substances, and buffers[9]. The saliva components neutralize the acids produced by bacterial metabolism in the plaque, raise the pH, and reverse the diffusion gradient for calcium and phosphate, thus returning calcium and phosphate into the subsurface lesion where these ions can regenerate new mineral on the surfaces of the crystal remnants that were produced by demineralization. These so-called remineralized crystals now have a veneer of much less soluble mineral. If fluoride is present in sufficient quantity, it enhances this remineralization process and is preferentially included in the new veneer on the subsurface crystals in the lesion in the form of a fluorapatite mineral, which has low solubility[8,10].

5.2 Conventional Treatment Methods

In the past, the primary caries preventive agents have been fluoride and fissure sealants[11]. Benefits from fluoride are derived from both topical and systemic uses. Fluoride can be found in dentifrices, oral rinses and professionally applied methods, as well as prescriptions (tablets or drops). Some individuals who receive fluoride still develop pit and fissure caries and this finding indicates that fluoride is apparently less effective for pits and fissures than it is for smooth surfaces on teeth. Pit and fissure sealant has been developed to overcome this problem. Sealants are used to fill in anatomical pits and fissures that normally are too narrow for the removal of bacteria plaque by the bristles of a toothbrush. However, complete or partial loss of sealant and secondary caries is common. Also, prevention and restorative treatment of root surface caries presents a poor prognosis for medically-compromised older adults. These facts emphasize the need for optimizing the caries preventive strategy.

From in vitro experiments, it is well established that low levels of fluoride in acidic buffer solutions may completely inhibit lesion development in enamel[12,13]. The in vivo situation is much more complex, as it is an open system where plaque fluid may exchange with saliva in periods when acid attacks occur. The optimum fluoride level that would inhibit caries development may therefore vary from individual to individual, and also most likely from site to site within the dentition (e.g., fissures, approximal surfaces).

5.3 Laser Application in Preventive Dentistry

5.3.1 Historical Aspects

Almost immediately after the development of the ruby laser by Maiman (1960), researchers postulated that it could be applied to dental treatment[14]. Stern and Sognnaes[15] began looking at the possible uses of the ruby laser in dentistry. They were the first in a long list of investigators looking for a better way to treat dental patients with lasers. They began their laser study on hard dental tissues by investigating the possible use of a ruby laser to reduce subsurface demineralization[16,17]. Early studies of the effects of lasers on hard dental tissues were based simply on the empirical use of available lasers and an examination of the modified tissue by various techniques. Even though these studies were primitive, i.e., the optical properties of dental tissues at the respective laser wavelengths and the laser pulse shape and characteristics were not investigated, they suggested the potential uses of lasers in preventive dentistry. Studies by Stern et al.[15,18] utilizing their ruby laser (λ = 693.4 nm) demonstrated that the laser could be used to heat the surface of human enamel, consequently increasing enamel resistance to subsurface demineralization in vitro.

Vahl[19] used electron microscopy and X-ray diffraction to study the effects of laser radiation on enamel. These studies clearly demonstrated ultrastructural and crystallographic changes in response to laser radiation. Later studies by Yamamoto et al.[20] showed the potential of an Nd:YAG laser (λ = 1064 nm) to fuse dental enamel at very high irradiation intensities (~1 GW/cm^2) and to make it highly resistant to subsequent dissolution.

The majority of the earliest studies were carried out using near-IR and visible light lasers at wavelengths that are weakly absorbed by dental hard tissues. Often very high irradiation intensities (> 107 W/cm^2) were used to generate the desired effects. Presumably the mechanism of coupling of the laser energy to the sample was by plasma formation at the high incident power densities applied. The high energies utilized, as well as the high transmission of these tissues in the visible and near-IR, would be expected to result in subsurface damage to the pulp.

5.3.2 Light Interactions with Dental Hard Tissues

For any procedures using lasers, the optical interactions between the laser and the tissue must be understood thoroughly to ensure safe, effective treatment[1]. The laser-tissue interaction is controlled by the irradiation parameters: wavelength, continuous or pulsed emission, repetition rate, pulse duration, pulse energy, beam size and delivery method, spatial and temporal characteristics of the laser beam, and optical properties of the tissue. The interaction of light with enamel and dentin is now well understood.

New observations together with earlier work have provided parameters from which dentists can choose appropriate wavelengths and other laser conditions to perform the desired tasks[21–25].

Whenever a dentist wants to alter tissue, e.g., to remove tissue by ablation, the tissue that is to be treated must absorb the laser wavelength, in order for ablation to occur[26,27]. If the dentist wants to heat a tissue to alter its composition or solubility (described in detail subsequently), the laser light must be strongly absorbed and converted efficiently to heat without damage to underlying or surrounding tissues[21,22,28–30]. Alternatively, extremely high power densities are needed.

The optical properties of specific interest for caries detection, caries removal by ablation, or prevention of caries progression, are transmission, scattering, and absorption. If light is transmitted mostly through the tissue with no interaction, it passes into underlying tissue. This is the case when absorption is minimal. If the light is scattered, it is no longer a coherent beam and is not delivered where needed. When light is absorbed, it interacts with the atoms in the tissue and generally is converted to heat. The degree of absorption determines the depth of penetration and the amount of heat deposited. Several workers have studied these properties in sound and carious enamel and dentin. The key results are summarized here in relation to the effects of lasers on hard tissues.

The optical properties are characterized by the refractive index of the tissue, the scattering coefficient (λ_s), the absorption coefficient (λ_a), and the scattering anisotropy[14,25,31]. The ultimate effects of laser irradiation on the tooth tissue depend on the distribution of the energy and how much is deposited in the tooth. The temperature rise at any point is a balance between energy deposited in a specific time and energy that is conducted away as heat. The temperature rise determines whether the morphology or chemical characteristics of the tissue at that point are changed[32–36].

5.3.3 Scattering and Absorption Parameters

Absorption and scattering coefficients are determined experimentally and are given values with units of reciprocal centimeters (cm^{-1}). For materials with high absorption coefficients (> 100 cm^{-1}), the laser energy is absorbed within about 100 µm of the surface and converted to heat[32–36]. In the case of a pulsed laser, if the pulse duration is short enough, nearly all the energy is deposited as heat in this region, whereas if it is longer, some heat is deposited in the upper layers, and the remaining energy is transmitted deeper into the tissue. Once the irradiation energy is transformed into heat, its further penetration into the tissue is done via heat conduction.

Energy transfer into the tissue as heat is by conduction of the heat. This transfer is determined by the thermal diffusivity and heat capacity of the tissue. Enamel and dentin are markedly different in these characteristics[33–35].

Wavelengths with high absorption correspond with specific components in the tissue. For example, the extremely high absorption coefficient for dental enamel at λ = 9.6 µm, one of the wavelengths that can be produced by a carbon dioxide (CO_2) laser, is due to the phosphate ions in the carbonated apatite mineral[22]. Another example is the Er:YAG laser (erbium:yttrium-aluminium-garnet) (2.94 µm), which coincides with the middle of the water absorption band in enamel (and even more so in dentin). The absorption coefficient is high and at this wavelength the laser irradiation couples rapidly and efficiently with the water, causing subsurface superheating, expansion, and explosion, resulting in removal of the tissue[25,37].

Weak Absorption in Visible and Near-Infrared. Enamel absorbs visible light weakly in the λ = 400–700 nm region (absorption coefficient < 1 cm^{-1}) and moderately (absorption coefficient about 10 cm^{-1}) in the UV (λ = 240–300 nm). The scattering coefficients decrease rapidly between λ = 240 and 700 nm and are even lower in the near-infrared, with values falling from 400 to 15 cm^{-1} over that range. In the region of the Nd:YAG laser at λ = 1.064 nm, the absorption coefficient in enamel is low (< 1 cm^{-1}), implying that light in the visible and near-infrared readily passes through enamel almost entirely, with minimal absorption and less scattering as the wavelength is increased.

Dentin has a much higher content of water and protein than enamel, decreasing the contribution of the mineral and emphasizing the water and protein contributions. Similarly to enamel, dentin absorption is low in the visible region (λ = 400–700 nm), but the tissue scatters much more than enamel. The tissue has low but measurable absorption at

Table 5-1 Approximate absorption and scattering coefficients for enamel and dentin (after Featherstone[1], Fried et al.[74]).

	ABSORPTION COEFFICIENT (cm^{-1})		SCATTERING COEFFICIENT (cm^{-1})	
WAVELENGTH	ENAMEL	DENTIN	ENAMEL	DENTIN
Visible Light Argon: λ = 488 nm λ = 514 nm	< 1	3–4	40–400	250–300
Near-infrared Nd:YAG: λ =1,064 nm	< 1	3–4	15	260
Mid-infrared Ho:YAG: λ = 2.10 µm CO_2: λ = 9.30 µm CO_2: λ = 9.60 µm CO_2: λ = 10.30 µm CO_2: λ = 10.60 µm	 < 20 5,500 8,000 1,125 825	 < 20 5,000 6,500 1,200 800	 no data approx. 0 approx. 0 approx. 0 approx. 0	 no data approx. 0 approx. 0 approx. 0 approx. 0

the Nd:YAG wavelength and scatters highly compared with enamel at this wavelength. Scattered Nd:YAG light continues to move through the tissue until it is all absorbed or transmitted to a surrounding tissue.

Strong Absorption at Specific Wavelengths in the Mid-Infrared. The mineral component of enamel and dentin is a carbonated hydroxyapatite and can be symbolized by the stylized formula $Ca_{10-x}Na_x(PO_4)_{6-y}(CO_3)_y(OH)_{2-u}F_u$ indicating that it contains calcium, sodium, phosphate, carbonate, hydroxyl, and fluoride ions. There are also many other substitutions in the mineral, but for the present purposes this formula suffices to understand the interactions of lasers with the mineral. Enamel and dentin also contain a substantial amount of water among the crystals, approximately 12% and 25% by volume, respectively[10,38]. The transmission spectrum of enamel clearly illustrates the absorption bands for water at approximately 3 µm, hydroxyl at approximately 2.8 µm, carbonate at approximately 7 µm, and phosphate at 9–11 µm.

The absorption coefficients at these wavelengths that coincide with the constituents of the tissue are high (800 to 8,000 cm^{-1}). For absorption values as high as this, transmission is low. For example, at λ = 9.6 µm, nearly all of the light is absorbed in the outer 1 µm. The scattering is not measurable. Consequently, the absorption coefficient becomes overriding, in predicting the laser-tissue interactions.

The Er:YAG laser (λ = 2.94 µm) and to a lesser extent the Er:YSGG laser (λ = 2.79 µm) overlap the absolute maximum of the water absorption band. Consequently, the principal absorber for the Er:YAG is the water in either enamel or dentin. This property explains the effectiveness of this laser for the removal of carious and sound, enamel and dentin. The Er:YSGG laser also overlaps the hydroxyl ion absorption in the mineral, heating the mineral as well as the water, contributing in two ways to the heating of the subsurface tissue and effective ablation.

The conventional CO_2 lasers used in medicine and dentistry emit light at λ = 10.6 µm, which is absorbed strongly by the mineral. There are four principal wavelengths of the CO_2 laser, each of which can be produced by appropriate changes in the laser configuration[22]. These four wavelengths are λ = 9.3, λ = 9.6, λ = 10.3 and λ = 10.6 µm. Light at wavelengths of λ = 9.3 and λ = 9.6 µm is

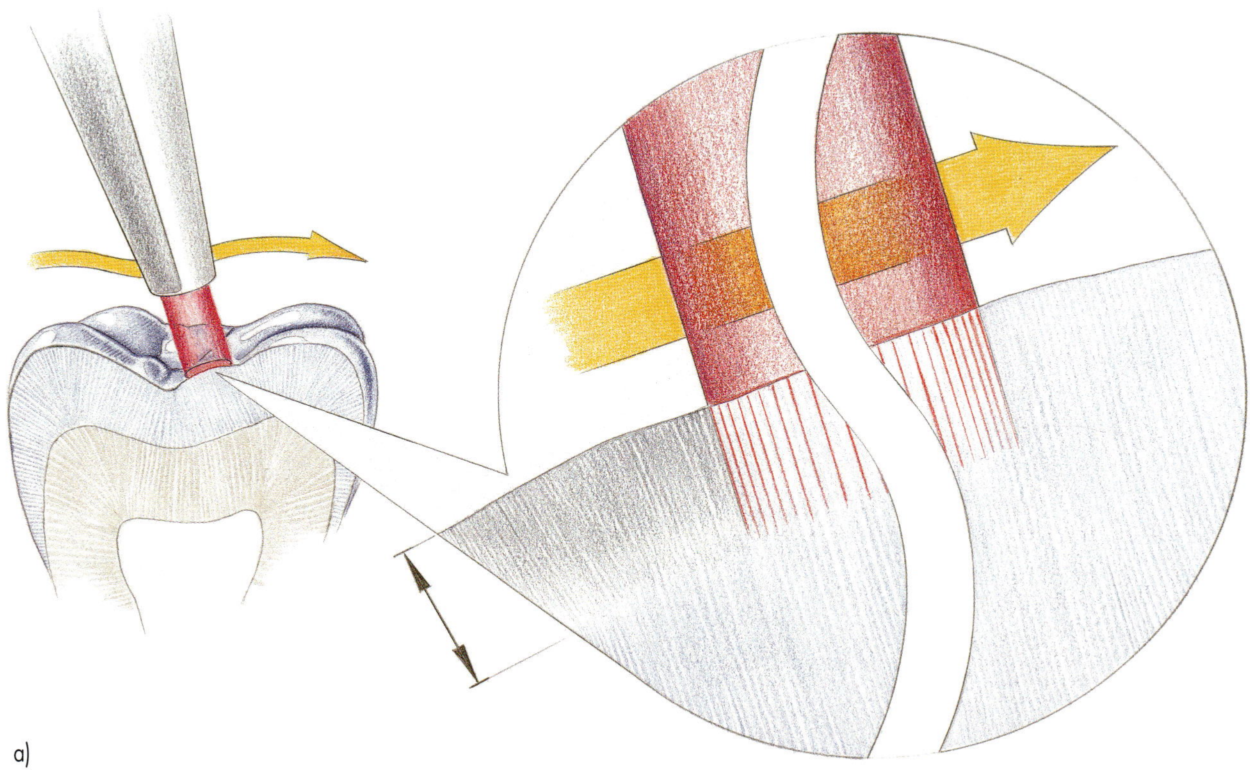

Fig 5-1a Laser treatment of occlusal fissures with magnification of the absorption depth in enamel by Er:YAG and CO_2 laser.

Fig 5-1 b Absorption in human enamel, dentin and cement.

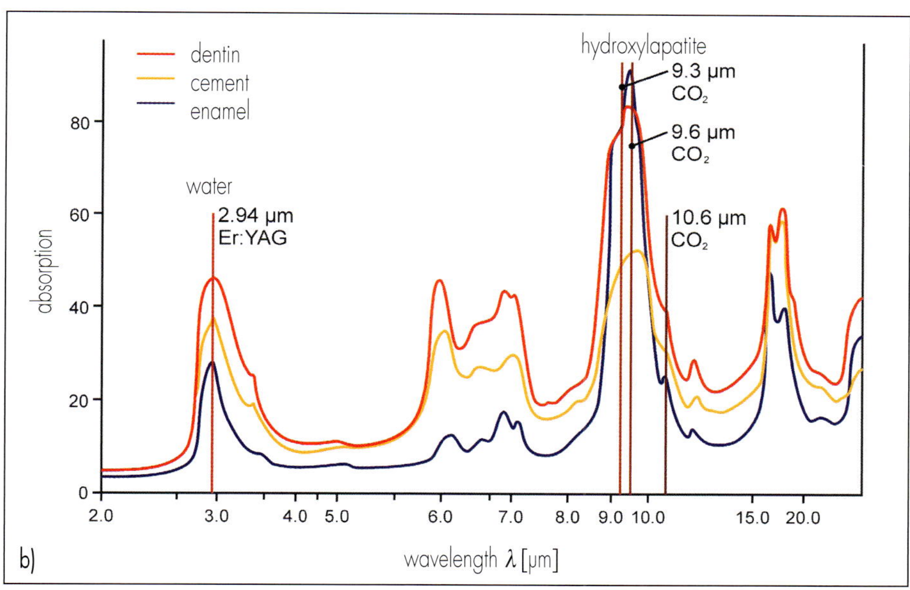

strongly absorbed by the mineral, with the absorption of these wavelengths being an order of magnitude higher than for the conventional 10.6 µm. The implications are, that if there is an application that requires efficient and short heating of the mineral, 9.3 and 9.6 µm would be the preferred wavelengths.

5.3.4 Mechanism of Laser Irradiation and Improved Caries Resistance

5.3.4.1 Changes in Enamel Composition

Theories regarding the mechanism by which laser irradiation enhances enamel resistance to artificial caries, range from a physical seal achieved by melting the surface through partial fusion and recrystallization of enamel prisms, to changes in enamel composition only[14]. It has been suggested by Stern et al.[18] and Lenz et al.[39] that the enamel surface is sealed by the laser and is less permeable for the subsequent diffusion of ions into and from the enamel.

Sato[40] reported that thermal treatment converts carbonated hydroxyapatite mineral to a less soluble mineral, and he found that the dissolution rate decreased after a 24-h heat treatment at 350°C. This change in solubility after low temperature treatment can be attributed to the thermal decomposition of the more soluble carbonated hydroxyapatite into the less soluble hydroxyapatite. At this time, the optimum temperature range for clinically applicable caries preventive treatments has not been determined. This is probably due to the complexity of the thermal decomposition of these materials. This complexity is compounded by several competing mechanisms that are optimized at different temperatures, e.g., high temperatures (>1,100°C) may lower the permeability of enamel; however, decomposition produces other phases that are more susceptible to acid dissolution. Lower temperature heat treatments (650°C) may increase the acid resistance by chemical changes (loss of organics and carbonate), even though the permeability has increased. With regard to subsurface enamel, it is believed that the laser-induced compositional changes of the enamel surface reduce its solubility and that changes below the surface will reduce the solubility beneath the surface.

SEM studies showed that enamel and dentin surfaces subjected to heat treatment by cw CO_2 laser (1, 2, 3 W) were sufficiently melted and the smear layer was solidified[41]. Even after acid demineralization the lased areas were unchanged. This corresponds to previous studies, which suggested that the reduced solubility is due to the laser-sealed enamel surface which is less permeable to the subsequent diffusion of ions into and from enamel[42,43].

SEM studies utilizing a pulsed CO_2 laser at $\lambda = 9.3$ and $\lambda = 9.6$ µm resulted in surface melting and recrystallization as polycrystalline masses, but conversely at $\lambda = 10.3$ µm and $\lambda = 10.6$ µm the original crystal size was observable with no fusion or recrystallization apparent[44]. The mineral content measurements made by Featherstone et al.[30] in the same range of laser conditions (1–12.5 J/cm^2) resulted in marked inhibition of dissolution which occurred in all cases (9.3 µm, 9.6 µm, 10.3 µm, 10.6 µm).

The combination of these two results indicate that the temperatures achieved by 10.3 and 10.6 µm were not sufficient to melt the surface, but were sufficient to have an effect on the chemical composition of the individual crystals making them less susceptible to acid dissolution. So the observations of Featherstone et al.[30] and McCormack et al.[44] are in agreement with the opinion that CO_2 laser-induced surface melting and fusion are not necessary to increase enamel resistance.

This result supports the theory of alteration in the composition of mineral phases with the decrease of carbonate, water and organic content which results in a reduction of lattice strain of hydroxyapatite and decreased solubility.

Dental material is a highly substituted form of hydroxyapatite and although many different elements are substituting the calcium, phosphate and hydroxy groups, the greatest substitution is that of the carbonate group (carbonate content in normal enamel 3–5%) and this carbonated apatite has a higher solubility than hydroxyapatite. Fowler and Kuroda[45] observed a reduction in the carbonate, water and apatite hydroxide content with a continuous wave CO_2 laser and they suggested that the laser treatment at temperatures < 650°C may convert sufficient acid phosphate HPO_4^{2-} to P_2O_7 to inhibit demineralization. Christofferson and Christofferson[46] reported that P_2O_7 concentrates reduced the hydroxyapatite dissolution rate to zero. Fowler and Kuroda[45] also hypothesized that heating to temperatures in excess of 1,200°C may actually increase the susceptibility of dental enamel to acid dissolution because the α- and β-$Ca_3(PO_4)_2$ and $Ca_4(PO_4)_2O$ phases formed at high temperature are more soluble than hydroxyapatite and dental enamel.

Featherstone et al.[28] proved that the lower the carbonate content, the lower the dissolution rate. The temperature range in which carbonate is driven from enamel is from 650 to 1,100°C[14] and Featherstone and Nelson[22] observed that the pulsed CO_2 laser produced a temperature rise (> 1,000°C) at the surface sufficient to fuse and melt enamel crystals, which are composed of carbonated apatite. This surface melt zone was no deeper than 5 µm, beneath which there was a region of interaction 10–40 µm deep, where the temperature rise was insufficient for the sintering process but sufficient for some compositional changes to the crystals. Subsequent infrared analysis[47] indicated that the carbonate content was dramatically reduced, and the surface phases were hydroxyapatite and tetracalcium diphosphate monoxide.

Zuerlein et al.[35] found in their bovine enamel studies with pulsed CO_2 laser, that the depth of carbonate loss (treatment depth) was consistent with a model that incorporates the absorption depth, the thermal relaxation time and also the pulse duration.

Comparable effects to those reported by Featherstone and Nelson[22] were reported, after heat treatment or laser treatment of human enamel, by Fowler and Kuroda[45]. These two scientists[48] observed a reduction in the carbonate content (66%), the water content, and apatite hydroxide content (33%) of enamel after irradiation with a continuous wave CO_2 laser (10,000 J/cm^2, 20 $W^{-1}s$). Analysis of the irradiated product using powder X-ray diffraction and infrared analyses indicated a mixture of minor phases of α-$Ca_3(PO_4)_2$ and $Ca_4(PO_4)_2O$ and modified hydroxyapatite. Fowler and Kuroda[45] categorized the chemical and morphological changes in dental enamel observed during heating (in a furnace) into three temperature zones: 100–650°C, 605–1,100°C and >1,100 °C.

All of the observed processes are dependent upon the rate and length of heating, which are of fundamental importance for the comparison of these observations with the effects of laser heating.

Table 5-2 Chemical and morphological changes in enamel during heating (Wigdor et al.[14]).

100–650 °C
1) Loss of H_2O (~ 30%)
2) CO_3^{2-}-loss (~ 66%) and rearrangement of carbonate to phosphate and OH^- positions
3) Acid phosphate HPO_4^{2-} condenses to pyrophosphate P_2O_7
4) Decomposition and denaturation of proteins
5) Contraction of a-axis lattice dimension at 250–300 °C
650–1,100 °C
1) Recrystallization, crystal growth of β-$Ca_3(PO_4)_2$, formed in tooth enamel
2) Decrease in OH^-
3) Conversion of OH^- to O^{2-}
4) Loss of H_2O and CO_3^{2-}
5) Loss of trapped CO_2 + NCO^-
> 1,100 °C
1) 1,450 °C: disproportionates α'-$Ca_3(PO_4)_2$ and $Ca_4(PO_4)_2O$, melting at 1 280 °C
2) 1,225 °C: β-$Ca_3(PO_4)_2$, converted to α-$Ca_3(PO_4)_2$
3) α'-$Ca_3(PO_4)_2$ and $Ca_4(PO_4)_2O$ melts at 1.600 °C, conversion of OH^- to O^{2-}

5.3.4.2 Creation of a Microsive or Micropore System

Some researchers suggest the creation of a microsive or micropore system[49–52] within the mineral structure (forming enamel, dentin and cementum) following laser treatment, and this provides a means for trapping calcium, phosphate and also fluoride ions released during demineralization. These micropores then act as sites for re-precipitation.

During the demineralization process, dissolution of mineral occurs with mobilization of the ions from the affected dental hard tissue. As mineral phases are released from the deeper layers of the hard tissue, re-precipitation in the more superficial or adjacent layers occurs and the surface remains intact.

Such a network has been described for lased enamel by quantitative polarized light techniques[52] and the trapped mineral phases inside it impede lesion formation and progression and cause enhanced resistance against demineralization.

So there is an enhanced uptake of fluoride, calcium and phosphate from endogenous and exogenous sources in lased dental hard tissue, due to the altered pore structure of enamel, cementum and dentin. In particular, the affinity for fluoride may result in redistribution of fluoride to root and enamel surfaces during demineralization, facilitating re-precipitation of the mineral phases into the tooth surface.

Additionally it has been shown that irradiation with an argon laser produces a change in the surface layer of the enamel by producing microporosities admixed with globular surface coating. This surface is rich in calcium, phosphate, and fluoride. The previously smooth surface enamel was transformed into a slightly roughened surface with fine porosities and discontinuous globular precipitates. All enamel surfaces in both low and higher fluence treatment groups were intact[53].

The presence of fine porosities with a confluent globular surface coating suggests that the effect of the argon laser at relatively low fluences (11.5 J/cm^2 and 100 J/cm^2) may alter or eliminate the organic material overlying and within the surface enamel. In addition, it appears as though the mineral phases previously embedded in this organic matrix may form globular precipitates, resembling calcium fluoride[54,55] confluent surface coatings. The surface enamel is known to contain an increased amount of fluoride compared to the underlying enamel, and mobilization of the mineral phases from the superficial enamel may result in a surface precipitate which is rich in fluoride, as well as calcium and phosphate[56].

The creation of such globular deposits with or without the formation of a confluent surface coating may provide a reservoir for mineral phases during a cariogenic attack. If the surface layer does indeed have an increased fluoride content in comparison with the adjacent underlying enamel, demineralization may be lessened and remineralization of the enamel surfaces by mineral phases acquired from the surface coatings, oral fluids and other exogenous sources may be facilitated.

Testing the argon laser also on root surfaces, Westerman et al.[57] found that the argon-lased root surfaces demonstrated alteration of root surfaces with creation of surface globular particulate material, microporosities and depressions. The globular deposits may provide readily mobilized tooth mineral, which may become redeposited into the underlying root surface during a cariogenic challenge and enhance resistance to caries formation.

Oho et al.[52] made a study in which they systematically investigated the argon laser effects. The birefringence for unlased enamel is the sum of a negative intrinsic birefringence, caused by the apatite crystals, and a positive form birefringence due to intercrystalline spaces[58,59]. The high positive birefringence of lased enamel observed in his study suggests that some additional spaces were formed by laser irradiation, which increased the positive form birefringence, resulting in the change of birefringence from negative to positive. The additional minute spaces are designated microspaces in his paper. No new products were found in lased enamel, though α-tricalcium phosphate and/or tetracalcium phosphate were reported in enamel treated with a CO_2 laser at a high energy density[48,60]. Such high temperature phases are not expected to be formed at the low energy densities of 67–160 J/cm^2 in his study.

Lattice strain was decreased after laser irradiation and this implies a better arrangement of ions in crystals of enamel. A slight contraction of the A-axis was observed but the C-axis was not altered by laser irradiation at an optimal energy density. The length of the A-axis is affected by the change of content and existing site (A or B site) of carbonate[61,62], and by a change of water content[63]. Reductions of water, carbonate and organic substances were revealed in lased enamel by infrared spectroscopy and thermal analyses. The reduction of carbonate and also the possible reduction of incorporated water from the crystals of enamel could have contributed to a slight contraction of the A-axis. The loss of water, carbonate and organic substances from enamel would have caused the formation of microspaces, which was suggested by the change of the optic character.

Fuchsin and fluoride clearly penetrated lased enamel, as did calcium and phosphorus. Tagomori and Morioka[64] also demonstrated a high fluoride uptake in lased enamel. The permeability of lased enamel was thus remarkably higher than that of unlased enamel, and this could be attributed to the existence of microspaces. The size of microspaces seems to be smaller than the micropores in caries lesions, because Thoulet's solution or quinoline did not enter the microspaces.

Reduction of carbonate content has been supposed to reduce the acid solubility of enamel[65,66], but Oho and Morioka[52] think that, although the carbonate reduction and the decrease of lattice strain would contribute to acid resistance, the role of microspaces in lased enamel should be taken into account when discussing the mechanism of acid resistance. In their study, the increased birefringence of lased enamel was reversed by the treatment with acid solutions such as lactate buffer, citrate buffer and perchloric acid. Acid resistance of lased enamel persisted during the reversal. When the birefringence had reached its original value, the acid resistance was at the same level as unlased enamel. A change of birefringence of human dental enamel was also observed during treatment with a calcifying fluid, and this was explained by remineralization of pores in dental enamel[59]. The change of birefringence in lased enamel during acid treatment could be attributed to the analogous mineralization process of microspaces.

So the hypothesis that laser irradiation might create microspaces would give an explanation for the observed acid resistance of dental enamel after laser irradiation.

5.4 The Caries Preventing Effect of CO_2 Lasers

Dental hard tissues strongly absorb[67] light in certain regions of the infrared spectrum, because of phosphate, carbonate and hydroxy groups in the crystal structure. The CO_2 laser produces radiation in the infrared regions that coincides closely with some of the apatite absorption bands[68]. This kind of laser can operate at discrete wavelengths between $\lambda = 9$ µm and $\lambda = 11$ µm. Those wavelengths correspond to specific rotational vibrational transitions in the ground state of the gas-phase CO_2 molecules. There are four principal vibrational emission bands which are centered at $\lambda = 9.3$ µm, $\lambda = 9.6$ µm, $\lambda = 10.3$ µm and $\lambda = 10.6$ µm, each consisting of several discrete rotational lines.

Commercially available CO_2 lasers are based on the wavelength of 10.6 µm and can be adapted to operate at the other wavelengths by various dispersive and nondispersive methods. The molecular groups mainly corresponding to the emitted CO_2 laser wavelengths in enamel are the phosphate groups with a strong absorption band near 1,000 cm^{-1} (=10 µm).

Table 5-3 Absorption coefficient and depth, reflectance and thermal relaxation time of enamel (Fried et al.[68]).

	$\lambda = 9.6$ µm	$\lambda = 10.6$ µm
Absorption coefficient (µ)	8,000 cm^{-1}	800 cm^{-1}
Absorption depth ($x = 1/\mu$)	1 µm	12 µm
Reflectance (R)	49%	13%
Thermal relaxation time (t)	1 µs	90 µs

In contrast to most other laser wavelengths, scattering is negligible in dental enamel at mid-IR wavelengths ($\lambda = 3$–12 µm), and so the energy deposition is determined by (a) the absorption coefficiency and (b) the tissue reflectance. The absorption coefficient of dental enamel at $\lambda = 9.6$ µm[36] is 8,000 cm^{-1} which is ~ 10 times higher than for a $\lambda = 10.6$ µm CO_2 laser wavelength (800 cm^{-1}) and also markedly higher than for any other wavelength throughout the visible and IR. Near resonance to the phosphate absorption band of carbonated hydroxyapatite, the imaginary component of the refractive index increases markedly and the magnitude of the Fresnel reflectance exceeds 50% for normal incidence at the air-tissue interface. Therefore the reflectance[25,69] can be very high, 49% at $\lambda = 9.6$ µm, 13% at $\lambda = 10.6$ µm.

A similar rise in reflectance does not occur in dental enamel near resonance to the strong absorption band of water at 3 µm.

Based on these facts, Featherstone and Nelson[22] suggested that using laser light would result in an effective energy deposition in the outer enamel layers.

Another suggestion they made was to use pulsed CO_2 lasers – rather than continuous wave lasers – to create high peak energy densities at the surface, while minimizing the cumulative energy deposition. It is preferable to use as little energy as possible because the cumulative energy determines the rise in pulp temperature[31].

They stated that the use of pulsed laser should allow surface changes without adversely affecting the underlying layers.

The laser treatment parameters that Featherstone et al.[21] investigated included: wavelength, pulse duration, pulse number, repetition rate, pulse energy and spot size. These studies[21,24,31,70] demonstrated that small changes in laser treatment parameters can sometimes result in a significant change in the caries inhibition achieved.

5.4.1 The Influence of Wavelength and Pulse Duration[6,35]

Dental mineral is a highly substituted form of hydroxyapatite, $Ca_{10}(PO_4)_6(OH)_2$, commonly referred to as carbonated apatite and represented by the simplified formula $Ca_{10-x}Na_x(PO_4)_{6-y}(CO_3)_y(OH)_{2-u}(F)_u$[6]. Although many different elements and functional groups have been found substituting for the hydroxyapatite components of the calcium, phosphate, and hydroxyl groups, three common substitutions are expressed in the formula. The most prevalent substitution is that of carbonate in place of the phosphate group. In normal enamel, the carbonate content is ~ 3–5% by weight[38]. At a given pH, the solubility of hydroxyapatite is approximately an order of magnitude below that of carbonated apatite. If the substitution of fluoride for the hydroxyl group is complete, fluorapatite results, ($Ca_{10}(PO_4)_6(F)_2$), which is another order of magnitude less soluble than hydroxyapatite.

Conventional heating experiments showed that ~ 30% of the carbonate was eliminated from dental enamel at temperatures between 400 and 600°C[62], and further carbonate loss occurred at higher temperatures. There is a correlation between carbonate loss in laser-treated dental enamel and a corresponding reduction in the rate of acid dissolution. The loss of carbonate results in a mineral phase that more closely resembles hydroxyapatite and is, therefore, less soluble than normal enamel at any given pH[29]. Previous studies showed a similar correlation in artificial apatites with varying carbonate content[6,71].

A major clinical concern with laser irradiation of teeth is the potential for overheating the tooth pulp that could lead to pulpal necrosis[72]. Carbon dioxide lasers are highly absorbed by enamel; therefore, the initial temperature rise occurs in a thin layer near the surface.

For temperature changes at the surface of the tooth, the duration of time over which the energy is delivered is equal in importance to the amount of energy delivered. To illustrate this, consider two extreme cases for a thermally-isolated enamel block. In the first example, assume all of the energy is delivered as an instantaneous pulse. The initial temperature rise at any depth will be dependent only upon the absorption properties of the enamel at the irradiating wavelength and on the energy delivered to the layer near the surface.

The temperature rise of the heated volume is $\Delta T = E/\rho cAz$, where E is the energy delivered, A is the surface area of heating, z is the depth of heating. The heat capacity of enamel is $c = 0.75$ J/g°C, and the density of enamel $\rho = 2.9$ g/cm^3. Subsequently the thermal energy diffuses to the remainder of the enamel block and heats the entire block to a more moderate temperature.

In the second case, if the same amount of energy is delivered continuously over an extended period of time, the layer and the entire block will have only a slight temperature rise.

So, in the first case, there would be a therapeutic effect in a thin layer near the surface, but the region that contains the pulp has a minimal temperature rise in the second case, and there will be no effect other than the slight temperature rise throughout the entire block. The aim is to maximize the benefit of laser treatment by heating a layer of the appropriate thickness to a sufficiently high temperature while causing minimal thermal insult to the deeper layers of the tooth.

The preceding two examples led to the concept of thermal relaxation time[68]. The relaxation time of the axial heat conduction (t) of the deposited energy in the tissue surface is representative for the length of time required for heat diffusion from the layer of tissue heated by the laser, and depends on both the thermal diffusivity (k) and the absorption coefficient (μ_a), at the respective laser wavelength. If the diameter of the laser beam is much greater than the absorption depth, radial conduction can be neglected. The relaxation time for the axial heat conduction is given by $t = 1/4\ k\mu_a^2$ or $x^2/4k$ (the absorption depth $x = 1/\mu$).

If pulse duration of the laser is of the order or less than the thermal relaxation time, the energy will remain in the volume where it was absorbed.

Since the energy is not leaving this region immediately, large temperature increases near the surface can be realized with low energy input similar to the case of instantaneous heating.

In this case, the absorption depth x correlates with the treatment depth and therefore the wavelength which determines the absorption depth can be changed and different depths can be treated (changing λ) in this manner, but the pulse duration limits the minimum depth.

If the pulse duration is much longer than the thermal relaxation time, a larger volume becomes heated to a lower temperature, which may or may not be effective enough for a therapeutic effect. In this way the pulse duration correlates positively to the depth of laser treatment, a shorter pulse will treat a thinner layer near the surface, but the minimum treatment depth is limited by the absorption depth (which correlates with the specific wavelength used).

Based on these theories, Zuerlein et al.[36] tried to determine the precise depth of modification and thermally-induced decomposition of dental enamel (carbonate loss), at the predicted optimum laser irradiation parameters. Bovine enamel blocks were irradiated at $\lambda = 9.6$ µm with 2-µs and 100-µs pulses and at $\lambda = 10.6$ µm with 2-µs pulses. Carbonate loss was calculated from infrared spectra as a function of depth and compared to numerical simulations of the maximum temperature rise.

After irradiating dental enamel at $\lambda = 9.6$ µm with either 2-µs or 100-µs (five pulses) pulses, the carbonate loss was calculated as a function of the depth. At the surface, complete carbonate loss was observed in dental enamel irradiated by either pulse duration. The carbonate loss first remained complete near the surface and then decreased as a function of depth until it was zero at 6 µm for the 2-µs pulse and zero at 11 µm for the 100-µs pulse.

Since the wavelength is equal for both different pulse durations, that are longer than the thermal relaxation time (1 µs), the treatment depth correlates positively to the pulse duration (6 µm and 11 µm for 2 µs and 100 µs).

After numerical calculations with the same laser parameters (but only one pulse) the temperature rise as a function of depth was modeled. The maximum temperature rise in dental enamel irradiated with 2-µs pulse duration is much higher than that of 100-µs but temperature rise also decays much more rapidly as a function of depth into the enamel.

For the two irradiation conditions (2 µs and 100 µs and 6 µm and 11 µm) the numerical calculation estimated the temperature at which carbonate is no longer lost (400–450°C). This temperature point is consistent with previous experiments using conventional heating. Complete carbonate loss was not obtained until temperatures greater than 800°C were reached, which coincides with the minimum melting point of carbonated hydroxyapatite[83].

The temperature at which carbonate loss begins is 400–450°C, the melting point of enamel occurs between 800 and 1,200°C, and vaporization occurs at temperatures above this.

After irradiating bovine enamel at the 2-µs pulse duration at $\lambda = 9.6$ µm or $\lambda = 10.6$ µm, the carbonate loss was calculated as a function of depth. The surface of the enamel irradiated at each of those two wavelengths was treated with five pulses or one pulse. The carbonate loss of enamel irradiated at $\lambda = 9.6$ µm with five pulses first remained at 76% and then decreased as a function of depth and fell to zero at 6 µm into the surface. The carbonate loss of enamel irradiated with $\lambda = 9.6$ µm for one pulse lost 40% and then decreased as a function of depth and fell to zero at 2 µm into the surface. The surface of enamel irradiated at 10.6 µm lost about 100% and 66% of the carbonate for five pulses and one pulse, respectively. The carbonate loss of enamel irradiated with five pulses remained at 100% and then decreased as a function of depth and at 8 µm the percent carbonate loss remained at almost 30%.

The carbonate loss of enamel irradiated with one pulse decreased as a function of depth and fell to zero at 5 µm into the surface. Since the pulse duration is equal for both wavelengths (2 µs), and with the thermal relaxation time of 1 µs, the treatment depth correlates to the absorption coefficient and therefore depends on the wavelength (2 µm and 5 µm depth for λ = 9.6 µm and λ = 10.6 µm at one pulse).

After numerical calculations with the same laser parameters as above, but only one pulse, the temperature rise as a function of depth was modeled. The maximum temperature rise in enamel irradiated at λ = 9.6 µm is much larger than that of 10.6 µm, but the temperature rise also decays much more rapidly as a function of depth in bovine enamel. At 20 µm depth, the calculated temperature of enamel irradiated with 10.6 µm wavelength is still almost 400° C (at this temperature carbonate loss is possible).

The maximum temperature rise at 9.6 µm is much larger than at 10.6 µm correlating to the higher absorption coefficient (8,000 cm^{-1} at λ = 9.6 µm, 800 cm^{-1} at λ = 10.6 µm).

Greater carbonate loss at the surface was expected for dental enamel irradiated with 9.6-µm light than for dental enamel irradiated with 10.6-µm light due to the greater maximum temperature rise. Experimentally, with either one pulse or five pulses the carbonate loss was greater at all depths for the enamel irradiated at 10.6 µm. Total carbonate loss at the surface was achieved in five pulses at 10.6 µm, but it took between 10–20 pulses for enamel irradiated at 9.6 µm. Since the duration for which the surface temperature is above the melting point is much greater for enamel irradiated at 10.6 µm than at 9.6 µm, carbonate loss is also greater.

5.4.2 The Influence of the Pulse Number

Previous experiments made by Kantorowitz et al.[67] have shown that the resistance of carbonate apatite achieved through laser treatment depends on the number of irradiation pulses used.

To isolate the effect of the number of laser pulses, they kept all other laser parameters constant while the number of pulses was varied. The additional samples were irradiated at two different wavelengths to determine whether the dependency of the number of pulses varied with wavelength.The laser parameters were:

– λ = 10.6 µm, 240 mJ/pulse, 12 J/cm^2/pulse and
– λ = 9.6 µm, 100 mJ/pulse, 5 J/cm^2/pulse.

For each wavelength the pulse duration was 100 µs, the frequency 10 Hz and the number of pulses 1, 5, 25 or 100. The different pulse energies selected for the wavelengths were because of the higher absorption at the 9.6-µm wavelength by enamel.

1. Fried et al. found that at both wavelengths the laser-treated groups had significantly smaller lesions. Compared with their control groups, a single pulse achieved some inhibition, but increasing the number of pulses increased the degree of inhibition to a level that changed little with additional laser pulses. At each of the two wavelengths tested, the optimal number of pulses was not more than 25 pulses. It seems that there is a point at which a further increase does not increase inhibition.
2. Laser irradiation at 10.6 µm achieved higher inhibition than 9.6 µm at each pulse number. At 25 pulses there was 87% inhibition for λ = 10.6 µm compared with 59% inhibition for λ = 9.6 µm.
   Although the laser irradiation at 10.6 µm achieved higher inhibition, from the pulpal safety point of view, it may not be the best wavelength to use for this purpose. Initial temperature measurements carried out 2 mm beneath the laser-irradiated surface indicate a 10°C rise for 25 pulses at 10.6 µm compared with a 1°C rise at 9.6 µm[70]. These differences probably result from the different optical interaction of these two wavelengths with enamel as evidenced by marked differences in the absorption coefficients.
3. In the study above[36], carbonate loss also was expected to depend upon the number of irradi-

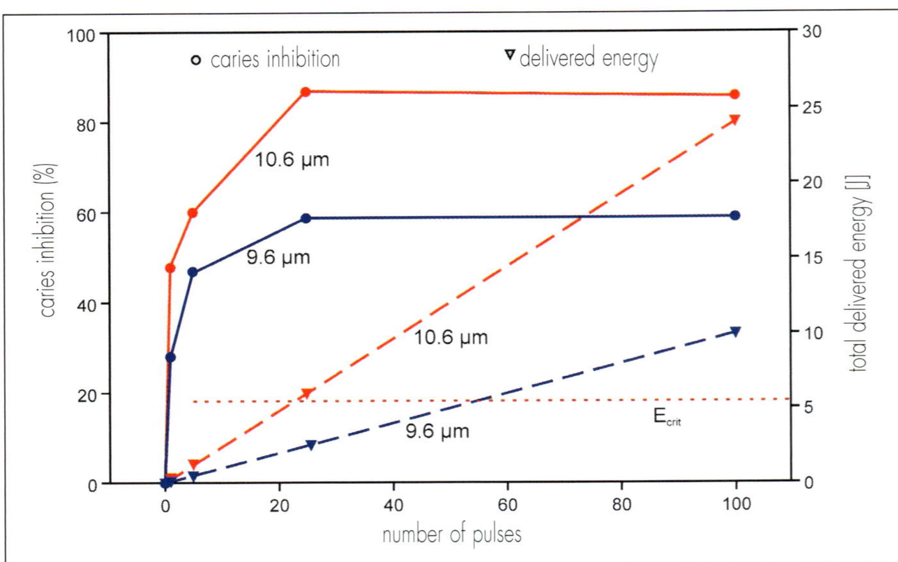

Fig 5-2 Influence of delivered energy amount on caries inhibition.

ating pulses. Carbonate loss was initiated at 400°C but complete carbonate loss did not occur until melting was achieved at temperatures greater than 800°C (melting point of enamel). To ensure carbonate loss, the enamel must be irradiated with a sufficient number of pulses which depends upon the fluence, pulse duration and the absorption coefficient.

4. The results of Lakshmi et al.[73] showed that CO_2 laser irradiation at $\lambda = 10.6$ µm can inhibit caries-like lesions up to 82.7% and it was optimal at 25 pulses, compared to 5, 15, 50 and 100 pulses.

5.4.3 The Influence of Wavelength and Fluence

To examine systematically the roles of wavelength and fluence, Featherstone et al.[29] used the four principal emission bands of the CO_2 laser.

Each wavelength was irradiated with 25, 150, 100, 200 or 250 mJ/pulse and the pulse number was 25 with a 100-µs pulse duration at 10 Hz and a beam diameter of 1.6 mm. The irradiated enamel window was 2 mm^2.

1. All the irradiation conditions tested in this study produced statistically significant inhibition of subsequent caries-like lesion formation. By using energy pulses in a range of 25–250 mJ/pulse the inhibition effect ranged from 42 to 85%.
2. The comparable caries inhibitory effect of 25 mJ/pulse of incident energy at 9.6 µm with 200 mJ/pulse at 10.6 µm indicates an eightfold difference in incident energy for the two wavelengths to produce similar caries inhibitory effects (= 60% caries inhibition, 57% caries inhibition). Previous studies of Featherstone and Nelson[22] indicated that $\lambda = 9.3$ µm and $\lambda = 9.6$ µm light was much more efficiently

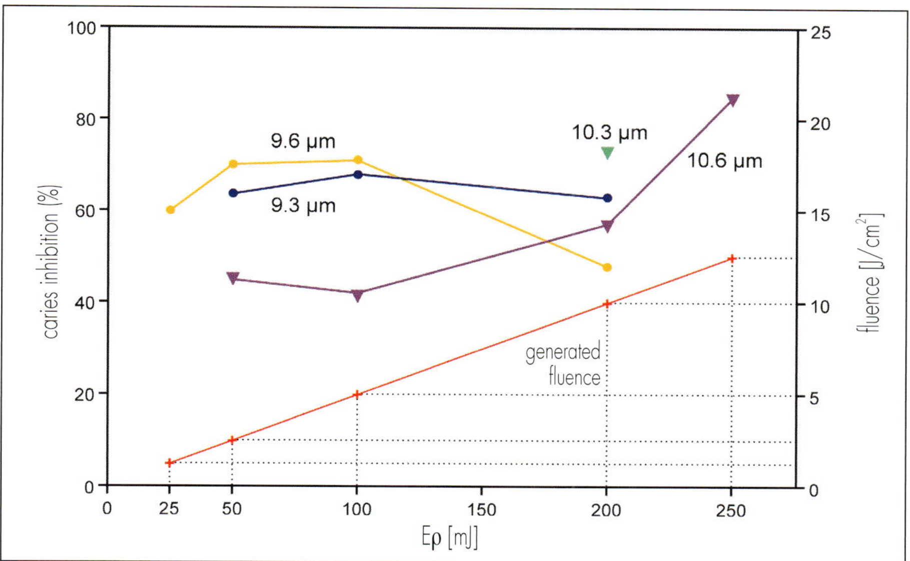

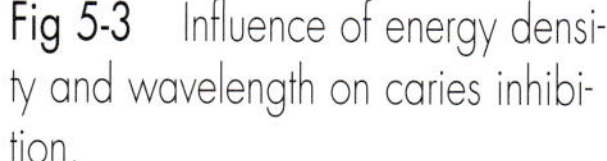
Fig 5-3 Influence of energy density and wavelength on caries inhibition.

absorbed than the $\lambda = 10.3$ µm and $\lambda = 10.6$ µm wavelengths. These conclusions are confirmed by the absorption coefficients of Duplain et al.[69], namely 18,500, 30,000, 6,500 and 5,000 cm^{-1} for the $\lambda = 9.3$ µm, $\lambda = 9.6$ µm, $\lambda = 10.3$ µm and $\lambda = 10.6$ µm wavelengths, respectively. The different absorption coefficients provide an explanation as to why it is possible for one eighth of the energy to produce an inhibition comparable to that at $\lambda = 10.6$ µm. The transformation of light to heat when it is absorbed into enamel mineral is more effective at $\lambda = 9.3$ µm and $\lambda = 9.6$ µm, than it is at $\lambda = 10.6$ µm[22]. Light may be reflected, absorbed, scattered or transmitted by tissue. For the wavelengths studied here, absorption occurs in the outer few micrometers and therefore scattering and transmission are essentially zero. The high absorption coefficients for all four CO_2 wavelengths indicate a very effective transformation of light to heat at these wavelengths. Reflectance at the surface, however, must also be considered. Reflectance studies by Duplain et al.[69] using bovine enamel, and recently confirmed using human enamel by Fried et al.[25], indicate that at $\lambda = 9.6$ µm ~ 50% of the added energy is reflected, whereas at $\lambda = 10.6$ µm only 10% is reflected. So the comparable caries inhibitory effect of 25 mJ/pulse of incident energy at 9.6 µm with 200 mJ/pulse at 10.6 µm indicates approximately a 14-fold difference in absorbed energy for the two wavelengths to produce similar effects.

3. Surprisingly at the higher incident energy level of 200 mJ/pulse with $\lambda = 9.6$ µm, significantly less caries progression was found. In a separate study made by McCormack et al.[44], surface damage was observed by SEM, following irradiation at this energy level by the highly efficiently absorbed $\lambda = 9.6$ µm wavelength. The damaged surfaces apparently were detrimental and provided less resistance to acid challenge (see section 5.4.6).

5.4.4 Oral Safety Parameters

1. With regard to the study mentioned before[29], a wide range of incident energy conditions was compared for each of the λ = 9.6 µm and λ = 10.6 µm wavelengths. With the exception of the group irradiated at 250 mJ/pulse, all of the lower energy conditions (from 50–200 mJ/pulse) for 10.6 µm produced inhibition of less than 58%, in contrast to inhibition of the order of 70% achieved (by 50–100 mJ/pulse) with 9.6 µm. This indicates that less energy at 9.6 µm produces caries inhibition at a higher level than more incident energy at λ = 10.6 µm, which shows caries inhibition at a lower level. The group irradiated with 250 mJ/pulse at 10.6 µm produced an inhibition of 85% but this was not statistically significantly different from that of 70% produced at λ = 9.6 µm with 50 mJ/pulse. Temperature measurements by Fried et al.[31] showed that temperatures at the surface for a single pulse at 9.6 µm and a fluence of 5 J/cm^2 exceeded 900°C whereas those for λ =10.6 µm were of the order of 500°C. Thermocouple measurements by Fried et al.[31] at a depth of 2 mm from the surface of the enamel showed a temperature rise, following 25 pulses at 10 J/cm^2 at λ = 10.6 µm, of ~ 10°C and a corresponding rise at 2.5 J/cm^2 and λ = 9.6 µm of ~ 1°C. So, using the wavelength of λ = 9.6 µm provides more pulp safety. The above-mentioned surface temperature effect is related to the absorption coefficient whereas the ratio of these internal temperature rises corresponded to the ratio of the absorbed total energies.
2. As a first attempt at the direct comparison of wavelength effects, the results for 200 mJ/pulse (fluence 10 J/cm^2) for each of the four wavelengths can be compared from the table. It can be seen that at these energy levels, λ = 10.3 µm is apparently the most effective. However, as stated above, with λ = 9.6 µm at this relatively high fluence (10 J/cm^2), surface damage occurred. Therefore, a direct comparison of efficiency in this way is not appropriate. Rather, the comparison of percentage inhibition as the end result is more suitable, with an attempt at determining the energy conditions at wavelengths that are most likely to be effective. Generally, the optimum conditions for clinical use will be those which achieve the highest caries inhibition with the lowest detrimental energy deposition in the underlying tissues. From the table, it can be seen that relatively low fluences/pulse of the order of 2.5–5 J/cm^2 were effective at wavelengths of λ = 9.3 µm and λ = 9.6 µm (9.6 µm is more effective). These values, when reflectance is taken into consideration, indicate that absorbed fluences between 1 and 3 J/cm^2/pulse were effective at inhibiting caries-like progression at these wavelengths. These fluences at 10 Hz and 25 pulses produced temperature rises at a depth of 2 mm in the enamel of only ~ 1°C or less, as described above.

In a study by Fried et al.[74], the laser parameters for the efficient thermal modification of dentin with minimum heat deposition at CO_2 laser wavelengths were firmly established. The surface temperatures of dentin were markedly higher than those measured on enamel for similar irradiation intensities due to the lower reflectance losses of dentin and the lower thermal diffusivity of dentin at the respective wavelengths. Hence, lower fluences are required for the thermal decomposition of dentin. Ablation typically occurred with the first few laser pulses during multiple pulse irradiation and eventually ceased after modification of dentin to a more highly mineralized enamel-like tissue. The debris ejected during the initial laser pulses shielded the surface by as much as 60% at the low fluences employed in this study. Optical and electron microscopy and IR spectroscopy indicated that incident laser pulses with incident fluence as low as 0.5 J/cm^2 at λ = 9.3 µm and λ = 9.6 µm wavelengths with a duration of 5–8 µs were sufficient to induce chemical and morphological changes in dentin.

5.4.5 Surface Morphology

Hossain et al.[75] investigated the effect of λ = 10.6 µm cw laser irradiation on the acquired acid resistance of sound dentin and enamel to artificial caries-like formation, and evaluated the effect by spectrophotometry and SEM in vitro. Caries inhibition for enamel and dentin ranged from 54% at 1 W to 79% at 3 W.

In the SEM observation, the unlased enamel or dentin surfaces showed the presence of a smear layer that occluded the enamel rods and dentinal tubules.

The lased enamel and dentin surfaces were partially melted and solidified, thus the enamel rods or the dentinal tubules were not visible.

After demineralization with 0.1 M lactic acid, the control samples showed complete removal of the smear layer and the enamel rods or the dentinal tubules could be recognized. While the lased enamel and dentin surfaces were almost unchanged, the enamel root or the dentinal tubules could not be recognized.

The reason is that the lased areas were found to be melting with solidification of the smear layer. Even after demineralization the lased surfaces were almost unchanged and this suggests that a CO_2 laser could sufficiently melt and solidify the smear layer and thus enhance resistance to artificial caries-like formation.

This corresponds to other previous studies like that of Fox et al.[76] and Nelson et al.[43] who suggested that moderate heat treatment by a CO_2 laser reduced the solubility of dental enamel and carbonated apatite. It was suggested that the enamel surface is sealed by the laser and is less permeable to the subsequent diffusion of ions into and from the enamel.

With a similar aim, Featherstone and Nelson[22] observed that a pulsed CO_2 laser produced a temperature rise > 1,000°C at the subsurface, sufficient to fuse and melt the crystals.

The objective of a study made by Nammour et al.[77] was to determine the dependence of the sealing effect, and the smoothness of the lased dentin, on the applied energy density, and to verify whether sound dentin, once sealed (using the irradiation conditions applied in the dental practice), proves more resistant to acid than unlased dentin.

As a result of the SEM examination, the surface of the lased dentin appeared to be sealed at all four energy densities used, but a smooth surface was only obtained when the energy density did not exceed 425 J/cm^2. The sealed dentin contained no tubular structure, whereas in the underlying dentin the dentinal tubules retained their normal aspect. At energy densities of 565 and 715 J/cm^2, cracking of the surface increased. The number and the length of the cracks were variable from one place to another in the same sample, but no acid erosion could be detected on the sealed surface. However, between laser beam impacts, the unlased dentin had not been sealed and showed demineralization and widened tubules after acid exposure. So the results of the SEM observations suggest that the lased dentin is less permeable to acid.

Indeed microradiography showing the mineral content of each specimen from the surface towards the pulp, revealed that the sealed layer seemingly had not been demineralized but the underlying dentin had, but to a limited extent.

The photodensitometric evaluation showed that the thickness of the laser-sealed layer varied from 20 µm for an energy density of 280 J/cm^2, to 70 µm for 715 J/cm^2. The degree of acid penetration into the lased dentin did not vary with the energy density used and amounted to 250 µm. In unlased dentin the depth of lesion amounted to 450 µm and more. So sealing did not totally prevent progression in depth, but the demineralization in the underlying dentin remained lower than in unlased dentin. There are two interpretations possible:

1. Acid penetration occurs through unsealed dentin areas.
2. The microcracking provides diffusion pathways to the underlying sound dentin.

The sealed layer of dentin seemed to be acid resistant because the mineral content of the sealed layer was increased. These observations agree with the increased calcium and phosphate found in lased and recrystallized dentin by Kantola[78] who attributed this increased mineral content mainly to the burning of the organic matter from the tissue. (In melted dentin the water is evaporated, the organic material is combusted, the hydroxyapatite is fused). Compared with this, in the sections before, there is a newer carbonate loss theory, conforming to the results of Flower and Kuroda, who recognized in an earlier study[45] a reduction in the water, hydroxyapatite and also carbonate content in enamel after irradiation with a cw laser.

5.4.6 The Problem of Cracking

The irradiation conditions applied showed that the lower use of energy decreased the appearance of cracks in dentin. With tooth enamel irradiated under different conditions it has also been shown that the occurrence of cracks depended on the irradiation conditions[31]. No crack-inducing internal tension occurred during resolidification after irradiation at 13 J/cm^2, which is much lower than in this dentin study.

Fowler and Kuroda[45] hypothesized that heating to temperatures in excess of 1,200°C may actually increase the susceptibility of dental enamel to acid dissolution. Therefore CO_2 laser treatment requires wavelength specification for efficient conversion of laser energy with heat not more than 1,200°C at the enamel and dentin surfaces.

As an example of the effect of overheating, the reader can take a look at the Figure 5-3 in the section 5.4.3[29], in which it is shown that at the incident energy level of 200 mJ/pulse at $\lambda = 9.6$ µm, significantly less inhibition of caries progression was found in enamel compared with lower energy levels.

In the above-mentioned investigation made by Fried et al.[37] with a pulsed CO_2 laser, an SEM examination was also made.

In the samples irradiated with 240 mJ pulses at $\lambda = 10.6$ µm (12 J/cm^2 per pulse), the treated areas showed little or no morphological changes. Only a few hot spots within the affected area showed fusion, recrystallization, or exfoliation of the enamel.

On the other hand, in all the samples irradiated with 100 mJ pulses at $\lambda = 9.6$ µm (5 J/cm^2 per pulse), most of the treated area showed morphological surface changes. In these samples the surface appears to have been fused. Higher magnification (x 60,000) showed that the surface was composed of new crystals that were larger than normal enamel crystals. There were occasional spots in which exfoliation had occurred.

The SEM observations at $\lambda = 10.6$ µm did not show physical changes, although all the laser-treated groups tested at this wavelength demonstrated a high level of caries inhibition. This indicates that the temperatures achieved at 10.6 µm are not sufficient to melt the surface, but were sufficient to have an effect on the chemical composition of the crystals, making them less susceptible to acid dissemination. These observations show that surface melting and fusion are not necessary to increase enamel resistance.

Furthermore, in this study the phenomenon of microcracking was shown again≠. A cross section of a typical unlased control lesion about 75–100 µm deep appeared to be uniform across the acid-exposed enamel window. If the inhibitory effect of the laser was uniform, the decreased caries in the laser-treated teeth simply would be shallower.

But in the laser-treated tooth, in some areas there is no evidence of demineralization, in other areas the demineralization seems to be almost as deep as the control lesion.

The appearance of inhibited lesions repeated itself in both wavelengths investigated in this study.

At x 500 magnification the demineralization in these lesions occurred around microfractures descending 50–75 µm from the surfaces, while the surfaces between these fractures seem to be totally resistant to demineralization.

The question, how to avoid the undesirable effect of the fractures with the preventive potential of laser treatment, is answered by Kantorowitz et al.[80] who showed that fluoride application immediately after laser irradiation may circumvent these effects.

Zuerlein et al.[36] found, as described above, using optical microscopy of the surface of dental enamel irradiated five times with a 2-µs pulse at 9.6 µm with 2 J/cm^2, the appearance of wave-like structures.

After a single pulse the surface appeared smooth, but after 10 pulses the surface was modified with the wave-like structures to a much greater extent, and these increased with the number of pulses. The reason is, that at temperatures exceeding the melting point of enamel, some fraction of material will be ejected from the surface, resulting in a loss of deposited energy from the sample with a concomitant reduction in the thickness of the modified zone.

The rapid vaporization of mineral and spallation of molten mineral, due to laser-generated stress transients, are likely to result in the formation of the observed wave-like surface structures produced after several laser pulses incident on the same spot.

McCormack et al.[44] analyzed systematically the wavelength-dependent structural changes that are attributed to the different effects of the CO_2 laser (λ = 9.3 µm, λ = 9.6 µm, λ = 10.3 µm and λ = 10.6 µm) absorption coefficients at each of these wavelengths.

In this study, melting was defined as the initial stages of individual crystals beginning to coalesce. Fusion was defined as the stage when melting is complete, and individual crystals have fused together to form large, new crystals. The physical changes in crystal size and shape that occurred as melting and fusion progressed followed a distinct pattern. Until the threshold temperature for melting was reached, the enamel crystals retained the needle-like form and size (~ 40 nm diameter) of normal enamel. As surface temperatures reached the threshold for melting, the crystals coalesced into nondescript shapes and increased in diameter, and when they exceeded the threshold for melting, the enamel crystals fused into large (from 200–400 nm) polyhedral crystals. At even higher temperatures, the polyhedral crystals fused further, forming a solid mass in which crystal boundaries were barely discernible.

5.4.7 Polished Enamel

1. 10.6-µm effects: The 10.6-µm wavelength produced no observable surface melting at 5 or 10 J/cm^2 absorbed fluence per pulse, although distinct surface cracks associated with the thermal stress created by the heat of the laser beam interaction were present. Polishing scratches were still visible, as were individual unchanged enamel crystals, indistinguishable in size and shape from normal enamel, indicating that no melting or fusion had occurred. An absorbed fluence of 20 J/cm^2 per pulse was required to melt the enamel and fuse the crystals at 10.6 µm.
2. 10.3-µm effects: At 5 J/cm^2 absorbed fluence per pulse, the effect of the laser was barely visible except for surface micro-cracks and occasional small (~ 100 µm diameter) regions of preferential melting and crystal fusion. At 10 J/cm^2 absorbed fluence per pulse, the melt zone was distinct although non-uniform, and some small (from 4 to 20 µm) smooth-edged craters with solid bottoms were present. Within the areas of melting, individual enamel crystals had begun to coalesce into nondescript shapes. At 20 J/cm^2 absorbed fluence per pulse, surface melting occurred to a greater extent, and the surface was partially ablated, creating large, elongated craters. In these areas, the enamel crystals were beginning to fuse together.
3. 9.3-µm effects: At 5 and 10 J/cm^2 absorbed fluence per pulse, uniform surface melting occurred across the area of irradiation. Enamel

crystals were fused to various degrees, from the nondescript shape of early melting to the large (up to 500 nm diameter) polyhedral shape of later stages of fusion. Droplets of re-condensed enamel mineral surrounded the area of irradiation. Due to the low fluence threshold for melting at this wavelength, these samples were not irradiated with 20 J/cm^2 absorbed fluence per pulse.

4. 9.6-μm effects: At 5 and 10 J/cm^2 absorbed fluence per pulse, surface melting was extensive throughout the area of irradiation. Portions of the surface were ablated, and droplets of re-condensed enamel surrounded the area of irradiation. In many areas, enamel crystal fusion had progressed to the point that crystal definition was no longer visible. Due to the low fluence threshold for melting at this wavelength, these samples were not irradiated with 20 J/cm^2 absorbed fluence per pulse.

5.4.8 Unpolished Tooth Crowns

The number of laser pulses delivered did not appear to have a significant effect on the degree of crystal fusion observed, except at $\lambda = 10.3$ μm.

5.4.9 Pulse-Width Effects on Unpolished Human Enamel

To study surface modifications due to pulse width, an additional series of unpolished human tooth crowns with 25 pulses (5 J/cm^2 absorbed fluence per pulse) at each of the four pulse widths (50 μs, 100 μs, 200 μs, and 500 μs) were irradiated. Within each wavelength, at constant fluence and number of pulses, the degree of surface effect decreased as pulse width increased. To discuss the result of McCormack's study, the SEM observations can largely be explained by the absorption properties of tooth mineral in the IR region.

Dental enamel is primarily composed of carbonated hydroxyapatite, which has strong absorption bands in the IR region due to phosphate, carbonate, and hydroxyl groups in the crystal structure[6]. CO_2 laser emission (from 9–11 μm) overlaps the strong phosphate absorption bands of dental enamel apatite[22]. Specifically, the 9.3- and 9.6-μm wavelengths (1073 and 1045 cm^{-1}, respectively) and to a lesser extent, $\lambda = 10.3$ μm (973 cm^{-1}) are close to the transition frequencies (1,060, 1,032, 961 cm^{-1}) of the molecular vibrations of the phosphate ion in carbonated hydroxyapatite. This is manifested in the high absorption coefficients, shallow absorption depths, and high reflectance at these wavelengths.

The 10.3-μm (973 cm^{-1}) and 10.6-μm (945 cm^{-1}) wavelength are on the longer wavelength side of the absorption band and are further from weaker resonance frequencies resulting in lower absorption coefficients, higher absorption depths, and lower reflectance. Laser light at $\lambda = 9.3$ μm or $\lambda = 9.6$ μm and to a lesser extent, at 10.3 μm and 10.6 μm, would therefore be strongly absorbed very near to the enamel surface and rapidly transformed into heat, as demonstrated by surface temperature measurements[28,81,82]. The melting point of carbonated hydroxyapatite varies with carbonate content[83]. Surface enamel (~2% carbonate) should therefore begin to melt at about 1,100°C and fuse at or above the hydroxyapatite melting point of about 1,280°C[48]. Based on the temperature data, absorption coefficients and reflectance values, the surface modifications resulting from CO_2 laser irradiation should occur with absorbed energies (fluence = energy/surface area) in the order of 9.6 μm < 9.3 μm < 10.3μm < 10.6 μm. Although dental enamel is more reflective at $\lambda = 9.3$ μm and $\lambda = 9.6$ μm, the laser absorption at these wavelengths is more efficient than at $\lambda = 10.3$ μm and $\lambda = 10.6$ μm, making the actual energy absorbed per volume greater and the resulting surface temperatures higher at $\lambda = 9.3$ μm and $\lambda = 9.6$ μm.

SEM micrographs of surface changes resulting from CO_2 laser irradiation clearly demonstrated

Fig 5-4 Surface parameters: temperature measurements,[24,81] absorption coefficients,[69] and reflectance values[82] for polished enamel surfaces (Peak temperature ranges measured following surface irradiation of polished human enamel by CO_2 laser light with 100-μs pulse duration.)

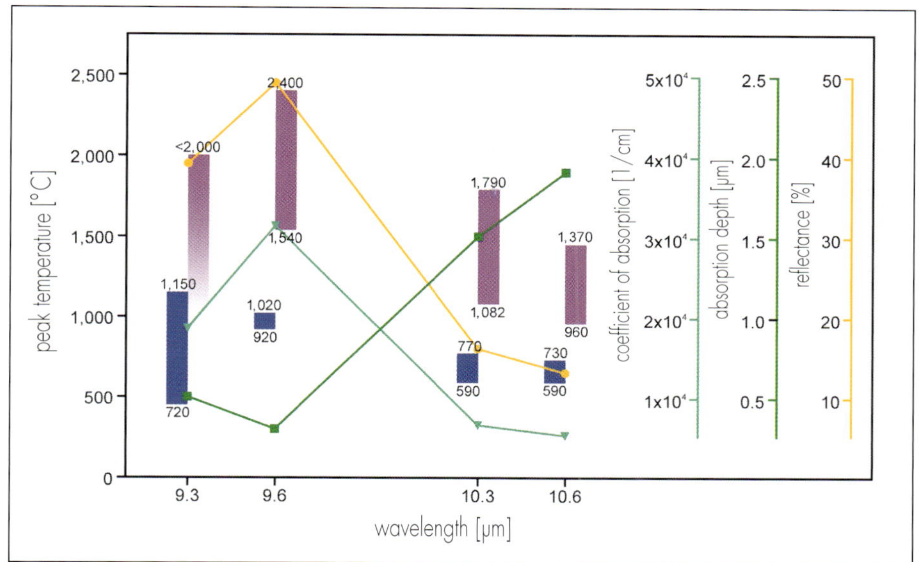

such a wavelength-dependent pattern. The heat generated by the CO_2 laser tuned to $\lambda = 9.3$ μm or $\lambda = 9.6$ μm and, to a lesser extent, 10.3 μm was sufficient to produce rapid surface melting and enamel crystal fusion at absorbed fluences as low as 5 J/cm^2 per pulse. At 10.6 μm, crystal fusion required fluences greater than 10 J/cm^2 on polished enamel surfaces. Previous studies[22,47] showed similar trends in surface effects and wavelength dependence with low-energy pulsed CO_2 laser irradiation of dental enamel but with irradiation intensities (1 MW/cm^2, from 100–200-ns pulse widths) much higher than those used in this study.

Although the overall effects on unpolished tooth crowns were similar to those observed on enamel polished to a flat surface, differences in detail were observed, which suggest that the actual temperatures generated by the CO_2 laser light at the surfaces of the tooth crowns may be different from temperatures measured on polished enamel. Geometrical considerations, primarily the surface roughness and curvature of tooth, reduce the absorbed energy density by increasing the total surface area being irradiated. In this study, it was possible to avoid highly curved surfaces; however, in a clinical situation, this aspect will need to be considered.

An effect of the laser observed exclusively on the unpolished human enamel was "exfoliational sputtering", where large pieces (from 1–5 μm in diameter) of material flaked off from the surface, leaving behind shallow craters. Exfoliational sputtering was not observed along with surface melting. Exfoliational sputtering can be expected to occur in systems of high thermal stress (i.e., materials rapidly heated by lasers, but to temperatures below the melting threshold), and has been observed previously for other materials that are subject to thermal stress during laser heating[84]. Thermal stress is strongly affected by absorption depth and the thermal relaxation time of a material. Exfoliation in this study was observed predominantly following irradiation at $\lambda = 10.6$ μm. It is possible that it occurred also at other wavelengths but was subsequently masked by surface melting. Exfoliational sputtering can also be caused by the rapid expansion of the gaseous decomposition products of heated enamel, such as water and CO_2. Exfoliational sputtering may have significant implications, depending upon the intended purpose of the laser treatment. During caries-preventive dental treatment, this effect could cause undesirable surface damage. Knowing the specific laser parameters to choose, or to avoid, to produce these effects is therefore desirable.

Within the possible wavelengths of the CO_2 laser, there were observed dramatic differences in the effects on dental enamel. Whereas the 9.3-, 9.6-, and 10.3-µm wavelengths produced significant surface melting and crystal fusion, with only a few laser pulses at low energies, λ = 10.6 µm appeared to chemically or structurally alter the composition of the enamel crystals, which would not be distinguishable by SEM. Changes in pulse width appeared to have little effect at fluences of 10 J/cm^2 per pulse, where surface temperatures for 10.3-, 9.3-, and 9.6-µm irradiation were well in excess of the melting point of the mineral. However, at the lower fluence of 5 J/cm^2 per pulse, a reduction in surface change was observed with longer pulse durations. Surface temperature measurements[82] showed that peak temperatures took longer to reach with a 500-µs pulse, and the maximum was ~100–200°C lower than with the 50- or 100-µs pulse widths. These thermal observations therefore provide an explanation for the SEM results.

If the more efficiently absorbed wavelengths of the CO_2 laser (λ = 9.3 µm and λ = 9.6 µm) and a carefully determined pulse width are used, it may be possible to alter the structure of the enamel crystals near the surface with only a few laser pulses at low energies, thus reducing the likelihood of heat conduction from the enamel surface to the pulp chamber.

As reported, laser has been used as a heat source for melting and recrystallization. Occurring at about 1,100°C, the melting of surface dental enamel along with recrystallization might have an assistant role in the therapy of a hypersensitive tooth, apical sealing of endodontic surgery in dentistry, preventive dentistry for pit and fissure sealing, and fluoridation. For laser to be accepted in clinical applications, studies must show that the incorporation of CaF_2 into hydroxyapatite could reduce the sintering temperature for the sake of safety. The results of Wu et al.[85], with a λ = 10.6-µm CO_2 laser, showed fusion between hexagonal shape crystals and cubic shape crystals (CaF_2) under SEM. Hexagonal shape crystals indicated the formation of fluorapatite under XRD (X-ray diffractometry) analysis. Under FTIR (Fourier transforming infrared spectroscopy) reductions of water (3,445 cm^{-1}) and hydroxyl bands (3,567 and 627 cm^{-1}) in irradiated compounds were examined. From the DTA (differential thermal analysis) pattern of the synthetic compound, it showed the endothermic reaction reaching its peak point around 1,180°C +/– 20°C. It was attributed to the phase transformation and/or initial melting. Wu et al.[85] proposed the interrelationship of the eutectics between initiator (CaF_2) and the reaction product (calcium hydroxide) that reduced the sintering temperature. It appeared that the co-eutectics interacted to reduce the sintering temperature of hydroxyapatite below 800°C and that the key eutectic was calcium hydroxide. The clinical feasibility of the melting and recrystallization of hydroxyapatite under a λ = 10.6-µm CO_2 laser would therefore be enhanced.

5.4.10 Combined Effect of CO_2 Laser Irradiation and Fluoride Treatment

Hsu et al.[86] evaluated the effects of CO_2 laser irradiation of dental enamel in enamel demineralization experiments in partially saturated solutions (i.e., solutions containing both calcium and phosphate ions) with and without fluoride ions.

Enamel blocks were irradiated with a continuous-wave CO_2 laser at a wavelength of λ = 10.6 µm using energy densities of from 42.5–170.0 J/cm^2.

A comparison between the lased and the unlased portions of enamel showed increased acid-resistance with increasing laser energy density, and at the highest energy density of 170.0 J/cm^2 there was little or no lesion development in the fluoride-free dissolution medium. The demineralization of enamel was reduced dramatically in the presence of 0.2 ppm fluoride for both lased and

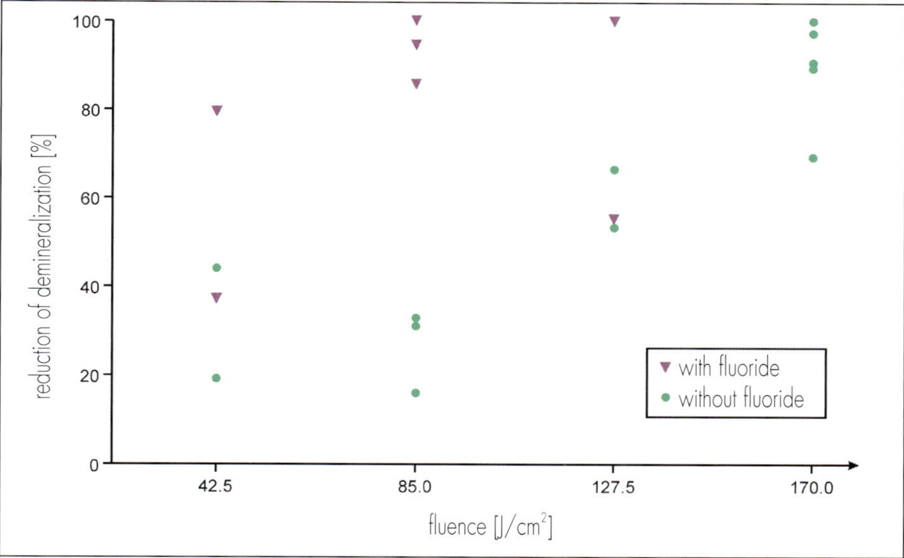

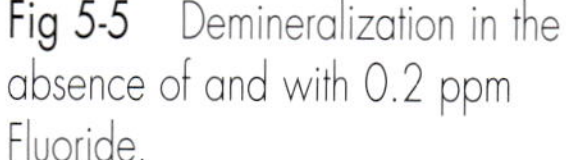
Fig 5-5 Demineralization in the absence of and with 0.2 ppm Fluoride.

unlased enamel; there was only modest lesion development observed for unlased enamel and, at an energy density as low as 85.0 J/cm^2, the surface of enamel was found to be completely protected. These findings were consistent with the mechanism that laser irradiation of dental enamel results in significant reduction of the effective solubility of enamel mineral and there is a significant synergism between laser irradiation and fluoride solution with regard to this effect.

Hossain et al.[87] investigated the caries-preventive effect of CO_2 laser irradiation with or without sodium fluoride (NaF) solution on human dental enamel and dentin in vitro. The lowest mean Ca^{2+} ppm was recorded at the enamel or dentin samples treated with NaF and laser. SEM observation showed that surfaces were changed to melted, smooth, and mirror-like appearances when CO_2 laser irradiation was applied with NaF solution. So it can be concluded that CO_2 laser irradiation with NaF solution has a greater caries-preventive effect than CO_2 laser irradiation only, at the enamel and dentin surfaces.

5.4.11 Clinical Aspects

Lasers can be used to effectively modify the chemical composition of the remaining mineral phase of enamel. This is possible because the mineral, hydroxyapatite, found in bone and teeth contains carbonate inclusions that makes it highly susceptible to acid dissolution by organic acids generated from bacteria in dental plaque. Featherstone and Nelson[22] demonstrated that transverse excited atmospheric pressure (TEA) CO_2 lasers operating at the $\lambda = 9.3$–10.6 µm wavelengths could be used effectively to inhibit enamel demineralization. Upon heating to temperatures in excess of 400° C, the mineral decomposes to form a new mineral phase that has increased resistance to acid dissolution.

Studies suggest that, as a side effect of laser ablation, the walls around the periphery of a cavity preparation will be transformed through laser heating into a more acid-resistant phase and have an enhanced resistance to future decay[88,89].

Lasers can be tightly focused to drill holes for micropreparations with very high aspect ratio (depth/diameter), well beyond the capability of the dental drill, which is limited by the size of the dental burr. This is of particular importance since early caries lesions are typically localized to the pit and fissures of the occlusal surfaces of the posterior dentition, and these fissures are of the order of 200–300 μm wide. Therefore, lasers have the potential to substantially reduce the amount of tissue that needs to be removed for cavity preparation.

5.5 The Caries Preventing Effect of Argon Lasers

The argon laser emitting at λ = 488 nm and λ = 514 nm has been effective in reducing loss of tooth structure and size of subsurface lesions on both root and enamel surfaces in vitro and in vivo at relatively low fluence levels (12 J/cm^2).

Westerman et al.[90] used, for the irradiation of root surface windows, an argon laser emitting primary wavelengths of λ = 488 nm and 514 nm. The lesions on the control surfaces were almost 30% deeper than those on the lased surfaces (188 µm vs. 132 µm) after the initiation period. After the first regression period the lesions on the control surfaces were 31% deeper than those on the lased surfaces (252 µm vs. 174 µm). There was a 35% decrease in lesion progression when comparing the lased and control group (64 µm vs. 42 µm). The second progression period showed that the lesions on the control surfaces were almost 35% deeper than those on the lased surfaces (302 µm vs. 197 µm) when comparing the lased and control groups. There was about a 50% lower progression rate (progression period II–progression period I) for the lased group compared with the control group (50 µm vs. 23 µm).

The same group of researchers[50] tested the effect of argon laser irradiation on artificial caries initiation and progression in enamel using the same laser conditions as before. The lesions on the control surfaces were almost 42% deeper than those on the lased surfaces (117 µm vs. 69 µm) after the initiation period. Progression period I resulted in 35% deeper lesion of the control surfaces than those of the lased surfaces (158 µm vs. 103 µm). There was a 17% decrease in lesion progression when comparing the lased and control group (41 µm vs. 34 µm). Progression period II: the lesions on the control surfaces were almost 39% deeper than those of the lased surfaces (221 µm vs. 135 µm) when comparing the lased and control groups. There was about a 49% lower progression rate (progression period II–progression period I) for the lased group compared with the control group (63 µm vs. 32 µm).

To evaluate also the clinical effectiveness of the argon laser[91], bilateral bicuspids scheduled for orthodontic extraction were used in vivo, utilizing a modified orthodontic band[92] to develop demineralization of human enamel in vivo. The researchers found in the teeth that were lased prior to band placement, an average of 29.1% reduction in lesion depth compared to the unlased teeth. Summarizing, clinical results as well as laboratory results showed a significant reduction of demineralization with low power irradiation (12 J/cm^2).

5.5.1 Oral Safety Parameters

The argon laser has been shown as a means of reducing demineralization of dental hard tissues. This procedure could inadvertently damage the teeth if proper precautions are not taken, or the parameters for damage not understood. Powel et al.[93] determined safety parameters for the intraoral use of the argon laser, such as how high an energy density can be applied to the enamel surface before irreversible damage occurs to the enamel or pulp tissues.

1.) Effects of argon laser on pulpal tissues: Teeth exposed to <600 J/cm^2 had a similar pulpal histology to that of the control teeth. There was an intact odontoblastic layer, normal vascularity without edema and extravascular blood cells. More than 600 J/cm^2 were required to cause evident damage to pulpal tissue and the damage observed between 600 and 800 J/cm^2 was judged to be minimal and was assured to be reversible with time (loss of odontoblastic orientation, edema, extravascular blood cells, no necrosis). In tooth lased with over 800 J/cm^2, focal necrosis in the odontoblastic layer, in

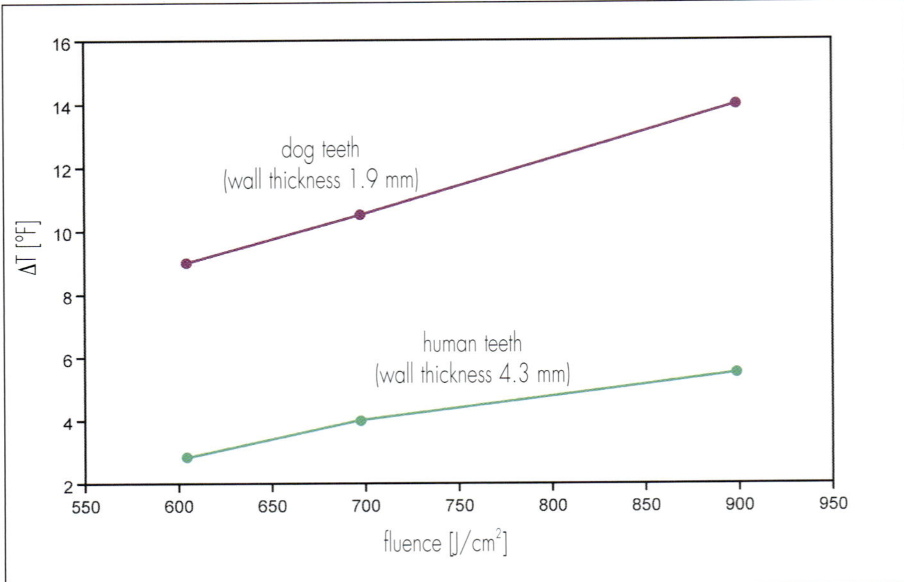

Fig 5-6 Pulpal temperature change.

addition to the edema and extravascular blood cells, occurred until generalized coagulation-type necrosis occurred at higher temperatures in all pulpal elements.

2. Changes in pulp chamber temperature: The temperature rises were proportional to the amount of energy applied to the enamel surface. The results were similar to those of Zach and Cohen[72] in which pulpal damage begins to take place at ~10°F increase in pulpal temperature. The argon laser parameters necessary to create 10°F pulpal temperature change in the dog teeth was similar to the energy density that created the first signs of pulpal damage of the dog's pulpal tissue (698 J/cm^2 = 10.5°F). It is anticipated that greater energy densities would be necessary to cause pulpal damage in human teeth because of their greater thickness. In addition, in the in vivo human tooth it is assumed that the surrounding tissue and blood flow through the pulp tissue would help dissipate generated heat. Thus it is hypothesized that the pulpal temperatures recorded in vitro in human extracted teeth would be higher than those that would be experienced in vivo.
3. Enamel surface damage: No visible enamel surface damage occurred at the energy levels applied in this study, not to the human eye, nor by light microscopy and magnified photographs.

The argon laser appears very safe for preventive procedures, if low limits of laser energy are used.

5.5.2 Surface Morphology

To compare the effects of argon laser irradiation at relatively low fluences (11.5 J/cm^2 and 100 J/cm^2) on enamel surface morphology, Westerman et al.[53] created a study using standard scanning electron microscopic techniques.

Sound unlased enamel surfaces possessed relatively smooth surface morphology with occasional depressions of 3–5 µm in diameter representing the prism end markings. The enamel surfaces were intact and without surface defects, crazing or fracture lines.

In contrast, following argon laser irradiation at both low and higher fluences (energy densities, 11.5 J/cm^2 and 100 J/cm^2) the surface morphology of sound enamel was altered substantially. The previously smooth surface enamel was transformed into a slightly roughened surface with fine surface porosities and discontinuous globular precipitates. The microporosities varied minimally in diameter, with the majority being less than 1 µm in maximum dimension. These fine porosities in the enamel surface were intermingled with islands of relatively dense surface precipitates. These islands of surface coatings appeared to be slightly elevated and more superficially located than the adjacent areas of microporosities. These fragmented surface coatings were composed of a coalescence of globular material ranging from ~500 nm to over 2 µm in dimension.

The surface alterations following argon laser irradiation of sound enamel were quite similar in both low and higher fluence argon-laser treatment groups. The only difference between these two groups was an increase in the area that was covered by the surface precipitates, and a decrease in areas characterized by micropores within the low fluence group (11.5 J/cm^2).

The lased surfaces lacked crazing, fracture lines, and exfoliative changes typically described for treatment with other laser types[44,94–97] and even the prism morphology was not exposed. The intact nature of the surface enamel is attested to by previous laboratory studies[98–102] which have shown intact surface layers using polarized light, following artificial caries formation in lased enamel and dentin. Surface disruptions in these studies were not found.

One mechanism of caries prevention hypothesizes that fine microporosities are created in tooth structure, building a microsieve network within the tooth structure. It is suggested that such a network would effectively "trap" and precipitate mineral phases mobilized by an acidogenic challenge, and thereby enhance caries resistance. Such a network has been shown to be present by quantitative polarized light studies[52]. The presence of fine porosities with a confluent globular surface coating suggests that the effect of the argon laser at relatively low fluences (both 11.5 J/cm^2 and 100 J/cm^2) may alter or eliminate the organic material overlying and within the surface enamel. In addition, it appears as though the mineral phases previously embedded in this organic matrix may form globular precipitates, resembling calcium fluoride[54,55], that partially occlude the microporosities and may form confluent surface coatings. The sound surface enamel is known to contain an increased amount of fluoride compared to the underlying enamel, and mobilization of the mineral phases (when pH falls) from the superficial enamel may result in a surface precipitate which is rich in fluoride as well as calcium and phosphate[56].

The laser-induced creation of globular deposits described above, with or without the formation of a confluent surface coating, may provide a reservoir for mineral phases during a cariogenic attack. If the surface layer does indeed have an increased fluoride content, in comparison with the adjacent underlying enamel, demineralization may be lessened, and remineralization of the enamel surfaces by mineral phases acquired from the surface coatings, oral fluids and other exogenous sources may be facilitated.

Supporting the idea that these surface coatings may have a caries protective effect, are prior cariology studies[98–102] which have shown an ~30–35% reduction in lesion depth in both lased enamel and dentin, when compared with matched nonlased enamel and dentin. The argon laser irradiation was used at a fluence of either 11.5 or 100 J/cm^2[98–102], and while providing surface alterations, the laser does not create the exfoliation (sloughing of layers of surface enamel), extensive crazing and cratering typically described with CO_2 lasers[44,94–97].

5.5.3 Combined Effect of Argon Laser Irradiation and Fluoride Treatment

Fluoride agents, like 1.23% acidulated phosphate fluoride APF-gel to be described later, can be utilized either before or after laser irradiation and result in a significant reduction in lesion depth. This fluoride treatment provides 12,300 ppm fluoride and results in both labile and bound fluoride retention within enamel[103]. Typically, fluoride agents at this concentration produce surface coatings that may[102] act as diffusion barriers, reduce enamel solubility in acid conditions, act as a reservoir for fluoride-rich reaction products such as calcium fluoride, and desorb proteins and microorganisms from the enamel surface[11,54,55,104].

Laser irradiation of enamel has been shown to reduce the threshold pH for enamel dissolution by 0.72 pH units, which corresponds to an almost fivefold increase in the amount of acetic acid normally required to initiate enamel dissolution[42,76]. Effectively, the dissolution threshold was lowered from pH 5.50 for non-treated enamel to 4.78 for lased enamel. In addition, the enamel solubility at pH 4.5 following laser treatment was reduced by fivefold for lased enamel, when compared with non-treated enamel[42,76].

The combination of fluoride and laser irradiation had a synergistic effect on caries formation. The addition of less than 0.1 ppm fluoride to demineralizing fluids resulted in a significant decrease in enamel solubility for both sound and lased enamel. In the presence of fluoride, the threshold for sound enamel dissolution was reduced from pH 5.50 to 5.14. Lased enamel in the presence of fluoride has an enamel dissolution threshold that was reduced from pH 4.78 to 4.31. Particularly interesting is the fact that lased enamel exposed to low levels of fluoride had a solubility that was sixfold less than that for nonlased enamel exposed to the same fluoride level. In this way, it was shown that laser irradiation combined with fluoride treatment has additive effects.

One proposed mechanism for the caries preventive effect of laser irradiation is, that the irradiation results in the creation of microspaces within enamel[43,47,52,105]. These microspaces may be of importance in reducing enamel solubility. During the demineralization phase of caries formation, various mineral phases like calcium, phosphate and fluoride ions become dissolved in acid solution and are released into the oral environment. It has been speculated that the microspaces, created by laser irradiation, may trap the released ions and act as sites for mineral re-precipitation. This deposition of released mineral phases may be connected with, and enhanced by, the lased enamel having an increased affinity for fluoride, phosphate and calcium ions from the oral environment, and this indicates an increasing amount of fluoride and other minerals in the dental hard tissue surface. The release of this greater amount of fluoride may be the critical factor in re-precipitation of mineral phases within lased enamel and overall reduction in enamel solubility.

Studies with the argon laser[100–102] demonstrated that combined with fluoride surface treatment, or fluoride in the demineralization solution, reduction in loss of tooth structure or size of lesion occurred.

Flaitz et al.[102] demonstrated a significant caries preventive effect in enamel when combining argon laser irradiation at a moderate fluence level (100 J/cm^2) with acidulated phosphate fluoride treatment prior to lesion formation. As a result, they found that when the argon laser was combined with acidulated phosphate fluoride APF-treatment, either before or after laser irradiation, the lesion depth was 51–55% (argon laser before acidulated phosphate fluoride, acidulated phosphate fluoride (APF) before argon laser) less than that of the control group.

The argon-laser-only group, compared with the control group, indicated a 34% reduction in lesion depth and combining the laser irradiation and fluoride treatment resulted in 26–32% greater reduction in lesion depth compared with the argon laser alone. The mean surface zone depths for all treatment groups were increased over that for the control group only (2–2.5 times). Not only the lesion depth has been affected but also certain qualitative differences in the degree of the birefringence within the body of the lesion were noticeable. With the combined laser irradiation and fluoride treatment groups, the body of lesions show a qualitatively decreased degree of positive birefringence (pore volume > 5%) and an increase in pseudoisotropy (pore volume = 5%) in contrast to the control lesion, which shows greater pore volume.

A follow-up study[100] in the same conditions, except with a lower fluence level (12 J/cm^2), resulted in a similar outcome: 10 weeks in a dialyzed reconstituted acidified gel significantly (31%) decreased lesion depth with argon laser treatment alone when compared with the control lesion. Acidulated phosphate fluoride treatment, either before or after argon laser exposure, provided over a 50% reduction in lesion depth compared with the control lesion, and a one-third decrease when compared with argon laser treatment alone.

So it is apparent that even low fluence laser treatment in combination with fluoride treatment provides a significant degree of protection against caries development and progression.

Fluoride treatment prior to laser irradiation, in both studies, provided the greatest reduction in lesion depth.

Fluoride preceding or following argon laser irradiation has not been shown to significantly affect lesion depths; however, there is a trend toward greater resistance to caries initiation and progression when fluoride treatment precedes argon laser exposure. Concerning the application time, Garcia et al.[106] demonstrated that either a 1- or 4-min acidulated phosphate fluoride treatment prior to caries-like lesion formation decreased the lesion depths in vitro by 37–49%.

Anderson et al.[107] compared the caries resistance of sound human enamel following argon laser irradiation, as well as the combination of topical fluoride, namely acidulated phosphate fluoride (APF) and sodium fluoride foam. After the 4 min of fluoride, the foams were rinsed off the enamel surfaces followed by the laser irradiation. The argon laser irradiation was 0.23 W, 11.5 J/cm^2 for 10 s. The argon laser irradiation alone reduced lesion depth by 15% compared with the control lesion after 96-h storage in demineralization solution. When argon laser irradiation was combined with 1.23% APF foam treatment, lesion depth decreased by 25% and by 29% when combined with 2.0% NaF foam.

Compared with the above-mentioned result of Hicks et al.[100] there are three reasons for the different reduction in lesion depth with APF treatment. Hicks et al.[100] used an APF gel, whereas this study used an APF foam; they used an acidified gelatin gel as the insulting medium, while this study used an acidified solution; they insulted the specimen for a longer time (3–6 weeks), while this study was for only 96 h. So one could speculate that a greater %-reduction in lesion deep would occur if the exposure time were extended.

If root caries reacts in a similar way, a simple preventive technique may be established[49]. When the argon laser was combined with APF treatment, either before or after laser irradiation, the lesion depth was 54–57% (argon laser before APF, APF before argon laser) less than that of the control group. The argon-laser-only group, compared with the control group, indicated a 24% reduction in lesion depth and combining the laser irradiation with fluoride treatment resulted in 40–43% reduction in lesion depth compared with the argon laser alone.

Whether fluoride precedes or follows argon laser irradiation has not shown to significantly affect lesion depth; however there is a trend towards greater resistance to caries development when fluoride treatment precedes argon laser exposure.

Caries development in root surfaces is initiated at a higher critical pH (pH 6) than that for enamel (pH 5.5), therefore the root surface has an increased affinity for uptake of fluoride when compared with sound enamel. This results in a greater amount of calcium fluoride deposition within the superficial layers of the root surface as well as on the root surface. So, with the addition of topical fluoride application to laser irradiation, the benefits of fluoride on caries resistance may be achieved in enamel and also on cementum and dentin forming the root surfaces.

The implication of the mentioned studies is that relatively low fluence argon laser irradiation in combination with topical fluoride treatment provides prevention of dental caries in artificial caries models. Argon laser irradiation and fluoride treatment enhances in vitro the resistance of sound enamel to a cariogenic challenge. The future may provide dental visits that include the services of an examination, prophylaxis, radiographs, sealants, and topical fluoride treatment in conjunction with laser irradiation.

5.5.4 Clinical Aspects

Investigation has shown that significant reduction in the extent of artificial caries formation and enamel solubility occur after laser irradiation of enamel and dentin, even with relatively low energy levels[52], and that the argon laser can be used for initiating the setting reaction with visible light-cured resins[108–110]. Argon-laser-curing of resin materials is a method which enhances the physical properties and degree of polymerization of the resin, while reducing the polymerization time by 75%.

A study examining the effect of argon laser curing of sealant material and microleakage resulted in interesting findings[111]. With argon laser-cured sealants, the incidence of wall lesions were similar at lesion initiation, but significantly different following lesion progression when compared with paired controls. An unexpected finding was that the lased surface enamel adjacent to the sealant material showed significant reductions in lesion depths both at lesion initiation and progression periods, when compared with paired, control surface enamel.

With the laser-cured sealant group, surface lesion depths were reduced by 36% after caries initiation and by 45% after caries progression, when compared with paired surface lesions adjacent to sealants.

It would appear that laser irradiation of sound enamel may be of considerable benefit in prevention of enamel caries. A significant caries-preventive effect has been demonstrated when combining argon laser irradiation at a low fluence level (12 J/cm^2) with acidulated phosphate fluoride treatment prior to lesion formation. Because it is possible to collimate the beam to a specific diameter and focus the beam to a selected depth, it may be possible to irradiate interproximal areas, especially beneath the contact area, which may be particularly susceptible to caries development[108–110]. The potential also exists for improving caries resistance in enamel forming pits and fissures. This may occur while one is actually utilizing an argon laser for polymerizing a visible light-cured sealant material.

5.6 The Caries Preventing Effect of Nd:YAG Lasers

The effect of laser radiation on tissues depends upon the interaction of the different wavelength photons with the target material, and is based for the Nd:YAG and the CO_2 laser on a photothermal mechanism[97]. The extent of the changes that occur within enamel and dentin is affected by the absorption characteristics of the substrate and the wavelength at which the laser operates. Considerable variation in the effects of different wavelengths of laser light on dental hard tissue has been observed. CO_2 laser radiation in the range of $\lambda = 10.6$ µm is absorbed very readily by tissue, with the color and structure of the tissue having little or no effect. This means that absorption and extinction of the radiation occurs within 0.1 mm of the surface[112]. Nd:YAG radiation at a wavelength of $\lambda = 1.06$ µm is affected to a much greater extent by the color and structure of the substrate and is not so readily absorbed.

One of the limitations of the application of Nd:YAG radiation to dental hard tissue is the variability in the color and composition of both enamel and in particular dentin. It has been reported that this can lead to considerable variations in the effect of this type of radiation when applied to different teeth[112]. The extent of this variation has not, however, been clearly defined. Enamel is a translucent tissue that readily allows the passage of visible and near IR light[113]. In order to produce an effect using Nd:YAG radiation, an energy absorbing initiator must be applied to the target surface to absorb the laser light[114]. The absorption of the beam by the initiator results in the conversion of the energy delivered to heat. This produces changes to the enamel surface. The efficacy of the initiator in conversion of the laser energy to heat is demonstrated by the intensity of the changes observed in the target tissue.

Dentin, a more opaque material, shows variable absorption characteristics depending on its color and translucency. Translucent sclerotic dentin will absorb little or no Nd:YAG radiation; instead it is transmitted to the underlying structure – usually the dental pulp[112]. Dark carious dentine will, however, absorb a large component of the energy and the tissue will be heated. These variations exist not only between different specimens but can also occur within a single tooth.

In the sections before, argon and CO_2 laser treatment were performed as an effective mechanism in elevating the resistance of enamel to the cariogenic challenge, reducing enamel solubility and inhibiting caries-like lesion formation. Additionally, Yamamoto and Sato[40] and Tooya[115] indicated that human enamel irradiated with an acousto-optically Q-switched Nd:YAG laser was more resistant to acid decalcification than an unlased control.

The prevention of caries in occlusal fissures is of practical importance, since pits and fissures are more susceptible to caries than any other area[116]. Day et al.[117], Barr et al.[118] and Backer Dirks[119] have all reported that the occlusal surface of molars and premolars, the lingual grooves and pits of upper molars and incisors, and the buccal pit of lower molars are particularly susceptible to caries attacks. Other investigations have also shown that occlusal surfaces are susceptible to dental decay, accounting for nearly 50% of all caries[120]. It is thus also necessary to develop an effective preventive measure against pit and fissure caries. Morioka et al.[121] suggested that a normal pulsed Nd:YAG laser is the most suitable for clinical use, because of the high resistance against acid decalcification and the smaller amount of damage caused to the enamel surface. Furthermore, Tagomori et al.[64] reported that an Nd:YAG laser can be guided to the patient through a flexible optical fiber. They showed that fluoride application after laser irradiation produces a greater fluoride uptake in the smooth enamel surface than fluoride application before laser irradiation.

Following this, the purpose of Bahar and Tagomori[122] was to investigate the effect of normal pulsed Nd:YAG laser irradiation (300 μs, 750 mJ/pulse, 20 Hz) on the acid resistance of pit and fissure enamel as well as on the cleaning of their contents. In addition, the fluoride uptake into the enamel of the pits and fissures treated with acidulated phosphate fluoride (APF) after laser irradiation was evaluated.

They found that the evaluation of acid resistance by comparing the amount of calcium dissolved per square millimeter of lased and unlased pit and fissure enamel indicated that the pit and fissure enamel exposed to the laser acquired a 30% higher acid resistance than the untreated controls. Similar results were reported in lased smooth surfaces of enamel[64, 123].

Myers and Myers[124] showed that an Nd:YAG laser has the potential to remove organic and inorganic debris from the pits and fissures without causing either pulpal or enamel injury. Cleaning with Nd:YAG laser irradiation was more effective in removing the pit and fissure contents than mechanical and chemico-mechanical methods[122]. However, the cleaning effect of laser irradiation showed that not all the fissure contents were removed. This is probably due to various factors, such as the narrow and deep shape of some fissures, air entrapment and consistency, and the application method of the black paint into the pits and fissures. The black paint, used as a removable absorptive coating, sometimes failed to penetrate deep into the pits and fissures. Because of the tip of the ultrasonic scaler used for cleaning, in the chemico-mechanical and mechanical methods, alteration of the shape of the pits and fissures as well as damage to the pit and fissure enamel were observed. These findings are thus considered to be attributable to the use of ultrasonic scaler tips. Regarding laser irradiation in combination with fluoride application, Yamamoto and Sato[125] found a reduction in the subsurface demineralization and the uptake of large amounts of fluoride in the enamel following exposure to a normal pulsed Nd:YAG laser after $Ag(NH_3)_2F$-treatment.

Tagomori and Morioka[64] also reported that APF application, after laser irradiation, produces a greater fluoride uptake in the enamel than APF application before laser irradiation. In their investigation, fluoride uptake at the pit and fissure entrance with a width of 200 μm in the teeth treated with APF, after laser irradiation, was higher than that treated with APF alone. Also, in the deep pits and fissures with a width of 60 μm, a higher fluoride uptake was found in the enamel in the teeth treated with APF application after laser irradiation, compared to APF application alone. These results suggest that a fluoride solution could penetrate deep into the pits and fissures and thus influence the fluoride uptake into the enamel after treatment with laser irradiation. Normal pulsed Nd:YAG laser irradiation is effective for increasing the acid resistance of the enamel of pits and fissures, as well as helping to remove the pit and fissure contents and increasing the fluoride uptake into the deep pit and fissure enamel.

5.6.1 Oral Safety Parameters

Laser systems operate in various modes, such as continuous wave, pulsed, chopped-wave, and Q-switched[126]. One purpose of using these different modes is to minimize the rise in tissue temperature within the target area[127]. The Nd:YAG laser has been used in various modes to alter the caries resistance of enamel[128].

The thermal effects of this kind of laser on the tooth must be considered, because an intrapulpal temperature rise of as little as 5.5°C can cause irreversible pulp damage[72]. In previous investigations, heat from irradiation with the Nd:YAG laser at continuous wave or long pulsed settings was often found to cause melting of the intertubular dentin[129]. Due to the proximity of heat-sensitive pulpal tissues to the dentin, it is important to minimize any temperature increase in dental hard tissue during irradiation. Thus, significant temperature increases in dentin can give rise to concerns regarding pulpal thermal damage. The Q-switched Nd:YAG laser system with nanosecond pulses may well offer significant advantages with regard to pulpal heating due to its short pulse duration and high peak powers.

So, Kimura and Wilder-Smith[126] tried to investigate the effects of Q-switched Nd:YAG laser irradiation with nanosecond pulses on crown and root dentin ablation, microstructure, and caries resistance characteristics. Thermal safety thresholds were also determined.

SEM results demonstrated microstructural damage at energy densities ~5.4 J/cm^2, and at similar energy densities, damage was greater with increasing pulse frequency. In the thermal investigation, a maximum increase of temperature exceeding 5.0°C was measured at energy densities > 2.0 J/cm^2. From these results, in order to remain within the range of useful microstructural alterations and below the threshold of thermal damage, the main investigation was performed at energy densities < 2.0 J/cm^2.

Light microscopic images of root dentin at 1 and 5 J/cm^2 showed no clear difference between artificial caries-like lesion depths in control and irradiated samples in either crown or root dentin.

However, duration of the temperature increase induced by a pulse of Nd:YAG laser irradiation was very short (less than 2 s). According to Zach and Cohen[72], temperature increases exceeding 5.5°C for 5–20 s can cause irreversible changes in the pulp. Thus, the temperature increases measured in this study appear to lie below the threshold of pulpal damage. However, in this investigation single pulses of laser irradiation were used.

These results were paralleled by measurements obtained using microhardness techniques, but there was no significant protective effect of nanosecond pulsed Nd:YAG laser irradiation.

Using SEM, the microstructural effects of artificially induced demineralization were clearly evident in all samples. After demineralization, surfaces of control samples were rough, and dentin tubules were open. In contrast, surfaces of irradiated samples after demineralization appeared partially melted and smoother than the control samples, and some dentin tubules were narrowed or occluded. According to previous reports[130,131], Nd:YAG laser irradiation of dentin with pulse durations longer than those used in this investigation caused the surface to melt, occluded dentin tubules, and also produced visible calcification structures. No such calcifications, however, were observed in another study. This is probably due to the different parameters used. In this investigation only a single pulse of laser irradiation was used at low energy densities. The long-duration irradiation in the continuous wave or long-pulsed mode used in most other investigations would induce far higher temperature rises in target tissues.

Kimura[126] was unable to detect any significant caries-preventive effect of nanosecond pulse duration Nd:YAG laser irradiation at moderate pulse energy parameters on crown and root dentin, but a range of microstructural effects was observed.

5.6.2 Surface Morphology

Cox et al.[132] tried to investigate the effects of short-term exposures of a pulsed Nd:YAG laser on enamel and dentin. In enamel the lesions had a defined round periphery with evidence of irregular areas of disrupted enamel within. Evidence of blister formation was apparent at all the energies evaluated. At the lower delivered energies (600–1,980 mJ total energy in 2 s) incipient melting was observed as well as irregular areas with loss of outer enamel. In a number of sites where blister formation had occurred, the blisters showed a ruptured center. This may be due to vaporization of the water in the depth of the enamel structure leading to a build up of pressure, which ruptures the enamel. The evidence of melting showed that temperature had risen to melting point temperature.

Increasing the energy delivered (7,200 mJ total energy in 2 s) produced lesions with more marked cratering, with rolled edges to the periphery of irradiated sites, and at higher magnification superficial melting and blistering became visible. The floor appeared porous and had microscopic vent holes for the release of vapor from the deeper parts of enamel. Reflex microscopic measurements showed that the dimensions of the affected areas remained constant. The diameters of the lesions were comparable with the dimensions of the handpiece tip at nearly all the energy values delivered. At pulse repetition rates of 20 pps there was an increase in the area of changed enamel.

On the other hand, on dentin, at the lowest energy density (600 mJ) SEM showed a smooth-walled cratering and disruption of the dentin structure, characterized by incipient melting with formation of globules of partially melted tissue. Increasing the energy led to deeper crater formation with loss of tissue, as a result of melting and finally vaporization of the constituent material. In this deeper lesion, the top of the wall was crazed with a number of globules apparent, whereas in deeper parts of the lesion wall the surface was amorphous (different cooling rates in different depths). The volume of dentin affected appeared to be greater than that observed for enamel when equal energies were delivered. The three constituents of dentin (water, collagen and hydroxyapatite) change state at different temperatures. Initially water and subsequently collagen would be lost, followed by melting and finally vaporization of hydroxyapatite.

The energy required to raise the temperature of the tissue sufficiently to displace the water and collagen would be less than that required to melt the same volume of hydroxyapatite. This may explain the greater loss of dentin when compared to enamel. The crazing of the wall of the lesion may be a result of rapid heating and cooling of the dentin, or its dehydration. There was a marked variation in the appearance and the depths of the lesions produced in dentin in different specimens when irradiated at the same fluence.

It may also be due to the variation in the composition of the constituent materials in different teeth, and also at different sites in the same tooth. This demonstrates the difficulties in predicting the effects of Nd:YAG radiation on dentin. It is apparent from these results that substantial changes in the enamel and dentin structure occur even at relatively low energy densities with this type of laser radiation. The extent of the changes surrounding the exposed area, which was visible optically, was only slightly greater than the width of the fiber delivering the beam. This suggests that the lateral spread of heat was limited. There must also be some concern at the crazing which occurred, as these cracks create potential pathways for the transmission of fluid to the underlying tooth tissue.

Fig 5-7 Combined effects of normal pulsed Nd:YAG laser irradiation (40 J/cm^2) and treatment with topical fluoride agents on the acid resistance of enamel: dissolved Ca^{2+} ratio with percent inhibition of Ca^{2+} release (%).

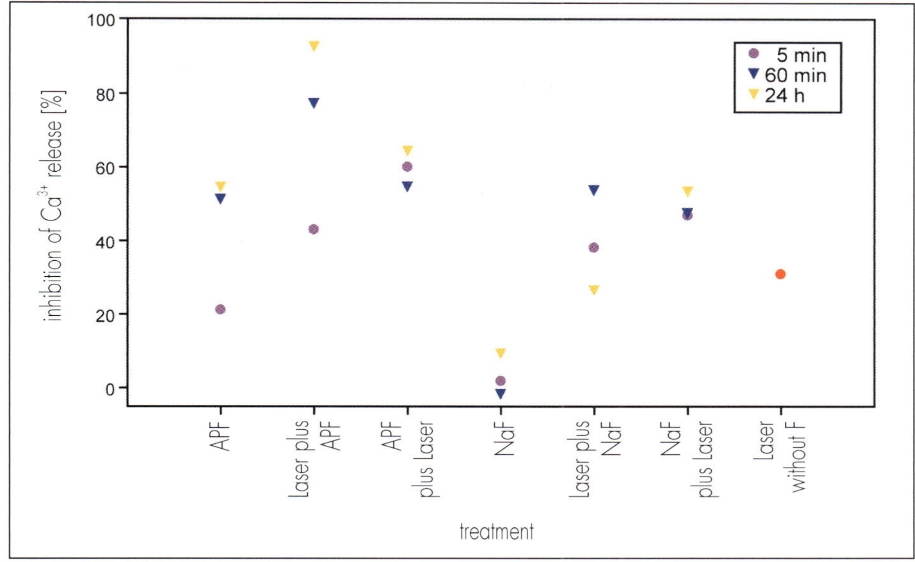

5.6.3 Combined Effect of Nd:YAG Laser and Fluoride Treatment

Combined laser and fluoride treatment has been successful in increasing the resistance against carious challenge[64,122].

It was found that in the case of combined treatment with laser irradiation and fluoride application, the enamel treated with APF and laser irradiation obtained the highest acid resistance compared to other treatments. The greatest combined effect was obtained when the APF incubation time was longer and the laser energy density was more than 30 J/cm^2. On the other hand, NaF treatment produced less impressive acid resistance, both before and after laser irradiation. In addition, longer incubation with NaF did not bring about a significant increase in acid resistance. Although the measurement of acid resistance and the time of APF application were not clinically relevant, this type of laser can be seen as a potential tool for caries prevention.

To prove the clinical relevance, Huang et al.[133] evaluated quantitatively the effectiveness of an Nd:YAG laser combined with a fluoride varnish on dental caries prevention at pit and fissure areas of teeth. Teeth were treated with the Nd:YAG laser followed by fluoride varnish, Nd:YAG laser only, fluoride varnish only or no treatment (control) (see table 5-4).

Comparing the results under a polarized light microscope on pit and fissure surfaces, in the control group 91% of the specimens developed lesions, in the F-varnish group (F-) 87%, the laser only group (L) 77% and in the group with fluoride following Nd:YAG laser irradiation (LF) 52%. The depth of lesion reduction compared with the control group was in the sequence C < F- (20%) < L (23%) < LF- (27%). On smooth surfaces, lesion formation appeared in 72% (C), 52% (F-), 39% (L) and 15% (LF-) and the lesion depth reduction was in the sequence of C < F- (33%) < L (34%) < LF- (49%).

From the parameters measured, the rank order of anticaries potential of the treatments was Nd:YAG laser combined with fluoride varnish, Nd:YAG laser alone, and fluoride varnish only.

During the microscopic evaluation of experimental carious lesions, it seemed that the laser corrected the anatomic defects of pits and fissures by cleansing, and odontoplasty-like effects. This finding was also observed by Bahar and Tagomori[122], along with the physical sealing of

Tab. 5-4 Synergistic effect of Nd:YAG laser combined with fluoride varnish on inhibition of caries formation in dental pits and fissures (Huang et al.[133]).

Treatment scheme	group	lesions at the pit and fissure area, examined under polarized light microscope	lesions on smooth surfaces
Nd:YAG laser followed by fluoride varnish	LF-	52% of specimens	59% of specimens
Nd:YAG laser only	L	77% of specimens	39% of specimens
fluoride varnish only	F-	87% of specimens	52% of specimens
no treatment (control group)	C	91% of specimens	72% of specimens
lesion depth reductions in dental pits and fissures compared with the control group		$C < F^- (20\%) < L (23\%) < LF^- (27\%)$	
lesion depth reductions on smooth surfaces compared with the control group		$C < F^- (33\%) < L (34\%) < LF^- (49\%)$	

pits and fissures by laser irradiation by Huang et al.[133]. This is another possible mechanism of caries inhibition. This effect is achieved by melting and resolidification of the enamel surface crystal at the pit and fissure area[67].

During Nd:YAG laser irradiation, many partially coalescent globular granules are produced by the process of melting and the subsequent resolidification of enamel crystals[64]. In this situation, fluoride can easily penetrate into the spaces between the granules. The microspaces formed by laser irradiation may trap the demineralized ions and provide space to allow them to combine with fluoride.

Other studies have shown that prolonged contact of fluoride varnish with tooth surfaces results in greater deposition of CaF_2-like material on the enamel surface, which may function as a fluoride reservoir[134,135]. The availability of fluoride ions from CaF_2-like material in the liquid phase around the apatite crystallites is thought to be more important in decreasing dissolution of crystallites than in incorporating fluoride into the crystal lattice[104,136]. The fluoride from enamel, treated with combined laser and fluoride varnish, undergoes prolonged release, resulting in greater deposition of CaF_2-like material, which facilitates remineralization of the lesion. Moreover, a less permeable enamel surface for ion diffusion results in inhibition of artificial lesion formation.

A reduced-energy Nd:YAG laser, immediately followed by high-concentration fluoride treatment, showed caries inhibition rates[133] comparable to those of Fox et al.[42]. Thus, the results also suggest that the clinically detectable damage to teeth, such as brown discoloration and friability, can be avoided with this treatment.

As mentioned at the beginning of this section, Tagomori and Morioka[64] demonstrated maximal inhibition of calcium dissolution from the enamel surface by prolonged fluoride treatment combined with Nd:YAG laser treatment. The experimental procedures in Huang's study[133] were reversed, but the lesion inhibition rate on smooth surfaces was consistent with theirs.

5.6.4 Clinical Aspects

Yamamoto and Sato[125] and Tooya[115] indicated that human enamel irradiated with an acousto-optically Q-switched Nd:YAG laser was more resistant to acid decalcification than an unlased control. Morioka et al.[121], Suzuki et al.[137] and Morita et al.[138], using various types of laser, suggested that the normal pulsed and acousto-optically Q-switched Nd:YAG lasers were suitable for clinical use. Normal pulse was found to be more suitable than acousto-optically Q-switch lasers because of the higher acid resistance and lower degree of damage to the enamel surface, when the two different kinds of laser beams were compared with an equal energy density.

Regarding laser irradiation in combination with fluoride application, Yamamoto and Sato[125] found a reduction in subsurface demineralization and an uptake of large amounts of fluoride in the enamel following exposure to normal pulsed Nd:YAG laser after $Ag(NH_3)_2F$-treatment. Remarkable acid resistance could not be found when the enamel was exposed to a normal pulsed Nd:YAG laser under different conditions of irradiation after NaF and APF treatment. In contrast, enamel treated with APF after laser irradiation became remarkably acid-resistant and it was supposed that the acid resistance might be caused by the morphological microscopic alterations which followed the uptake of fluoride into the enamel.

Another aspect is that high intensity infrared light from the pulsed Nd:YAG dental laser is absorbed by carious enamel and not absorbed by healthy enamel. Consequently, this system has potential for selective removal of surface enamel caries. The safety and efficacy of the clinical procedure was evaluated by Harris et al.[139]. Selective ablation was evaluated with FTIR spectroscopy. Caries were removed in all conditions. There were no adverse events and both clinical and histological evaluations of pulp vitality showed no abnormalities. The more conservative laser treatment removed the caries but not the sound enamel below the lesion. The pulsed Nd:YAG dental laser was found to be both safe and effective for surface caries removal.

5.7 The Caries Preventing Effect of Er:YAG, Er,Cr:YSGG, Ho:YAG and UV Lasers

Ceballos et al.[140] determined that an Er:YAG laser used instead of acid-etching influenced artificial secondary caries formation in enamel and root surfaces. Er:YAG laser irradiation resulted in a 56% reduction in primary enamel surface lesion depth when compared with the acid-etched group, and a 39% decrease in root surface lesion depth compared with that for acid-etching pretreatment. Wall lesion frequency was similar between treatment groups. Hossain et al.[141] suggest that Er:YAG laser irradiation with and without water mist appears to be more effective for caries prevention. SEM observation showed that the lased areas had melted and seemed to be thermally degenerated. Delbem et al.[142] concluded that the Er:YAG laser influenced the deposition of CaF_2 on the enamel after the application of acidulated phosphate fluoride and showed a superficial anticariogenic action, but not in depth. Based on in vitro tests, Apel et al.[143] did not assume that the use of Er:YAG (λ = 2,940 nm) or Er,Cr:YSGG laser (λ = 2,780 nm) for cavity preparation offers any advantages in terms of resistance to secondary caries in clinical practice. The Er:YAG laser cavities revealed demineralization to a depth of 133.9 µm, while the value observed with the Er,Cr:YSGG laser was 133.8 µm. The depth of demineralization in the control groups was only 77.4 and 79.3 µm! A significantly lower calcium content was found in the demineralization solution after fluoridation of the specimens. Additional laser radiation had no further effect on this result[144].

Ho:YAG laser (λ = 2,120 nm) energy irradiation after application of resin/NaF to restorative margins and adjacent areas showed a significant increased resistance to acid/mechanical destruction on cementum-dentin root surfaces. The integrity of the restorative/dentin margins was maintained after extended exposures to formic acid and mechanical challenges[145]. SEM examinations of the dentinal root surfaces showed consistently smooth surfaces with tubule closures when using topical resin with fluoride and Ho:YAG laser treatment; in contrast, Ho:YAG laser energy treatment alone exhibited increased roughness of root surfaces. Alone, topical fluoride applications presented surfaces similar to untreated control sites. Toluidine blue dye penetration into root surfaces of the fluoride/laser-treated root surfaces showed significantly less dye penetration after acid exposures than controls. The results indicate that the resin–fluoride application and Ho:YAG irradiation effectively produced increased smoothness and increased resistance to destruction of root surfaces in human extracted teeth under these in vitro conditions[146].

Wheeler et al.[147] hypothesize that the short UV laser pulses are primarily absorbed by protein and lipid localized between the enamel prisms, resulting in removal of intact mineral effectively etching the surface without thermal modification of the mineral phase. Such modification is likely to increase the permeability of the enamel surface and the subsequent absorption of fluoride. In addition, there is an increase in surface roughness without the formation of a layer of loosely adherent, thermally-modified enamel that increases the bond strength to composite restorative materials. Surface treatments with a near-UV laser, operating with λ = 355-nm laser and pulses of 3–5 ns duration, significantly increased the shear-bond strength of enamel to composite, to a level exceeding 20 MPa, which was significantly more than the non-irradiated control samples, and significantly less than the acid etch. Laser irradiation alone and topical fluoride application alone did not significantly increase the resistance to acid dissolution. The laser treatment followed by topical application of fluoride significantly increased the resistance to acid dissolution to a level of over 50% versus the control samples.

5.8 Conclusion

Lasers available for utilization in dentistry include CO_2, Er:YAG, Er:YSGG, Ho:YAG, Nd:YAG and argon lasers, and in the near future also KTP and UV lasers.

The argon laser may occupy a prominent role in both caries prevention and restoration in the near future. This laser can significantly affect the susceptibility of dental surfaces to caries initiation and caries progression, and there is also the possibility of laser polymerization of light-cured surface restorations. This may reduce secondary caries and provide additional protection for the adjacent root surface. Finally, the argon laser may have certain advantages over other lasers. Argon lasers operate at relatively low energy levels that are well tolerated by hard and soft tissues, as well as the dental pulp. A flexible fiberoptic delivery system allows easy adaptability for intraoral use. For these reasons, the clinical use of the argon laser in prevention and restoration of surface caries seems feasible.

On the other hand, it is also possible to utilize CO_2 laser irradiation at wavelengths of $\lambda = 9.3\ \mu m$ and $\lambda = 9.6\ \mu m$ to alter dental enamel to make it markedly more resistant to subsequent acid attack, without producing elevated temperatures in the underlying tissue that could lead to pulpal damage. The advantages of the CO_2 lasers are that they not only inhibit caries, they also can be used to remove caries and inhibit thereby the decalcification of the cavity wall.

The possibility to remove dental caries and inhibit secondary caries may offer significant advantages over the other laser types. Additionally, the possibility to precisely control the treatment depth with a (pulsed) CO_2 laser – changing pulse duration or wavelength – makes this kind of laser a promising instrument for medical use.

The exposure of dental hard tissues to Nd:YAG laser irradiation also showed remarkable acid resistance as well as increased fluoride uptake in the irradiated tissues. The limitation of the application of Nd:YAG laser to dental hard tissue is the need for an energy-absorbing initiator to absorb the laser light on the enamel surface. There is also a marked variation in the color of the dentin of different teeth and also within a single tooth, which alters the degree of absorption of the Nd:YAG laser radiation and in this way the caries-preventive effect.

Which type of laser will be found suitable in dentistry in the future will depend on the following: safety for the oral tissues, especially the pulp, the efficiency and precision of the laser, and finally the cost.

5.9 References

1. Featherstone J D B: Caries detection and prevention with laser energy. Dent Clin North Am 44: 955–969, 2000
2. Loesche W J: Role of *Streptococcus mutans* in human dental decay. Microbiol Rev 50: 353–380, 1986
3. Featherstone J D B, Rodgers B E: The effect of acetic, lactic and other organic acids on the formation of artificial carious lesions. Caries Res 15: 377–385, 1981
4. Leverett D H, Featherstone J D B, Proskin H M: Caries risk assessment by a cross-sectional discrimination model. J Dent Res 72: 529–537, 1993
5. Leverett D H, Proskin H M, Featherstone J D B: Caries risk assessment in a longitudinal discrimination study. J Dent Res 72: 538–543, 1993
6. Nelson D G A, Featherstone J D B: Preparation, analysis and characterization of carbonated apatites, 1982
7. LeGeros R Z: Calcium phosphates in oral biology and medicine. In: Myers H M (ed.): Monographs in Oral Science. Karger Verlag, Basel 1991
8. ten Cate J M, Featherstone J D B: Mechanistic aspects of the interactions between fluoride and dental enamel. CRC Crit Rev Oral Biol 2: 283–296, 1991
9. Lamkin M S, Oppenheim F G: Structural features of salivary function. Crit Rev Oral Biol Med 4: 251–259, 1993
10. Featherstone J D B: Prevention and reversal of dental caries. Role of low level fluoride. Community Dent Oral Epidemiol 27: 31–40, 1999
11. Ogaard B: Effects of fluoride on caries development and progression in vitro. J Dent Res 69 (Spec. Iss.): 813–823, 1990
12. Christoffersen J, Arends J: Progress of artificial carious lesions in enamel. Caries Res 16: 433–439, 1982
13. Larsen, M J: Chemical events during tooth dissolution. J Dent Res 69 (Spec. Iss.): 575–580, 1990
14. Wigdor H A, Walsh J T, Featherstone J D B, Visuri S R, Fried D, Waldvogel J L: Lasers in dentistry. Lasers Surg Med 16, 103–133, 1995
15. Stern R H, Sognnaes R F: Laser beam effect on hard dental tissues. J Dent Res 43: 873, 1964
16. Stern R H, Renger H L, Howell F V: Laser effects on vital dental pulps. Br Dent J 26–28, 1969
17. Stern R H, Vahl J, Sognnaes R F: Laser enamel: Ultrastructural observations of pulsed carbon dioxide laser effects. J Dent Res 51: 455–460, 1972
18. Stern R H, Sognnaes R F, Goodman F: Laser effect on in vitro enamel permeability and solubility. J Am Dent Assoc 78: 838–843, 1966
19. Vahl J: Electron microscopical and X-ray crystallographic investigations of teeth exposed to laser rays. Caries Res 28: 10–18, 1968
20. Yamamoto H, Ooya K: Potential of yttrium-aluminium-garnet laser in caries prevention. J Oral Pathol 38: 7–15, 1974
21. Featherstone J D B, Barrett-Vespone N A, Fried D, Kantorowitz Z, Lofthouse J, Seka W: CO_2 laser inhibition of artificial caries like lesion progression (Abstract 470). J Dent Res 74: 70, 1995
22. Featherstone J D B, Nelson D G A: Laser effects on dental hard tissues. Adv Dent Res 1: 21–26, 1987
23. Fried D, Featherstone J D B, Glena R E: The light scattering properties of dentin and enamel at 543, 632 and 1053 nm. Presented at Lasers in Orthopedic, Dental and Veterinary Medicine II. SPIE 240–245, 1993
24. Fried D, Featherstone J D B, Glena R E: The nature of light scattering in dental enamel and dentin at visible and near-IR wavelengths. Appl Optics 34: 1278–1285, 1995
25. Fried D, Glena R E, Featherstone J D B, Seka W: Permanent and transient changes in the reflectance of CO_2 laser irradiated dental hard tissues of lambda = 9.3, 9.6, 10.3 and 10.6 microns and at fluences of 1–20 J/cm^2. Lasers Surg Med 20: 22–31, 1997
26. Hibst R, Keller U: Experimental studies of the application of the Er:YAG laser on dental hard substances: I. Measurement of the ablation rate. Lasers Surg Med 9: 338–344, 1989
27. Hibst R, Keller U: Heat effect of pulsed Er:YAG laser radiation. In: Joffe S N (ed.): Laser Surgery: Advanced Characterization, Therapeutics and Systems II. Presented at SPIE, Bellingham, WA 379–386, 1990
28. Featherstone J D B, Rechmann P: Lasers in dentistry III (proceedings). Presented at SPIE, Bellingham, WA 112–116, 1997
29. Featherstone J D B, Barrett-Vespone N A, Fried D, Kantorowitz Z, Seka W: CO_2 laser inhibition of artificial caries-like lesion progression in dental enamel. J Dent Res 77: 1397–1403, 1998
30. Featherstone J D B, Fried D, Duhn C: Surface dissolution kinetics of dental hard tissue irradiated over a fluence range of 1–8 J/cm^2. Proc SPIE Lasers Dent IV 3248: 146–151, 1998
31. Fried D, Seka W, Glena R E, Featherstone J D B: Thermal response of hard dental tissues to 9–11 μm CO_2 laser irradiation. Opt Eng 35: 1976–1984, 1996
32. Zijp JR, ten Bosch J J: Theoretical model for the scattering of light by dentin and comparison with measurements. Appl Optics 32: 411–415, 1993
33. Zuerlein M J, Fried D, Seka W et al.: Absorption coefficients of dental enamel in the infrared: A solution to a seemingly straight forward problem. Presented at Lasers in Dentistry IV, SPIE, Bellingham, WA 137–145, 1998
34. Zuerlein M J, Fried D, Seka W et al.: Modeling thermal emission in dental enamel induced by 9–11 μm laser light. Appl Surf Sci 127–129: 863–868, 1998
35. Zuerlein M J, Fried D, Featherstone J D B: Modeling the modification depth of carbon dioxide laser-treated dental enamel. Lasers Surg Med 25: 335–347, 1999

36. Zuerlein M J, Fried D, Featherstone J D B et al.: Optical properties of dental enamel in the mid-IR determined by pulsed photothermal radiometry. J Selected Topics in Quantum Electronics 5: 1083–1089, 1999
37. Fried D, Zuerlein M J, Featherstone J D B: IR laser ablation of dental enamel: Mechanistic dependence on the primary absorber. Appl Surf Sci 127–129: 852–856, 1998
38. Curzon M E J, Featherstone J D B: Chemical composition of enamel. In: Lazzari E P (ed.): Handbook of Experimental Aspects of Oral Biochemistry. CRC Press, Boca Raton 1983, 123–135
39. Lenz P, Glide H, Walz R: Studies on enamel sealing with the CO_2 laser. Dtsch Zahnärztl Z 37: 469–478, 1982
40. Sato K: Relation between acid dissolution and histological alteration of heated tooth enamel. Caries Res 17: 490–495, 1983
41. Mozammal H, Yukio N, Yuichi K, Mitsuhiro I, Yoshishige Y, Koukichi M: Acquired acid resistance of dental hard tissues by CO_2 laser irradiation. J Clin Laser Med Surg 17(5), 223–226, 1999
42. Fox J L, Yu D, Otsuka M, Higuchi W I, Wong J, Powell G: Combined effects of laser irradiation and chemical inhibitors on the dissolution of dental enamel. Caries Res 26: 333–339, 1992
43. Nelson D G A, Shariati M, Glena R, Shields C P, Featherstone J D B: Effect of pulsed low-energy infrared laser irradiation on artificial caries-like lesion formation. Caries Res 20: 289–299, 1986
44. McCormack S M, Fried D, Featherstone J D B, Glena R E, Seka W: Scanning electron microscope observations of CO_2 laser effects on dental enamel. J Dent Res 74: 1702–1708, 1995
45. Fowler B O, Kuroda S: Changes in heated and in laser-irradiated human tooth enamel and their probable effects on solubility. Calcif Tissue Int 38: 197–208, 1986
46. Christofferson J, Christofferson M R: Kinetics of dissolution of calcium hydroxyapatite IV. The effect of some biologically important inhibitors. J Crystal Growth 53: 42–54, 1981
47. Nelson D G A, Wefel J S, Jongebloed W L, Featherstone J D B: Morphology, histology and crystallography of human dental enamel treated with pulsed low-energy infrared laser radiation. Caries Res 21: 411–426, 1987
48. Kuroda S, Fowler B O: Compositional, structural and phase changes in in vitro laser-irradiated human tooth enamel. Calcif Tissue Int 36: 361–369, 1984
49. Westerman G H, Hicks M J, Flaitz C M, Blankenau R J, Berg J H, Powell G L: Argon laser irradiation in root surface caries in vitro. J Dent Res 71: 210, 1992
50. Hicks M J, Flaitz C M, Westerman G H, Berg J H, Blankenau R J, Powell G L: Caries-like lesion initiation and progression in sound enamel following Argon laser irradiation. ASDC J Dent Child 60: 201–206, 1993
51. Clarkson B H, Wefel J S, Silverstone L M: Redestribution of enamel fluoride during white spot lesion formation; an in vitro study on human dental enamel. Caries Res 15: 158–165, 1981
52. Oho T, Morioka T: A possible mechanism of acquired acid resistance of human dental enamel by laser irradiation. Caries Res 24: 86–92, 1990
53. Westerman G H, Hicks M J, Flaitz C M: Surface morphology of sound enamel after Argon laser irradiation: an in vitro scanning electron microscopic study. J Clin Pediat Dent 21: 55–59, 1996
54. Rolla G: On the role of calcium fluoride in the cariostatic mechanism of fluoride. Acta Odontol Scand 46: 341–345, 1988
55. Rolla G, Ogaard B, De Almeida Cruz R: Topical application of fluorides on teeth. New concepts of mechanism of interaction. J Clin Periodontol 20: 105–108, 1993
56. Silverstone L M, Hicks M J, Featherstone M J: Dynamic factors affecting lesion initiation and progression in human dental enamel. Quintessence Int 19: 683–711, 773–785, 1988
57. Westerman G H, Hicks M J, Flaitz C M, Blankenau R J, Powell G L: Argon laser irradiation effects on sound root surfaces: in vitro scanning electron microscopic observations. J Clin Laser Med Surg 16: 111–115, 1998
58. Carlström D, Glas J E: Studies on the ultrastructure of dental enamel III. J Ultrastruct Res 8: 1–11, 1963
59. Silverstone L M, Johnson N W, Hardie J M: Enamel caries. In: Silverstone L M, Johnson N W, Hardie J M et al. (eds.): Dental Caries Aetiology, Pathology and Prevention. MacMillan, London 1981, 133–161
60. Kantola S, Laine E, Tarna T: Laser-induced effects on tooth structure VI. Acta Odontol Scand 31: 369–379, 1973
61. LeGeros R Z: Effect of carbonate on the lattice parameters of apatite. Nature 206: 403–404, 1965
62. Holcomb D W, Young R A: Thermal decomposition of human tooth enamel. Calcif Tissue Int 31: 189–201, 1980
63. LeGeros R Z, Bonel G, Legros R: Types of H_2O in human enamel and in precipitated apatites. Calcif Tissue Res 26: 111–118, 1978
64. Tagomori S, Morioka T: Combined effect of laser and fluoride on acid resistance of human dental enamel. Caries Res 23: 225–231, 1989
65. Neuman W F, Mulryan B J: Synthetic hydroxyapatite crystals IV. Calcif Tissue Res 7: 133–138, 1971
66. Ingram G S: The role of carbonate in dental mineral. Caries 7: 217–230, 1973
67. Kantorowitz K, Featherstone J D B, Fried D: Caries prevention by CO_2 laser treatment: dependence on the nubmer of pulses used. J Am Dent Assoc 129: 585–591, 1998
68. Fried D, Ragadio J, Akrivou M, Featherstone J D B: Dental hard tissue modification and removal using sealed transverse excited atmospheric-pressure lasers operating at $\lambda = 9.6$ and 10.6 µm. J Biomed Optics 6(2): 231–328, 2001
69. Duplain G, Boulay R, Belanger P A: Complex index of refraction of dental enamel at CO_2 wavelengths. Appl Optics 26: 4447–4451, 1987
70. Featherstone J D B, Barrett-Vespone N A, Fried D et al.: Rational choice of laser conditions for inhibition of caries progression. Presented at SPIE, Bellingham, WA 57–67, 1995
71. Featherstone J D B, ten Cate J M, Shariati M, Arends J: Comparison of artificial caries-like lesions by quantitative microradiography and microhardness profiles. Caries Res 17(5): 385–391, 1983

72. Zach L, Cohen G: Pulp response to externally applied heat. Oral Surg Oral Med Oral Pathol 19: 515–530, 1965
73. Lakshmi A, Shobha D, Lakshminarayanan L: Prevention of caries by pulsed CO_2 laser pre-treatment of enamel: an in-vitro study. J Indian Soc Pedod Prev Dent 19(4): 152–156, 2001
74. Fried D, Zuerlein M J, Le C Q, Featherstone J D B: Thermal and chemical modification of dentin by 9–11-micron CO_2 laser pulses of 5–100-micros duration. Lasers Surg Med 31(4): 275–282, 2002
75. Hossain M, Nakamura Y, Kimura Y, Ito M, Yamada Y, Matsumoto K: Acquired acid resistance of dental hard tissues by CO_2 laser irradiation. J Clin Laser Med Surg 17(5): 223–226, 1999
76. Fox J L, Yu D, Otsuka M, Higuchi W I, Wong J, Powell G L: Initial dissolution rate studies on dental enamel after CO_2 laser irradiation. J Dent Res 71: 1389–1398, 1992
77. Nammour S, Renneboog-Squilbin C, Nyssen-Behets C: Increased resistance to artificial caries-like lesions in dentin treated with CO_2 laser. Caries Res 26: 170–175, 1992
78. Kantola S: Laser induced effects on tooth structure IV. A study of changes in the calcium and phosphorus contents in dentine by electronprobe microanalysis. Acta Odontol Scand 30: 463–474, 1972
79. Böhm R F, Rich J, Webster J: Thermal stress effects and surface cracking associated with laser use on human teeth. J Biomech Eng 99: 189–194, 1997
80. Kantorowitz Z, Featherstone J D B, Fried D: Augmentation of CO_2-laser inhibition of in vitro-caries by fluoride (Abstract 63). J Dent Res 75 (Spec. Iss.): 25, 1996
81. Fried D, Glena R, Featherstone J D B, Seka W: Multiple pulse irradiation of dental hard tissues at CO_2 laser wavelengths. In: Lasers in dentistry. Vol. 2394. SPIE 41–50 for Fried et al. and 56–56 for Seka et al., Bellingham, WA 1995a
82. Fried D, Borzillary S F, McCormack S M, Glena R, Featherstone J D B: The thermal effects on CO_2 laser irradiated dental enamel at 9.3, 9.6, 10.3 and 10.6 µm. In: Laser surgery, Advanced characterization, therapeutics and systems IV. Vol. 2128. SPIE 319–328, Bellingham, WA 1994
83. Ellies L G, Nelson D G A, Featherstone J D B: Crystallographic structure and surface morphology of sintered carbonated apatites. J Biomed Mater Res 22: 541–553, 1988
84. Kelly R, Cuomo J J, Leary P A, Rothenberg J E, Braren B E, Aliotta C F: Laser sputtering: Part 1. On the existence of rapid laser sputtering at 193 nm. Nucl Instr Meth B7: 319–340, 1984
85. Wu C C, Roan R T, Chen J H Sintering mechanism of the CaF_2 on hydroxyapatite by a 10.6-l microm CO_2 laser. Lasers Surg Med 31(5): 333–338, 2002
86. Hsu J, Fox J L, Wang Z et al.: Combined effects of laser irradiation/solution fluoride ion on enamel demineralization. J Clin Laser Med Surg 16: 93–105, 1998
87. Hossain M M, Hossain M, Kimura Y, Kinoshita J, Yamada Y, Matsumoto K: Acquired acid resistance of enamel and dentin by CO_2 laser irradiation with sodium fluoride solution. J Clin Laser Med Surg 20(2): 77–82, 2002
88. Konishi N, Fried D, Featherstone J D B, Staninec M: Inhibition of secondary caries by CO_2 laser treatment. Am J Dent 12(5): 213–216, 1999
89. Young D A, Fried D, Featherstone J D B: Ablation and caries inhibition of pits and fissures by IR laser irradiation. Lasers in Dentistry VI, Proc SPIE 3910: 247–253, 2000
90. Westerman G H, Hicks M J, Flaitz C M, Blankenau R J, Powell G L, Berg J H: Argon laser irradiation in root surface caries: in vitro study examines laser's effects. J Am Dent Assoc 125: 401–407, 1994
91. Blankenau R J, Powell G L, Ellis R W, Westerman G H: In vivo caries like lesion prevention with Argonlaser: Pilot Study
92. Ogaard B, Rolla G: The in vivo orthodontic banding model for vital teeth and the in situ orthodontic banding model for hard-tissue slabs. J Dent Res 71 (Spec. Iss.): 832–835, 1992
93. Powell G L, Morton T H, Whisenant B K: Argon laser oral safety parameters for teeth, Lasers Surg Med 13: 548–552, 1993
94. Pogrel M A, Muff D F, Marshal G W: Structural changes in dental enamel induced by high energy continuous wave carbon dioxide laser. Lasers Surg Med 13: 89–96, 1993
95. Ferreira J M, Palamara J, Phakey P P: Effects of cw-CO_2 laser on the ultrastructure of human dental enamel. Arch Oral Biol 34: 551–562, 1989
96. Cernavin I: A comparison of the effects of Nd:YAG and Ho:YAG laser irradiation on dentine and enamel. Aust Dent J 40: 79–84, 1995
97. Cox C J, Pearson G J, Palmer G: Preliminary in vitro investigation of the effects of pulsed Nd:YAG laser radiation on enamel and dentine. Bio Materials 15: 1145–1151, 1994
98. Hicks M J, Flaitz C M, Westerman G H, Berg J H, Blankenau R J, Powell G L: Caries-like lesion initiation and progression in sound enamel following Argon laser irradiation. ASDC J Dent Child 60: 201–206, 1993
99. Westermann G H, Hicks M J, Flaitz C M, Berg J H, Blankenau R J, Powell G: Argon laser irradiation in root surface caries in vitro study examines laser´s effect. J Am Dent Assoc 125: 401–407, 1993
100. Hicks M J, Flaitz C M, Westerman G H, Blankenau R J, Powell G L, Berg J H: Enamel caries initiation and progression following low fluence (energy) Argon laser and fluoride treatment. J Clin Pediat Dent 20: 91–93, 1995
101. Hicks M J, Westerman G H, Flaitz C M, Blankenau R J, Powell G L, Berg J H: Effects of Argon laser irradiation and acidulated phosphate fluoride on root surface caries. Am J Dent 8: 10–14, 1995
102. Flaitz C M, Hicks M J, Westerman G H, Berg J H, Blankenau R J, Powell G L: Argon laser irradiation and acidulated phosphate fluoride treatment in caries-like lesion formation in enamel. Pediat Dent 17: 31–35, 1995
103. ten Cate J M, Simons M Y, van Strijp A J, Exterkate R A M: Relation between enamel fluoride retention and time of topical fluoride application. J Dent Res 67: 114 (Abstract 12), 1988
104. ten Cate J M: In vitro studies on the effect of fluoride on de- and remineralization. J Dent Res 69 (Spec. Iss.): 614–619, 1990

105. Haider S M, White G E, Rich A: Combined effects of argon laser irradiation and fluoride treatments in prevention of caries like lesion formation in enamel. J Clin Pediat Dent 23(3): 247–257, 1999
106. Garcia-Godoy F, Hicks M J, Flaitz C M: Acidulated phosphate fluoride treatment and formation of caries-like lesions in enamel: effect of application time. J Clin Pediat Dent 19: 105–110, 1995
107. Anderson J R, Ellis R W, Blankenau R J, Beiraghi S M, Westerman G H: Caries resistance in enamel by laser irradiation and topical fluoride treatment. J Clin Laser Med Surg 18(1): 33–36, 2000
108. Powell G L, Kelsey W P, Blankenau R J: The use of Argon laser for polymerization of composite resin. J Esthet Dent I: 34–37, 1989
109. Kelsey W P, Blankenau R J, Powell G L, Barkmeier W W, Cavel W T, Whisenant B K: Enhancement of physical properties of resin restorative materials by laser polymerization. Lasers Surg Med 9: 623–627, 1989
110. Blankenau R L, Kelsey W P, Powell G L et al.: Degree of composite resin polymerization with visible light and Argon laser. Am J Dent 4: 40–44, 1991
111. Flaitz C M, Hicks M J, Blankenau R J et al.: Caries-like lesion initiation and progression around laser-cured sealants. Pediat Dent 13: 391–392, 1991
112. Dederich D N: Laser/tissue interactions. J Am Dent Assoc 124: 57–61, 1993
113. Spitzer D, ten Bosch J J: The absorption and scattering of light in bovine and human dental enamel. Calcif Tissue Res 17: 129–137, 1975
114. Morioko T, Tagamori S: Effects of beam absorption mediators and acid resistance of surface enamel by Nd:YAG radiation. J Dent Health 34: 40–44, 1984
115. Tooya Y: Acousto-optically Q-switched Nd:YAG laser effect on resistance of human deciduous enamel to demineralization in vitro and in vivo. Jap J Oral Biol 24: 442–452, 1982
116. Hennon D K, Stookey G K, Muhler J C: Prevalence and distribution of dental caries in preschool children. J Am Dent Assoc 79: 1406, 1969
117. Day C D M, Sedwick H J: Studies on the incidence of dental caries. Dent Cosmos 77: 442–452, 1935
118. Barr J H, Diodati R R, Stephen R G L: Incidence of caries at different locations on the teeth. J Dent Res 36: 536–545, 1957
119. Backer Dirks O: The distribution of caries resistance in relation to tooth surfaces. In: Wolstenholme G E W, O'Connor M (eds.): Ciba Found Caries Resistant Teeth. Churchill, London 1965
120. Kemper R N: Pit and fissure sealant. In: Menaker L (ed.): The biologic basis of dental caries. Harper & Row, Hagerstown 1980, 461–481
121. Morioka T, Morita E, Suzuki K: An increment of acid-resistance of dental enamel with the irradiation of various types of laser beam. J Jap Soc Laser Med 3: 605–612, 1982
122. Bahar A, Tagomori S: The effect of normal pulsed Nd:YAG laser irradiation on pits and fissures in human teeth. Caries Res 28: 460–467, 1994
123. Morioka T, Tagomori S, Nara Y: Application of Nd:YAG laser and fluoride in the prevention of dental caries. Laser Dent: 55–61, 1989
124. Myers T D, Myers W D: The use of a laser for debridement of incipient caries. J Prosthet Dent 53(6), 776–779, 1985
125. Yamamoto H, Sato K: Prevention of dental caries by Nd:YAG laser irradiation. J Dent Res 59: 2171–2177, 1980
126. Kimura Y, Wilder-Smith P: Effects of nanosecond pulsed Nd:YAG laser irradiation on dentine resistence to artificial caries-like lesions. Lasers Surg Med 20: 15–21, 1997
127. Arcoria C J, Steele R E, Wagner M J, Judy M M, Mathews J L, Hults D F: Enamel surface roughness and dental pulp response to coaxial carbondioxide-neodymium YAG-laser irradiation. J Dent 19: 85–91, 1991
128. Morioka T, Tagomori S, Oho T: Acid resistence of lased human enamel with erbium:YAG laser. J Clin Laser Med Surg: 215–217, 1991
129. Widgor H A: Study investigates effects of three lasers on dental hard tissue. Biomed Optics 1: 1, 1992
130. Dederich D N, Zakariasen K L, Tlip J: Scanning electron microscopic analysis of canal wall dentin following Nd:YAG laser irradiation. J Endod 10(9): 428–431, 1984
131. Levy G: Cleaning and shaping the root canal with Nd:YAG laser beam: a cooperative study. J Endod 18: 123–127, 1992
132. Cox C J M, Pearson G J, Palmer G: Preliminary in vitro investigation of the effects of pulsed Nd:YAG laser radiation on enamel and dentine. Biomaterials 15(14): 1145–1151, 1994
133. Huang Guay-Fen, Wan-Hong Lan, Ming-Kuang Guo, Chun-Pin Chiang: Synergistic effect of Nd:YAG laser combined with fluoride varnish on inhibition of caries formation in dental pits and fissures in vitro. J Formos Med Assoc 100(3): 181–185, 2001
134. Nellson D G A, Jongebloed W L, Arends J: Crystallographic structure of enamel surface treated with topical fluoride agents. TEM and XRD considerations. J Dent Res 63: 6–12, 1984
135. Arends J, Christoffersen J: Nature and role of loosely bound fluoride in dental caries. J Dent Res 69: 601–605, 1990
136. Arends J, Christoffersen J: The nature of early carious lesion in enamel. J Dent Res 65: 2–11, 1986
137. Suzuki K, Morita K, Morioka T: An increment of acid-resistance of dental enamel with the irradiation of various types of laser beam (2nd report). J Jap Soc Laser Med 3: 613–618, 1982
138. Morita E, Suzuki K, Morioka T: An increment of acid-resistance on dental enamel with the irradiation of various types of laser beam (3rd report). J Jap Soc Laser Med 3: 619–624, 1982
139. Harris D M, White J M, Goodis H, Arcoria C J, Simon J, Carpenter W M, Fried D, Burkart J, Yessik M, Myers T: Selective ablation of surface enamel caries with a pulsed Nd:YAG dental laser. Lasers Surg Med 30(5): 342–350, 2002
140. Ceballos L, Toledano M, Osorio R, Garcia-Godoy F, Flaitz C, Hicks J: Er:YAG laser pretreatment effect on in vitro secondary caries formation around composite restorations. Am J Dent 14(1): 46–49, 2001

141. Hossain M, Nakamura Y, Kimura Y, Yamada Y, Ito M, Matsumoto K: Caries-preventive Effect of Er:YAG Laser Irradiation with or without Water Mist. J Clin Laser Med Surg 18(2): 61–65, 2000
142. Delbem A C, Cury J A, Nakassima C K, Gouveia V G, Theodoro L H: Effect of Er:YAG laser on CaF_2 formation and its anti-cariogenic action on human enamel: an in vitro study. J Clin Laser Med Surg 21(4): 197–201, 2003
143. Apel C, Schafer C, Gutknecht N: Demineralization of Er:YAG and Er,Cr:YSGG laser-prepared enamel cavities in vitro. Caries Res 37(1): 34–37, 2003
144. Apel C, Meister J, Schmitt N, Graber H G, Gutknecht N: Calcium solubility of dental enamel following sub-ablative Er:YAG and Er:YSGG laser irradiation in vitro. Lasers Surg Med 30(5): 337–341, 2002
145. Holt R A, Nordquist R E: Effect of resin/fluoride and holmium:YAG laser irradiation on the resistance to the formation of caries-like lesions. J Prosthod 6: 11–19, 1997
146. Holt R A, Nordquist R E: Holmium:YAG Laser: Effects of various treatments on root surface topography and acid resistance. J Biomed Optics 1(2): 230–236, 1996
147. Wheeler C R, Fried D, Featherstone J D B, Watanabe L G, Le C Q: Irradiation of dental enamel with Q-switched lambda = 355-nm laser pulses: surface morphology, fluoride adsorption, and adhesion to composite resin. Lasers Surg Med 32(4): 310–317, 2003

6

Lasers in Endodontics

A. Moritz, U. Schoop
with contributions from J. Klimscha, S. Patruta, I. Terpotiz, W. Kluger

6.1 Introduction

6.1.1 The Importance of Endodontics in Dentistry

Endodontic treatment in modern dentistry has become increasingly important. Patients are asking dentists to save their teeth and expect that the results will be permanent, with no following complications. Many teeth that are endodontically treated are subsequently crowned, or involved in expensive reconstruction procedures, so that it is imperative that endodontic techniques can be relied upon for a satisfactory long-term prognosis.

The standards of endodontics have been constantly raised in the last 25 years by research and interest among practitioners, particularly at universities. Preparation techniques, both manual and by machines, have been refined, along with filling materials and their placement in the root canals.

Among the more important advances in endodontics have been the microscope, and electronic devices for measuring root-canal length.

However, many consider the recent development and use of lasers as the most exciting advance in endodontic treatment.

Different lasers are being used in root canal preparation, cleaning of the canal walls, disinfection of canals and surrounding dentinal tubules, removal of the smear layer and debris, and sealing of tubules. Thus, the laser is effective in eliminating bacterial infection and preventing its recurrence, and when used in conjunction with traditional techniques, will significantly enhance the long-term success of endodontic treatment.

6.1.2 Identifying Endodontic Problems

Endodontic treatment continually presents us with problems, which lead to failure in the therapy. Conventional methods, even if carried out with the utmost care, and following set procedures, will not always be successful.

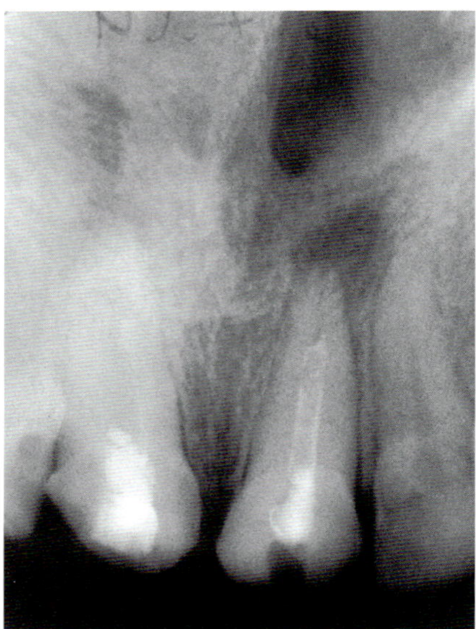

Fig 6-1 Periapical translucency.

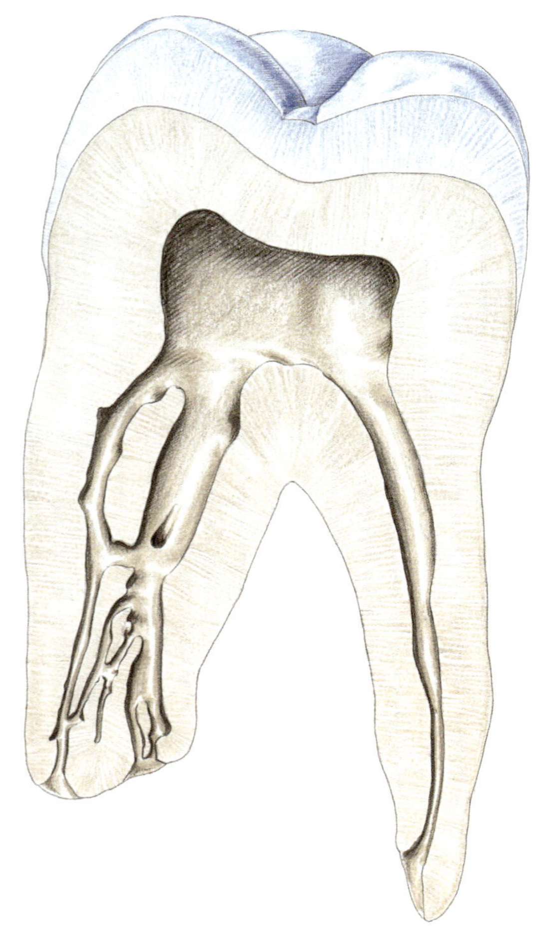

Fig 6-2 Representation of the macroanatomic variety within the root canal system.

Bacteria and their toxins that spread from the root canal and contaminate the apical region cause inflammation, infection and bone resorption.

The therapeutic goal of each root treatment has to be decontamination of the root canal and accessory canals, along with the dentinal tubules. Also, the periapical tissues have to be included, in case they are involved. We must create a sterile, bacteria-free environment both in the tooth and at the apex, including the periodontal membrane and the surrounding apical bone. Only then will osteoblasts in the apical area be able to complete the healing process.

There are three factors that complicate achieving sterility in the tooth

- The anatomical root configuration
- The special characteristics of the resident bacterial flora

6.1.2.1 Anatomical Root Configuration

6.1.2.1.1 Macro Anatomy

Macro anatomy shows a very complex root canal system, which is difficult to see with our present diagnostic procedures, e.g., X-rays, CT. We can find a lot of different structures – e.g., ampullae, denticals, and lateral canals branching off the main canal and ending in accessory foramina.

Thus, the presence of a single root canal cannot be assumed. The enormous variability in the configuration of the root canal system includes the number, cross section and courses of the canals. The greatest anatomical variety can be found in the area of the apical delta where the main canal may be connected to the apical area with one or many foramina.

With the aging of the tooth there is also considerable change taking place in the apical delta by apposition and resorption within the canals and externally. Also, with the aging process the

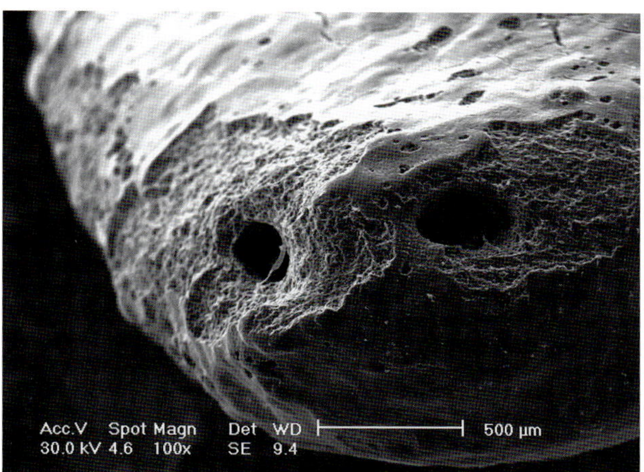

Fig 6-3 Accessory foramina.

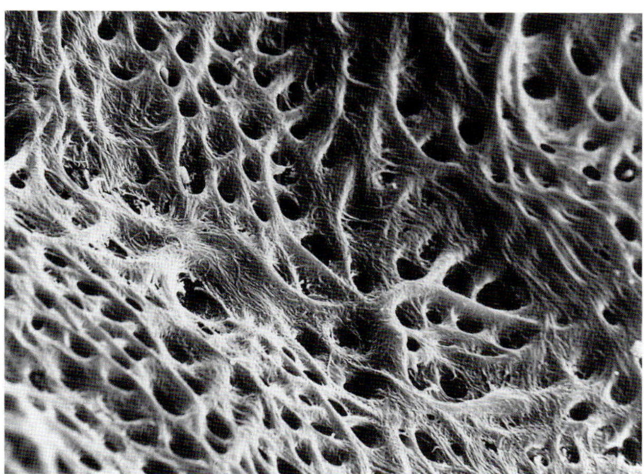

Fig 6-4 Complex three-dimensional network of dentinal tubules.

canal system is narrowed by the deposition of secondary dentin. This is most obvious at the base of the pulpal cavity and on the lateral walls of the pulp horns. In addition, the sidewalls of the canal close in. This secondary dentin production causes both the canal entrances to become smaller and the diameter of the canals to decrease. It is these changes that make the mechanical preparation of the root canals much more difficult.

In the more coronal portion of the root canal system, the mark canals are found. These lead perpendicularly from central to the periodontal gap. They are usually lined with connective tissue and communicate from endodontic tissue to paradontal tissue.

Similar connections may be found in the bi- and tri-furcations of deciduous and permanent molars. Finally, blind ending canals, called diverticels, pass through the root dentin, in irregular patterns. All these anatomical features predispose towards ideal conditions for bacteria to reside in and flourish. From all these protected macro and micro sites, bacteria and their byproducts along with infection, can easily spread to periapical and paradontal tissues. The criterion for success, therefore, is to completely eliminate all the bacteria within the complex canal system.

With existing methods of mechanical preparation we can create an entrance into the main root canals and also into the branching foramina. Removal of the canal debris follows and enlargement of the canals will remove bacteria residing in the infected dentin walls.

But despite mechanical removal, irrigation and disinfection of the canals, the bacteria can still persist in the complex network of dentinal tubules and micro-canals, which cannot be reached by conventional techniques.

6.1.2.1.2 Micro Anatomy

The entire dentin area of the tooth is composed of a system of fine small canals – the dentinal tubules – containing a nervous system. This nervous system is made up of the processes of the odontoblasts.

Using light microscopy, it has been shown that the structure of dentin has s-shaped canals in the crown and more straight-lined canals in the root dentin.

Ketterl[1] found a substantial biological range in the diameter and number of dentinal tubuli in different dentin areas of the tooth in different age groups (see table 6-1).

The author concluded that the number of dentin tubules remained constant throughout life. The lumens, however, experienced a decrease in diameter, up to complete obliteration with in-

Table 6-1 Biological variability of the diameter (µm) and number of tubules in different dentinal areas (after Ketterl[1]).

Age	Close to pulp	Middle of dentin	Periphery	Close to pulp	Middle of dentin	Periphery
16–30 years	4.0	3.1	1.7	61,000	34,000	13,000
30–50 years	3.1	2.6	1.7	68,000	40,000	16,000
50–75 years	2.9	2.4	1.7	64,000	35,000	18,000
average				64,000	36,000	16,000

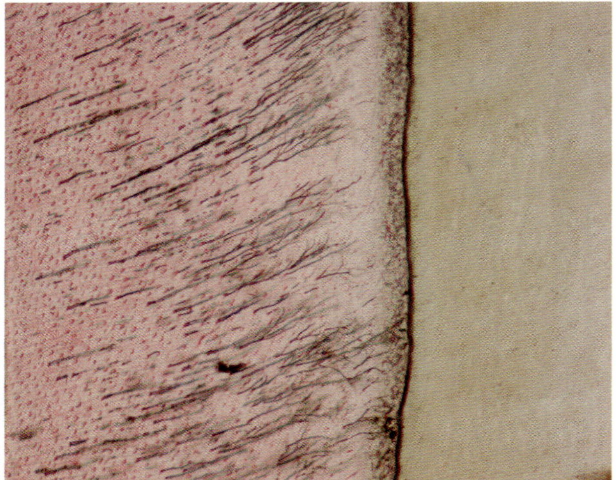
Fig 6-5 Histology of the tooth at the enamel-cementum border.

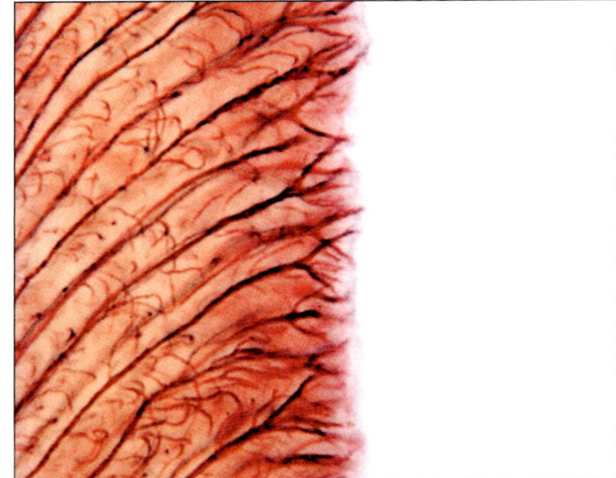
Fig 6-6 Lateral connection between dentinal tubules and peripheral branches.

creasing age. In each age group the tubule density in the apical root area was smaller (10,000–7000 tubules/mm^2) compared to the root center and cervical area.

Ketterl, using decalcified cuts, found that the sum of all dentin tubule lumens in upper juvenile canines was 93 mm^3, with older canines being 54 mm^3. These results were compared to lower first molars, which were 250 mm^3 and 150 mm^3.

The study further showed that more than 2/3 of the small tubules at the periphery were furcated several times and that these furcations merge about 0.5 mm in the direction of the pulp.

All dentin tubules split into innumerable, very fine, side branches.

Sauerwein[2] noted (1957) that the majority of the tubules showed repeated branching, with also straight tubules present. There were furcated tubules at the dentin-enamel and dentin-cement borders. Tubules with 3–7 branches were present. He also found small side branches. He described it as a "maze arrangement." Sauerwein also stated that a substantial part of the branching leads back towards the pulp. The small tubules were found to anastomose among themselves, sometimes even going around a neighboring tubule, and then continue with their end branches into the next tubule.

The presence of the small side branches and the furcations were explained by the primary configuration of the odontoblasts. Their cytoplasmic appendices extend into the tubules, first at a diameter of some µm and then, caused by branching, even thinner further into the dentin. While the cell retracts itself towards the pulp chamber, the cytoplasmic appendices become embedded in the dentinal matrix and their lumina stay intact.

Density and percentage by volume of the dentinal tubules are of fundamental importance in the understanding of the dentin structure and the dentinal wound. The dentin tubules cover 45% of the surface close to the pulp. In the teeth of juveniles, this percentage rises to 60% so that the nearby pulpal surface has a honeycomb structure.

At the border of the pulp there are up to 65,000 tubules per mm^2 and ~15,000 per mm^2 in the transitional area between dentin and enamel[3].

A large number of studies were made to measure the tubules, with a noticeable difference in results. This may be because of the different types of measured teeth or because of the way the teeth were stored, and preparation technology. Peritubular dentin dissolves to a large extent with acidic pretreatment, with the result that the measured tubule diameter is too large. Therefore, all calculations of the volume relationship between soft tissues (cytoplasm of the odontoblast extensions) and hard tissue, will lead to different results when using decalcified and non-decalcified dentin.

Even the carious process can change the measurement results. Arends et al.[4] showed that the demineralized process primarily began in the peritubular dentin and that the diameters of the dentin tubules subsequently increased by ~30%.

According to Fromme and Riedel[5], the maximum diameter of the tubules was 2.006 µm and the minimum was 0.737 µm. Their study also confirmed that tubules of juvenile teeth are substantially wider than those of adult teeth. Closer to the pulp, the lumen of the tubule is wider than at the periphery.

Tronstad[6] found that the number of tubules in the crown dentin was 60,000 per mm^2 surrounding the pulp, but only 7000 per mm^2 in the periphery. The average diameter was between 2 and 3 µm, decreasing to 0.5 µm close to the enamel.

Garberoglio and Brännström[7] measured the tubules of healthy teeth in different age groups. Their results are summarized in Table 6-2:

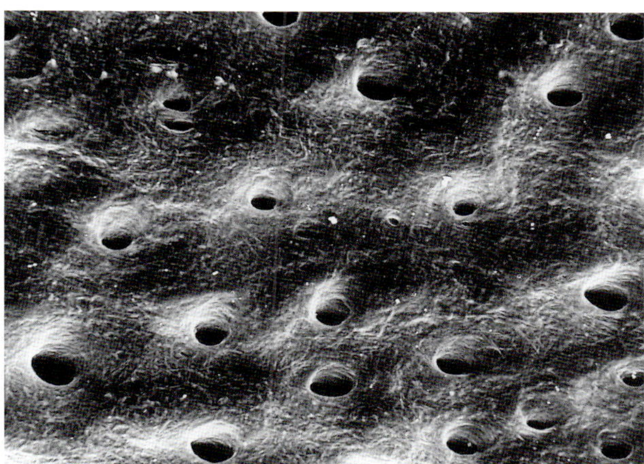

Fig 6-7 Representation of the dentinal tubules.

Table 6-2 Tubules of the healthy teeth in different age groups (Garberolglio and Brannström[7]).

Distance to pulp (mm)	Average number of tubuli in $1{,}000/mm^2$	Average diameter (µm)
Root canal wall	45	2.5
0.1–0.5	43	1.9
0.6–1.0	38	1.6
1.1–1.5	35	1.2
1.6–2.0	30	1.1
2.1–2.5	23	0.9
2.6–3.0	20	0.8
3.1–3.5	19	0.8

The reduction in the diameter of the tubules with increasing distance from the actual root canal is caused by the peritubular dentin. The authors calculated that the dentin tubules near the pulp were 28% of the total volume, but in the coronal dentin they were only 10% of the total volume.

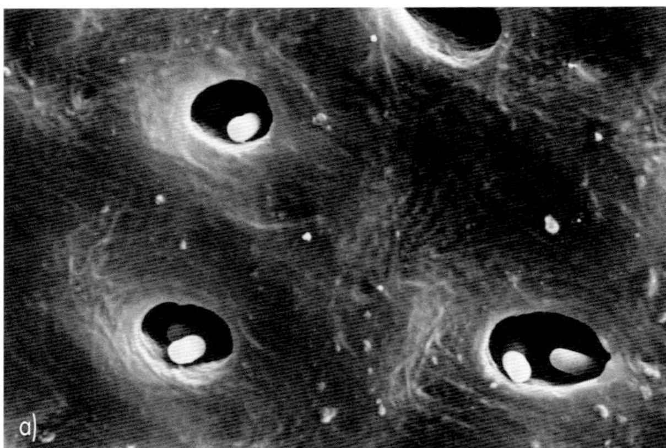

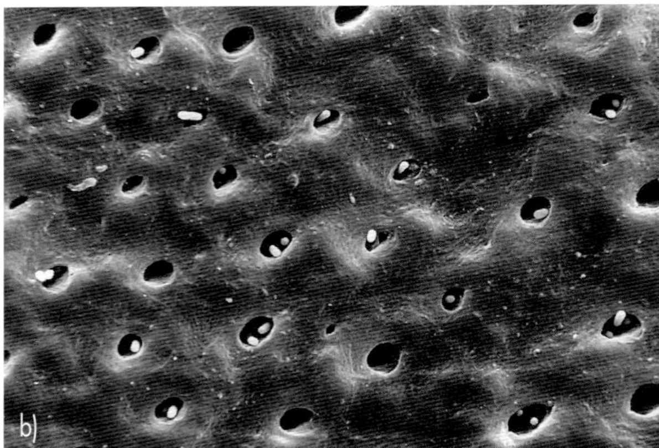

Fig 6-8a and b Scanning electron microscopic picture of bacteria penetrating into the dentinal tubules.

Goracci and Mori[8] found that the diameter was much larger. Near the pulp it was 4 μm and after 1 mm distance it narrowed to ~2 μm. At 2 mm from the pulp it narrowed to 1 μm. They also showed that the tubules bifurcate at the enamel–dentin border. The inner wall of the tubules appeared to be smooth and even, except for the presence of small branching accessory tubules.

One of the most extensive studies on the dentin and its branching tubule pattern was made by Mjör and Nordahl[9]. They analyzed the average number of tubules per 100 μm in different sections of dentin.

On the basis of size, direction and localization they divided the branching of the tubules into the following groups.

1. *Main small branches*:
   diameter of 0.5–1.0 μm. Found in dense numbers in the peripheral 250 μm of the dentin. Their y-form is typical and they correspond to the "end branching tubules" that were previously mentioned in earlier work. They are found more frequently in crown dentin than in root dentin.
2. *Side branches*:
   diameter of 300–700 nm. These are branches of the main small tubules and occur every 3–5 μm, penetrating the intertubular dentin at an angle of 45°. They form numerous anastomoses with other side tubules particularly in the central area of the root dentin. They are frequently present in those areas of the root dentin where the density of dentin tubules is rather small.
3. *Micro small branches*:
   diameter of 50–100 nm. They branch perpendicularly from the dentin tubules and run by the peritubular dentin into the intertubular matrix. They then continue to fan out and reunite with other micro small branches. Thus the intertubular dentin appears to be nerved with the finest small channels. This type of branching is found everywhere in the dentin but is particularly plentiful in the crown.

In the course of an infection the dentin tubules are penetrated by microorganisms. The tubule system forms a bacteria reservoir, which offers ideal conditions for their growth (constant warmth, humidity and nutrients). The entire root dentin becomes a perfect incubator, in which the bacteria are safe from the body's own defenses[10–14].

6.1.2.2 Special Quality of the Bacterial Colonization

Antoni van Leuwenhoek (1632–1723) was the first to describe the bacteria that exist in the root canal. In 1697, using a simple microscope, he observed "small animals" in the pulpal tissue derived from an extracted tooth. Up until the 19th century it was still believed, however, that these "small animals" were resulting from "abiogenesis" (generatio spontanea).

Willoughby Dayton Miller (1853–1907) was the first to recognize the inter-relation between microorganisms and the pulp, and also paradontal diseases.

Around the same time Miller was carrying out his scientific analyses in the laboratory of Robert Koch (1843–1910) and was studying the oral flora, Koch himself developed methods to color bacteria contained in smears. In 1881 he developed the solid media technique with which it was possible to cultivate single bacteria cultures derived from mixed infections.

Miller (1894) microscopically examined dyed smear tests of inflamed pulp tissue and observed a rich diversity of bacterial forms, including spirochetes. He found, however, that only a small number of bacteria could be cultivated and stated that most bacteria occurring in the pulp were difficult to cultivate.

It is only recently that bacteriological techniques have been developed that make it possible to cultivate the majority of microorganisms that are found in the oral cavity. The break-through came with the introduction of accurate anaerobic methods, where bacteria in different phases of laboratory testing could survive under oxygen exclusion.

These procedures were introduced into the general medical research programmes around 1960 and into endodontics about 1974 after Engström and Frostell[15], and Berg and Nord[16], had shown that special methods were necessary to detect bacteria in the pulp (Wittgow and Sabiston[17], Carlsson and Sundquist[18]).

The bacterial flora of root canals consisted predominantly of aerobic and facultative anaerobic bacteria, which partly originated from the oral cavity. Due to the introduction of improved bacteriological techniques, it is possible today to cultivate all kinds of bacteria isolated from infected root canals. And it has been shown that bacteria cause most endodontic diseases.

Today, we know that over 300 types of bacteria are found in the human oral cavity, under normal conditions. Apart from these bacteria we also have yeasts, mycoplasma and spirochetes, together with passing oral cavity inhabitants from the skin, gut flora and external contaminants.

Mostly only qualitative microbiology has been done on all these organisms and nothing definitive is known of the etiology of these bacteria.

In the last years, numerous types of bacteria have been described, but many colonizing the oral cavity and the root canal have to be reclassified.

Although difficult and expensive to classify, an exact identification is necessary to determine which bacteria are causing the contamination. To control the progress of the infection it is thus important to find out the bacteria that resist conventional root canal treatment and contribute to treatment failures.

In contrast to the oral cavity, which has up to 300 types of microorganisms, a selected bacterial spectrum of 1–12 species is found in the root canal. Only a few species (*Pseudomonas*, *Enterococcus*) are able to survive as a mono-infection (see *Enterococcus*).

Generally root infections are mixed infections, which contain eight or more species of bacteria. Typically the polybiotic flora contains approximately the same proportion of gram-positive and gram-negative bacteria, mainly anaerobes. The number of individual bacteria can vary between 10^2 and 10^7 [19–25].

Adhesion to the dentin surface is an important process for the settling of gram-positive cocci in the root canal. Firstly, there is a weak physical binding between the bacteria and the dentin. This is then intensified by adhesions of the cell wall, together with superficial complimentary receptors of the hard tooth tissue.

The bacteria are in a nutritious environment and can interact with the existing flora either competitively or in cooperation. Proliferation soon occurs after overcoming the local immune

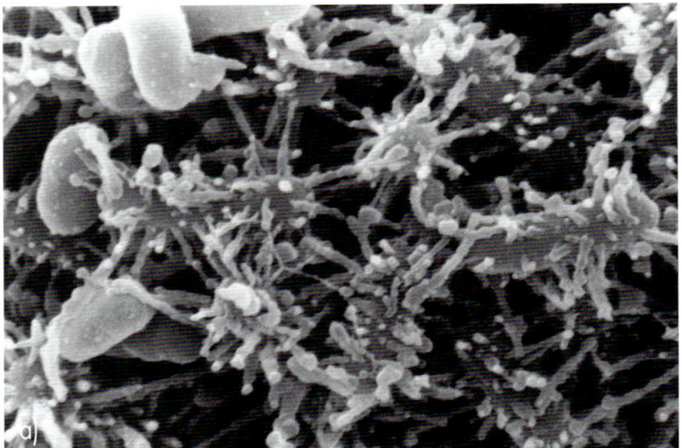

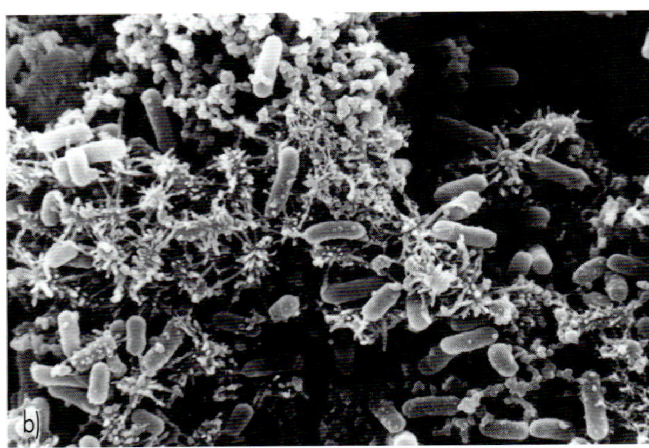

Fig 6-9a and b Oral flora (two overlapping SEM pictures).

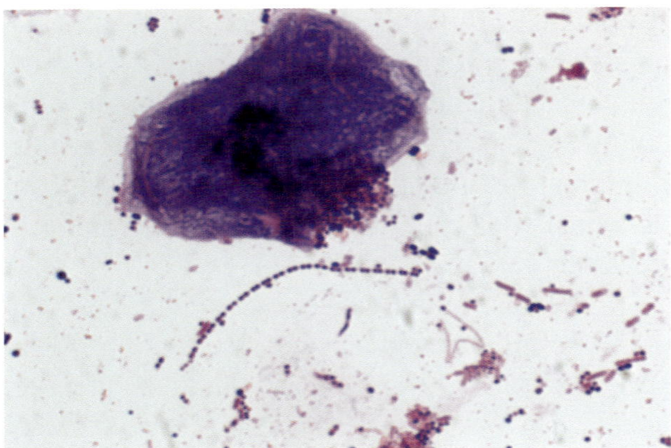

Fig 6-10 Oral flora. Light microscopic picture of scraped epithelium cells with different bacterial germs discernible.

defenses. Once these steps have taken place in several places, then bacterial colonization is completed[26].

Kantz and Henry[20] identified 377 types of bacteria in 24 non-vital teeth that had intact pulp cavities. They also succeeded in cultivating a high percentage of the microscopically-visible bacteria. On average, the infected pulps each contained 10^7 bacteria.

Utilizing intransigent bacteriological techniques and comprehensive taxonomic methods, the thesis of Sundqvist[27] proved the connection between the presence of bacteria in the pulp and clinically-defined endodontic symptoms.

There is a correlation between the extent of the periapical lesion and the number of different types of bacteria, and the specific type of bacteria present within the root canal. Teeth with large periapical lesions include more types of bacteria and a higher bacteria density within their root canal, than do teeth with small periapical lesions[27,28].

Environmental changes in the root canal can seriously affect the interaction of the individual types of bacteria. Therefore, we can expect that in the course of time, specific changes to the bacterial flora will occur.

A completely different flora will be found in already started or unsuccessfully treated canals, compared to freshly infected teeth. Bacteria will be found that are resistant to root canal rinsing solvents and bactericidal root canal solutions and inserts.

The dominant bacteria are gram-positive cocci that can also survive as a mono-infection, and these have a high resistance to anti-microbiological intervention. Gram-positive cocci are characterized by a simply developed cell wall, which is one reason for this high resistance (see Figs 6-21 and 6-23).

Sundqvist et al.[25] studied persisting infections in root canals. They examined the microbial flora in root canals after failed endodontic treatment. This flora differed clearly from that found in untreated root canals with necrotic pulps.

Table 6-3 Bacteria which could be isolated after the removal of the root canal filling (Sundqvist et al.[25]).

Isolated Mircoorganism	Number of Cases
Enterococcus faecalis	9
Streptococcus anginosus	2
Streptococcus constellatus	1
Streptococcus intermedius	1
Streptococcus mitis	1
Streptococcus parasanguis	1
Peptostreptococcus micros	2
Actinomyces israelii	3
Eubacterium alactolyticum	1
Eubacterium timidum	1
Lactobacillus catenaforme	1
Propionibacterium acnes	1
Propionibacterium propionicum	1
Fusobacterium nucleatum	1
Bacteriodes gracilis	3
Candida albicans	2

The above table lists (see table 6-3) the bacteria that could be isolated after the removal of the root canal filling.

In 19 cases, a single isolate was found, in four cases two isolates and only in one case a polymicrobial colonization consisting of four different species was found. The most frequently isolated bacterium was *Enterococcus faecalis* – see section 6.1.2.2.1.

Enterococcus faecalis is a gram-positive facultative anaerobe and inhabits the human gastrointestinal system and ranks among the main representatives of enterococci in the human body, i.e., 80–90%[29].

At the beginning of a bacterial settlement in the root canal, *E. faecalis* can be isolated initially, but only represents a small percentage of the predominantly gram-negative mixed infection[27,30]. In contrast, *E. faecalis* is present in a majority, in root canal treated teeth with chronic apical pathology[25,31].

The high resistance of *E. faecalis* against active antibacterial substances explains its persistence in an environment in which other bacteria could hardly survive, due to a lack of nutrition or the presence of antimicrobial agents, such as endodontically-treated teeth. In addition, *E. faecalis* has the ability to prevail against concurring microorganisms and to manipulate the immunologic response[32] or the local cell environment of the host organism[33,34].

Isolated from chronically infected canals, *E. faecalis* is often a mono-infection[25,35], and has the ability to survive in the extremely nutrient-poor environment of a treated root canal (see section 6.1.2.2.1.1).

6.1.2.2.1 The Dentinal Tubules as Bacterial Reservoirs

In an existing infection of the pulp, the bacteria not only settle on the entire root canal walls, branching canals, and apical delta canals, but they also penetrate the surrounding dentinal tubules.

It represents a hideout where the microorganisms are able to survive against the conventional endodontic instrumentation and disinfection procedures.

It is the presence of bacteria in the dentinal tubules that is considered by many authors to be one of the main causes of root canal failures[36–39].

These findings are supported by the fact that certain bacteria are able to penetrate and colonize the small dentinal tubules very effectively in a short time.

Perez et al.[12] found that *Streptococcus sanguis* penetrated up to a depth of 792 µm within 28 days, but could not penetrate where peritubular dentin blocked the tubules.

Kouchi et al.[40] in 1980 studied 76 extracted teeth whose root canals had been lying partly exposed and found that *Streptococcus mutans* had penetrated up to 509 µm. Certain sero-groups of *Streptococcus mutans* even reached peak values around 1,150 µm.

Sen et al.[41] examined molar teeth with periapical lesions and stated that substantial amounts of cocci and rods had penetrated only to 150 µm. They also determined the presence of yeast. In

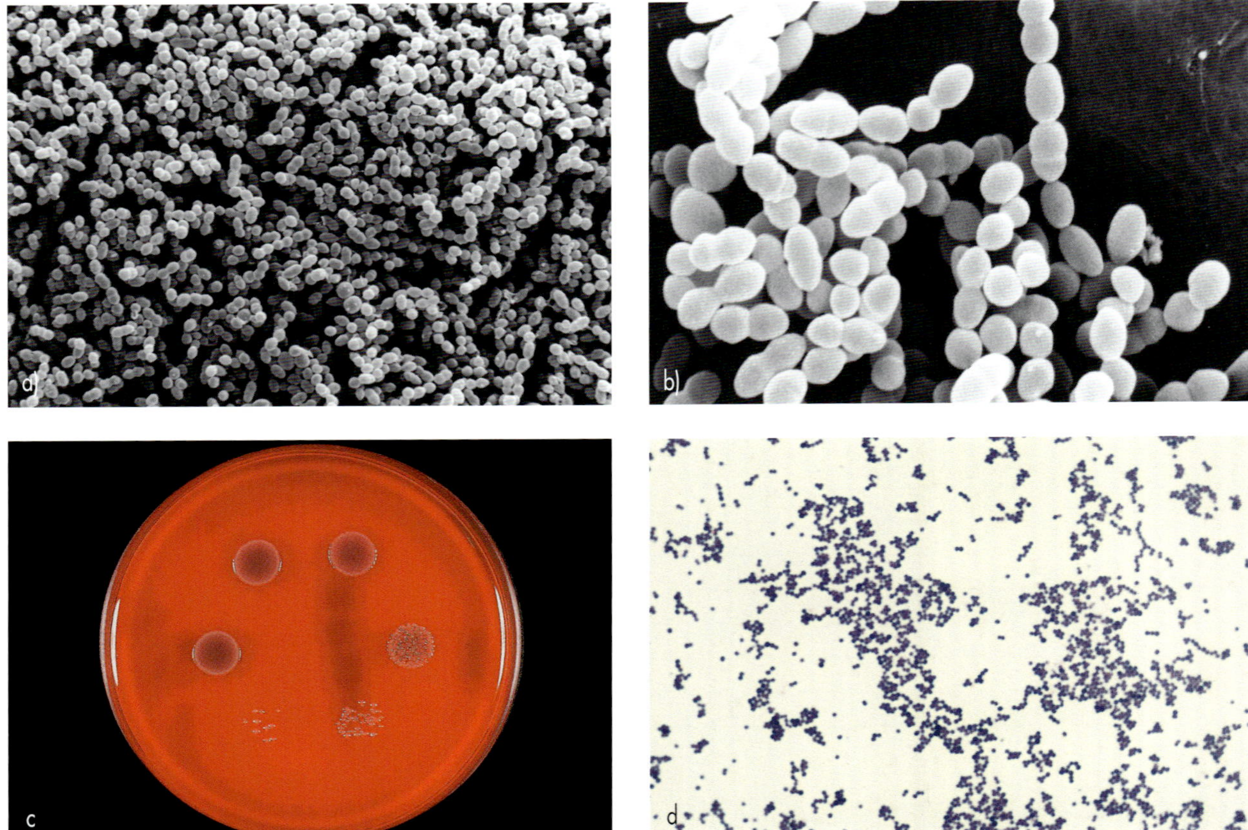

Figs 6-11a–d *Enterococcus faecalis*: a) low magnification, b) high magnification, c) semi-quantitative evaluation of an *E. faecalis* culture, d) light microscopic picture.

1997, they showed unequivocally that fungal hyphae, too, can penetrate into the dentin[42].

Siqueira et al.[38] proved that test bacteria of *Propionibacterium endodontalis*, *Fusobacterium nucleatum*, *Actinomyces israeli*, *P. gingivalis*, *P. acnes*, and *E. faecalis*, had all infiltrated the dentin tubules after 21 days. However, no accurate measurement of the depth was possible for the authors, except to state that *P. gingivalis* penetrated particularly deeply.

Siqueira also concluded from REM examinations, that the bacteria deep in the dentin could not be accessed by conventional endodontic methods.

Streptococcus sanguis, Actinomyces viscosus, and *Corynebacteria* spp., were able to reach a depth of 500 µm through the tubules within 72 h. Since a monolayer of fibroblasts was present on the dentin platelet of the experimental assembly, the cytotoxicity of the individual strains could be examined and it was also shown that *Streptococcus sanguis* caused major cell destruction[43].

The dentin of juvenile teeth is colonized extraordinarily quickly. Under incipient caries, bacteria have been seen to penetrate to a depth of 1.5 mm from the enamel-dentin border[44].

Bacterial infiltration can also take place in the opposite direction, i.e., not from the root canal but from the paradontal pockets where bacteria populate the area between the remaining Sharpey's fibers and root cement. Adriaens et al.[45] determined that most bacteria passed through the outside 300 µm thickness of dentin and may penetrate the dentinal tubules until they reach the pulp cavity. He also concluded that colonized dentinal tubules are to be regarded as bacterial reservoirs. From these reservoirs, the

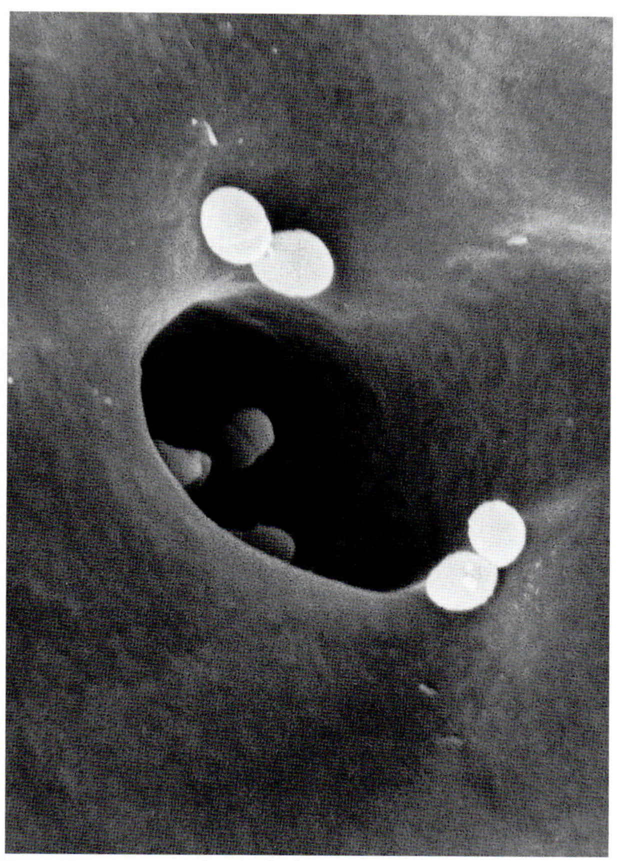
Fig 6-12 Bacteria in the depth of dentin.

already-treated root canal surfaces may be recolonized at any time.

In vitro it is found that it is the obligatory anaerobic bacteria that will migrate into the deep layers of the dentin. Ando and Hoshino[46] found, at distances of 0.5–2 mm from the root canal wall, *Lactobacillus, Streptococcus* and *Propionobacterium* and that this bacterial flora was similar to the flora in the deep carious lesions of the crown dentin.

The data of different authors varies substantially regarding the penetration depth of bacteria. The different test results may be attributed to the fact that each individual type of bacterium seemed to have a specific spreading mode in the dentin. The condition of the dentin also plays a relevant role. It has been proven that increased mineralization of the dentin, and the associated loss of diameter of the tubules, will stop the spread of bacteria[47,48]. On the other hand, it has been shown that the demineralization processes, by uncovering the collagen matrix, will help the penetration of the bacteria[49].

6.1.2.2.1.1 *Enterococcus faecalis*: the Problem Germ in Endodontics

E. faecalis penetrates very easily and rapidly into the lateral dentinal tubules[36,50,51].

As previously stated, the infection is inaccessible to conventional chemo-mechanical cleaning and disinfection, and the effectiveness of canal preparation is greatly reduced. And from this reservoir within the dentinal tubules, reinfection of the obturated canal can occur. Even with the changed nutrient conditions, proliferation of *Enterococcus* takes place, exhibiting a multiplicity of virulence factors, e.g., adherence to host cells[52], and the exprimation of protein, thus ensuring the survival of the bacteria despite the reduced nutrition.

E. faecalis also possesses a special ability to compete successfully against other microorganisms, succeeds against the immune defense system[32] and manipulates the cell milieu of the host[34].

E. faecalis probably uses the interstitial tissue fluid from the surrounding paradontal tissues and alveolar bone to survive in deeper dentin layers. This fluid can penetrate the root dentin and is similar in composition to serum.

The plentiful non-mineralized collagen in the dentin tubules acts as a suitable substrate for adhesion, and induces growth in the bacteria cell after adhesion[53].

Streptococcus gordonii has been shown to use diaphragm receptors (SspA and SspB) to attach themselves to the type 1 collagen of dentin. The propagation of these bacteria in the tubules correlates directly with their ability to attach to the collagen. This process functions as a growth stimulus and leads to extensive chain formation[54].

In addition, Love[55] could prove that *E. faecalis* remains viable in the presence of human serum and that its ability to penetrate into the dentinal

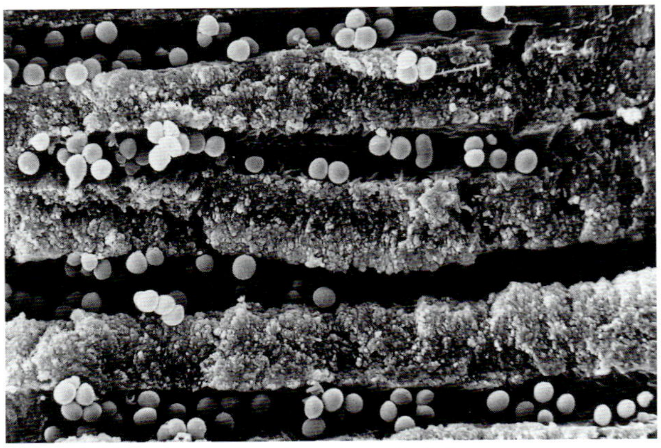

Fig 6-13 *Enterococcus faecalis* in dentinal tubules.

tubuli is restricted only to a small extent. The binding to collagen is increased – in contrast to other bacteria investigated (*Streptococcus gordonii* and *Streptococcus mutans*) in which serum inhibited the binding to collagen.

Hubbel et al.[56] investigated the influence of cellular enzymes and proteins which are responsible for the adherence to dentin. The bacterial serin protease and the collagen binding protein (ACE) proved to be important binding components and act as virulence factors.

These mechanisms of transportation of nutrition and adhesion explain the ability of *E. faecalis* to initiate apical periodontitis even after an endodontic treatment has been accomplished.

The aim of a root canal treatment is the reduction or elimination of bacteria in the main canal and the adjacent dentin.

6.2 Conventional Working Methods

6.2.1 Chemo-mechanical Disinfections

Classical root treatment involves cleaning the root canals using mechanical preparation and rinsing with antibacterial solutions and solvents. These should remove the bacteria from the canal system.

The mechanical preparation with flexible drills and files serves primarily to create an entrance to the apical third of the root canal by removal of the infected periluminal dentin. The preparation of side canals and other branching is impossible (see section 6.1.2.1.1). Using this bio-chemical preparation technique always produces a smear layer.

The smear layer is composed of organic components and consists of dentin chips, remnants of the pulp, predentin- and odontoblast appendices. Additionally the infected pulp remnants will contain bacteria and their by-products. To remove this smear layer and pathogens, various rinsing solutions are used.

The rinsing of the root canal with antibacterial and tissue-solvent substances represents a substantial component of the chemo-mechanical preparation.

The goals of chemo-mechanical disinfection are

- Killing of the bacteria
- Removal of dentinal debris
- Dissolving of organic and inorganic canal contents which are not accessible to mechanical removal
- Lubrication

The following materials are used for chemo-mechanical preparation

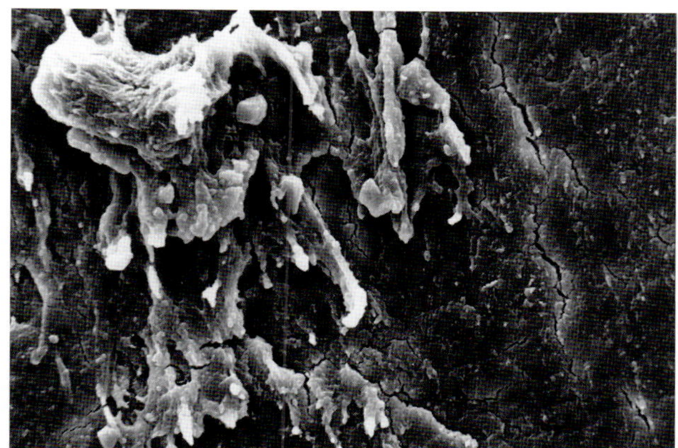

Fig 6-14 Smear layer in an SEM picture.

- NaOCl – dissolves necrotic and vital tissue and exhibits a strong anti-microbial effect. The optimal concentration used in endodontics is still disputed but varies between 0.5 and 5.25%
- H_2O_2 – a faintly acidic fluid, which disintegrates as an aqueous solution into water and oxygen. The tissue-dissolving effect is less that NaOCl. H_2O_2 can be combined with NaOCl thereby releasing oxygen and giving a bubbling rinsing solvent. This helps with the evacuation of the dentin and tissue remnants from the apical area. Further, the nascent oxygen is able to kill the strictly anaerobic bacteria. However, as a final rinse, NaOCl should be used, since any H_2O_2 remaining in the canal could react with the peroxidase of the blood. The resulting production of O_2 could lead to an increase in pressure in the canal causing pain.
- Chlorhexidine – has a broad antimicrobial spectrum, but the disadvantage of no tissue-solvent effect.
- EDTA – has no antibacterial effect but is the solution of choice when removing the smear layer. It binds calcium of the dentin to itself, and softens the dentin, facilitating the preparation of narrow curved canals.

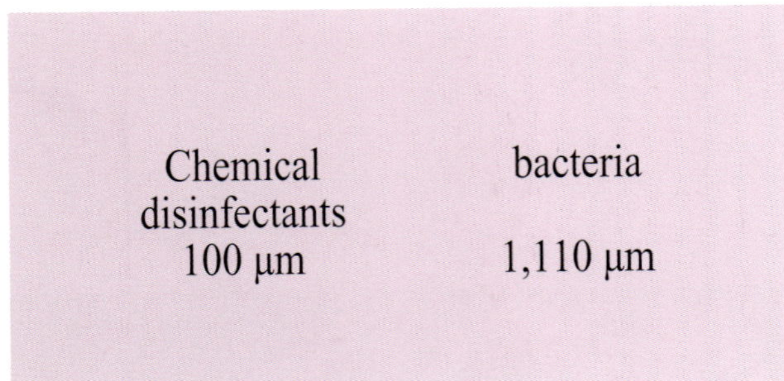

Fig 6-15 Penetration depths of chemical disinfectants and bacteria into dentin.

With the above usually-used root canal disinfectants, a sufficient removal of dentin remnants from the root canal can be accomplished. The concentration-dependent antimicrobial effect of these agents has been described in numerous studies indicating their partially effective efficiency[23,51,57–62].

The crucial disadvantage of the rinsing solutions is that their bactericidal effect is limited to the root canal. Because of the narrow diameter of the dentinal tubules and the high surface tension of the liquid solutions, they are able to penetrate only a small distance down the tubules. The penetration depth of chemical disinfectants only reaches 100 µm into the adjacent dentinal tubules[63].

On the other hand, the bacteria can penetrate over 1000 µm from the canal lumen, as described by Kouchi et al.[40], and Ando and Hoshino[46], and are therefore protected in the deeper layers of dentin. In this protected area we find the gram-negative bacteria (see section 6.1.2.2). The gram-negative bacteria are characterized by their unusual migration qualities and also their actual resistance to the chemical rinsing solutions. They maintain their virulence against conventional endodontic techniques. And we find that from this bacterial reservoir, the bacteria will spread to the periapical areas of the tooth causing inflammation and infection.

Today lasers are being used in endodontics to dramatically improve the prognosis of root-filled teeth. Using suitable wavelengths, together with conventional methods, canal, dentin and periapical regions are being effectively sterilized.

6.2.2 Laser-supported Root Canal Sterilization

The disinfecting effect of laser radiation has been well known for a long time but has only recently been used in dentistry.

Zakariasen et al.[64] showed the anti-bacterial potential of the CO_2 laser in root canals. Attempts by Pini et al.[65] and Frentzen and Koort[66] first showed that the Xe–Cl excimer laser had a good bactericidal effect using a wavelength of $\lambda = 308$ nm. Hardee et al.[67] and Rooney et al.[68] then described the high bactericidal effect of the Nd:YAG laser. In the late 1990s increasing numbers of in vitro studies were completed, using different laser types, stating the efficacy, security in application and overall practicability. Supplemented by further clinical studies, the results supported the use of laser-associated endodontic procedures as a standardized therapy concept[69]. In addition, further wavelengths, i.e., diode laser[70] and the Er:YAG laser[71,72], were examined with respect to their antibacterial effect.

Only lasers can be used which deliver their power through extremely fine flexible fiber optic systems. In particular, these include lasers in the near infrared range.

And only lasers with a wavelength that can penetrate dentin to a depth that can eliminate bacteria are applicable.

To understand how laser energy contributes to the disinfection of the tooth we must consider the physical phenomena of laser radiation within the root canal and surrounding dentin.

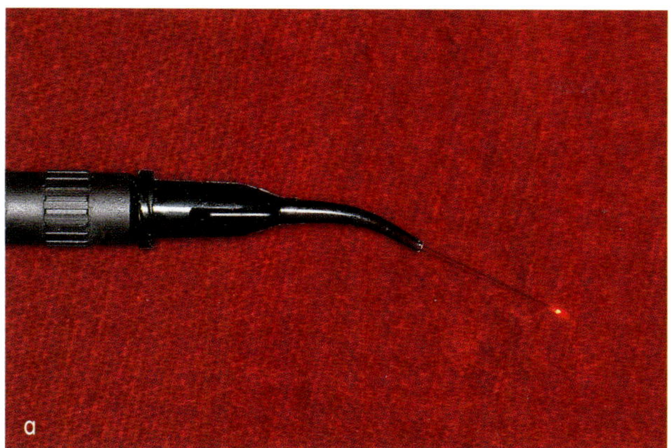

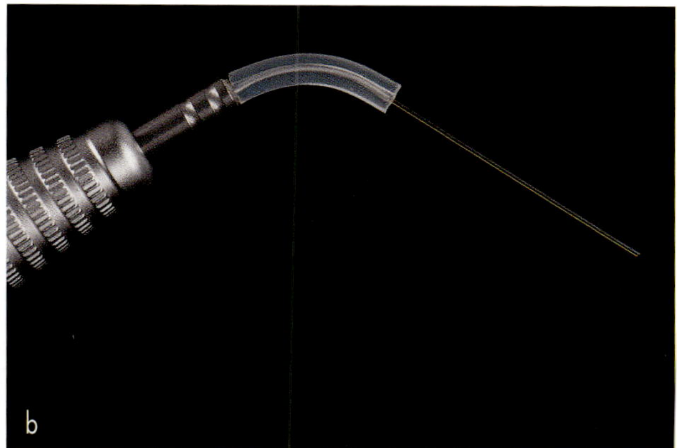

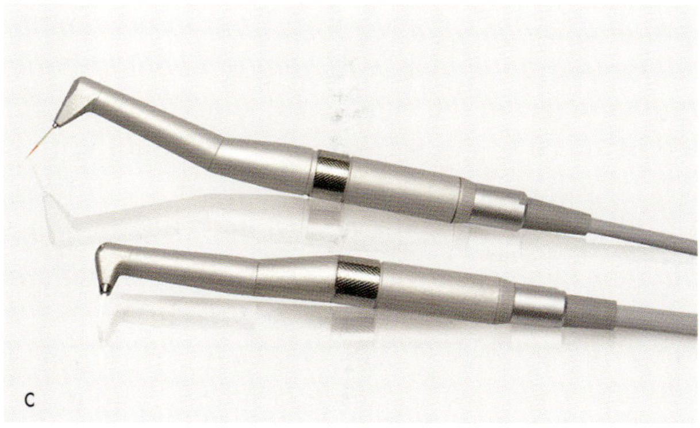

Figs 6-16a–c Different laser systems.

6.2.2.1 Distribution of Light in the Tubular Network

As we know, the impact of the laser light depends on the interaction of the light quanta and the molecules and the molecular formations in the target material. When bacteria in the depths of the dentin are irradiated, we must consider that the laser light may have had an interaction with the dentin it has passed through, and have different qualities. The laser light that attacks the bacteria may therefore differ strongly from the light emitted by the fiber tip.

6.2.2.2 Optical Characteristics

Dentin has a complex tissue architecture composed of organic and inorganic material. The incident light is partly reflected and refracted but its main propagation is scattering, i.e., the splitting of the light by repeated directional diversion.

Thus the original parallel beam of light loses its parallelism, the illuminating volume changes its form, and it becomes larger. The light emitted by the laser thereby creates a "light fog" in the dentin, and does not have the characteristic of a concentrated beam anymore[73–75].

Coherent light exhibits the phenomenon of interference. When two light beams merge, the peaks and the troughs of their waves interfere with each other, then mutually strengthen themselves. Thereby the amplitude of the total wave increases. If the wave peak of one beam overlaps the troughs of the second light jet, then they extinguish each other, and the wave disappears. In the case where a laser beam is directed towards an opaque plate with parallel slots, the slots act as light sources. Light beams fan out, interacting with one another. This effect is used in mode chemistry to selectively crack chemical compounds[76].

The hard tissue of teeth seems to be the most suitable tissue for research in laser propagation.

Firstly, the optical-physical characteristics of the tooth are very similar in vivo and in vitro, and secondly, the tooth is solid, with a polycrystalline structure very similar to other structures examined in optics.

Nevertheless, the description of the optical characteristics of the tooth in general terms is an extremely difficult task. We must understand in detail the tooth structure, otherwise the use of optics and laser methods is unsatisfactory.

Although the light propagation and dispersion by the hydroxyapatite crystals of the enamel have often been described, there are only a few studies which discuss the optical characteristics. Zijp and Bosch[77], and Ten Bosch et al.[78] described in 1993 a theoretical model of light refraction in dentin. The authors pointed out that the micro heterogenicity of the material has to be considered for all the computations and that it leads to scattering phenomena. They further pointed out that the bulk of the dentin consists of peritubular dentin that surrounds the tubules, together with the intertubular dentin, which again consists of collagen fibers and interfibrillic material. They calculated the density of the tubules to be 15–65 × 10^3 per mm^2 with an average diameter of 1.58 µm. Tubules are surrounded by peritubular dentin with a mineral content of 90%. The mineral content of the intertubular dentin was only 40%. The tropocollagen molecule has a dimension of 280 × 1.5 nm and a molecular weight of 360,000.

The fibrils have a diameter of 50–150 nm and are irregularly arranged. All dentin tissues, with the exception of the tubules, contain needle-shaped hydroxyapatite crystals that are 0.5 nm wide and 20 nm long. These data served as a basis for their work.

They differentiate between two kinds of refraction superimposed in the dentin.

a. Symmetrical processes around the incoming laser beam, caused by the irregularly arranged mineral crystals and collagen fibrils and
b. Asymmetrical processes caused by the tubuli.

The authors came to the conclusion that neither the mineral crystals nor the collagen fibrils substantially contribute to the light scattering in the dentin. The scattering was caused mainly by the tubules. However the peritubular dentin was not referred to in their calculations. They also assumed that the demineralization progress in the carious dentin changes the optical characteristics substantially.

In a comparative study on micro-porous glass, Altshuler and Grisimov[79] determined that the light transmission consists of a directed and a diffuse component. They justified the emergence of the directed component by the presence of optical light conductors and therefore proposed a wholly new approach. The appropriate experiments show, that beside this deviation, still another partial light capture in the light conductor took place, i.e., in the enamel prisms, and in the dentin in the amorphously mineralized substance between the small dentin canals. The experiments showed large anisotropy of the light propagation in the dentin, whose transparency can be very different, according to whether the light conductors (tubuli) are met parallel or at a 90° angle by the beam. Within a layer thickness of 1 mm the anisotropy differed by up to a factor of 30. The authors also pointed out that incipient caries significantly changes the optical characteristics of the hard tissue.

In the following study in 1991, Altshuler et al.[73] expanded the previous findings about the tooth as an optical medium. They confirmed how the laser light scatters and spreads in the tooth, and found that the light propagation was independent of the angle of the incoming beam.

Altshuler et al. concluded that this was due to the closely arranged light conductors in the tooth – the enamel prisms and/or the intertubular areas. The optical information is led from the enamel surface to the pulpal cavity in this way. Every point on the surface of the tooth corresponds to a defined point on the surface of the root canal, decreasing the picture information.

On this basis, Altshuler et al. provided an optical model of the tooth, with respect to its irregular structure. Despite the strong scattering resulting from the different structures within the tooth, light can be led over long distances in this medium. This is possible because the scattered light parts are recaptured by the numerous light-conducting structures.

Similar observations were made by Vaarkamp et al.[80], who stated in the context of diaphanoscopy, that the transmission in a tooth depends on

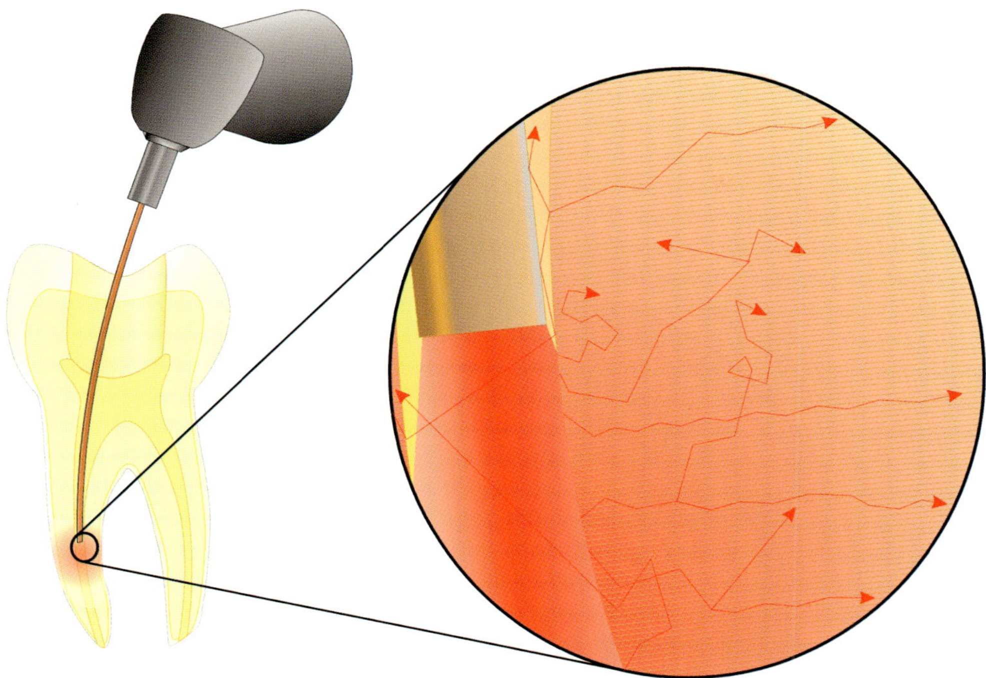

Fig 6-17 Diagrammatic view of the light propagation in the depth of dentin.

whether the surface of the sample is met by the laser beam at a 90° angle or parallel. The deviation in the enamel was caused by hydroxyapatite crystals, while in the dentin the tubuli are the main cause for this phenomenon.

It cannot be excluded that the tubules also cause an interference phenomenon leading to both local intensity enhancement and attenuation, but detailed examinations are still missing.

By reflection, refraction and scattering, photons can pass through a material, without interfering with it. Only if photons are absorbed, can one expect physical or chemical effects. Laser light in the near infrared range is absorbed by dentin only to a small extent.

This characteristic is used for root canal sterilization since we do not want superficial absorption in the dentin – but a deep penetration into the intertubular tissue, in order to produce a sufficient bactericidal effect in the deep layers.

Because of the physical conditions present in a tooth, the Nd:YAG and the diode laser wavelengths are not absorbed in the hard dental substances and are thus able to be effective in the deep layers.

The Er:YAG laser acquires its efficiency by the photoablative effect. Hydroxyapatite has its absorption maximum at a wavelength of $\lambda = 2940$ nm. The result of using the laser is that the water within the crystals turns into steam and explodes, splitting off parts of the dental hard tissue. The antibacterial effect of this laser is effective[72] but restricted to a small area surrounding the root canal (see section 6.2.2.3.1).

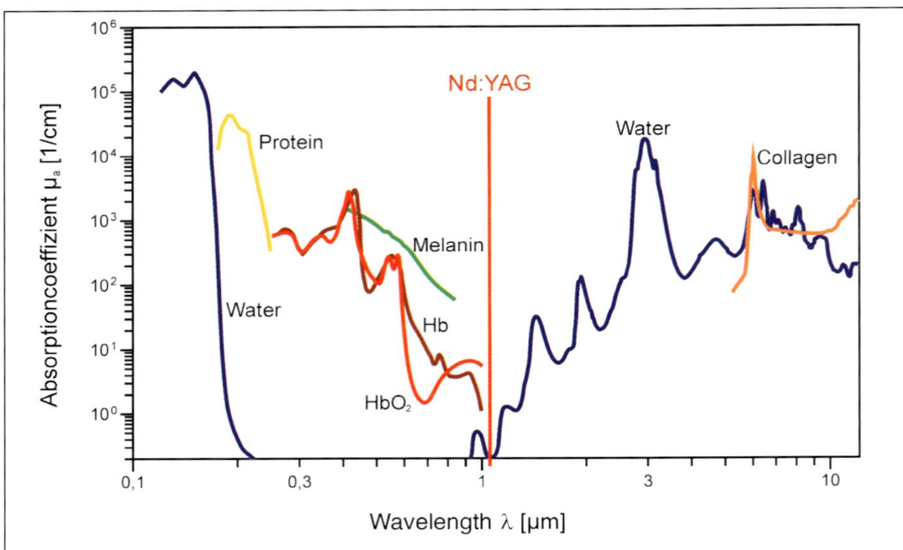

Fig 6-18 Absorption spectrum of the Nd-YAG laser.

6.2.2.3 Reaction of the Bacteria to Laser Light

Under the use of laser light both biological tissues and individual cell systems change their structure. The reactions between photons and molecules have not yet been explained in detail. The kind and the development of the reactions depend on the condition of the irradiated cells as well as the wavelength, power density and duration of application.

The absorption of UV or visible light by organic molecules leads to the stimulation of π-electrons (the double and triple bonds) or n-electrons (non-binding pairs of electrons of oxygen, sulfur or nitrogen atoms), and thus to photochemical reactions; the power consumption of the absorbed light quanta of the near-IR range causes molecular oscillations, i.e., mechanical oscillations between the atoms of a molecule. This can cause deformation of the binding angle and the deformation vibration can weaken or break up chemical compounds.

Laser radiation has a bactericidal effect by causing changes in the bacterial cell wall. These changes can be seen with laser beams used in root canal treatment (Nd:YAG, diode and Er:YAG laser). The bactericidal effects in the deep dentin layers differ because of the different absorption of the different wavelengths of the lasers (this is mentioned in the following section).

The structural characteristics of gram-positive and gram-negative bacteria differ substantially in their cell walls. For this reason, the structure of the cell walls wiall be discussed.

The cell wall of gram-negative bacteria shows a three-layer structure typical for this group of microorganisms.

The most important component of the cell coat of both gram-positive and gram-negative bacteria is the murein (latin: murus = wall) or peptidoglycan layer, which the cytoplasmic membrane rests upon. It encloses the bacterial cell as a kind of giant molecule and its form and mechanical stability is important, in relation to the high osmotic pressure inside the cell (up to 25 atm!). Without murein the bacterial cell would explode immediately in most surroundings. The murein-net of gram-negative bacteria has one layer (5–10 nm thick) and is less than 10% of the cell wall's dry weight.

Beside this strong supporting sac around the cell, large quantities of lipoproteins, lipopolysaccharides and other lipids are present, which seem

Fig 6-19 Cell walls – differences in the structure of gram⁺ and gram⁻ cell walls caused by different concentration and arrangement of murein.

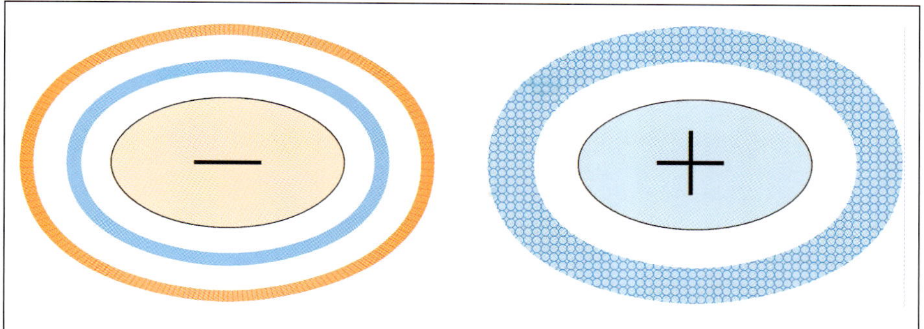

to be glued on the outside of the murein cage. They are bound covalently and constitute up to 80% of the dry weight of the cell wall.

This so-called outer membrane is the outstanding feature of gram-negative bacteria. It is asymmetric in comparison to the cytoplasmic membrane regarding their lipid matrix: while the internal half of their double layer is composed of phospholipids, one finds the lipopolysaccharides and the typical component of this auxiliary membrane in the outside lamella. The outer membrane has both mechanical and substantial physiological functions.

The murein layer directly borders the cytoplasmic membrane. Within the murein layer the hydrophilic ends of the lipoproteins are linked covalently. These extend their lipophilic ends into a lipid double layer, which contains phospholipids and the lipid A zones of the lipopolysaccharides.

The lipoproteins take a key position: they are the main part of the protein of the gram-negative cells – up to 700,000 molecules per cell. Their function is the stabilization of the outer membrane and the connection to the murein layer. The "bound form" is with its protein component linked to the peptide part of the murein, while the lipid component is stored in the outer membrane[81–83].

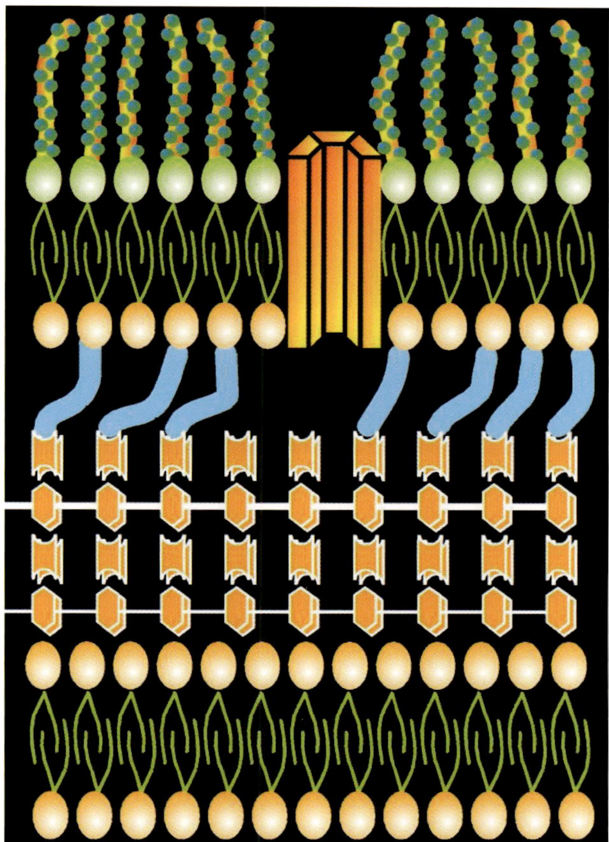

Fig 6-20 Model of the cell wall structure of gram-negative bacteria.

The inner membrane of the triple layer corresponds to the cytoplasmic membrane. It forms a double-layer structure out of lipids, with hydrophobic lipid acid chains in the center and hydrophilic lipid borders outwardly. Numerous transportation proteins are integrated in the structure. The triple layer is the seat of the enzymes for electron transportation and for oxidative phosphorylation — thus the cell membrane takes the place of the cell mitochondria to a certain extent.

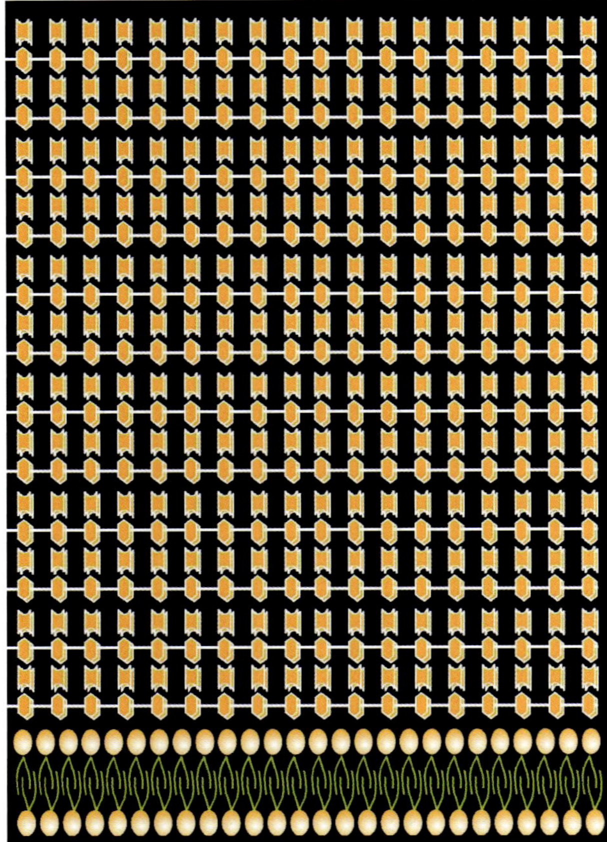

Fig 6-21 Cell wall structure of gram-positive microorganisms.

The bacterial cytoplasm membrane can in-fold itself in certain places to form complex diaphragm bodies, the mesosomes. These have an important role during the cell's mitotic division. The cytoplasmic membrane is not only a selective permeability barrier but also contains enzymes and carrier molecules for the synthesis of the DNA and the cell wall, components which are of fundamental importance for the survival of the bacterium cell[84].

The cell membrane of the gram-positive bacteria is much more simply developed and appears as a one-layer structure.

The peptidoglycan layer of the gram-positive bacteria is rather thick and has a very high rate of criss-cross bondings. Similar to the gram-negative bacteria, the cell coat of the peptidoglycan layer is made up of two major components: N-acetyl-glucosamine and N-acetyl-muramine, which produce a polymer structure with covalent binding. Up to 40 layers of these sugars can be found in gram-positive bacteria. This murein layer makes up 50–70% of the bacteria mass. The cell coat itself consists of up to 90% high bonded peptidoglycans. They reach a wall thickness up to 80 nm and have a very even, flat cell surface.

One further binding component between the different murein layers is teichon acid, which is a polymer of glycerin with phosphoric acid bridges. The appearance of the teichon acid is responsible for the gram-positive cell walls being hydrophilic and also gives the surface of the bacterium a negative charge. In contrast to gram$^-$ microorganisms, lipopolysaccharides are missing completely in the cell wall, and lipids (and lipoproteins) are only present in traces (<3% by weight).

The criss-cross bonding of these three layers is responsible for the stiffness and stability of the cell wall of gram-positive bacteria. They have a higher resistance to drying out, anionic detergents, and alkalis such as sodium hydroxide and sodium hypochlorite. The enormous thickness of the murein layer also gives them a high resistance against mechanical and physical treatment in comparison with gram-negative bacteria. Only the antibiotics of the β-lactam type (Penicillin, Cephalosporin, and Carbapeneme) that selectively disable the synthesis of the peptidoglycans, have a bigger effect on the gram-positive bacteria (streptococci and staphylococci). These antibiotics effectively stop the formation of the protective cellular coat.

The real problem in endodontics lies, as described before, in the penetration depth of the rinsing detergents (100 μm).

Laser light, however, penetrates up to >1000 μm into the dentin (see Fig 6-22).

This provides a distinct advantage, since bacteria can immigrate up to 1000 μm into the tubules. Different studies have shown that laser radiation is weakened as it penetrates the dentin, but the bactericidal effect is still effective even to

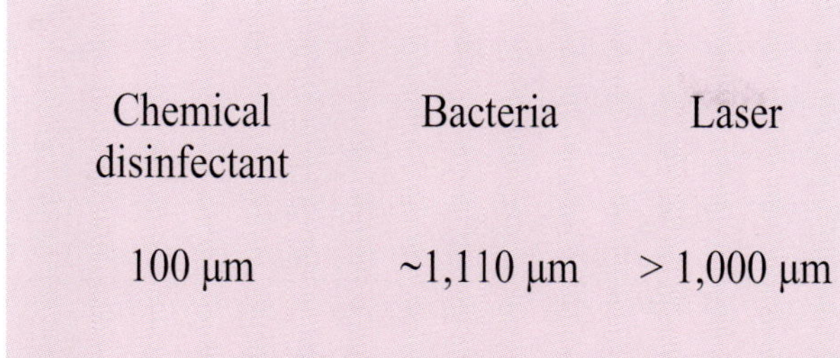

Chemical disinfectant	Bacteria	Laser
100 µm	~1,110 µm	> 1,000 µm

Fig 6-22 Penetration depths of chemical disinfectants, bacteria and laser light.

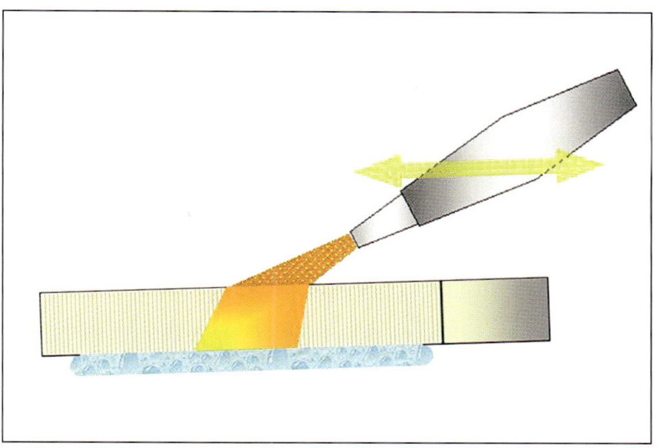

Fig 6-23 Indirect irradiation modus.

a depth thickness of 1000 µm or more. Klinke et al.[85], Vaarkamp et al.[80], as well as Odor et al.[86] were able to show that enamel prisms and dentin tubules act as light conductors.

The following describes how bacteria react to irradiation in the depth of the dentin. The cell coat not only has a mechanical function (holding the cell together), but also is one of the most important cell organelles. It is a very complex, dynamic structure that regulates all exchanges between the bacterium and its surroundings. Any change to the membrane brings even bigger changes to the whole cell.

Moritz et al.[87] showed that this structure was substantially changed by laser irradiation.

In this study bacteria were irradiated indirectly with an Nd:YAG laser. The bacteria showed changes in the cell morphology and correlating cell membrane damage, depending on the dose. This was an indication that the main damage caused by laser light in the near-IR range is done to the cell membrane.

Because of the complex three-layer membrane, gram-negative bacteria are very sensitive to irradiation, and only very small densities of energy result in severe damage to the cell membrane.

An indirect irradiation with ~ 1.0 W causes obvious changes to the cell membrane. A number of large, vesicle formations of different sizes can be observed (so-called membrane blebbing) which cover the bacteria totally or partly. Even bacteria where the cell membrane is not destroyed at higher energy (>1.5 W) show this phenomenon.

The blebbing phenomenon probably is the result of the inner layer of the membrane splitting from the two outer layers.

Microbiologists talk about a permanent destruction of the cell membrane, which is commonly in connection with direct heat having an impact on the bacteria. This damage is enough to stop the growth of the cells and can be reached with very small doses of heat.

The microbiological literature describes blistering on the surface of *E. coli* in connection with heat impact. Hitchener and Egan[88] heated *E. coli K-12* to 48°C and observed structural changes before the death of the bacteria. The slow heating over 60 min led to a release of 20% of the lipopolysaccharide. By adding EDTA, the percentage increased to 50%; however, the authors did not regard this as the direct cause of cell death.

Yatvin[89], during cancer therapy research, using the *E. coli Mutante K 1060*, showed how increased installation of unsaturated fatty acids into the cell wall under heat impact affected the

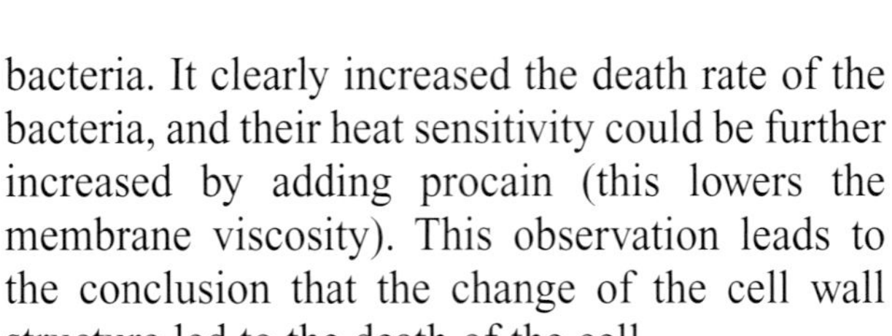

Fig 6-24 "Membrane blebbing".

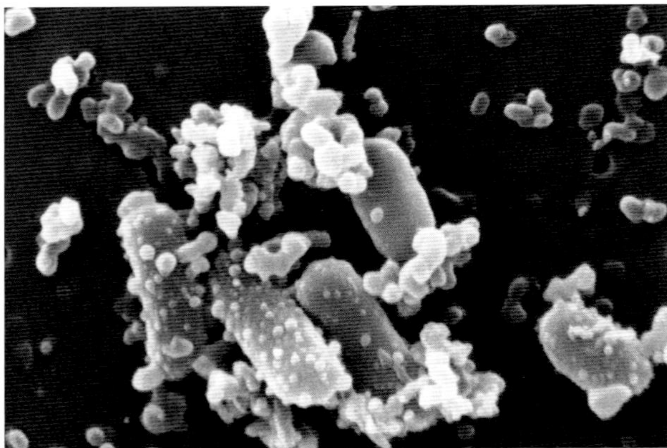

Fig 6-25 Blisters/vesicles: bacteria with an overall intact cell wall show larger and smaller vesicles on their surface. In part, these vesicles are separated from the cell and have been scattered in the direct vicinity ("membrane blebbing").

bacteria. It clearly increased the death rate of the bacteria, and their heat sensitivity could be further increased by adding procain (this lowers the membrane viscosity). This observation leads to the conclusion that the change of the cell wall structure led to the death of the cell.

Katsui et al.[90] indicated that heating of *E. coli W-3110* to 55°C in a buffered solution led to blistering in the area of the division septum of the cell. Enzymatic analyses proved there was withdrawal of periplasmatic, but not cytoplasmatic, enzymes: they concluded that the vesicles consist exclusively of components of the outer membrane. The author further assumed that the outer parts of the membrane separate from the murein layer, because of the heat. Nevertheless, further investigation will be necessary.

Also, Tsuchida et al.[91] described the heating of *E. coli wild type* to 55°C. Lipopolysaccharides loosened themselves from within the membrane and the permeability of the cell coat clearly increased. The damage could be accelerated by adding Tris.

The linking structures that connect the outside layer with the murein layer covalently are the lipoproteins. They attach the two layers like push-buttons. A change of their α-helical conformation by thermal effect, i.e., "melting", leads to the lifting of the outside layer and vesicle formation. Spectrometric analyses proved that the α-helical structure of the lipoproteins changes at 79.4°C, whereupon the outside layer loses its connection to the murein sacculus[92]. This change of the cell membrane impacts upon the barrier function and since the cell coat is also the site of a most diverse enzyme system, one can also assume that a slight restructuring of the membrane disturbs the cell's metabolism substantially.

In the literature, it is controversially discussed whether the described membrane changes alone are sufficient, in order to lower the vitality of the cells. Studies on defect mutants, which were not able to synthesize the lipoprotein of the outside layer, show that this structural defect does not directly have an effect on the vital processes of growth and the cell ability to split. However, the strength of the bacteria in relation to external influences of a physical and chemical nature is strongly reduced[93].

The physiology of structure-defective *E. coli* mutants was also examined by Yem and Wu[94]. The changes of the murein-lipoproteins increased the sensitivity against EDTA and various detergents, and changes also caused the loss, through the membrane, of periplasmatic enzymes like ribonuclease (this enzyme is involved in the reduplication and repair synthesis of the DNA).

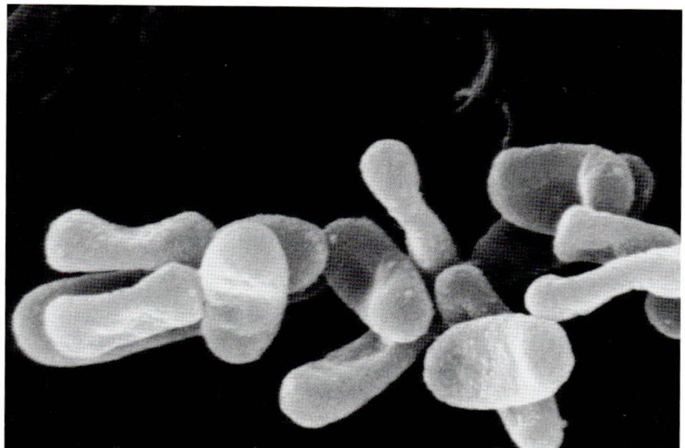

Fig 6-26 Shrinking: the size of individual bacteria is only half of the normal size or even lower, the cell shape appears rounded.

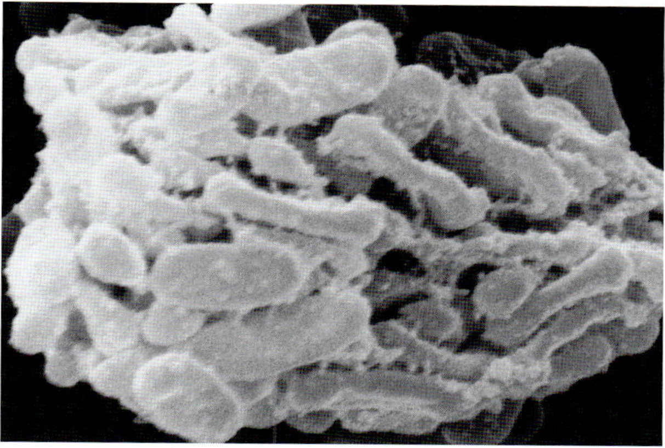

Fig 6-27 Coagulation: agglomerated, agglutinated structures of different size can be seen. The cell morphology of the individual bacteria has been completely destroyed. The bacteria seem to be fused together.

These analyses were proved by Sonntag et al.[95]. Mutants in which lipoprotein and protein II were missing built spherical shapes with superficial blistering, since the murein layer had no further connection to the outside diaphragm. Also, these mutants were extraordinarily sensitive to the influence of antibiotics and detergents. They also needed increased electrolyte concentrations in the growth medium, in order to be able to grow.

With increased laser energy, the full effect can be seen. Numerous varieties of cell damage can be found in gram-negative bacteria: from forms that show an open hole, to remaining parts of the cell that are partly melted. Finally we see total cell destruction, as illustrated in the figures 6-25 to 6-31.

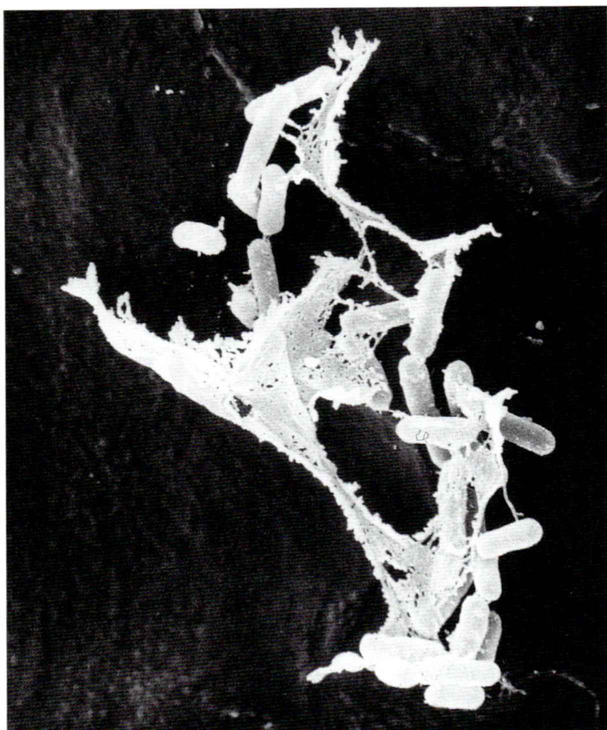

Fig 6-28 Ropy structures: between morphologically intact bacteria ropy structures can be found, probably remnants of the cell walls from destroyed bacteria.

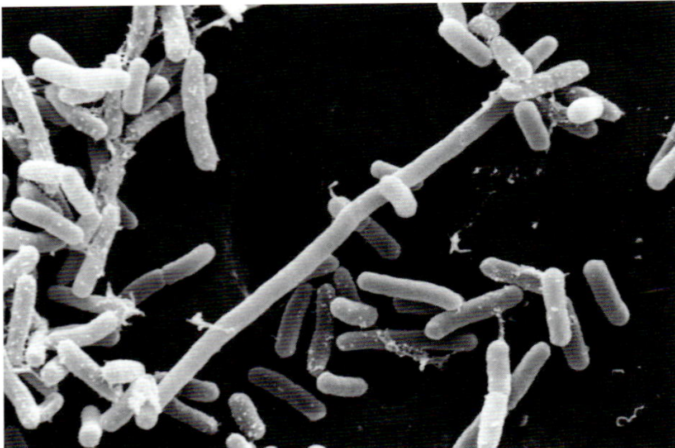

Fig 6-29 Bacteria arrested in mitosis: the length of the filament formations averages 20 μm; no invaginations are discernible.

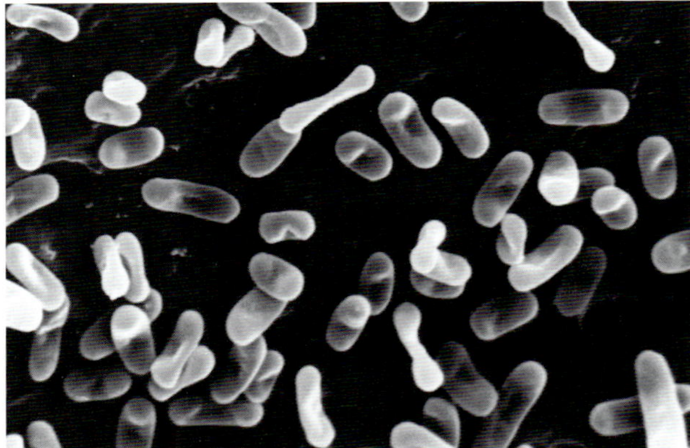

Fig 6-30 Empty cell bodies: the bacteria show partly clearly visible perforations of the cell walls. The cell bodies appear to be shrunken and empty to a different extent.

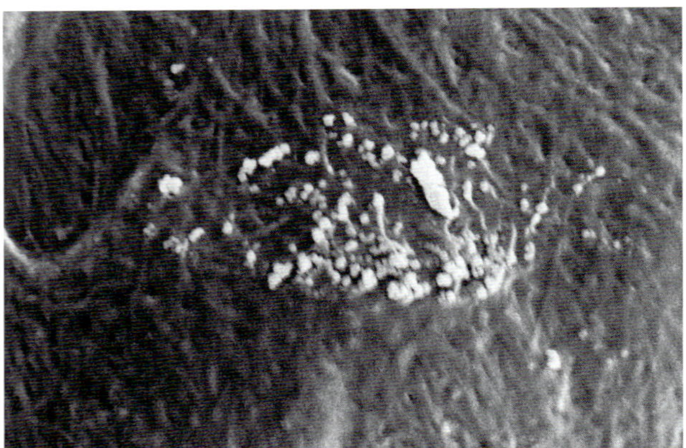

Fig 6-31 Fragmentation: it is a total, "explosively" appearing destruction of the cell body. Only fragments of the cell bodies are discernible. They bear resemblance to "ghosts", which are created when bacteria are introduced in a hypotonic medium.

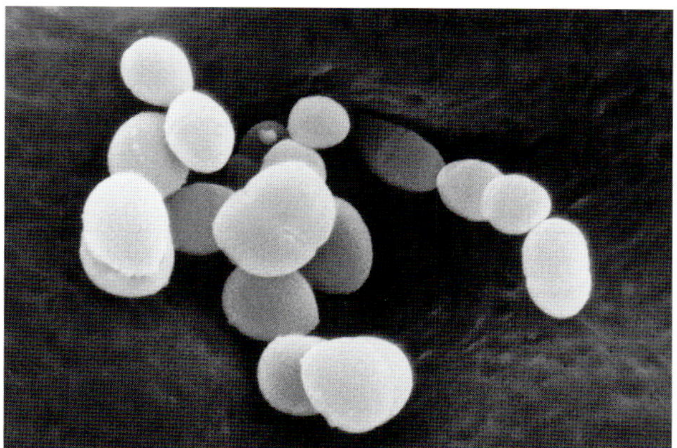

Fig 6-32 Megalospheres.

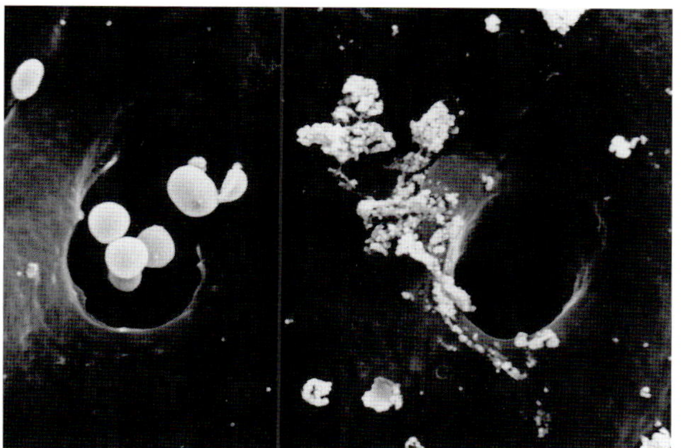

Fig 6-33 Cell debris of gram-positive bacteria.

6.2.2.3.1 Comparison of different wavelengths

In comparison, the gram-positive microorganisms showed a higher resistance against irradiation. The reason therefore seems to be the simple structure of the cell membrane. The cell wall of the gram-positive *E. faecalis* shows an astonishingly high resistance against the laser irradiation. Low energies (~ 1 W) show almost no changes to those problem bacteria. At higher energy (> 1.5 W) there are cells that become very obvious because of their higher volumetric size (megalospheres). These are alongside the regular cells. This bigger size seems to be caused by cell wall damage. Because of that damage there is an osmotic gradient that results in cell swelling. Quantitative studies showed a difference of growth when this type of cell wall damage occurs.

With the application of multiple irradiations, visible damage of the bacteria can be detected, but there can still be a few unaltered cells. However, the quantitative bacteria death increases steadily, and the damage seems to depend on a cumulative effect, as proved through the mathematical model of cell damage by Jung[96]. A cellular stress factor leads to sublethal, reversible changes, but when the cell is hit again by the irradiation it dies. This mechanism is called the "knock on" effect (see section 6.8).

These changes can be seen as a reaction to the irradiation by most of the lasers that are used in endodontics (Nd:YAG, diode and Er:YAG laser). The bactericidal effect in the depth of the dentin has to be different because of the different absorption of the different wavelengths (this shall be illustrated in the following section).

To illustrate this, the Nd:YAG and the Er:YAG laser were compared in a study[97], using a slightly different design to directly evaluate the bactericidal effect in the deep dentin.

Four different irradiation distances were used for the direct comparison (0.25, 0.5, 0.75 and 1 mm). The same power settings were applied for the Nd:YAG and the Er:YAG laser (70 mJ, 15 Hz measured directly at the fiber tip).

Again, *E. coli* and *E. faecalis* were taken as test bacteria. On the bases of morphological changes detected by the electron microscope, it was shown that both lasers had a good bactericidal effect (see Fig 6-35a and b, distance 0.25 mm).

The Er:YAG laser loses its effect with increasing layers of dentin between the laser and the bacteria. From a distance of 0.5 mm it seems to have very little effect (especially with the irradiation of *E. faecalis*).

In contrast, the Nd:YAG laser is convincing even at large distances through its excellent bactericidal effect on both test germs. Even when the

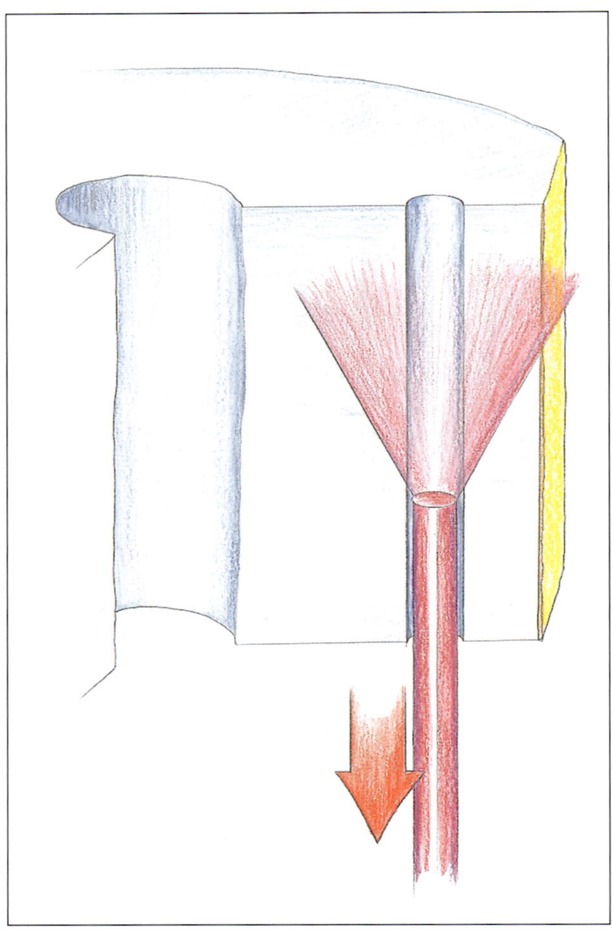

Fig 6-34 The figure shows the irradiation mode. Parallel to the root canal a hole was drilled at defined distances to the inoculation site (yellow), from where the laser irradiation was carried out.

distance between the irradiation and the inoculation site measures more than 1 mm, a nearly complete elimination of the problem bacterium *E. faecalis* can be achieved from a morphological point of view.

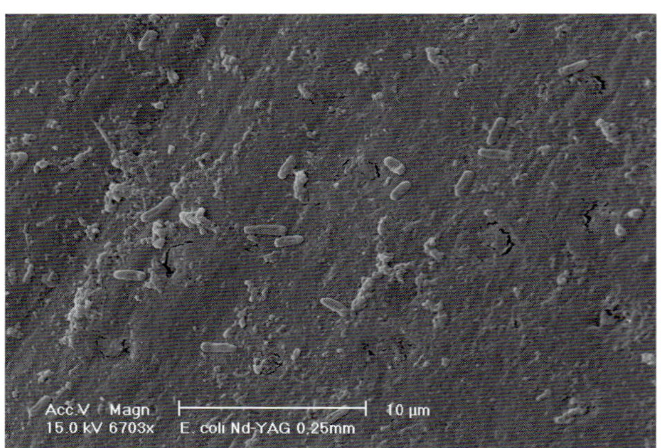

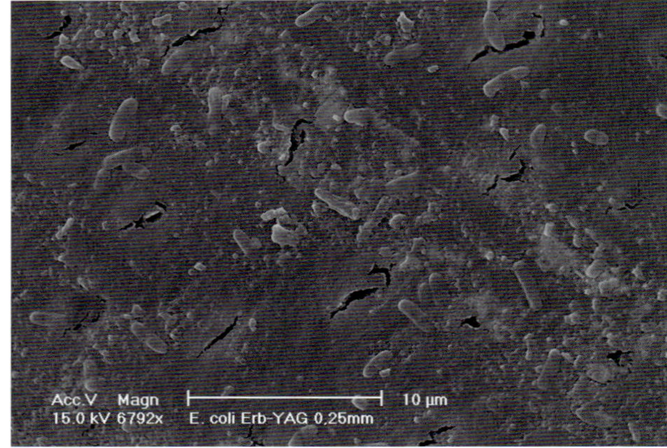

Fig 6-35 At a distance of 0.25 mm the Nd:YAG and the Er:YAG laser produce total cell destruction (germ used: *E. coli*).

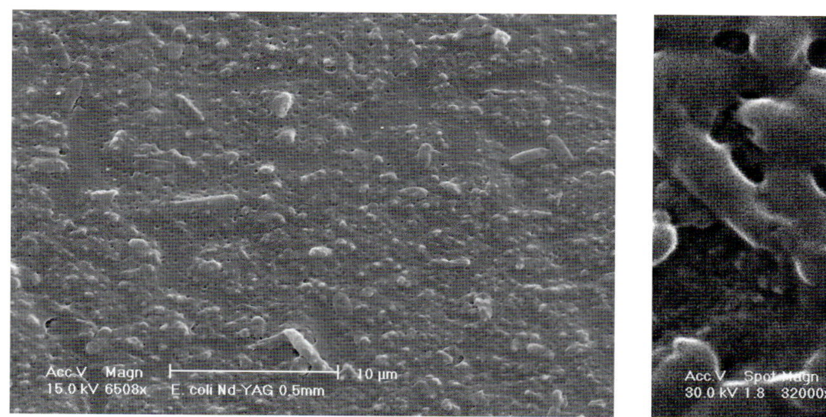

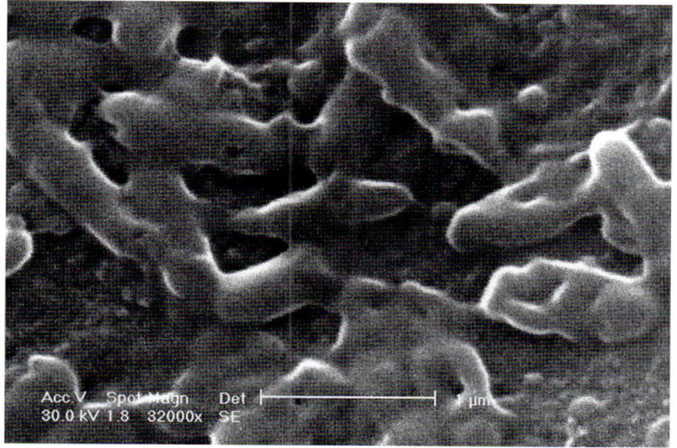

Fig 6-36 At a distance of 0.5 mm the Nd:YAG laser shows a pronounced bactericidal effect, the Er:YAG laser decreases in efficacy (germ used: *E. coli*).

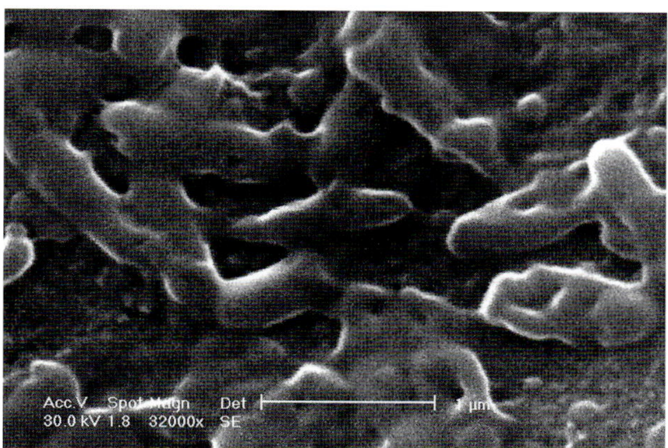

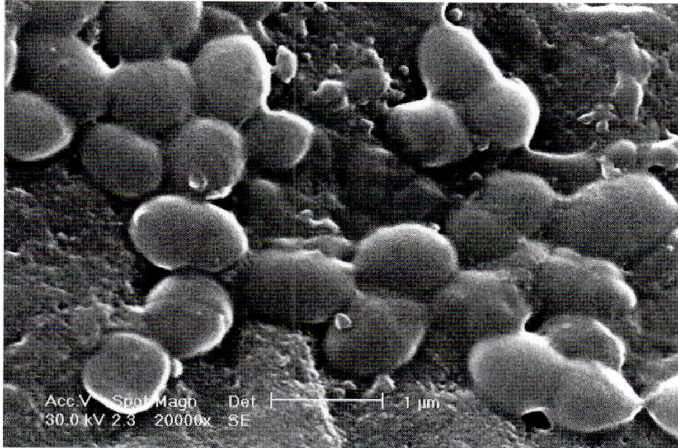

Fig 6-37 A similar picture as in Fig 6-35 can be seen in the test bacterium *E. faecalis*. Cell destruction on the left (Nd:YAG), numerous morphologically unaltered cells on the right hand side (Er:YAG).

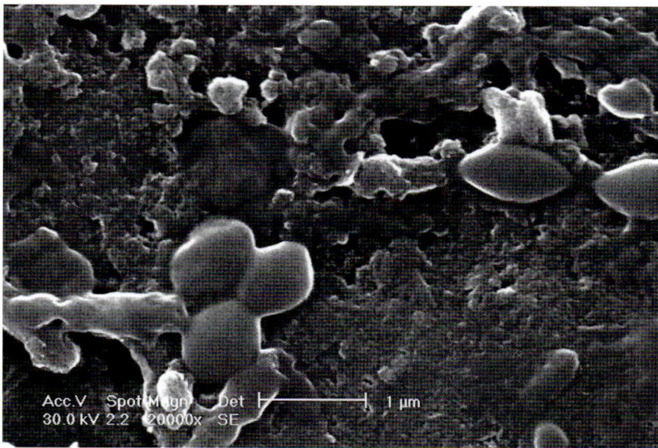

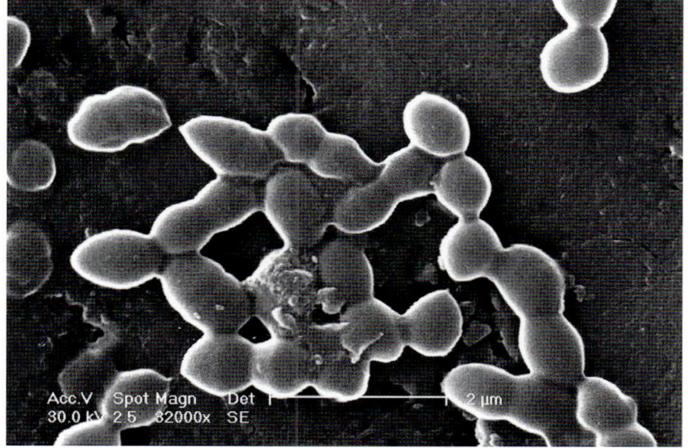

Fig 6-38 Regarding the test bacterium *E. faecalis*, total cell destruction can be found in the Nd:YAG group (left) at a distance of 1 mm. The Er:YAG laser (right) appears to be nearly ineffective. Unaltered cultures and chain formations can be seen.

6.3 Description of the Different Wavelengths

6.3.1 The Nd:YAG Laser

This seems to be the laser of choice in root canal treatment. It is also the best-documented laser in the literature for root canal sterilization. Most of the studies concerned with the Nd:YAG laser in endodontics deal with the quantitative evaluation of bacteria reduction.

Midda and Renton-Harper[98] were the first to refer to the bactericidal effect of the Nd:YAG laser and recommended its use in endodontics. The first studies in this field were made in 1995 by Rooney et al.[68] and Hardee et al.[67]. Rooney et al. assessed the impacts of the Nd:YAG laser at different settings between 0.3 W and 3 W in vitro. For their evaluations, a 350 µm fiber was used. An excellent bactericidal effect was achieved. By adding a black photo absorber, a bacterial reduction could be reached at lower energies. In the work of Hardee et al. that came out a few months later, a reduction of *Bacillus stearothermophilus* in the range of two log-levels, in comparison to the control group, was observed.

In a study by Fegan and Steiman[99] comparing conventional NaOCl-solution, ultrasound instruments, and Nd:YAG laser, and using the same bacterium (*Bacillus stearothermophilus*), it was proved that when using the laser, bacterial growth could be decreased. Moshonov et al.[100] in an in vitro study also achieved a positive bactericidal effect with the Nd:YAG laser against the resistant problematic *E. faecalis*.

In an in vivo study with patients that had endodontic treatment without laser (long time therapy without success, or patients with root treatment that could not be finished) Gutknecht et al.[101] showed that 82% of these patients could be treated successfully with the Nd:YAG laser. He also imputes these positive results to the elimination of bacteria in the root canal.

Moritz et al.[102] showed that it was possible to almost totally eradicate streptococci and staphylococci with Nd:YAG laser treatment. Ramskold et al.[103], at the same time, looked at the correlation between the radiation cycles and the thermal side effects of the Nd:YAG laser used in root canal treatment. By using pigmented test bacteria, they found out that with the number of radiation cycles the bactericidal effect increased, and without thermal side effects to the surrounding structures.

Berkiten et al.[104] used *Streptococcus sanguis* and *Prevotella intermedia* as contaminating bacteria in the root canal. At two different energy levels, 1.8 W and 2.4 W, at 30 s irradiation time, the Nd:YAG laser caused total elimination of *Petrovella*, though the less sensitive *Streptococcus* could only be eliminated by 98.5%. In another, more diversified study by Piccolomini et al.[105], the different energy levels of the Nd:YAG laser were compared with 5.25% NaOCl. However, the result showed better bactericidal effects for the highly concentrated NaOCl than for the laser groups. Folwaczny et al.[106] used the Nd:YAG laser at 100–200 mJ, showing a bactericidal effect against *E. coli* and *Staphylococcus aureus*. He noted particularly the big temperature changes at energy levels between 100–200 mJ.

In a previously cited study by Moritz et al.[87], it was shown that the Nd:YAG laser still had a bactericidal effect, even after passing through a dentin layer of 1 mm (1 W, 1.5 W). The death of the bacteria at higher energy resulted from total membrane destruction. At lower energy, where the morphological change is not that big, a parallel quantitative study showed that there is almost no more cell growth. This only holds true if a number of irradiation cycles are done, especially with *E. faecalis*.

Further, the study showed that there is no relation between the bactericidal effect in the near-IR range and the increase of the temperature in the dentin. The laser has its effect selectively at the membrane structures of the gram-negative bacte-

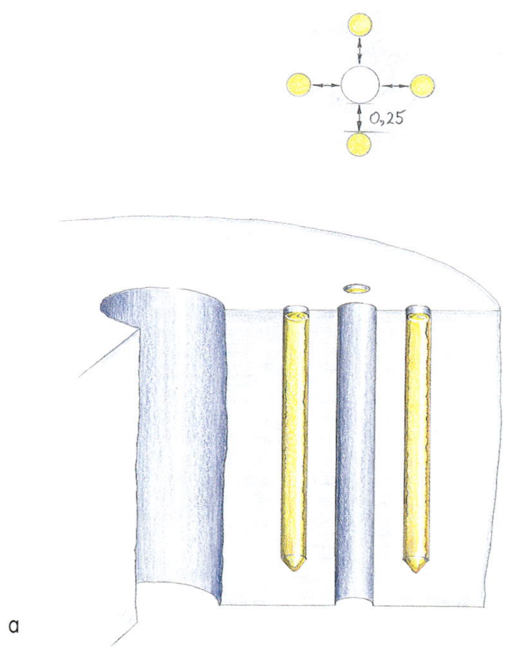

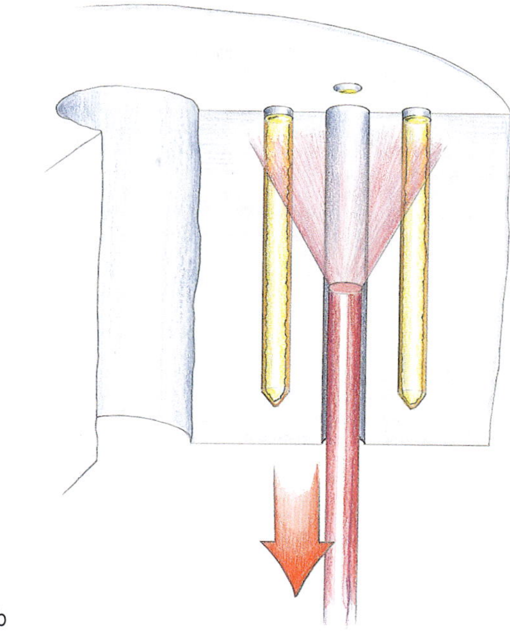

Figs 6-39a and b Test 1 and test 2.

ria, with the dentin only absorbing a small percentage of the radiation. This was shown through parallel temperature measurements (see section 6.6).

One further advantage of the Nd:YAG laser is that bacteria lying in clinical, but not radiologically-verified side canals, especially the apical delta, can be reached by the penetration depth of the laser (see section 6.1.2.1.1.).

In a recent study by Moritz et al.[97] it was shown that the Nd:YAG laser has a bactericidal effect in accessory side canals. Artificial canals in the root dentin were incubated with *E. coli* and *E. faecalis*. Through the artificial central canal the parallel micro burrings (0.25, 0.5, 0.75, 1 mm) were indirectly irradiated.

A bactericidal effect was obtained that was inversely proportional to the distance between the main canal and the accessory canal. Even at longer distances, i.e., 1 mm, the Nd:YAG laser caused almost total bacterial eradication (three log-steps). In comparison, the Er:YAG laser could only reduce bacteria within a distance of 0.25 mm. At longer distances no difference was seen compared to the control group.

As a result of all these studies it was shown that the Nd:YAG laser, because of its wavelength and pulsed action, had the highest bactericidal effect of all lasers presently available on the market. It is a very effective tool for disinfecting the root canal after mechanical root canal treatment, since it is in the near-IR range, and has sufficient penetration depth (see section 6.2.2.3).

With these types of lasers, the energy can be transported by thin, flexible fibers which exist even with diameters of only 200 µm. The radiation of bent and curved canals is possible and the laser tip can also be placed in critical apical areas. It seems that the Nd:YAG laser not only eradicates the microbial flora of the root canal but also has the same effect on the surrounding dentin and its tubules, without affecting the surrounding tissues (see section 6.6).

The Nd:YAG laser is used not only for canal disinfection but also to modify the morphology of the root canal. With the laser, a sealing effect on

Bacterial counts – *E. Coli*, CFU/ml

	• ND:YAG	• Er:YAG
←0.25→	0	0
←0.50→	0	5.5×10^2
←0.75→	0	4.5×10^3
←1.00→	6×10^2	2.4×10^3

• control – 1.2×10^5

a)

Bacterial counts – *E. faecalis*, CFU/ml

	• ND:YAG	• Er:YAG
←0.25→	0	3.5×10^2
←0.50→	0	1.3×10^4
←0.75→	1.6×10^2	0.6×10^5
←1.00→	3.5×10^2	3.0×10^5

• control – 5.5×10^5

b)

Fig 6-40 Bactericidal effects of Nd:YAG and Er:YAG lasers.

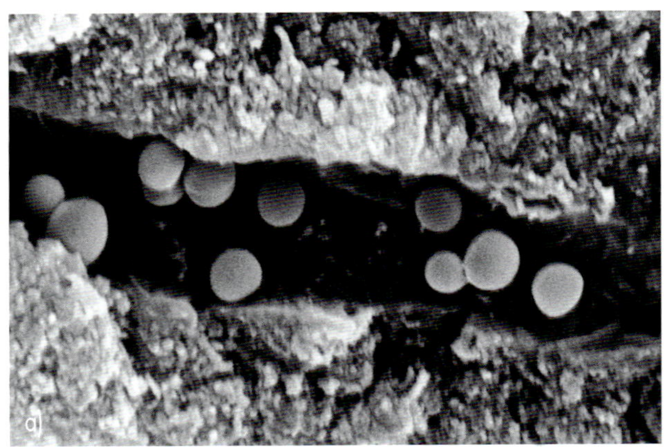

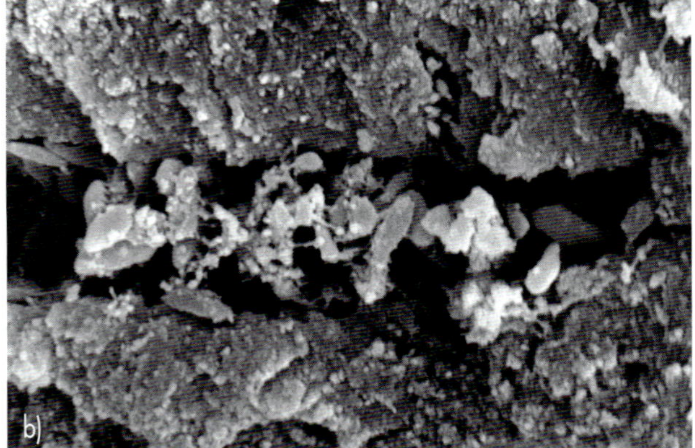

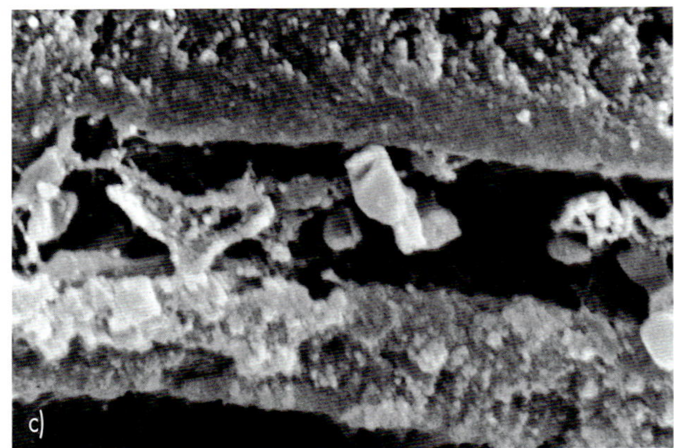

Fig 6-41a–c Bacteria in the dentinal tubules (a) before and (b,c) after laser irradiation.

the root canal wall can be reached, using the right parameters. With the melting together of the root canal surface with the smear layer, a new homogenous flat and recrystallized layer can be produced. The open dentin tubules become closed and sealed.

In the electron microscopic pictures, it can be seen that following Nd:YAG laser radiation, the dentin tubules are closed, and at least part of the canal wall surface is sealed (Fig 6-42). The difference is obvious when compared to a mechanically-prepared root canal wall that was cleaned with EDTA (Fig 6-43). Without using the EDTA, the laser irradiation melts and recrystallizes the smear layer parts, and assists in closing up the tubules (Fig 6-44). The color penetration test proved these results: in a two-rooted tooth, one of the root canals was irradiated with the Nd:YAG laser, and the other one was used for comparison.

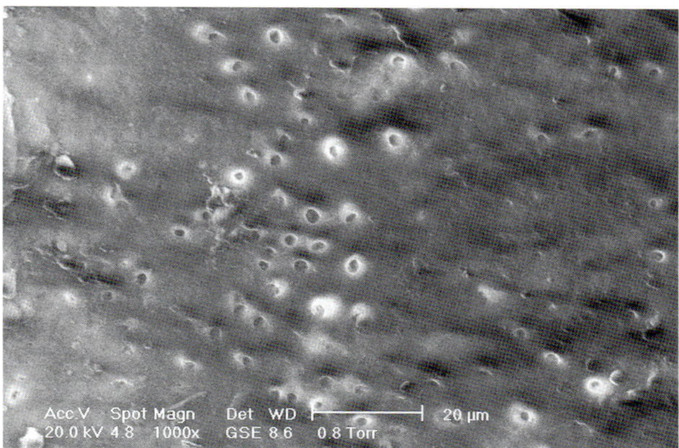

Fig 6-42 Root canal wall, Nd:YAG, after EDTA. The orifices of the dentinal tubules were partly sealed by laser irradiation.

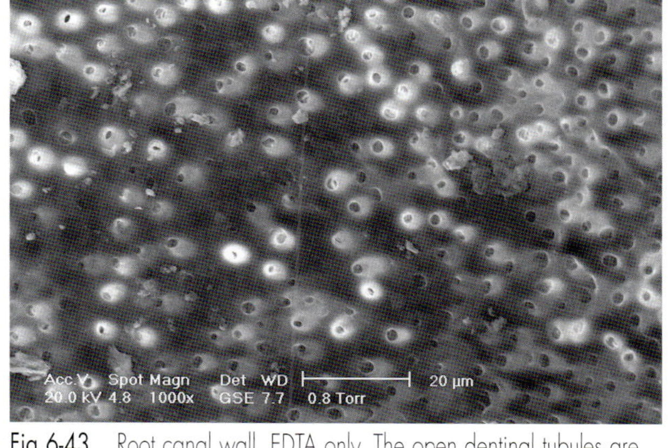

Fig 6-43 Root canal wall, EDTA only. The open dentinal tubules are clearly discernible.

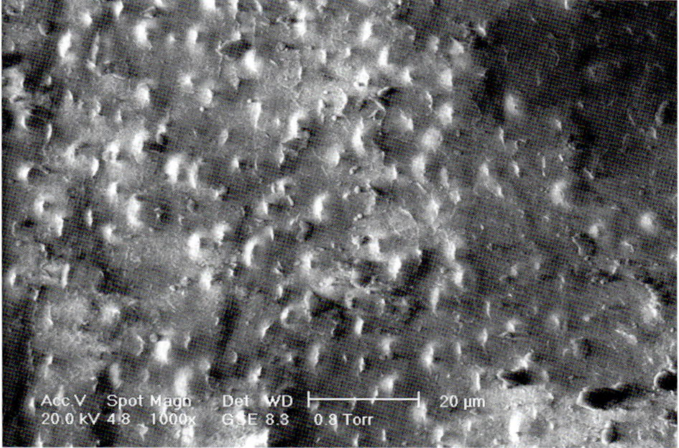

Fig 6-44 Root canal wall, no EDTA. The orifices of the tubules are closed by recrystallized parts of the smear layer to a large extent.

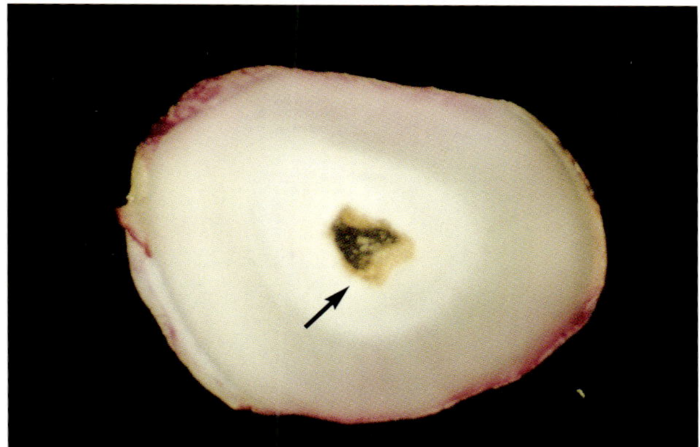

Fig 6-45 Color penetration Nd:YAG. In the irradiated canal the dye does not penetrate to the periphery.

In the irradiated canal the color is not seen in the periphery (Fig 6-45).

A study on this effect was done by Goya et al.[107]. They compared the loss of the smear layer in the apical stop, following pulsed Nd:YAG laser radiation. They used black ink or no black ink, and sealed off the apical ending after obturation, in vitro. The study included conventional preparation, and laser treatment, SEM observation and evaluation of the apical permeability through stereoscopy.

They found that the smear layer is significantly better removed in the laser group than in the control group. Additionally, the cleansing effect of the laser was improved by the application of black ink. The stereoscopy did not find any permeability in the area of the apex of the teeth treated with black ink, and the canals where only the laser was used also showed decreased permeability compared to the control group.

Other authors found differing results concerning the cleansing capacity of lasers. Some studies even suggested that debris and the smear layer could be an advantage in closing up the dentin tubules to stop the invasion of the bacteria.

Other studies find that the smear layer is a disadvantage, because it can decrease the penetration of rinsing solutions and filling material into the dentin tubules and even reduce the contact of the solutions with the canal walls.

Studies about the cleansing effects of a pulsed Nd:YAG laser and formation of a molten apex sealing (see section 6.5) were done by Saunders et al.[108]. The laser was used in vitro to define whether different laser energies, 0.75–1.7 W, at a pulse frequency of 15 pps were able to remove debris and pulp tissue from the prepared canal wall. An almost total removal of the debris and the remaining pulp tissue was observed.

Harashima et al.[109] showed that the Nd:YAG laser can be used for removing the smear layer and the debris. At 2 W/20 pps, a clean root canal surface was found and the dentin was melted and recrystallized.

Goodis et al.[110] compared the canal cleansing effect of a cw and a pulsed Nd:YAG laser. In the study, the smear layer, organic parts and microorganisms were removed completely. A modification of the canal wall morphology was also observed.

Kaitas et al.[111] showed that the smear layer could be removed after Nd:YAG laser irradiation. The root canal wall appeared as a clean glazed surface, with a number of open tubules and craters with gaps. The control group treated by conventional methods showed an area of remaining debris and a smear layer that covered the entrances of the dentin tubules.

A similar study by Zhang et al.[112] compared the morphological changes in the root canal after Nd:YAG laser irradiation (2 W, 20 pps) without any absorber, with irradiation and two different absorption increasing materials, i.e., 38% $Ag(NH_3)_2F$ and black ink (four groups), and without laser treatment. The treatment showed a statistically relevant difference of the permeability in the apical regions between the control group and the two groups where an absorber was used. The electron microscope showed that there was little change in the group using no absorber. In the two groups using laser and absorber, melting, evaporation of the smear layer and open dentin tubules appeared. The black ink appeared to be more effective.

Crespi et al.[113] looked at the cleansing effect of the Nd:YAG laser within the root canal at different energy levels, on histological preparations. Energies from 0.5 to 1.5 W at 20 pps showed that debris, smear layer and recrystallization were present, similar to the control group. At energy levels of 2.0–2.5 W at 20 pps, very clean canal walls without debris and with molten and recrystallized smear layer were observed. At higher energy (3 W and above), total removal of all tissue remnants, structural changes, carbonizations and cracks, were found.

Altamura et al.[114] using the electron microscope compared manual and laser-supported instrumentation. In this study extremely high energy levels were used (up to 6 W). The electron microscope results showed a very thick debris layer on the surface in the non-irradiated control group. At low energy levels, glazed surfaces with reduced debris and closed canals were found compared to the control group, but the groups that were irradiated using higher energy showed a higher percentage of debris, whether on the openings of the dentin canals or in the intertubular regions.

Blum and Abadie[115] compared electron microscope groups: (a) only Nd:YAP laser prepared group, (b) manual and Nd:YAP laser prepared, (c) manual and ultrasound prepared, (d) manual, ultrasound and Nd:YAP laser prepared, (e) control group with only conventional manual preparation. The best results of the cleansing effect of the canal were reached with the combination of laser and ultrasound — there was almost no debris and the debris remnants were of very small particle size. Open tubules were also present. From these results Blum indicated the usefulness of using the Nd:YAP laser for canal cleansing.

In another study, Barbakow et al.[116], using different energy levels (159, 239 and 318 J/cm^2) and a control group, could not find any difference in the reduction of the smear layer. Carbonization was observed in the apical parts of the canal – though this did not seem obvious to the authors, if only electron microscopic images were used.

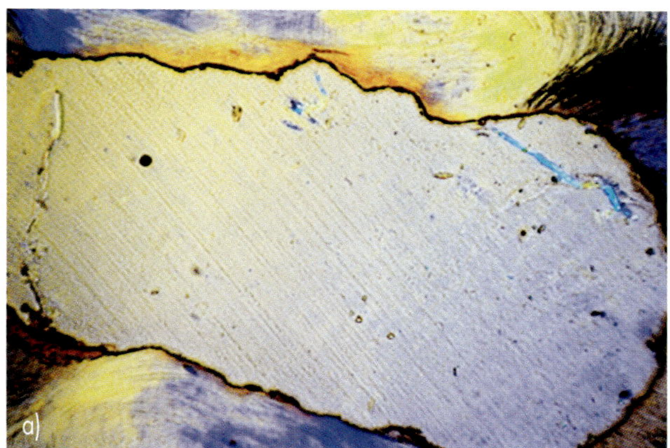

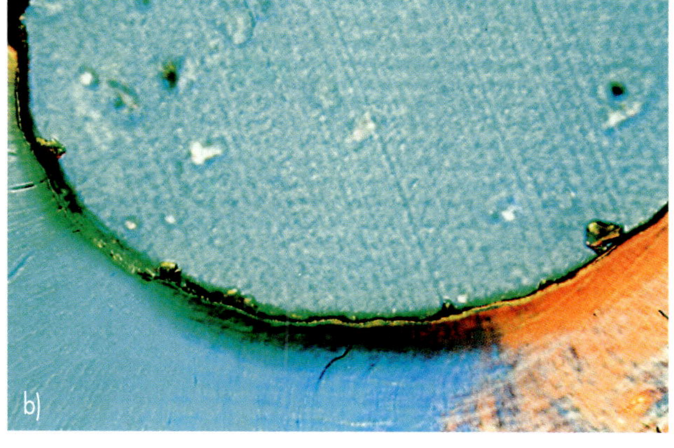

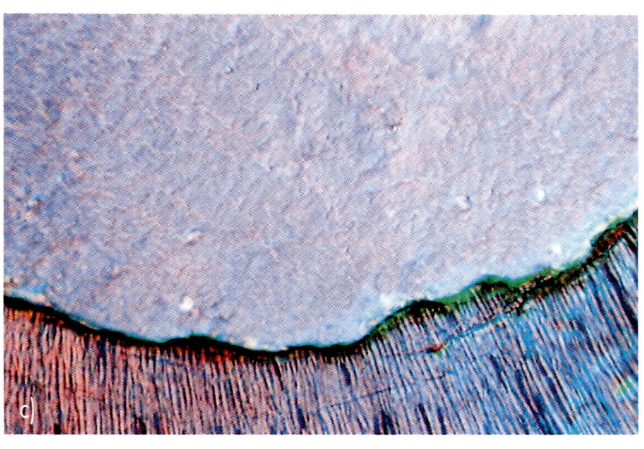

Figs 6-46a–c Histological pictures.

A study by Schaller et al.[117] looked at the effects of Nd:YAG laser irradiation on the permeability of the dentin. Dentin slices were examined. It was shown that the laser treatment increased the permeability of the smear layer-covered dentin, but on the other hand lowered the permeability after etching. This is partly important for root canal treatment.

Dederich et al.[118] described in 1984 how Nd:YAG laser irradiation caused a melted and recrystallized root canal wall. He suggested that this form of changed canal wall dentin is less permeable.

The same opinion was presented by Miserendino et al.[119]. They described reduced permeability for methylene blue after Nd:YAG laser irradiation and a bridge of glazed material was present that partly closed up the lateral canals (tubules).

6.3.2 The Diode Laser

In recent years the diode laser has gained more importance in root canal sterilization. It has an unquestionable bactericidal effect, similar to the Nd:YAG laser, and this has been proved in numerous in vitro and in vivo studies. The penetration depth of the diode laser, which is lower in the case of endodontics than that of the Nd:YAG laser, also lowers the risk of an unwanted temperature rise[120]. At the same time, however, this means less efficiency in the case of very deep infections. Since most diode lasers are chopped lasers, no pulse noise is to be heard and thus during application the valuable answer regarding the condition of the canal (damp or dry) is missing. For daily practice however, the diode laser is suitable because of its safe application (small rise in temperature) (see section 6.6). In addition, diode lasers have a broad application spectrum. These qualities and a reasonable price will increase their use in general practice[121].

It is crucial that shorter-wave laser radiation penetrates the entire root dentin, and has a bactericidal effect at depths that are not accessible in conventional therapy, as mentioned before.

In the last few years, research has proven that the sterilization effect of the diode laser resembles that of the Nd:YAG laser.

Moritz et al.[70] showed in an in vitro study, the effect of the diode laser on extracted teeth that were incubated with *E. coli* and *E. faecalis*. They found that an extraordinarily high reduction of bacteria could be achieved.

The same results were found by Gutknecht et al.[122], in endodontically prepared teeth incubated with *E. faecalis*. They obtained a general reduction of 99.91% in the bacteria using diode laser irradiation.

In an in vivo study by Moritz et al.[120], the antibacterial effect of the diode laser was compared to conventional root canal disinfection methods. Forty root canals were treated with the laser (2 W, 20 ms pulse duration, 50 Hz) and 10 root canals were used as a control group. At three appointments per patient, microbiological tests were made. After the first procedure a significant bacterial reduction was found. The maximum logarithmic reduction factor in the laser group was 4.22 for streptococci and 3.33 for staphylococci whereas in the conventionally treated control group only a small bacterial reduction was reached (1.37 for streptococci, 1.0 for staphylococci).

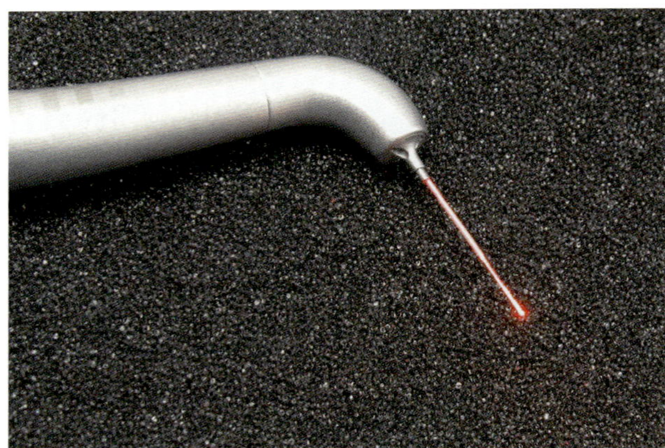
Fig 6-47 Hand piece diode laser.

A clinical study by Gutknecht et al.[123] showed that root canal disinfection by the diode laser, and 5% hypochlorite, are equal. A slightly better result was reached through irradiation with the diode laser but the difference from pure NaOCl rinsing was not significant.

Because of the similar wavelength, the effect of the diode laser on the root canal wall differs only slightly from the Nd:YAG laser. Therefore similar effects are to be expected during root canal treatment, e.g., the closing effect of the openings of the tubules. This is confirmed by several studies.

In an in vitro study, root canals (without the removal of the smear layer) were irradiated with 2, 3 and 4 W and then stored in 1% fuchsin solution. The porosity of the dentin results in a typical staining pattern, which makes it possible to draw conclusions on the permeability due to the penetration depth and the staining intensity. The color

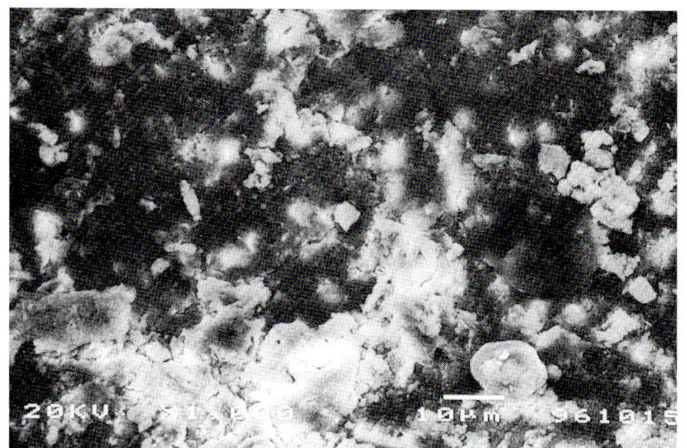

Fig 6-48 SEM evaluation after irradiation with the diode laser.

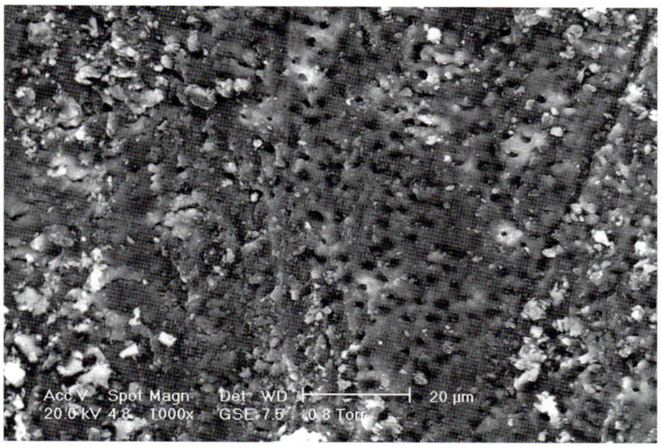

Fig 6-49 Canal wall, diode, after EDTA rinsing. The open dentinal tubules are partly closed by laser irradiation.

penetration test showed a complete sealing of the dentinal tubules achieved by an irradiation at 4 W. Using an output power of 2 or 3 W, distinct color penetration from the canal lumen into the tubules was found, restricted to some areas. The electron microscopic evaluation also showed a complete closure of the tubules at 4 W.

In the electron microscope pictures it is seen that the diode laser also closes up the dentin tubules (Fig 6-49). If the smear layer is not removed during mechanical preparation and EDTA rinsing, the effect on the tubules seems to be even bigger (Fig 6-50). The color penetration test proves these results: using a two-rooted tooth, one root canal was irradiated with the diode laser, and the other one remained untreated. In the irradiated canal the color did not diffuse to the periphery (Fig 6-51).

In addition, a bio-stimulative effect is attributed to the diode laser, which could gain extraordinary importance in the future of laser-assisted endodontics. From different studies[124,125], it is known that the diode laser stimulates cell proliferation and that it shows an inhibiting effect on inflammation-propagating enzymes (see section 6.10).

6.3.3 The Er:YAG and Er,Cr:YSGG Lasers

Some authors have suggested the Er:YAG laser as an alternative to rotary instruments in the root apex resection. Paghdiwala[126] and Komori et al.[127,128] showed that apicoectomies could be performed efficiently with this wavelength, with better postoperational conditions prevailing (see chapter 11).

With the development of flexible light conductors for the Er:YAG laser, this wavelength was tried in conservative endodontics.

For solitary root canal sterilization, the Er:YAG laser is not really suitable. It has a bactericidal effect through the removal of the smear layer in the root canal (see section 6.8.2) and is therefore comparable with the chemical rinsing solutions. It could be described as a "physical rinsing".

However, the bactericidal effect in the depth of the dentin as described in the section above, is not as good as achieved with the Nd:YAG or diode laser.

It can only penetrate the areas closer to the canal lumen because of its wavelength and surface absorption by the dentin, and develop an effect on the bacteria.

A bactericidal effect in the depth of the dentin is hardly conceivable for physical reasons and

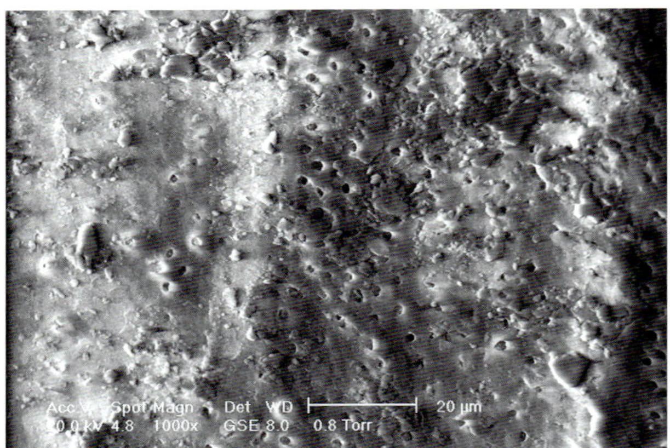

Fig 6-50 Root canal wall after diode laser irradiation. No rinsing with EDTA prior to laser treatment. The orifices of the dentinal tubules are obturated to a high extent by recrystallized portions of the smear layer.

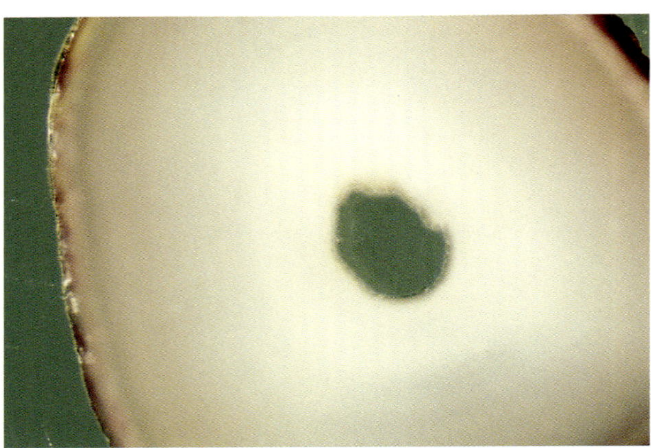

Fig 6-51 Colour penetration, diode. No dye penetration is discernible in the irradiated canal.

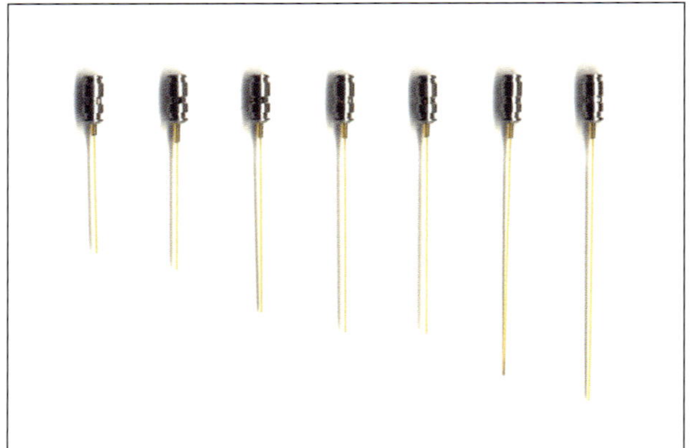

Fig 6-52a Special flexible waveguide for endodontics (example: Er,Cr:YSGG laser).

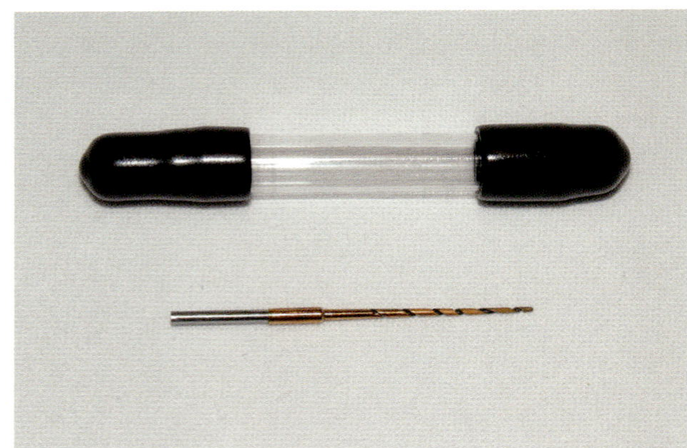

Fig 6-52b Picture of a "side-firing-fiber" for the Er:YAG laser. The fundamental idea is to apply the radiation perpendicular to the fiber at the root canal wall.

could only be achieved through an unwanted temperature rise.

Some of the recent studies using the wavelength of the Er:YAG have proved this (see section 6.2.2.3.1).

Mehl et al.[71] showed that with *E. coli* and *Staphylococcus aureus* a bacterial reduction to 0.034–0.06% of the initial number in the root canal can be reached depending upon the irradiation duration. They compared in-vitro results with conventional 1.25% NaOCl rinsing solutions and found that the Er:YAG exhibits a comparable sterilization effect. To what extent thermal damage occurs through the increase of the irradiation duration is not described.

In a study of the Nd:YAG, the Er:YAG and the Ho:YAG laser, the Er:YAG laser did quite well in bacterial reduction. Moritz et al.[129] used *E. coli* and *E. faecalis* to contaminate prepared root canals in vitro, and tested different wavelengths in the root canal. The depth effect of the lasers could not be determined in this study.

In this connection, Jelinkova et al.[130] attempted to determine the tissue effect in contaminated tooth roots on the basis of an alexandrite and an Er:YAG laser. They found almost complete bacterial eradication for the Er:YAG, granted however that the sterilization was limited to the superficial dentin layers.

Schoop et al.[131] investigated the Er:YAG laser in root canal treatment comprehensively. They also found a bactericidal effect in the root canal, when they used different pigmented and non-pigmented bacteria in vitro. They proved with thermographs that with bactericidal energy levels, no temperature damages of the paradontal tissues were to be expected, and the root canal wall changed by photo ablation.

Another study by Schoop et al.[132] was aimed at a comparison of the bactericidal effect between the Nd:YAG, diode, Er:YAG, and Er,Cr:YSGG lasers. The highest bactericidal effect was yielded with the Er:YAG laser; however, only restricted volumes of dentin (slices measuring 6 × 2 × 1 mm) were assessed.

In an already mentioned study, the Nd:YAG and the Er:YAG laser were directly compared concerning their antibacterial effect (*E. coli* and *E. faecalis*). The Er:YAG was able to produce a bacterial reducing effect in dentin areas close to the root canal, especially for the radiation-sensitive *E. coli*, but in comparison with the Nd:YAG laser, its effect was much lower against the bacteria.

6.4 Root Canal Shaping

Nowadays the Er:YAG laser is mostly used for canal preparation and shaping the root canal. It uses a photoablative action similar to that of cavity preparation (thermomechanical).

As already mentioned, the smear layer that develops during canal preparation has to be removed.

During treatment, organic debris adheres to the root canal wall. This smear layer contains microorganisms and bacterial toxins, and should be removed completely. This is a particular difficulty in side canals when using conventional rinsing solutions. With the laser, however, different effects can be produced on the smear layer.

The Er:YAG laser has the ability to open the tubules completely and remove the smear layer in toto. Because of that, the canal sealant can easily penetrate the canal wall following root canal filling, and seal it with optimum results. Thus an unstable layer of debris is avoided.

Looking at electron microscope pictures of a root canal that has been irradiated with the Er:YAG laser, the ablative effect of the wavelength is recognizable. The wall seems to be rough and the entrances of the tubules are open. Ablative products and parts of the smear layer are melted and recrystallized. In the color penetration test, the fuchsin solution diffuses easily into the periphery of the root.

Additionally, the Er:YAG laser enlarges and extends the root canal lumen without any tension so that the definitive filling is a lot easier to place.

Some authors regard the combination of root canal treatment and sterilization as particularly useful. Chen[133] describes in a case study the possibility of accomplishing a complete endodontic treatment by using a hard laser. From the cavity preparation, up to the canal extension and disinfection, they document the advantages of this method, in particular, less pain and the favorable prognosis of the procedure because of complete smear layer removal and bacterial reduction. In their study they used the Er,Cr:YSGG laser which is closely related to the Er:YAG laser. Matsuoka[134], Takeda[135], and Shoji et al.[136] studied in detail the canal cleansing effect of the Er:YAG laser and came to the conclusion that this is sufficiently attained using the Er:YAG laser.

Other groups of researchers also thought it possible that apex sealing and/or the sealing of the dentin openings in the canal lumen by irradiation with this wavelength is more effective, and

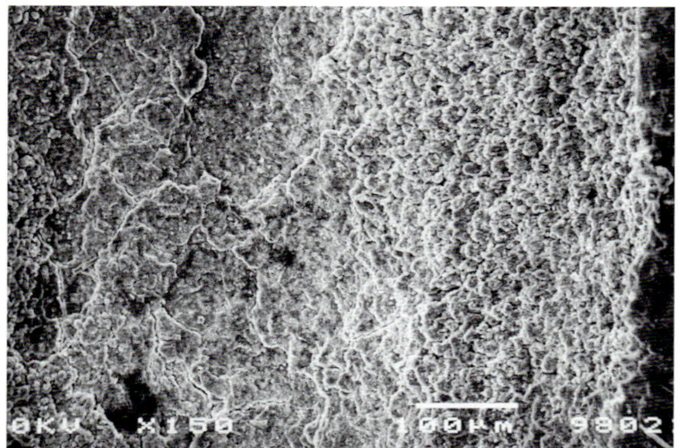
Fig 6-53 Overview of the Er:YAG: the rough surface structure of the canal wall is clearly discernible.

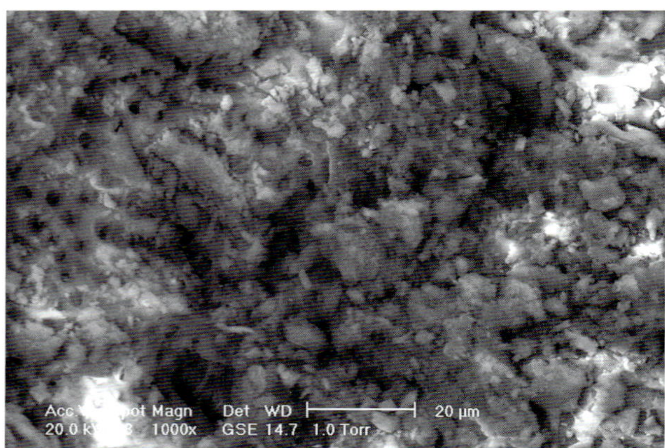

Fig 6-54 Detail Er:YAG: the very rough structure of the surface caused by the ablative action of the wavelength can be seen in this picture, too.

offers a better prognosis for endodontic treatment.

A comparative study by Takeda[137] showed that with the Er:YAG laser an evaporation of the smear layer and opening of the dentin tubules in the middle and apical area was obtainable to a high degree, but the argon and/or the Nd:YAG laser could not obtain the same results in cleaning the canal.

In another study by Takeda et al.[135], the Er:YAG was compared with a CO_2 laser. The Er:YAG laser could remove the smear layer, but caused melted, glazed and recrystallized canal walls with carbonization. However, the Er:YAG laser proved to be effective for this indication.

Yamazaki et al.[138] describes in a study the positive effect of water cooling during the treatment of canal walls. In the study, an Er:YSGG laser with and without water spray was used. Without water, cooling crackings and carbonization occurred with rises in temperature around 37°C. With water cooling, however, rises in temperature of only 8°C were measured with no carbonization, and there was complete removal of the smear layer.

Kesler et al.[139] used special microfibers of 200–400 µm, for the canal preparation. SEM photographs of extracted front teeth showed uniform canal preparations with a large number of open dentin tubules. The canals were free from debris – no further smear layer was present. Kesler claims that the Er:YAG laser in combination with the special fibers is very effective in shaping, cleaning and enlarging the root canal and it seems to be superior in speed and efficiency to the traditional methods.

Matzuoka et al.[134] observed a significant reduction of debris in the apical portions of the root canal of extracted front teeth using radiation energy of 2 W (SEM + fibrescope).

A similar study showed contradictory results, when an Er:YAG laser was used. Matsumoto et al.[140] examined the effects of the Er:YAG on the root canal wall of human teeth using an electron microscope. According to his opinion the laser irradiation can give promising results in endodontic treatment. The Er:YAG laser seems to be very effective in cleaning prepared root canals. According to this study non-irradiated teeth showed debris as a compound of pulp tissue remnants and dentin, as well as a smear layer that covered the dentinal tubules. In contrast to that, teeth that were irradiated for 3 s had a majority of the debris and smear layer evaporated, with discernible openings of the dentin tubules remaining. The teeth that were irradiated for 5 s were completely free of smear layer and debris and showed open dentinal tubules.

Numerous comparative studies, which examined different lasers for their effects on the canal wall, were done. Kimura et al.[141] examined the

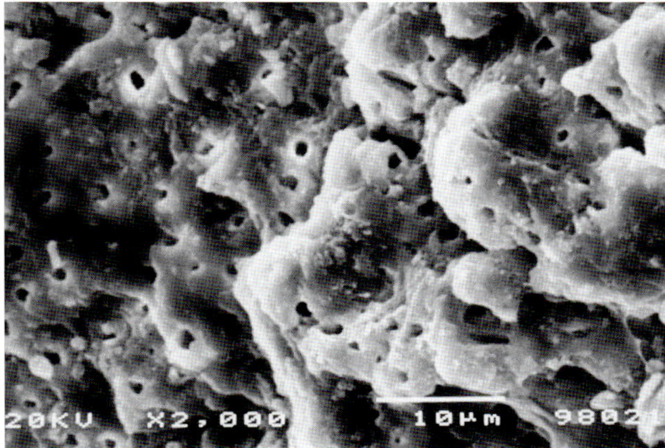

Fig 6-55 Detail Er:YAG: the openings of the dentinal tubules and recrystallized ablation products can be discerned.

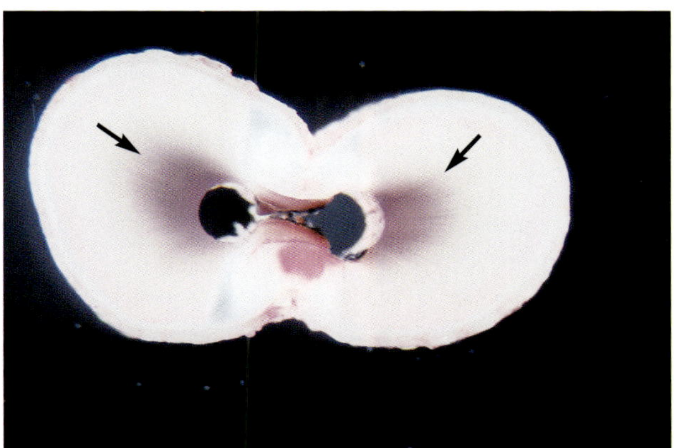

Fig 6-56 Dye penetration Er:YAG. The dye solution penetrates into the periphery of the root dentin.

effect of Er:YAG and CO_2 laser concerning the removal of the smear layer in vitro, in the middle and apical part of the root canal. The tests showed that in the control group, which was treated only with EDTA, the smear layer could not be removed completely. The CO_2 laser showed good smear-layer removing effects, but in the apical third there were portions with carbonized, melted, recrystallized and glazed surfaces. The study showed that EDTA could not produce a smear-layer-free surface. The Er:YAG laser proved extremely effective in the cleaning of the prepared root canal.

6.5 Apex Sealing

Different wavelengths of lasers are capable of sealing surfaces and making them impermeable to bacteria and their toxins, so the concept of sealing the apical stop with laser radiation would be obvious. Sealing of the root tubule system is one of the most important factors for a successful prognosis for endodontic treatment and this includes the apical region.

The Nd:YAG laser and the argon laser have been described in detail in the literature. Here, generally smaller energy levels than for the conventional sterilization of the root canal are used. Since the fiber remains stationary at the apex for some seconds, thermal stress of the paradontal tissues is avoided. But the parameters for energies used to potentially seal the apex vary widely.

One of the first studies in this field was done by Saunders et al.[108] with an Nd:YAG laser in vitro. Among other aspects, they investigated the possibility of bringing in dentin chips, hydroxyapatite, or ceramic powder, and producing a sealed closure with the Nd:YAG laser. At 1 W and 15 Hz it was only possible to harden the hydroxyapatite and the ceramic powder to a certain extent, and no comment was made on the quality of the sealing.

Kimura et al.[141] showed using an Nd:YAG laser with 2 W power and 20 Hz pulse, that within the range of the apical deltas the smear layer could not only be removed, but also melting and recrystallization were observed. According to his opinion, the melting process of the apical canal walls and apices that are treated with the laser seems to be responsible for a decreased dye penetration in comparison with conventionally treated samples.

As well, with a pulsed Nd:YAG laser and using 2 W power, Goya et al.[107] found a substantially closer apical sealing, than in the untreated control group. In this test a photo absorber (ink) was used.

Park et al.[142] examined in vitro prepared root canals, using potential difference measurements to see how tight the apical sealing was after Nd:YAG laser irradiation. They were able to show that with the use of 5 W and 20 Hz, a reduction of apical leakage was present.

The influence of dentin residues to produce apical sealing, using an Nd:YAG laser, was tested by Gekelman et al.[143]. The best results were reached with irradiation of root canals that were prepared and clean of debris at 1 W, 10 Hz and an apical irradiation duration of 3 s. In the presence of debris and condensed dentin powder, a smaller sealing effect was found.

In contrast to that, Yamakazi et al[144] used an argon laser in continuous wave mode with only 0.3 W energy and an irradiation duration of 3 s maximum. Using this possibly too-low energy level, he could only find an insignificant increase in the canal apical seal.

In a following study, Kimura et al.[145] looked at the quantity of apical leakage after using an Er:YAG laser for root canal preparation (laser group) in comparison to conventional K-file-prepared root canals (control group). The preparation was done with 170–230 mJ at 2 Hz. The analysis of the root canals by stereoscope and REM methods showed a rough, non-homogenous surface, but no significant difference in the apical leakage compared with the control group.

A similar study by Khan et al.[146], on the effect of laser treatment on human root canals, showed with an electron microscope, that the laser energy evaporated the debris, forming a glazed surface. Different ablative effects of the root canal were observed which showed as cracks, carbonization, glazed surfaces and melted dentin tubules and these were directly proportional to the applied energy and irradiation parameters. Because of the reduced diameter and the number of opened dentin tubules, a decrease in permeability was found in the apical region. The author interprets this as an advantage in endodontic therapy. In his work he found that the Nd:YAG laser brought the best results at 2 W and 20 pps in the removal of debris, without changing the root canal shape; this also holds true regarding the decreased permeability of the apex.

Schoop et al.[147] compared the possibilities and limits of four different laser wavelengths in the fields of apex sealing. In an in vitro study, 85 extracted human teeth were prepared endodontically, up to a width of ISO 70. From the roots of other teeth, a dentin powder was made which was brought into the apical region of the root canals, and sealed with a plugger.

In groups of 10 teeth, an irradiation with a corresponding wavelength was done. An Nd:YAG, diode, Er:YAG and an Er,Cr:YSGG laser were used. The parameters of each laser were chosen in such a way as to have energy of 1–1.5 W available at the fiber tip. Following the irradiation, a color penetration test with fuchsin was done to obtain information about the changes of permeability in the apical region of the canal. The stained samples were examined under the light microscope. The teeth that looked tight in the light microscope were again looked at in an E-SEM.

It was shown that an apex sealing, in the mechanical meaning, was reached with all four wavelengths. But the desired decrease of permeability in the apical region was only reachable using parameters that would harm the paradontal structures in vivo because of the high temperature rise. Further studies have been done to find out if there are more suitable filling materials, which can be used in combination with the laser.

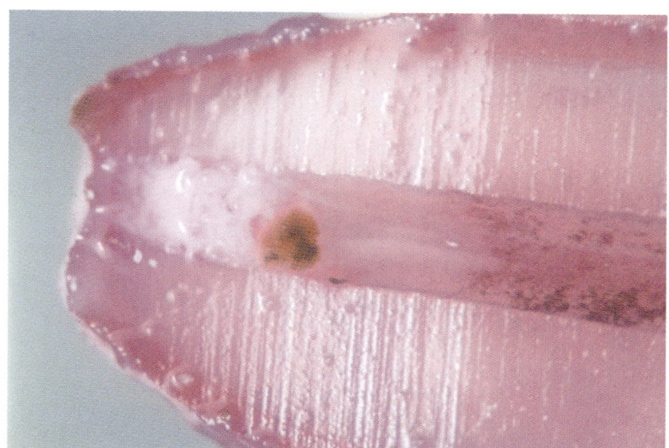

Fig 6-57 Apical sealing: irradiation with the Nd:YAG laser at 1.5 W. The sealing appears to be complete in light microscopy.

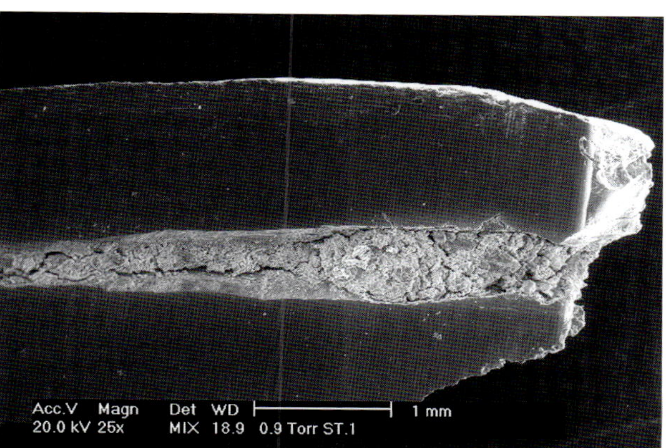

Fig 6-58 Apical sealing: irradiation with the Nd:YAG laser at 1.5 W. Scanning electron microscopy reveals gaps.

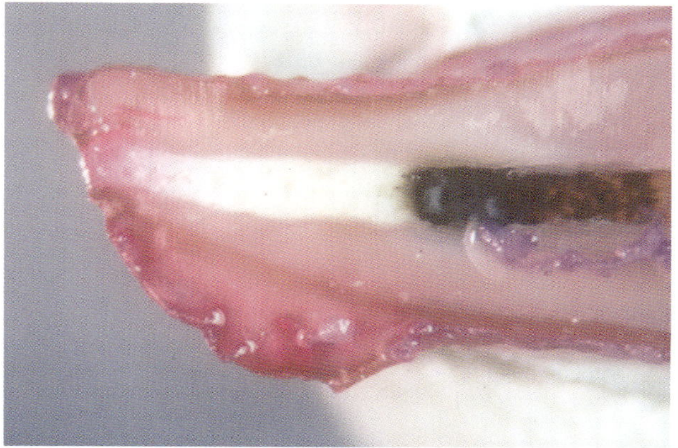

Fig 6-59 Apical sealing using the Er,Cr:YSGG laser at 1.5 W. In light microscopy, no dye penetration into the apical plug can be seen, but severe carbonization occurs.

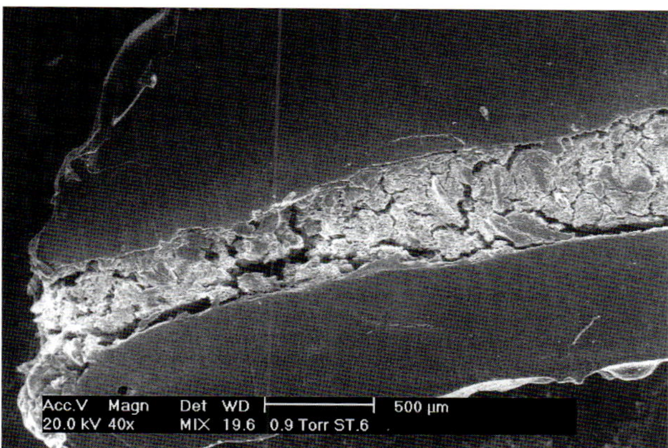

Fig 6-60 Apical sealing: Scanning electron microscopy shows sealed areas beside discrete gap formations.

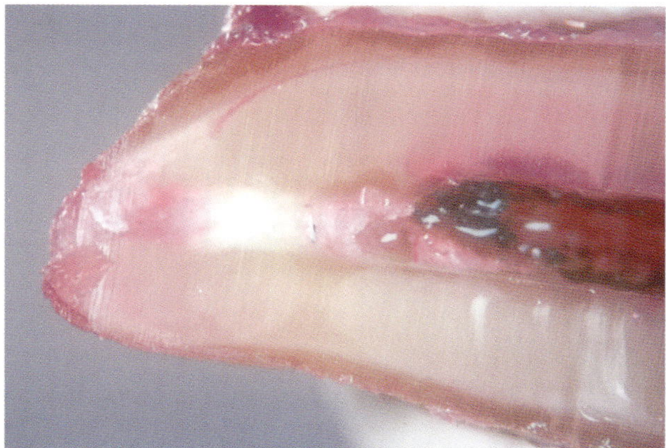

Fig 6-61 Apical sealing: The sample was irradiated with the Er:YAG laser at 1.5W. The central area of the dentin plug is not stained, but ablations can be seen in the more coronal portion of the root canal wall.

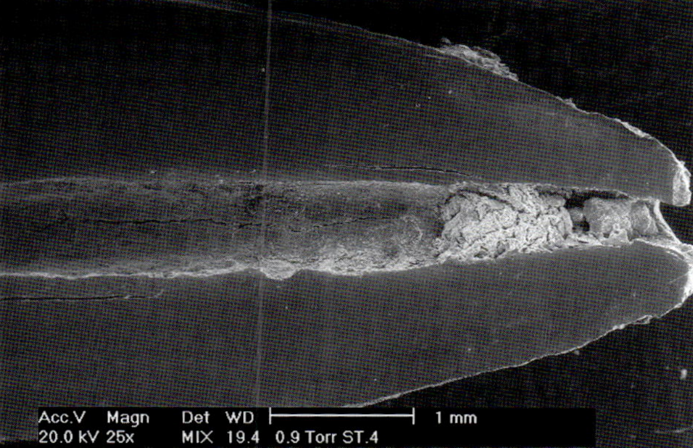

Fig 6-62 Apical sealing: Scanning electron microscopy reveals the tight connection between the dentin plug and the root canal wall. Nevertheless, ablations in the more coronal portion are visible.

6.6 Safety in Laser Treatment

The high energies that are delivered to surrounding tissues by medical lasers can lead to irreversible thermal damage to neighboring structures. In endodontics there is always the question whether any damage to the paradontal tissues occurs during the irradiation of the root canal. This was investigated in in-vitro analyses by Moritz et al.[70] and other authors, using different wavelengths and laser parameters, to exclude the rise in temperature at the root surface (temperature sonde, thermal camera, finite elements; Fig 6-63).

The development of the temperature at the root surface during the irradiation of the root canal with the Nd:YAG laser was calculated with a standard tooth model using the finite element method. The illustrations demonstrate that we need not be concerned about the temperature rise caused by laser irradiation, as long as the correct parameters are used.

An in vitro study on irradiation effects in the root canal using the diode laser showed a harmless temperature rise in standard settings. The infrared spectral analysis showed temperature rises in the apex of 6°C after 1 s, 12°C after 2 s but an alarming 18°C after 3 s. These temperature rises occurred only after stationary irradiation. If the treatment was done with circular movements of the fiber, the temperature rises stopped at 6°C, even after 10 s.

One of the first studies dealing with the problem of the temperature rise in the narrow area of the root canal was done with the argon laser by Blankenau et al.[148]. With pulsed (0.1-s pulse duration) and with pulse breaks of 1 s, they reached an average temperature rise of 2.6°C at the highest energy of 2 W. With these results, the authors concluded that one can safely remove the pulpal tissue with the argon laser.

Two years later, Anic et al.[149] compared the temperature rise in the root canal using the argon, Nd:YAG, and CO_2 lasers. They measured the apical temperature difference of about 55°C at

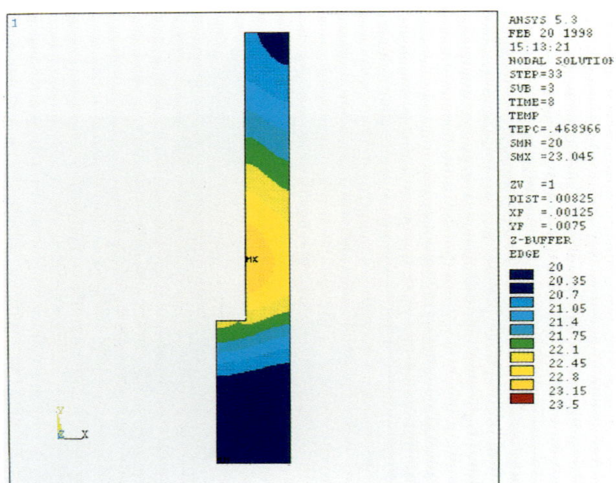

Fig 6-63 Calculation of the temperature distribution in a tooth model using finite elements. The figure shows the temperature distribution in the dentin after an irradiation time of 5 seconds. The temperature rise at the surface can be regarded as harmless.

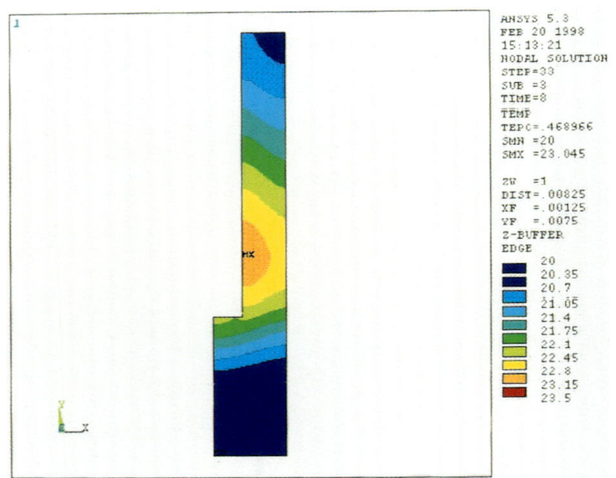

Fig 6-64 The figure shows the temperature model after additional 5 seconds.

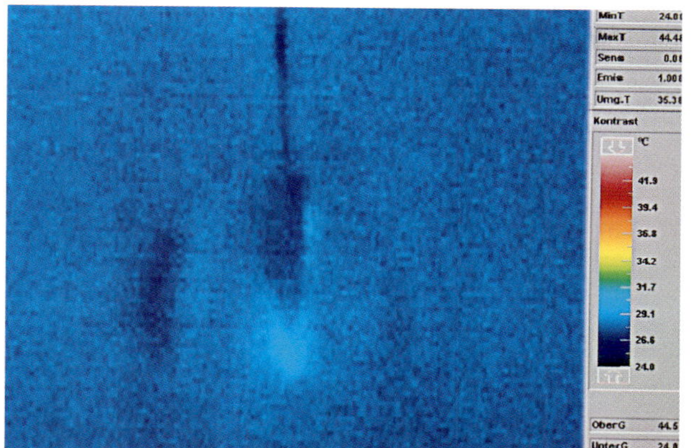

Fig 6-65 Laser activation at the apex for 1 second without moving the fiber.

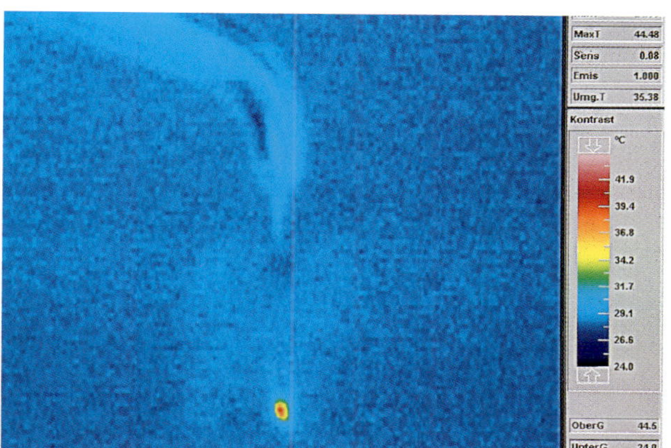

Fig 6-66 Laser activation at the apex for 2 seconds without moving the fiber.

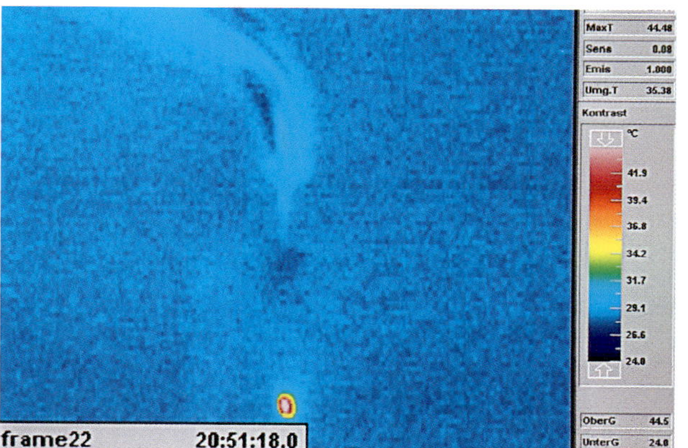

Fig 6-67 Laser activation at the apex for 3 seconds without moving the fiber.

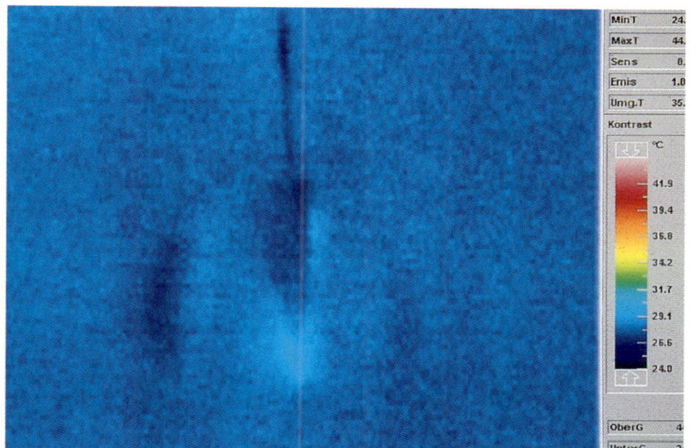

Fig 6-68 Irradiation of the canal wall under circling movements of the fiber for 5 seconds.

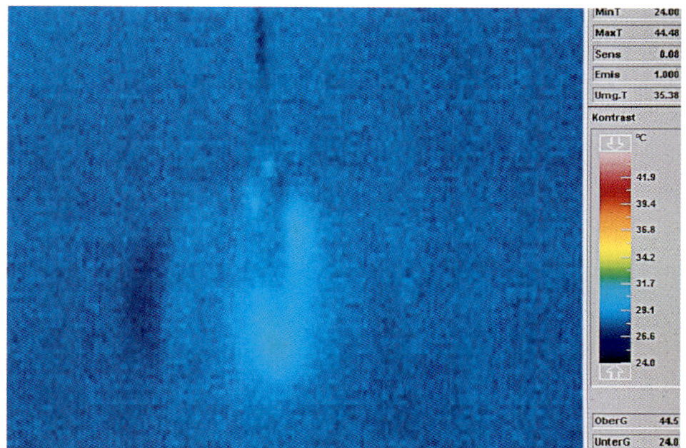

Fig 6-69 Irradiation of the canal wall under circling movements of the fiber for 8 seconds.

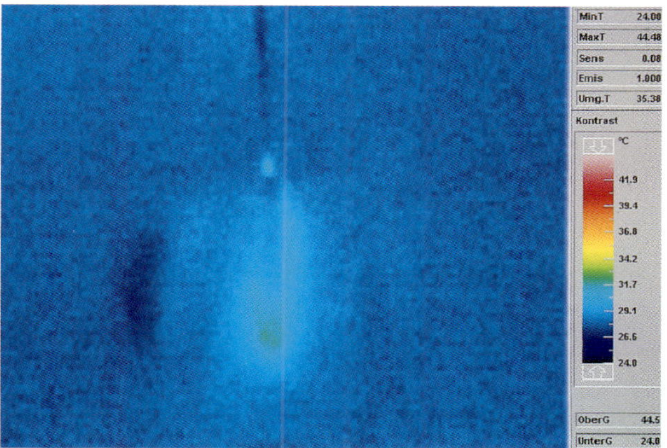

Fig 6-70 Irradiation of the canal wall under circling movements of the fiber for 10 seconds.

higher energy levels with the argon laser, which was very harmful to the paradontal tissues. For the CO_2 laser they found results were 10°C. These results can probably be explained by the incommensurable experimental set-up.

Khan et al.[146] reached in 1997 similar conclusions concerning temperature rises, when they compared the same three lasers in vitro. The highest temperatures in the tissues were smaller than those observed by Anic et al.[149] but once again the argon laser had the highest results. Even so, all the temperatures were described as tolerable for the periodontal tissues.

Kesler et al. did a detailed study with the CO_2 laser, which had a special endodontic delivery system. They were able to measure the temperature development at the apex in vivo, using thermal sensors deep in the gingival pockets of periodontally compromised teeth. During the laser irradiation they found temperatures around 38°C which gave apical sterilization and pulpal removal. They also used energies that caused necrosis of the apical pulp seen in the following histological cuts.

The Ho:YAG laser was also suggested for root canal preparation and Cohen et al.[150,151] made two studies on the efficiency of the system. They could only find a slight temperature rise with different fiber diameters and energy levels. The authors showed that at a level up to 1 W, the maximum temperature development on the root surface did not rise over 5°C and the application of the laser can be regarded as safe.

Machida et al.[152] used a KTP laser for root canal preparation. This showed a harmless paradontal temperature rise on an endodontic in vitro model. The authors concentrated on parameters up to 3 W and proved that even at higher energies (and with the complete removal of smear layer and debris) no harm is to be expected for the paradontal tissues.

In one of the first studies on endodontic prepared root canals and temperature changes in endodontic laser use, Ramskold et al.[103] observed the optimal energy level of the Nd:YAG laser for harmless irradiation of the root canal system. They suggested a 15-s irradiation interval to reduce the thermal stress.

Before, Behrens et al.[153] used dentin platelets in an in vitro study to define the energy parameters at which the Nd:YAG laser did not cause any damage to the paradontal tissues.

In a morphological study, Moritz et al.[87] looked at Nd:YAG laser-irradiated bacteria. They investigated and compared temperature and energy levels that would preserve the paradontium but still have a reasonable bactericidal effect. In a test using a thermal sensor, and a dentin thickness of 1 mm, a temperature rise of 4.3°C at 1.5 W was seen, on the opposite side of the dentin platelet. This was considered to be harmless to the neighboring structures.

With an Nd:YAP (similar to the Nd:YAG, slightly higher wavelength of $\lambda = 1340$ nm) laser at energies of 200 mJ/20 Hz, Farge et al.[154] found no critical increase in periodontal temperatures. Lan[155] looked at temperature rises in the apical third of the root after Nd:YAG laser irradiation at different levels (50–200 mJ/20–30 Hz). The temperature did not rise by more than 10°C, but only if levels under 100 mJ and 20 pps were used.

Nevertheless, Folwaczny et al.[106] found out that there were high temperature rises using the Nd:YAG laser. At a very high level of 200 mJ and 20 Hz (effective 4 W) they found a temperature rise around 62°C (!) in the root canal and at 100 mJ/20 Hz (2 W) there was still a rise of 24.3°C.

In a study, mentioned before, by Moritz et al.[70], the authors looked at the bactericidal effect of the diode laser and the temperature rise during irradiation of the root canal. They made pictures with an infrared camera to document the temperature on the root surface of endodontically prepared extracted teeth during laser irradiation. At an energy level of 4 W they found a maximum temperature rise of 6°C on the surface and came to the conclusion that the diode laser can be used in vivo without danger.

Kreisler et al.[156] were concerned with the temperature rise during canal sterilization with the diode laser in a bacteriological in vitro study. They came to the conclusion, that even at high energy use (4.5 W), the thermal stress to the periodont is acceptable.

In an in-vitro study, using a pulsed Er:YAG and energies under 1.5 W, Schoop et al.[131] observed a maximum temperature rise of 3.5° C. So it is seen that using the Er:YAG laser, temperature rises can be discounted, providing standardized energies are used for canal sterilization.

Similar results on a study using an Er:YAG laser in the root canals and higher energies (up to 230 mJ, 2 Hz) were reported by Kimura et al.[157]. They looked at the preparation possibilities of the Er:YAG laser and made parallel temperature measurements. During this study maximum temperature rises of 6° C were found in the apical part of the root surface, so that no periodontal thermal stress is caused.

One of the few studies using an Er,Cr:YSGG laser in endodontics was also concerned with the temperature rise during canal preparation. The use of water spray was absolutely necessary (see before). In these results the temperature rise was less than 8° C[138].

Therefore, we may conclude that as long as accepted international standards of energy parameters are used with individual lasers, then the resulting endodontic procedures are harmless to the paradontal tissues and yet provide the optimal bactericidal effect (table 6-4).

The parameters recommended in today's clinical use of lasers form the basis for the continually updated use of lasers in endodontics.

Table 6-4 International standardized laser settings.

Nd:YAG laser	Er:YAG laser	Diode laser
≤ 100 mJ/15 Hz	≤ 75 mJ/15 Hz	≤ 150 mJ/15 Hz

6.7 Indications

For laser endodontics the same guidelines apply as in conventional root treatment. The question whether the tooth is worth preserving from prosthetic and esthetic considerations has to be answered. It has to be considered as well: can we successfully restore the tooth after endodontics and will there be a satisfactory prognosis? Finally, is the patient willing and physically able to partake in the whole procedure?
After clarification of all these fundamental conditions, laser-supported endodontics can be used in the following cases:

- *Chronic apical parodontitis*
  Bacteria located in the infected dentin and the toxins they produce are responsible for inflammation. The laser gives the possibility of a bactericidal effect; a fundamental therapy overcoming the inflammation and associated bone resorption.
- *Acute apical parodontitis*
  Virulent bacteria present during acute pulpitis or the spread of bacteria by iatrogenic treatment (by instruments), result in penetration of bacteria into the periapical tissues, causing acute inflammation. Also possible is the spread of bacteria and inflammation through an exacerbation of chronic apical parodontitis. Since the bactericidal effect of the laser reaches the periapical tissues, the success of laser therapy can be expected.
- *Purulent pulpitis and pulp necrosis*
- *Gangrenous pulpitis*
  (of the crown pulp and of the entire root canal)
- *Periapical abscess*
  In these cases the highly porous dentin tissues are invaded by bacteria, which cannot be reached with conventional chemical disinfecting methods. The bactericidal effect of the laser guarantees secure and fast therapy success. In the case of a periapical abscess one has to look at the drainage of the pus and the exudates, in a combination therapy approach.
- *Apical resorption (inflammatory)*
  With lasers, the apical resorption area can be irradiated and the inflammatory process stopped.
- *Therapy-resistant long-term failure, i.e., root canal treatment of more than 4 months without improvement of the subjective or objective symptoms*
  Long-term endodontic failure can often be caused by persisting pathogens. These bacteria resist conventional disinfection (see above) and the inflammation continues. Through laser irradiation, successful therapy is achieved.
- *Combined periodontal–endodontic pathology (e.g., the consequence of side canals)*
  High penetration depths to all parts of the root dentin are reached. Even bacteria in side canals can be killed. In some cases a parallel irradiation of corresponding paradontal pockets seems to be successful, because the laser has a very high bactericidal effect in this area as well.
- *Partly sclerosed canals*
  Often mechanical instrumentation of the root canal for reaching the physiological apex is not possible, because of sclerosis. The high penetration depth of the laser reaches bacteria even in cases where the mechanical preparation has to stop 2–3 mm above the apex.

Laser-supported endodontics is only limited by inaccessible root canals. It is therefore contraindicated in case of non-removable foreign bodies and where there is complete obliteration of the root canals. Deep root fractures, as in conventional endodontics, will still require surgery.

Finally, we may say that modern laser technology has brought crucial advantages to successful techniques, beyond those of conventional endodontics. Since laser-supported endodontics provides an excellent prognosis with substantial bacterial reduction, the patient may in many cases be saved from an invasive, surgical intervention (root apex resection, retrograde dressing and abjuration).

6.8 Practical Procedure

After enquiry about the medical history, and a precise clinical examination with X-ray analysis, the decision about laser treatment is made. The preparation for laser-supported endodontics does not differ substantially from the conventional steps in endodontics.

From the X-rays, the anatomy of the tooth to be treated can be studied. The approximate working length is calculated. And this is the measured length from the root tip to the selected point of reference. To avoid over-instrumentation, this length is reduced by 1–2 mm.

After placing the rubber-dam, the actual root canal treatment starts.

The laser-supported root canal treatment can be arranged into four sections 6.8.1 to 6.8.4.

6.8.1 Preparation of the Entrance Cavity

For preparation of the entrance cavity, the pulp cavity roof with its overhanging parts, and the crown pulp, are removed and the root canal entrances are prepared.

The preparation of the entrance cavity depends on the particular anatomy of the tooth that is being treated. A correctly selected entrance is an important condition for a good preparation. With anterior teeth and canines, the entrance is chosen from the lingual and/or palatal approach, the incisal edge remaining untouched. The outline form of the entrance cavity corresponds in form to the dentin shape. Pre-molars and molars are entered from the central occlusal surface. Here the outline form also corresponds to the tooth profile.

By using conical rounded diamond burs, the cavity is prepared to the correct depth (Fig 6-71). After opening up the pulp cavity, the pulp roof and the surrounding tooth parts – if forming an obstacle for root canal preparation – from the central to peripheral parts are taken away with a rose drill (Fig 6-72). After that the canal entrances are searched for with a pointed probe without using pressure. If the operator is working without optical assistance, hard-to-find entrances can be found using methylene-blue dye.

6.8.2 Root Canal Preparation

The next step of the root canal treatment is the preparation.

According to the German Society for Tooth Conservation (August 1999) the definition of root canal preparation, means preparing the root canal for a root canal filling, i.e., removal of tissue remnants and bacteria, and extension and shaping of the root canal.

We differentiate the biomechanical preparation (use of instruments to uncover, clean, extend and shape a root canal, usually in connection with rinsing solutions) from the chemo-mechanical preparation (intra-canal use of chemicals for rinsing, eliminating and neutralizing bacteria, tissue remnants and toxins in combination with the biomechanical preparation).

Preparation can be done manually or mechanically.

The preparation differs depending upon the root canal curvature.

For straight canals, manual preparation is chosen and for moderate to strongly curved canals, a combined mechanical–manual method is used.

6.8.2.1 Manual Preparation

The manual preparation can be divided into two areas depending on the method of preparation.

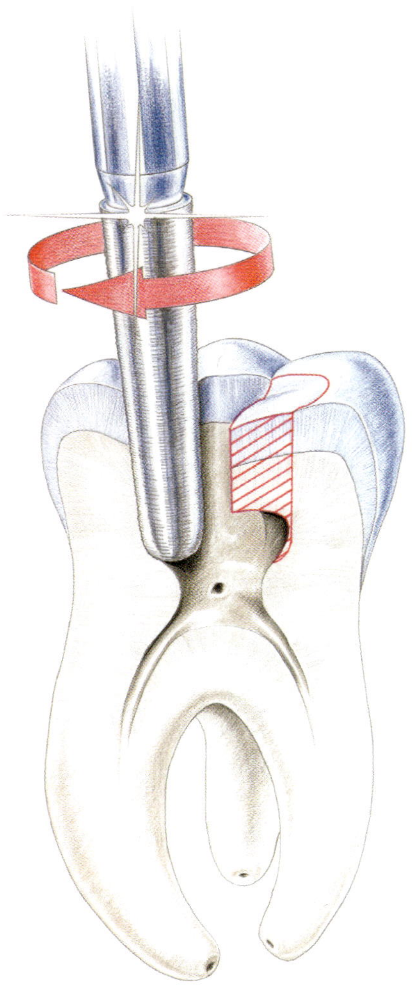

Fig 6-71 The preparation down to the pulp chamber is done with conical rounded diamond burs.

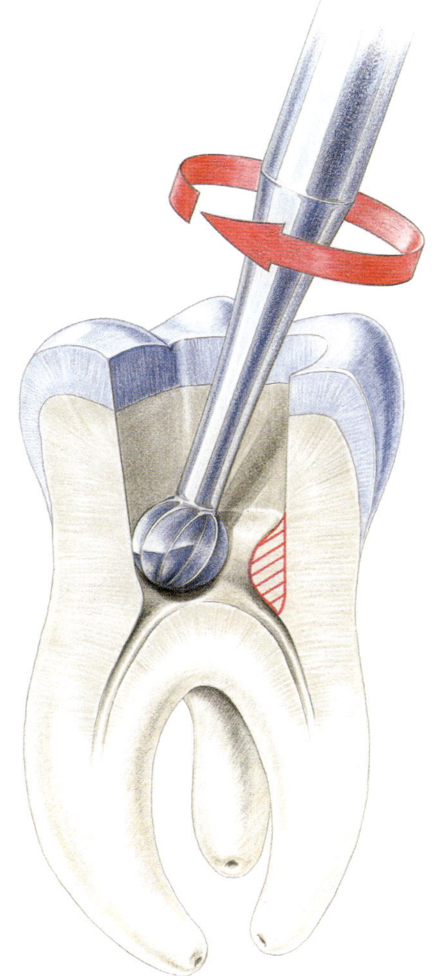

Fig 6-72 After opening up the pulp cavity, the pulp roof and the surrounding tooth parts – if forming an obstacle for root canal preparation – from the central to peripheral parts are taken away with a rose drill.

- *The apical–coronal method* – setting of the work length and conical preparation of the root canal in the coronal direction.
- *The coronal–apical method* — conical extension of the coronal root canal portion, setting of the working length and conical extension in an apical direction.

6.8.2.1.1 Apical-Coronal Methods

- *Step back technique* – the goal of this technique is to accentuate the conicity of the canal. The obturation is facilitated by this reshaping and a lateral condensation technique is possible. Risk of perforation and step formation is reduced, because less flexible instruments of increasing diameter are not used in the area of the largest curvature.
  Procedure: preparation of the canal entrances, removal of the pulp tissue with an extirpation needle and setting of the working length. The first instrument that has friction on its full length in the canal is called the initial apical file (IAF). Designated extension of the canal is around 3–5 ISO sizes. The last file that is brought into full working length is called the master apical file (MAF).

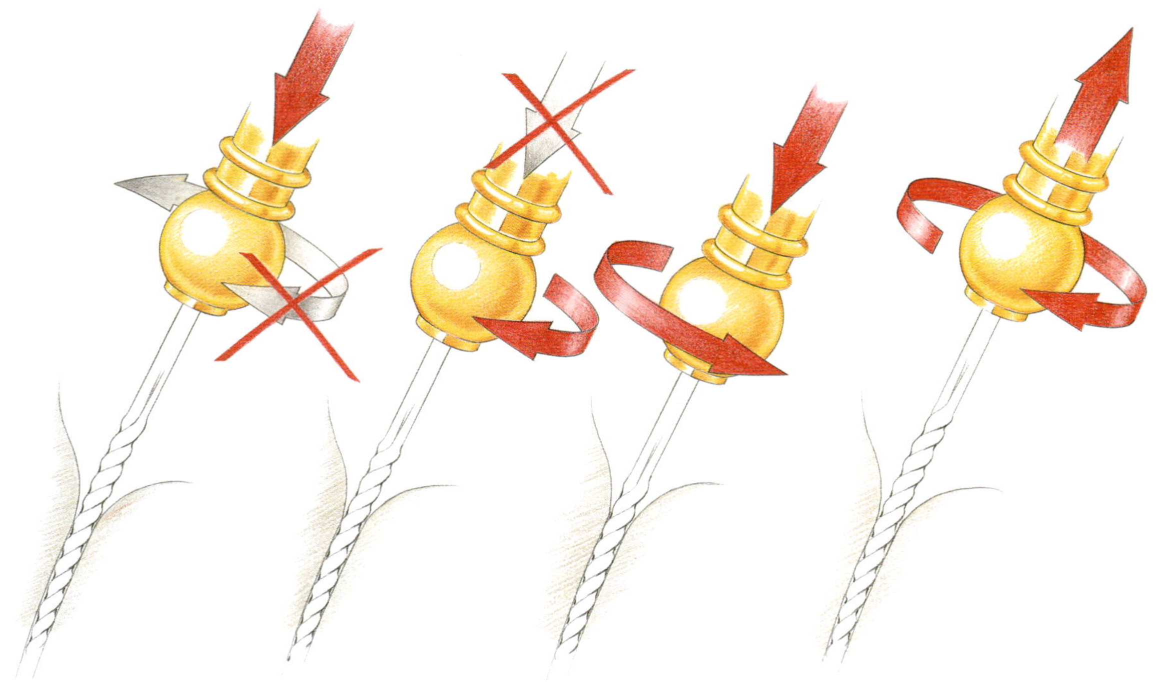

Abb. 6-73 Balanced force method.
Enter the canal with a file without rotating movement until the first signs of friction. Turn the instrument clockwise without apical pressure. Turn the file towards the apex by 90°C counter-clockwise. Finally the file is withdrawn from the canal by a clockwise rotation in the coronal direction.

Depending upon the canal curvature the apical root canal third is extended conically by means of the step back technique. With straight canals, instruments of ascending size are shortened by 0.5 mm below working length and in curved canals, around 1 mm.
The instrument used last is called the final file (FF). Between changing of instruments, the MAF should be inserted to working length and the canal should be rinsed thoroughly with NaOCl.

- *Balanced force method* – the application of this technique needs files with triangular cross section and a non-cutting point, so-called Flex R files. The advantage of this technique is that there is hardly any preparation-conditioned deviation, especially in the apical third of the canal. Procedure: the file with the non-cutting point is inserted into the canal up to the first sign of friction. A clockwise quarter-turn, followed by an apically-directed rotational movement of 180° counter-clockwise are carried out (Fig 6-73). Afterwards the instrument is removed by a clockwise rotation in a coronal direction. The canal is then cleaned and rinsed thoroughly with NaOCl.

6.8.2.1.2 Coronal-Apical Methods

The fundamental advantage of these methods is that with coronally-limited instrumentation, inflamed pulpal tissue and bacteria are not brought into the apical region.

Further, the coronal extension facilitates the cleansing of the canal, and because of this, the danger of blockage by broken off dentin splinters is reduced.

- *Step down technique*

Procedure: there is initial preparation of the coronal and middle third of the canal or up to the beginning of the canal curvature by gradually increasing the diameter of the instruments. Afterwards the canal entrance is shaped with Gates-Glidden instruments. The working length is then established and the preparation continued into the apical third of the canal, with instruments of smaller diameter.

The advantage of this technology is that with the initial extension, the instruments used in the coronal portion have smaller wall contact and because of that they can be used more efficiently in the apical region. The risk of a canal straightening is thereby minimized.

- Crown down pressureless technique

  With this technique a straight entrance is first created with Gates-Glidden drills. Following that, the canal is extended by rotation without apical pressure, with a file of ISO size 35, which is inserted up to the friction point. This procedure is repeated with instruments of decreasing diameter up to the point where the working length is reached. After radiological control of the working length, the apical third is extended, in the next cycle.

- Double flared technique

  Here a combination of the step down and step back technique is used and the efficiency is improved by Gates-Glidden drills.

  Procedure: with instruments of relatively large diameter, e.g., ISO 80, the canal is gradually prepared from coronal towards the apex. That diameter decreases step by step until the working length is reached. Following that, the canal is prepared conically with the help of the step back technique, so that the conicity increases.

  If there is a straight canal (measured by the Schneider Method) the possibility of passing down the canal has to be proved with a file (ISO 0.08 or 0.10) (Fig 6-74) and afterwards the entrance is extended with a Gates-Glidden drill (Fig 6-75).

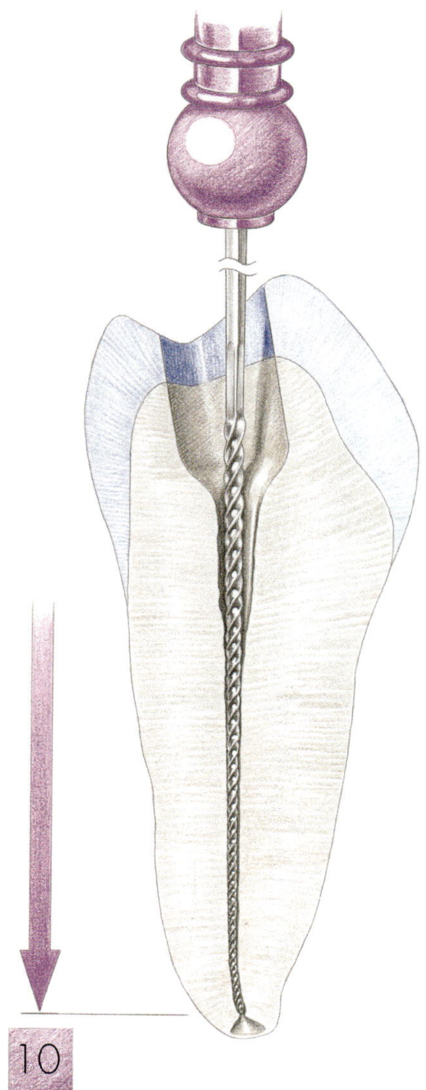

Fig 6-74 The possibility of passing down the canal is proved with a file (ISO 0.08 or 0.10).

- *Method of measuring by Schneider (1971)*

  On a small X-ray, a line is drawn through a point A and B referring to the root axis (longitudinally). Point A is the canal entrance and point B is where the canal moves out of the straight line. The angle enclosed by those two lines with the angle point B equals the curvature of the canal. Schneider divides them in three categories:

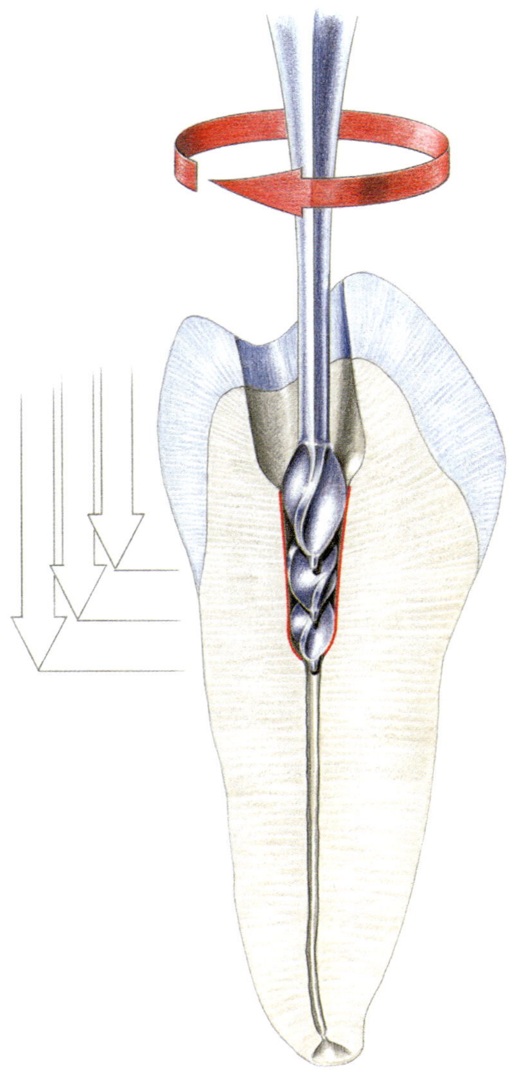

Fig 6-75 Enlargement and rectification of the canal entrance using Gates-Glidden drills. This facilitates further instrumentation, because the following instruments have to manage less curvature.

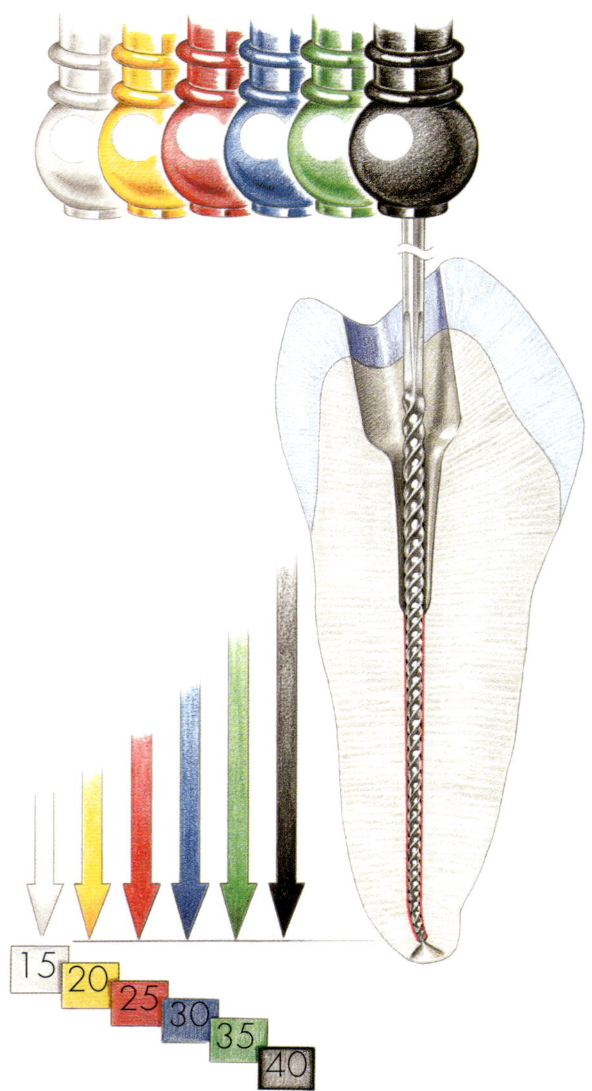

Fig 6-76 Using a file of ISO 15 and the balanced force technique, an attempt is made to make the canal accessible up to the full working length. Preparation of the canal with instruments of increasing diameter until the working length is reached. Laser treatment requires an enlargement to ISO 40.

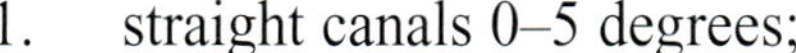

1. straight canals 0–5 degrees;
2. moderately curved canals 10–20 degrees;
3. strongly curved canals 25–70 degrees.

The remaining root pulp in the canal is removed with an extirpation needle and NaOCl rinsing. Now the working length is measured, and confirmed with an X-ray. This is done with a file of ISO 15 that is connected to an electrical length-measuring tool and with the balanced force technique; the total working length of the root canal is prepared. After putting the rubber stops on the reference points, a measurement by X-ray is made.

After radiological confirmation, and fixing the definitive working length, the canal is prepared with instruments of increasing size, using the balanced force technique (Fig 6-76).

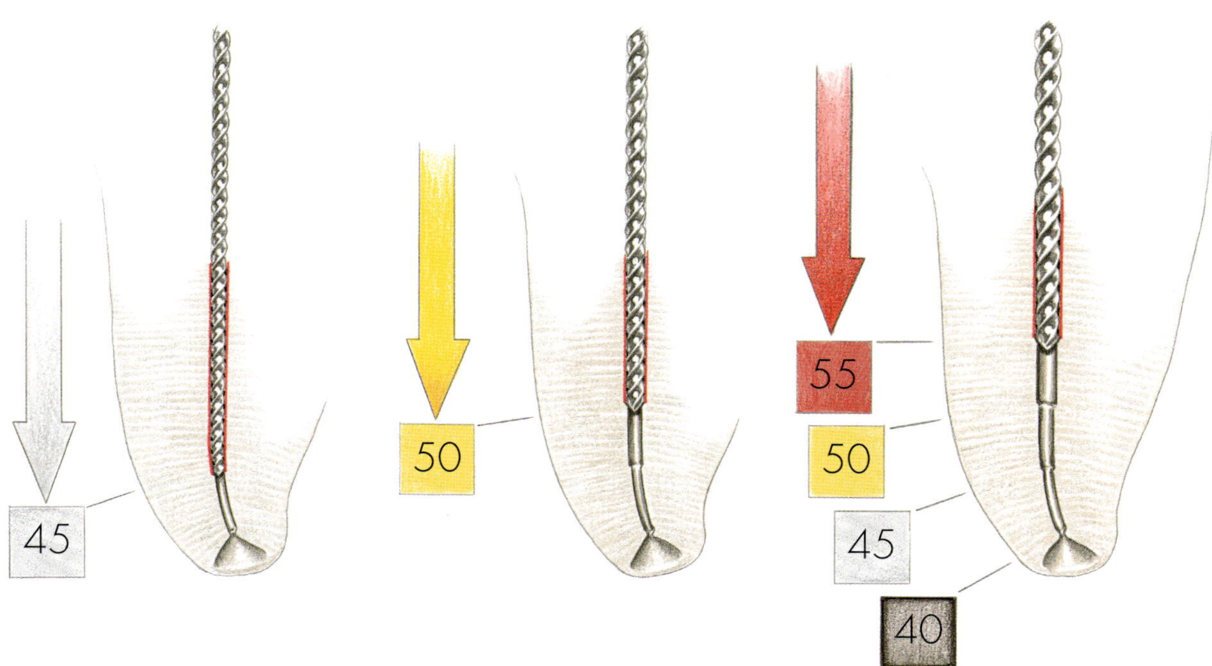

Fig 6-77 After the canal has been instrumented to a width of ISO 40 at full working length, the following instruments are introduced in the canal to a working length reduced by 0.5 mm. Step back technique.

The laser treatment can only be done after apical extension using the minimum size of ISO 30–40, so that a friction-free insertion of the fiber up to the apical stop is possible even in strongly curved canals.

After the canal is extended to the size of ISO 30–40 (for fiber diameters of 200 or 300 μm), all further instruments are shortened 0.5 mm before being inserted into the canal (step-back technique) (Fig 6-77).

To prevent clogging of the canal with dentin debris, a lubricant (EDTA) should be used and the canal also rinsed with NaOCl. The effect of the rinsing only reaches a few millimeters from the needle tip and sufficient penetration depth is important. It may be helpful to put a silicon stop on the rinsing needle to control the penetration depth.

6.8.2.2 Combined Mechanical – Manual Preparation

The preparation of a canal that is curved to a moderate or high degree (according to Schneider) is more complex. Although the sequence of treatment may be the same as in straight canals, a combined mechanical–manual technique is suggested. The reason for this is not only the time-saving component, which only has to be taken into account for an experienced user.

The actual mechanical preparation is done with nickel–titanium instruments, which are able to follow the curvature of the root canal because of the flexibility characteristics of this material. Also the higher conicity of these instruments enables a quick extension of the canal and the circular removal of dentin, because they are used in a rotational manner.

It is tried first to see whether one can pass a file (ISO 0.08 or 0.10) down the canal (Fig 6-78) and then the entrance is extended and straight-

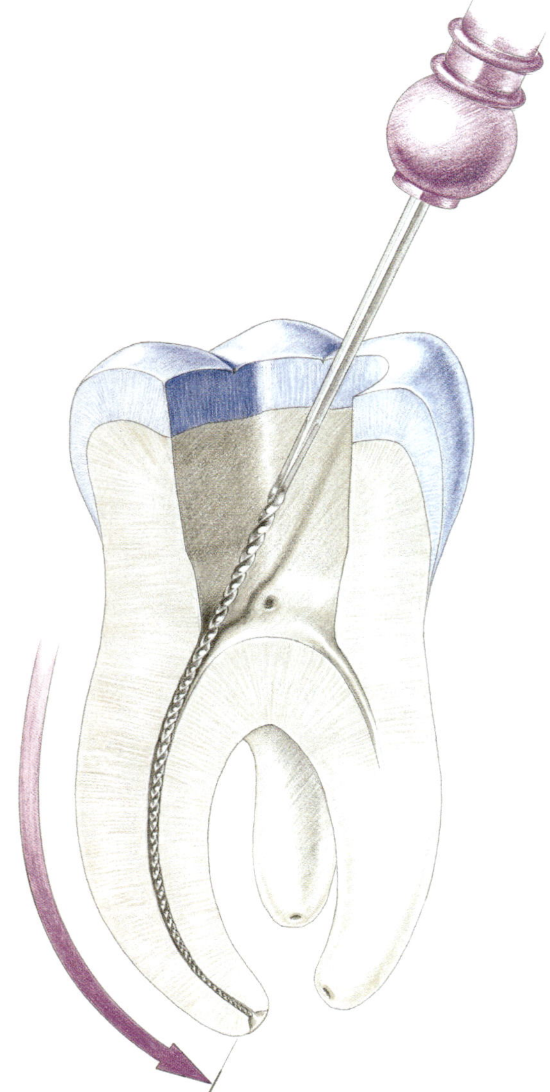

Fig 6-78 Passage control with a 0.10 file.

ened mechanically with an intro file. A special hand piece in a torque-control steered motor is recommended. For mechanical preparation a chelator is used to reduce the smear layer that is produced during preparation, and it also lubricates the instruments. The electronically specified and radiologically verified working length is adjusted using a rubberstop on the nickel-titanium instruments.

The next step is the preparation of the coronal canal portion, and this is done with an instrument of size 06/30. After another rinsing with NaOCl and a change of instruments to size 06/25, the penetration advances to the apical third of the canal (Fig 6-79). This should be done without using any pressure, and the canal always kept damp with a chelator.

The preparation of the apical third is now done mechanically–manually. Up to 3 mm before the *Foramen physiologicum*, the canal is prepared mechanically, with an instrument of size 04/30. The lower conicity of this size instrument means that there is no friction over the full length of the canal wall.

The last unprepared part of the canal is now done manually (Fig 6-80). Starting with a file ISO 15, the canal is penetrated to working length and extended to a minimum of ISO 30. All further instruments are now reduced in length (1 mm) and inserted into the canal to extend the apical region conically, using the step back technique.

After finishing the conventional preparation and rinsing the canal, it is dried with sterile paper points. The laser treatment can now begin.

6.8.3 Laser Treatment

After having finished the conventional preparation, extensive rinsing and drying of the canal with sterile paper points, all prerequisites are given for the laser treatment.

The laser fiber is inserted into the canal, after the working length has been marked with a rubber stop at the fiber and the laser activated. Special care should be exercised so that the fiber does not remain at the apical stop for longer than 1 s, since the temperature will rise to critical levels (see standard settings).

Subsequently, the fiber is pulled from apical to coronal in circling movements to cover the whole root dentin (Fig 6-81). This procedure is repeated at least five times.

An experienced dentist can "feel" the laser, i.e., with the pulsed laser one can differentiate the

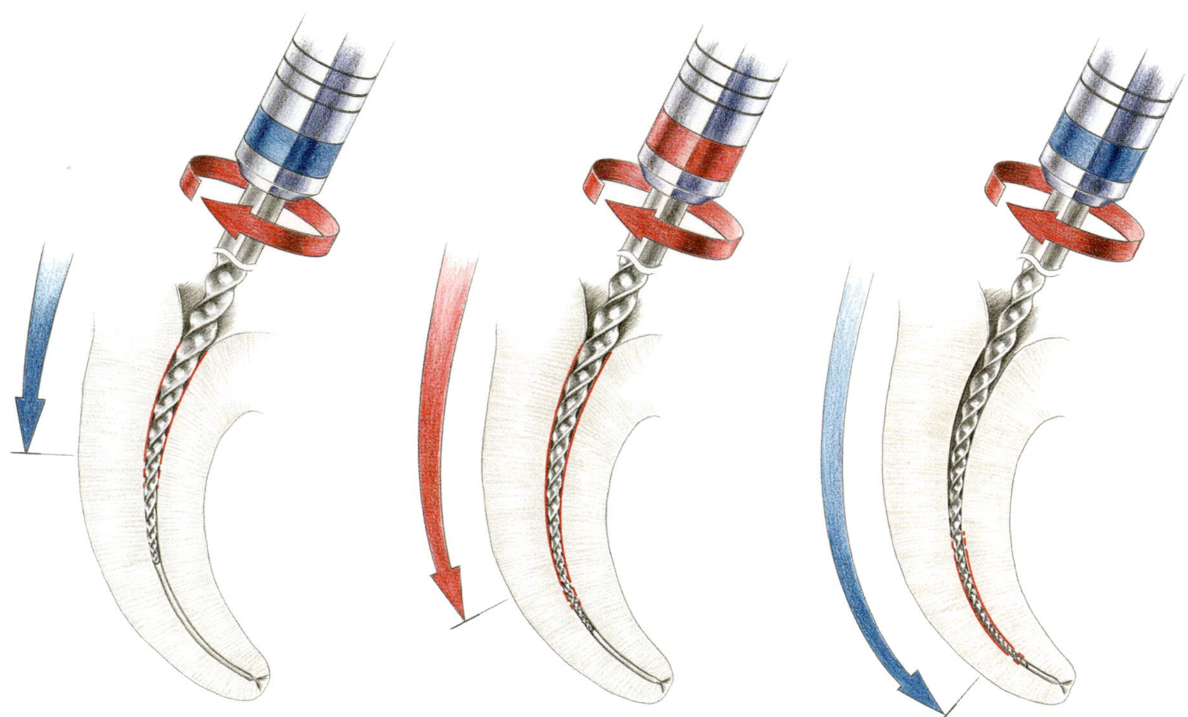

Fig 6-79 Preparation of the upper canal portions until 3 mm away from the expected apex.

Fig 6-80 Preparation of the remaining canal portions with hand instruments.

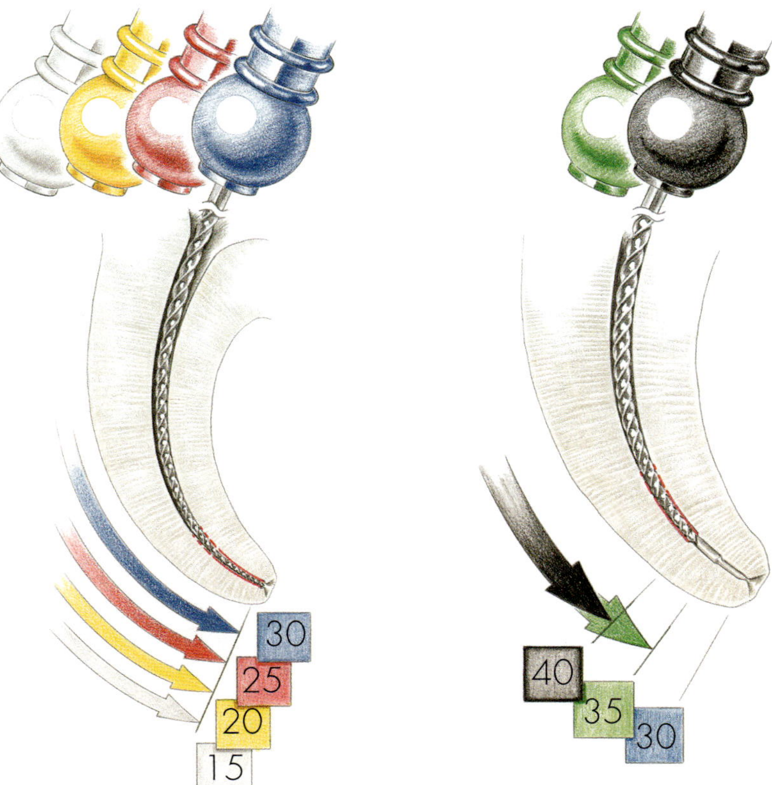

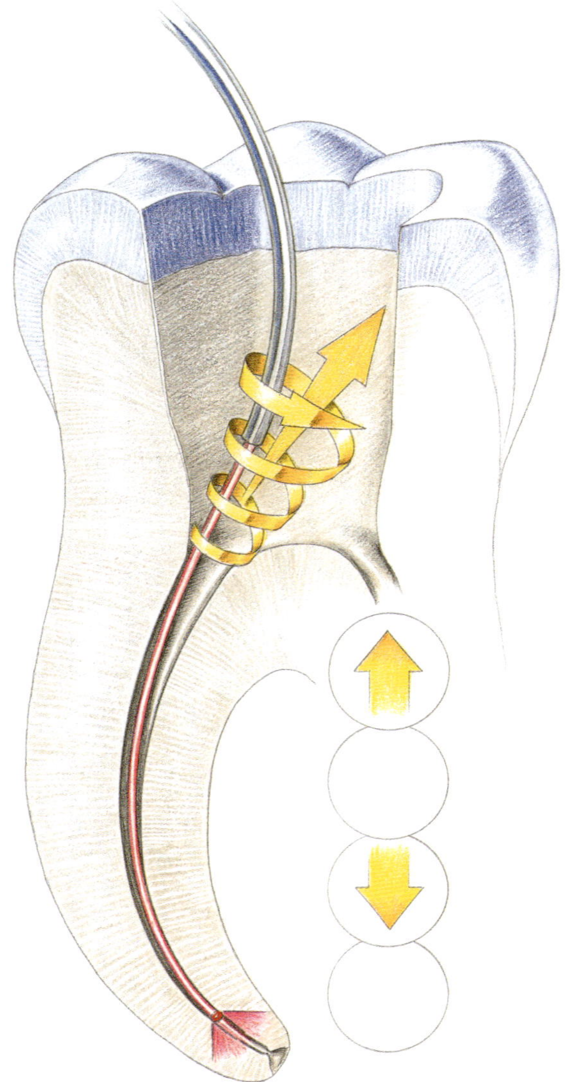

Fig 6-81 The fiber is pulled evenly in a circling motion from apical to coronal, in order to reach the entire root dentin. This procedure is repeated at least three times.

pulse noise between a wet or dry canal and if there was any incorrect movement (e.g., over-instrumentation) of the fiber.

After finishing the laser treatment, the canal is filled up with calcium hydroxide and sealed with Cavit or Glass Ionomer Cement to prevent bacterial invasion until the next appointment. Clinical experience has shown that at least two sessions are needed for optimal laser-supported root canal treatment. With only one treatment session, there is the risk of not sufficiently sterilizing the canals and surrounding dentin. In some cases the bacteria may actually increase after the first treatment, but after a second session of irradiation, clinical sterilization is achieved.

It is highly probable that one can expect an after-effect following laser irradiation (this "post-laser-effect" can be compared with the "post-antibiotics-effect"). Bacteria that are irradiated with lower light intensities show cell membrane damage. Even if this does not result in the cell death it has an effect on the survival of the bacteria. Their general resistance towards changes of their environments is reduced and their sensitivity towards chemical disinfectants, which are used synergistically, is increased. With numerous irradiations, a cumulative bactericidal effect is reached (see section 6.2.2.3).

6.8.4 Root Canal Filling

A definitive root filling after the third irradiation treatment is suggested (an interval of 3 days is recommended between the appointments). In extremely difficult cases extra sessions may be necessary.

The ISO size of the MAF is the size chosen for the gutta-percha point. The master point is slightly covered with sealer and brought into the canal up to the full working length. With lateral condensation of the master point using a spreader, space is created for the extra points. The size of the spreader will also determine the ISO size of the extra points, and the coronal third of the root canal should be filled with these extra points.

Finally, the excess gutta-percha points extending from the canal are removed with a warm excavator and the coronal part of the canal is sealed by vertical condensation.

The goal of a root canal filling according to the ESE is:

– to exclude the passage of microorganisms and liquids along the root canal

– to fill out the entire duct system, not only the main canal to the apex but also to close the dentin tubules and accessory canals.

The requirements of a root canal filling material are extensive, as follows:
- biocompatibility
- dimensional stability
- water insolubility
- small moisture absorption
- X-ray opacity
- easily applied and
- easily removed.

At the present time, these requirements are best fulfilled by gutta-percha.

Gutta-percha is the dried up milk of the gutta-percha tree. Besides the gutta-percha matrix, the points also contain barium sulfate as a roentgen contrast medium, and as fillers there are waxes, zinc oxide, coloring materials and trace elements.

To compensate for small irregularities, and for sealing the tubule system, the gutta-percha points are inserted with a sealer, into the canal. The sealer also acts as cement.

After the treatment, a complete X-ray documentation is carried out, to begin a radiographic record monitoring the periapical healing in the bone and paradontal tissues.

6.9 Clinical Cases

Case 1

A 39-year-old patient, tooth 36 endodontically treated 5 years ago and had a crown as restoration. In the mesial root channels, fractured root channel instruments were detected radiologically, CAP and the tooth generated pain. In one of the mesial root canals the broken instrument could be removed, in the second channel this was not possible, but instrumentation was carried out until 1 mm from the radiological apex. After endodontic laser therapy the patient was symptom-free and the tooth could be filled.

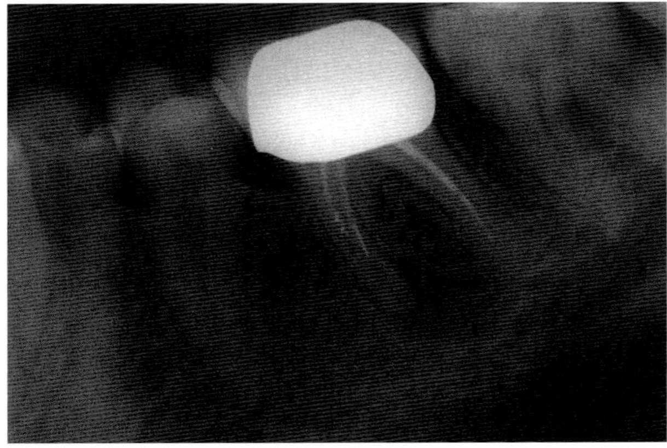

Fig 6-82 X-ray. CAP in tooth 36. Mesial, two fractured root canal instruments are discernible.

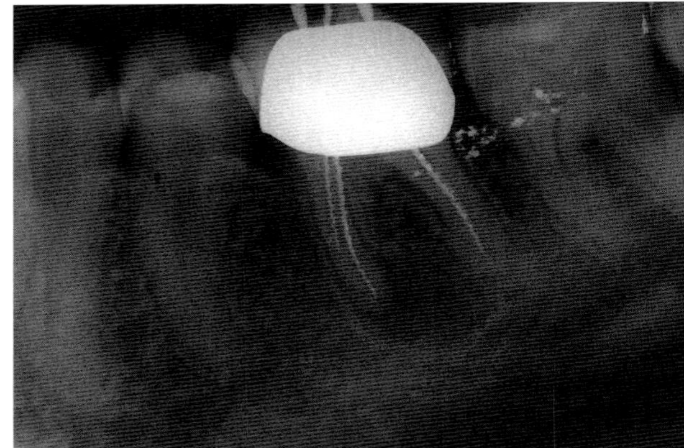

Fig 6-83 Measuring X-ray. Despite the fact that one instrument could not be removed, the instrumentation of all canals to the apex was accomplished.

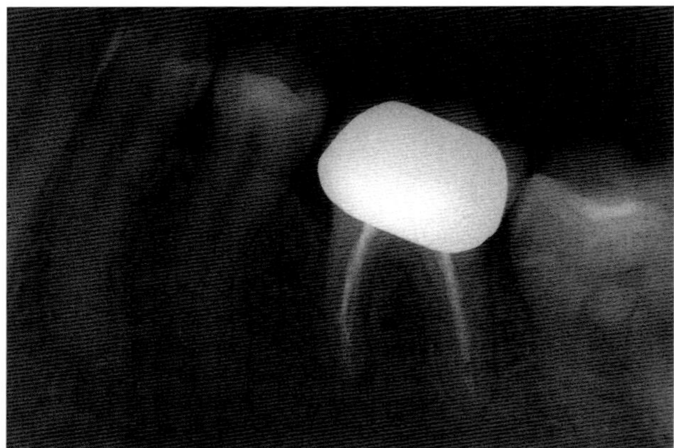

Fig 6-84 Situation after laser treatment and filling of the canals.

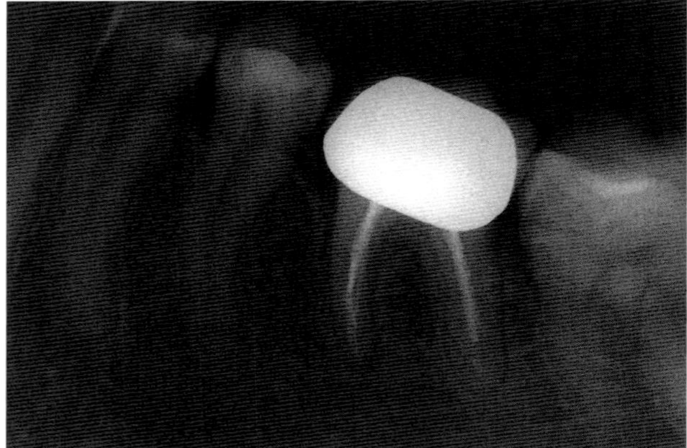

Fig 6-85 Control X-ray after 5 months. The defect healing is discernible.

Case 2

A 46-year-old patient. Tooth 15 was endodontically treated 20 years ago, later a crown with postal fixation was built. Later, a huge radiolucency in the apical region of 15 was detected and the tooth showed a mobility of degree II. After endodontic retreatment laser therapy was used. Four months later the tooth was restored with a fiber post and a ceramic-coated crown. The apical radiolucency of 15 disappeared and the patient was symptom-free.

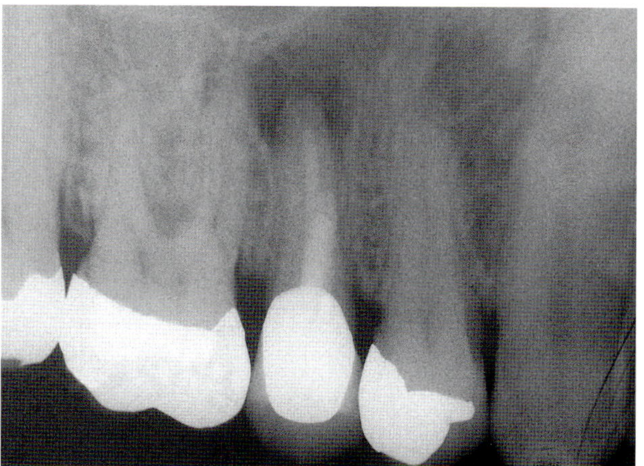

Fig 6-86 X-ray. The huge focus on tooth 15 can be discerned.

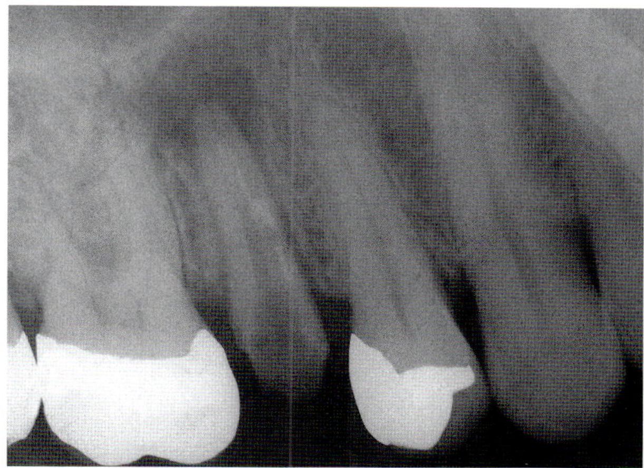

Fig 6-87 Situation after the removal of the screw post and old root canal filling.

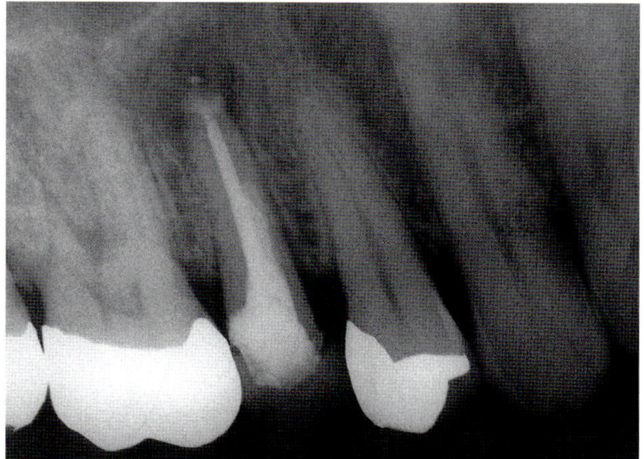

Fig 6-88 Control X-ray after laser therapy and new root canal filling.

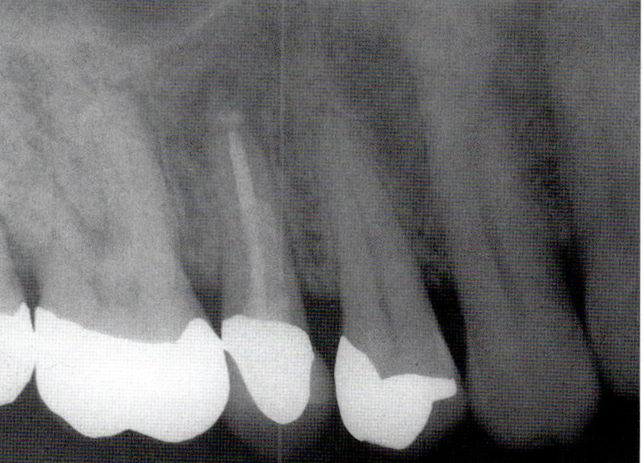

Fig 6-89 Situation 3 months after the definitive restoration of the tooth with a glass fiber post and a crown.

Case 3

A 29-year-old patient with interradicular radiolucency 36, without visible periodontal involvement. After three laser therapy sessions for bactericidal purposes and two diode laser therapy sessions using a diode laser with 1 W for osteoblast stimulation, the interradicular radiolucency disappeared. With completed radiologic interradicular bone regeneration, the root canals were filled and the tooth is now symptom free for 2 years

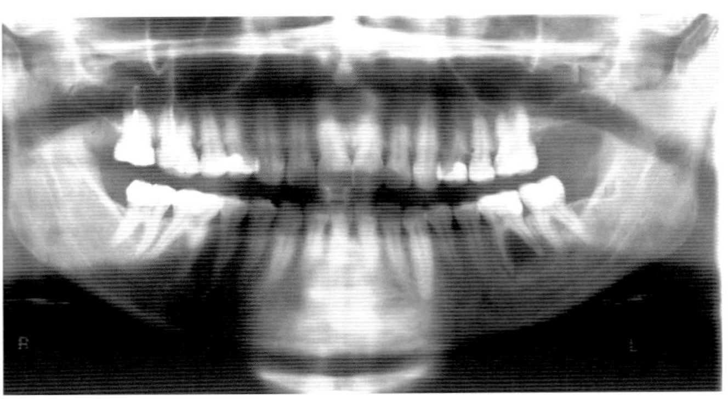

Fig 6-90 Panoramic X-ray.

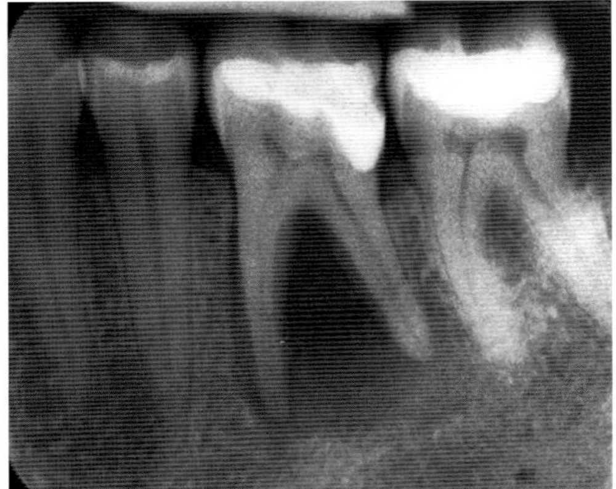

Fig 6-91 A large bone defect on tooth 36 can be discerned, which extends to the whole interradicular space.

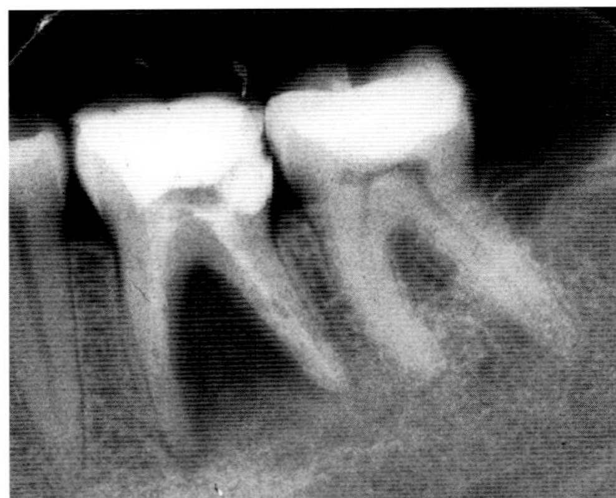

Fig 6-92 Situation after laser therapy and temporary root canal filling. A partial build-up of bone can be seen.

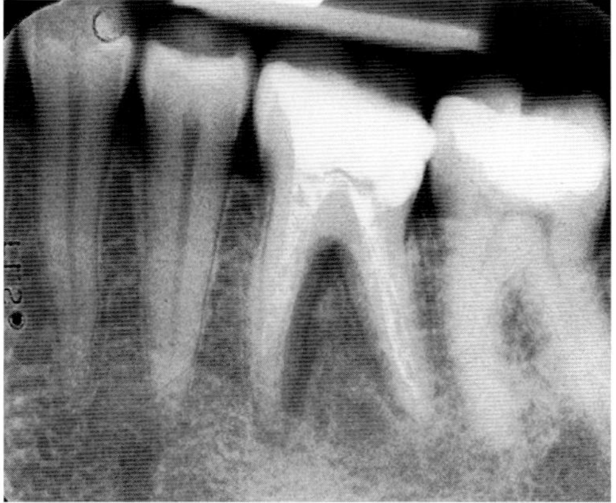

Fig 6-93 After repeated laser irradiation and temporary filling, the full extent of bone formation is clearly discernible.

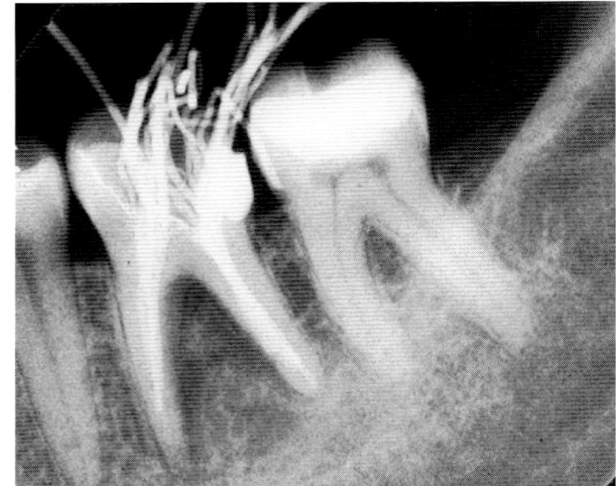

Fig 6-94 Control X-ray of the definitive root canal filling.

Case 4

A 43-year-old patient with a bridge 45, 46/2, 47. Huge radiolucency apical 47. After three conventional laser therapy sessions for bactericidal purposes the patient became symptom-free and after five laser therapy sessions with a diode laser (1 W) the tooth could be filled endodontically.

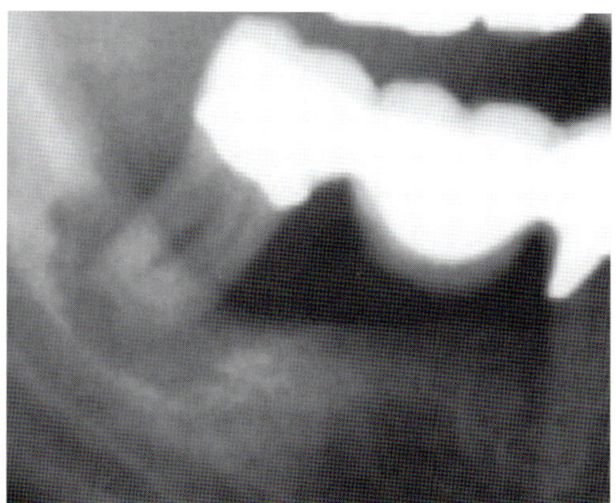

Fig 6-95 X-ray. A large focus, extending over both roots can be seen.

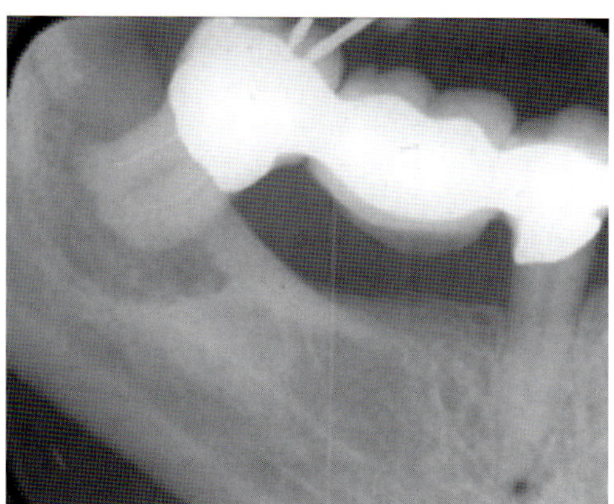

Fig 6-96 Measuring X-ray.

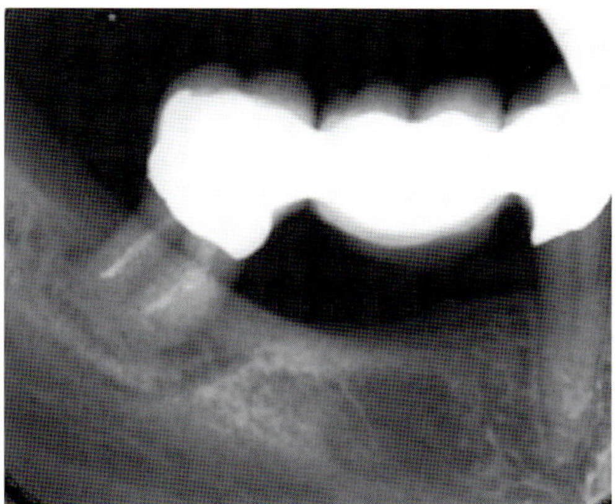

Fig 6-97 Situation after laser irradiation and temporary root canal filling with calxyl.

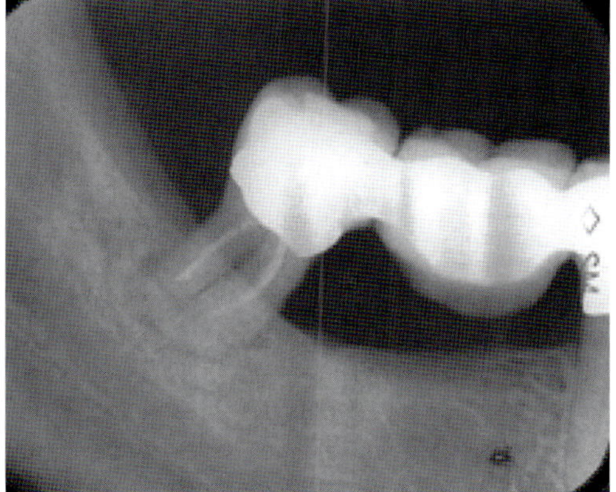

Fig 6-98 Control after 6 months, nearly normal circumstances. A pronounced regression of the bone resorption can be discerned.

Case 5

A 56-year-old patient with postal restoration and insufficient root canal filling in tooth 11. After the removal of the post and revision of the root canal filling, irradiation with the Nd:YAG laser was carried out. After 5 months, the tooth could be restored with post and crown.

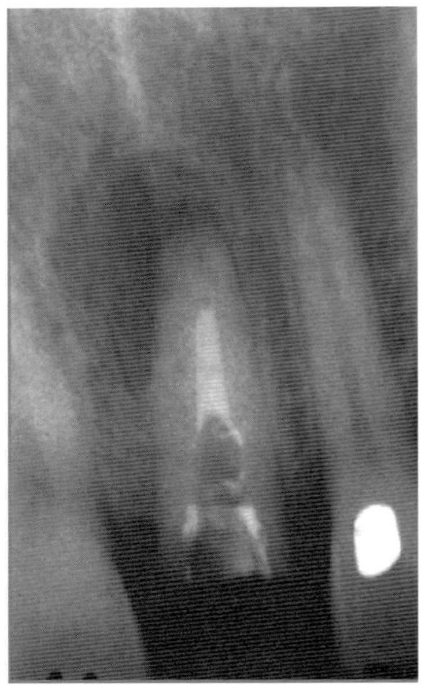

Fig 6-99 Situation after the removal of the post. The apical bone resorption can be discerned.

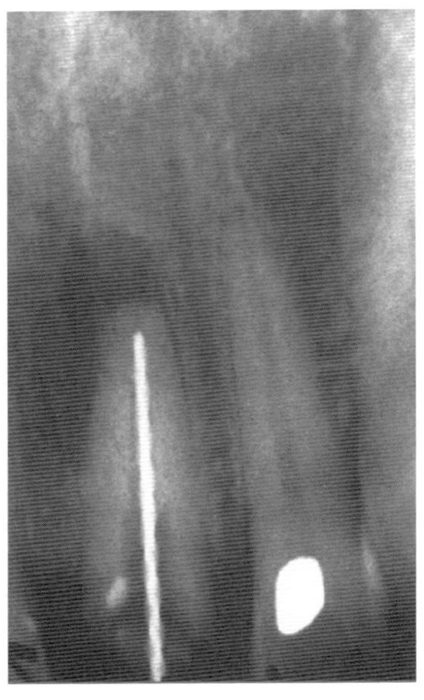

Fig 6-100 Measuring X-ray.

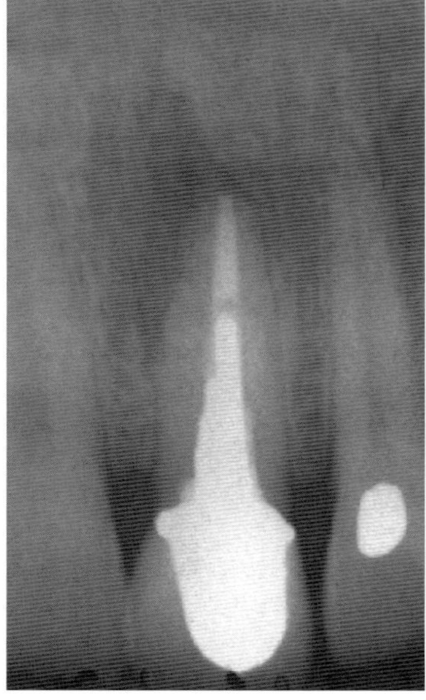

Fig 6-101 Five months after the laser treatment, the tooth could be restored definitively with post and crown.

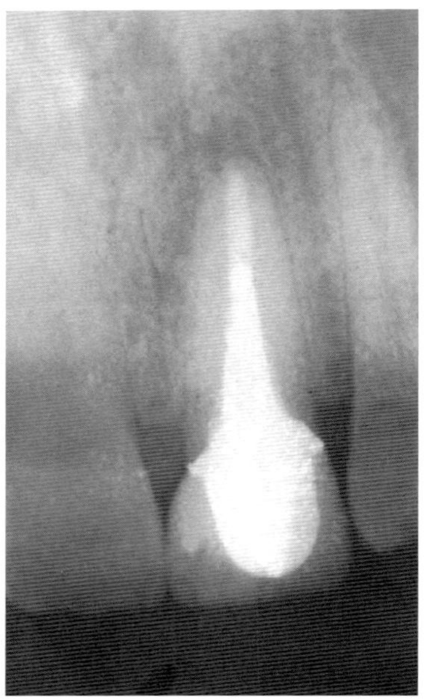

Fig 6-102 A control X-ray reveals the complete healing of the bone destruction.

Case 6

A 58-year-old patient with distal-paro-lesion at tooth 35, 8 month after triming of the bridge. After three preceding laser treatments the defect healed within 3 months.

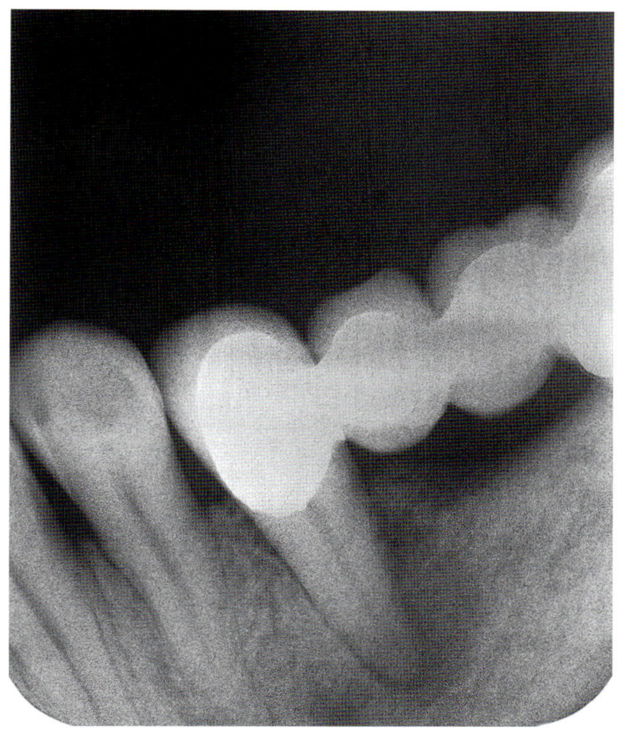

Fig 6-103 X-ray. A large focus on tooth 35 is discernible.

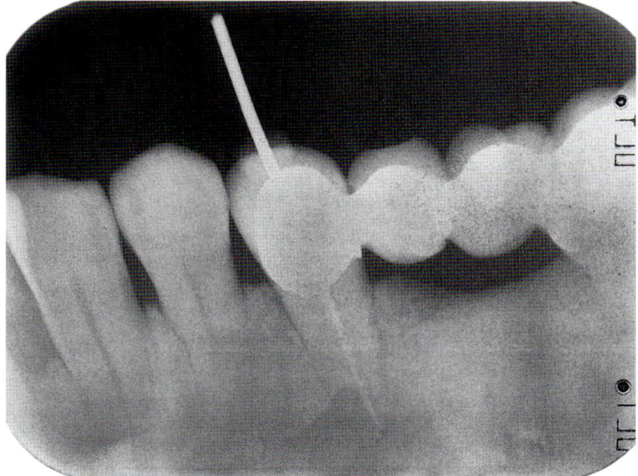

Fig 6-104 The point X-ray 2 months after the first laser treatment reveals a remarkable healing tendency of the focus.

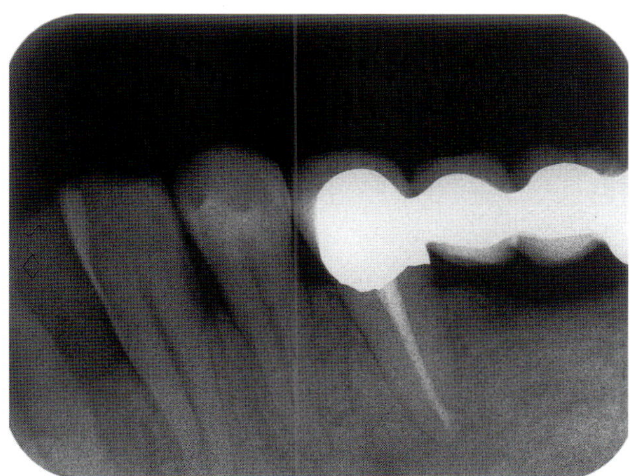

Fig 6-105 Control X-ray 3 months after the first laser treatment. A filled lateral canal in the apical area can be discerned on the side of the former focus.

6.10 Future Perspectives

As already cited above, cell stimulating properties are ascribed to the diode laser. This effect could be of great importance in regard to the healing of periapical lesions. Future strategies in the prevention and treatment of oral diseases should also biologically regulate fibroblast activities, implicated in periapical regeneration in endodontics.

Fibroblasts, which are responsible for the assembly of the extracellular matrix, are capable of responding directly to oral microbial challenges, or indirectly following activation of the host immune response, and can alter the composition of connective tissue in several ways: synthesis of inflammatory mediators, their receptors or antagonists, fibroblast proliferation, collagen synthesis, phagocytosis of collagen fibrils and synthesis of proteolytic enzymes, including matrix metalloproteinases and their corresponding inhibitors[158].

Human gingival fibroblast cells reside in oral tissues, which are challenged frequently by pathogenic bacteria. Progenitors for gingival fibroblast-developing tissues derive both from odontogenic and non-odontogenic mesenchyme, while in wounded tissues, gingival fibroblasts are derived from gingival connective tissue and comprise a heterogeneous cell population, with diverse properties and functions[159].

Studies of immunological aspects in addition to the structural components of gingival fibroblasts showed that these cells actively participate in immune and inflammatory events in oral diseases[158]. Since fibroblasts are the predominant cell type in soft connective tissue matrices, regulation of their proliferative, synthetic and degradative behavior is likely to be important in tissue physiology and pathology.

Among the many physiological effects of laser irradiation for therapeutic purposes, anti-inflammation and stimulation of wound healing have been reported[160]. However, little is known about the biological mechanisms of the anti-inflammatory effect of laser irradiation in oral diseases.

The anti-inflammatory effects of low-laser irradiation in an in vivo experimental model in rats have been reported[161]. In vitro studies proved low level laser irradiation to inhibit LPS-increased prostaglandin E2 production in human gingival fibroblasts. The inhibitory effects on PG-E2 production were laser irradiation time-dependent, with almost complete inhibition found after 10 min irradiation and the underlying mechanism was the reduction of COX-2 gene expression[162]. COX is the rate-limiting enzyme which catalyzes the conversion of arachidonic acid to prostaglandin endoperoxide and is involved in many inflammatory states.

Soluble proteins that serve as mediators of cell function and are produced by various cell types, such as structural and inflammatory cells, are collectively called cytokines.

LPS from periodontal pathogens can penetrate gingival tissues and stimulate the production of cytokines and interleukins. So, fibroblasts are surrounded by leukocyte-derived proinflammatory cytokines such as interleukin 1β (IL-1β), tumor necrosis factor alpha (TNF-α) and lymphocyte-derived interleukin-6 in inflamed gingival tissue. IL-1β and TNF-α are thought to be therapeutic targets, because these cytokines are essential for the initiation of inflammatory immune reactions and are produced for prolonged periods in inflammatory diseases. IL-1β is also implicated in bone resorption. In an in vitro study, low laser irradiation inhibited interleukin 1b production and gene expression in a dose-dependent manner[163].

A comparison was made of the low level laser therapy effects on cultured human gingival fibroblast proliferation, using different irradiance and the same fluence. When irradiated, fibroblasts in nutritional deficit presented cell growth similar to or higher than that of the control cells

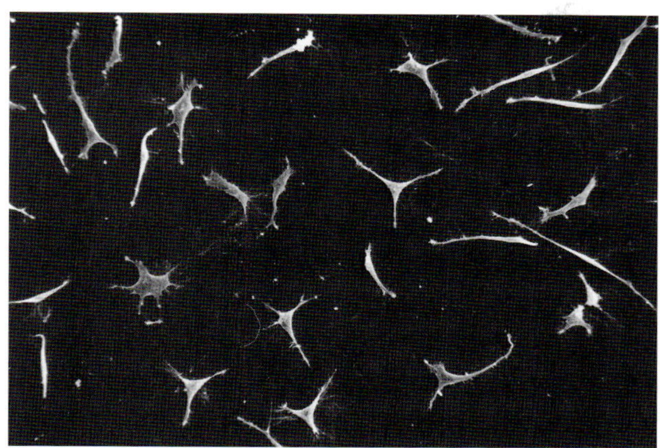

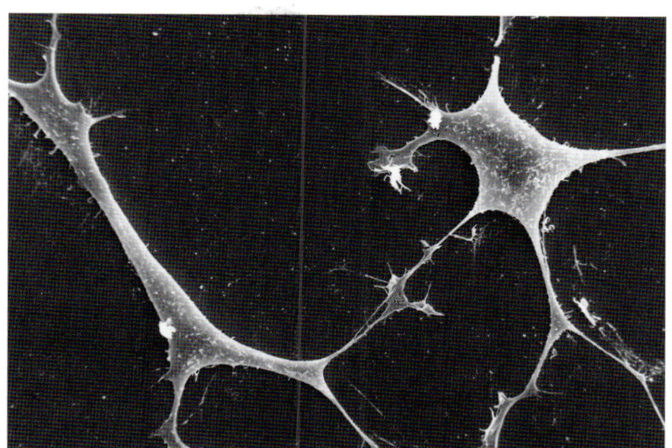

Fig 6-106 and 6-107 Fibroblasts from an unirradiated control group.

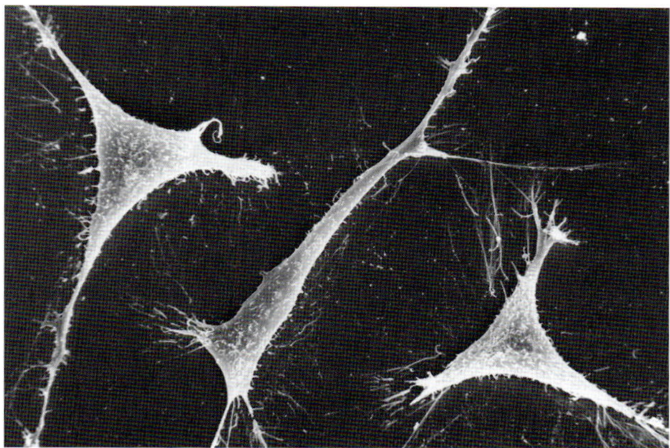

Fig 6-108 Fibroblast 48h after irradiation. Enhanced cell activity can be discerned.

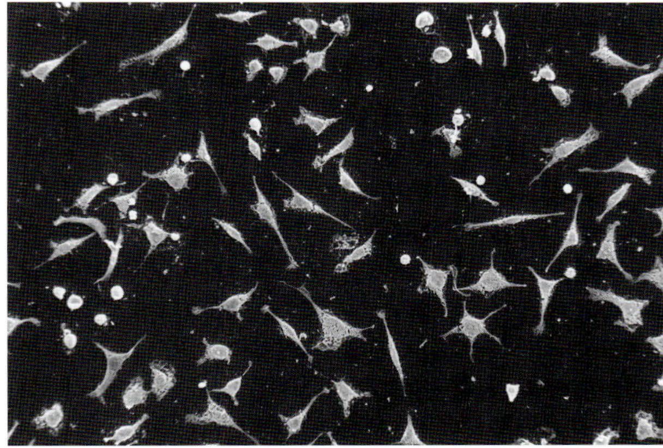

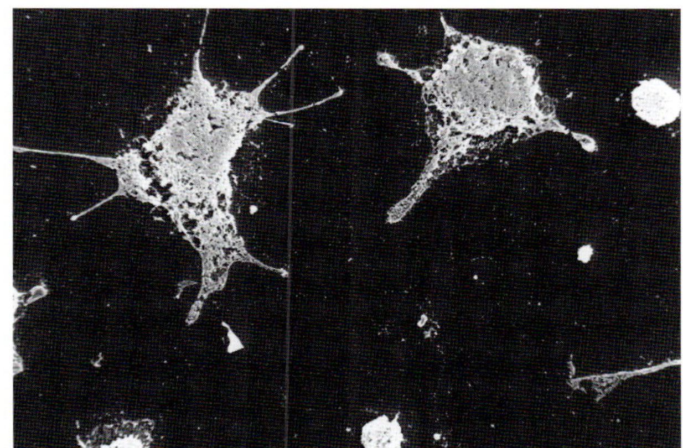

Fig 6-109 and 6-110 Cells destroyed by too high irradiation energy.

grown in normal culture conditions. Lasers of equal power output presented similar effects on cell growth, independently of their wavelengths. Low laser therapy acts by improving the in vitro fibroblast proliferation and a smaller laser exposure time results in higher proliferation. A similar study demonstrated a considerably higher proliferation activity of low level laser irradiated cells. The differences were highly significant 24 h after irradiation but decreased in an energy-dependent manner after 48 and 72 h[164].

These findings might be clinically relevant, indicating that repeated treatments are necessary to achieve a positive laser effect in clinical applications.

Moritz et al.[125] investigated the proliferation response of human gingival fibroblasts, after in vitro irradiation with a diode-laser (5 × 5 s, cw, non-contact, spot diameter 5 mm, 300–1000 mW). Cell proliferation was tested using the [^{3}H]thymidine incorporation test, 24, 48 and 72 h after irradiation. A highly significant increase in fibroblast proliferation was found after 48 h in the cell group irradiated with 700 mW.

In a second study, the effect of diode-laser irradiation (0.5–1.5 W, spot size 5 mm) on the in vitro production of the tissue inhibitor of matrix metalloproteinases 1 (TIMP-1) by human gingival fibroblasts by ELISA was investigated by Patruta et al.[124]. Preliminary results indicate that diode laser irradiation using 0.5 W significantly stimulated the production of TIMP-1, which blocks matrix metalloproteinases implicated in tissue destruction.

Adhesion and growth of cultured gingival fibroblasts on dental root surfaces treated by either irradiation with Er:YAG laser or curette were compared. The surfaces treated with 60 mJ/pulse Er:YAG laser irradiation promoted faster adhesion and growth than surfaces treated with either root planing or 100 mJ/pulse Er:YAG[165].

Negative effects have been reported using Nd:YAG laser irradiation and diode laser irradiation on in vitro fibroblast growth and proliferation[165]. Degenerative cytomorphometric changes to cell death were proven on human gingival fibroblasts using this type of laser energy on soft tissue. If the energy output is enough for clinical purposes, a laser with low pulse energy and corresponding pulse rate should be selected to minimize the damage on adjacent soft tissue.

6.11 References

1. Ketterl W: Morphologic studies on the dentin of deciduous teeth. Dtsch Zahnärztl Z 20: 652–657, 1965
2. Sauerwein E: Alterszahnheilkunde. Thieme Verlag 1993
3. Stock C et al.: Atlas der Endodontie. Ullstein-Mosby Verlag 1996
4. Arends J, Ruben J, Jongebloed W L: Dentine caries in vivo. Combined scanning electron microscopic and microradiographic investigation. Caries Res 36–41, 1989
5. Fromme H G, Riedel H: Measurements of the width of the dentin tubules in non demineralized permanent and deciduous teeth. Dtsch Zahnärztl Z 25(3): 401–405, 1970
6. Tronstad L: Ultrastructural observations on human coronal dentin. Scand J Dent Res 81(2): 101–111, 1973
7. Garberoglio R, Brännström M: Scanning electron microscopic investigation of human dentin tubules. Arch Oral Biol 21(6): 355–362, 1976
8. Goracci G, Mori G: Micromorphological aspects of dentin. Minerva Stomatol 44 (9): 377–387, 1995
9. Mjör I A, Nordahl I: The density and branching of dentinal tubules in human teeth. Arch Oral Biol 41(5): 401–412, 1996
10. Nagaoka S, Miyazaki Y, Liu H J, Iwamoto Y, Kitano M, Kawagoe M: Bacterial invasion into dentinal tubules of human vital and nonvital teeth. J Endod 21(2): 70–73, 1995
11. Nair P N et al.: Intraradicular bacteria and fungi in root-filled, asymptomatic human teeth with therapy-resistant periapical lesions: a long-term light and electron microscopic follow-up study. J Endod 16(12): 580–588, 1990
12. Perez F, Rochd T, Lodter J P, Calaos P, Michel G: In vitro study of the penetration of three bacterial strains into root dentine. Oral Surg Oral Med Oral Pathol 76(1): 97–103, 1993
13. Ramachandran Nair P N: Light and electron microscopic studies of root canal flora and periapical lesions. J Endod 13 (1): 29–39, 1987
14. Shovelton D S: The presence and distribution of microorgansisms within non-vital teeth. Br Dent J 117: 101–107, 1964
15. Engstrom B, Frostell G.: Bacteriological studies of the non-vital pulp in cases with intact pulp cavities. Acta Odontol Scand 19: 23–39, 1961
16. Berg und Nord 1973: ?
17. Wittgow W C Jr, Sabiston C B Jr.: Microorganisms from pulpal chambers of intact teeth with necrotic pulps. J Endod 1(5): 168–171, 1961
18. Carlsson J, Sundqvist G: Evaluation of methods of transport and cultivation of bacterial specimens from infected dental root canals. Oral Surg Oral Med Oral Pathol 49(5): 451–454, 1980
19. Sundqvist G, Johansson E, Sjogren U: Prevalence of black-pigmented *Bacteroides* species in root canal infections. J Endod 15(1): 131–139, 1989
20. Kantz W E, Henry C A: Isolation and classification of anaerobeic bacteria from intact chambers of non-vital teeth in man. Arch Oral Biol 19(1): 91–96, 1974
21. Zavistoski J, Dzink J, Onderdonk A, Bartlett J: Quantitative bacteriology of endodontic infections. Oral Surg Oral Med Oral Pathol 49(2): 171–174, 1980
22. Bystrom A, Sundqvist G: Bacteriologic evaluation of the efficacy of mechical root canal instrumentation in endodontic therapy. Scand J Dent Res 89(4): 321–328, 1981
23. Bystrom A, Sundqvist G: Bacteriologic evaluation of the effect of 0.5 percent sodium hypochlorite in endodontic therapy. Oral Surg Oral Med Oral Pathol 55(3): 307–312, 1983
24. Chaudhry R, Kalra N, Talwar V, Thakur R: Anaerobic flora in endodontic infections. Indian J Med Res 105: 262–265, 1997
25. Sundqvist G: Microbiologic analysis of teeth with failed endodontic treatment and the outcome of conservative re-treatment. Oral Surg Oral Med Oral Pathol Oral Radiol Endod 85(1): 86–93, 1998
26. Jenkinson H F, Lamont R J: Streptococcal adhesion and solonization. Crit Rev Oral Biol Med 8(2): 175–200, 1997
27. Sundqvist G: Bacteriologic studies of necrotic dental pulps. Odontological Dissertation 7, University of Umea 1976
28. Bystrom A, Happonen R P, Sjogren U, Sundqvist G: Healing of periapical lesions of pulpless teeth after endodontic treatment with controlled asepsis. Endod Dent Traumatol 3(2): 58–63, 1987
29. Ruoff K L, de la Maza L, Murtagh M J, Spargo J D, Ferraro M J: Species identities of enteroccocci isolated from clinical specimen. J Clin Microbiol 28(3): 435–437, 1990
30. Le Goff A, Bunetel L, Mouton C, Bonnaure-Mallet M: Evaluation of root canal bacteria and their antimicrobial susceptibility in teeth with necrotic pulp. Oral Microbiol Immunol 12(5): 318–322, 1997
31. Molander A, Reit C, Dahlen G, Kvist T: Microbiological status of root-filled teeth with apical periodontitis. Int Endod J 31(1): 1–7, 1998
32. Miyazaki S, Ohno A, Kobayashi I, Uji T, Yamaguchi K, Goto S: Cytotoxic effect of haemolytic culture supernatant from *Enterococcus faecalis* on mouse polymorphonuclear neutrophages and macrophages. Microbiol Immunol 37(4): 265–270, 1993
33. Rosan B, Williams N B: Hyaluronidase production by oral enterococci. Arch Oral Biol 11: 291–298, 1964
34. Hase C C, Finkelstein R A: Bacterial extracellular zinc-containing metalloproteases. Microbiol Rev 57(4): 823–837, 1993
35. Dahlen G, Samuelsson W, Molander A, Reit C: Identification and antimicrobial susceptibility of enterococci isolated from the root canal. Oral Microbiol Immunol 15(5): 309–312, 2000
36. Haapasalo M, Orstavik D: In vitro infection and disinfection of dentinal tubules. J Dent Res 66(8): 1375–1379, 1987
37. Fukushima H, Yamamoto K, Hirohata K, Sagawa H, Leung K P, Walker C B: Localization and identification of root canal bacteria in clinically asymptomatic periapical pathosis. J Endod 16(11): 534–538, 1990

38. Siqueira J F Jr, De Uzeda M, Fonseca M E: A scanning electron microscopic evaluation of in vitro dentinal tubules penetration by selected anaerobic bacteria. J Endod 22(6): 308–310, 1996
39. Giulana G, Ammatuna P, Pizzo G, Capone F, d'Angelo M: Occurrence of invading bacteria in radicular dentin of periodontally diseased teeth: microbiological findings. J Clin Periodontol 24(7): 478–485, 1997
40. Kouchi Y, Ninomiya J, Yasuda H, Fukui K, Moriyama T, Okamoto H: Location of Streptococcus mutans in the dentinal tubules of open infected root canals. J Dent Res 59 (12): 2038–2046, 1980
41. Sen B H, Piskin B, Demirci T: Observation of bacteria and fungi in infected root canals and dentinal tubules by SEM. Endod Dent Traumatol 11: 6–9, 1995
42. Sen B H, Safavi K E, Spangberg L S: Growth patterns of Candida ablicans in relation to redicular dentin. Oral Surg Oral Med Oral Pathol Oral Radiol Endod 84(1): 68–73, 1997
43. Meryon S D, Brook A M: Penetration of dentine by three oral bacteria in vitro and their associated cytotoxicity. Int Endod J 23(4): 196–202, 1990
44. Mejare I, Brannstrom M: Deep bacterial penetration of early proximal caries lesions in young human premolars. ASDC J Dent Child 52(2): 103–110, 1985
45. Adriaens P A, De Boever J A, Loesche W J: Bacterial invasion in root cementum and radicular dentin of periodontally diseased teeth in humans. A reservoir of periodontopathic bacteria. J Periodontol 59(4): 222–230, 1988
46. Ando N, Hoshino E: Predominant obligate anaerobes invading the deep layers of root canal dentin. Int Endod J 23 (1): 20–27, 1990
47. Love R M: Adherence of streptococcus gordonii to smeared and nonsmeared dentind. Int Endod J 26(2): 108–112, 1996
48. Love R M: Clinical Mangement of infected root canal dentin. Pract Periodont Aesthet Dent 8(6): 581–584
49. Van Strijp A J, Van Steenbergen T J, Ten Cate J M: Bacterial colonization of mineralized and completely demineralized dentine in situ. Caries Res 31(5): 349–355, 1997
50. Akpata E S, Blechmann H: Bacterial invasion of pulpal dentin wall in vitro. J Dent Res 61(2): 435–438, 1982
51. Orstavik D, Haapasalo M: Disinfection by endodontic irrigants and dressings of experimentally infected dentinal tubules. Endod Dent Traumatol 6(4): 142–149, 1990
52. Kreft B, Marre R, Schramm U, Wirth R: Aggregation substance of Enterococcus faecalis mediates adhesion to cultured renal tubular cells. Infect Immun 60 (1): 25–30, 1992
53. Dai X F, Ten Cate A R; Limeback H: The extent and distribution of intratubular collagen fibrils in human dentine. Arch Oral Biol 36(10): 775–778, 1991
54. Love R M, McMillan M D, Jenkinson H F: Invasion of dentinal tubules by oral streptococci is associated with collagen recognition mediated by the antigen I/II family polypeptides. Infect Immun 65(12): 5157–5164, 1997
55. Love R M: Enterococcus faecalis – a mechanism for its role in endodontic failure. Int Endod J 34(5): 399–405, 2001
56. Hubble T S, Hatton J F, Nallapareddy S R, Murray B E, Gillespie M J: Influence of Enterococcus faecalis proteases and the collagen-binding protein, Ace, on adhesion to dentin. Oral Microbiol Immunol 18(2): 121–126, 2003
57. Buck R, Eleazor P D, Staat R H: In vitro disinfection of dentinal tubules by various endodontic irrigants. J Endod 25(12): 786–788, 1999
58. Bystrom A, Sunqvist G: The antibacterial action of sodium hypochlorite and EDTA in 60 cases of endodontic therapy. Int Endod J 18(1): 35–40, 1985
59. D'Arcangelo C, Varvara G, De Fazio P: An evaluation of the action of different root canal irrigants on facultative aerobic-anaerobic, obligate anaerobic, and microaerophilic bacteria. J Endod 25(5): 351–353, 1999
60. Harrison J W: Irrigation of the root canal system. Dent Clin North Am 28(4): 797–808, 1984
61. Siqueira J F Jr, de Uzeda M: Influence of different vehicles on the antibacterial effects of calcium hydroxide. J Endod 24(10): 663–665, 1998
62. Yoshida T, Shibata T, Shinohara T, Gomyo S, Sekine I: Clinical evaluation of the efficacy of EDTA solution as an endodontic irrigant. J Endod 21(12): 592–593, 1995
63. Berutti E, Marini R, Angeretti A: Penetration ability of different irrigants into dentinal tubules. J Endod 23(12): 725 –727, 1997
64. Zakariasen K L, Dederich D N, Tulip J, DeCoste S, Jensen S E, Pickard M A: Bactericidal action of carbon dioxide laser radiation in experimental dental root canals. Can J Microbiol 32(12): 942–946, 1986
65. Pini R, Salimbeni R, Vannini M, Barone R, Clauser C: Laser dentistry: a new application of excimer laser in root canal therapy. Lasers Surg Med 9(4): 352–357, 1989
66. Frentzen M, Koort H J: Lasers in dentistry: new possibilities with advancing laser technology? Int Dent J 40(6): 323–332, 1990
67. Hardee M W, Miserendino L J, Kos W, Walia H: Evaluation of the antibacterial effects of intracanal Nd:YAG laser irradiation. J Endod 20(8): 377–380, 1994
68. Rooney J, Midda M, Leeming J: A laboratory investigation of the bactericidal effect of a Nd:YAG laser. Br Dent J 22; 176(2): 61–64, 1994
69. Gutknecht N, Moritz A, Conrads G, Sievert T, Lampert F: Bactericidal effect of the Nd:YAG laser in in vitro root canals. J Clin Laser Med Surg 14 (2): 77–80, 1996
70. Moritz A, Gutknecht N, Goharkhay K, Schoop U, Wernisch J, Sperr W: In vitro irradiation of infected root canals with a diode laser: results of microbiologic, infrared spectrometric, and stain penetration examinations. Quintessence Int 28(3): 205–209, 1997
71. Mehl A, Folwaczny M, Haffner C, Hickel R: Bactericidal effects of 2.94 microns Er:YAG-laser radiation in dental root canals. J Endod 25(7): 490–493, 1999
72. Schoop U, Moritz A, Goharkhay K, Rehart A, Enislidis C, Doertbudak O, Wernisch J, Sperr W: Die Anwendung des Er:YAG-Lasers in der Endodontie – eine In-vitro-Studie. Stomatologie 96(2): 23–27, 1999

73. Altshuler G B, Grisimov V N, Ermolaev V, Vityaz I: Human tooth as an optical device. SPIE 1429 Holography. Interferometry and Optical Pattern Recognition in Biomedicine 95–105, 1991
74. Grisimov V N: Refractive index of bulk dentin. Proc. SPIE Advanced Laser Dentristry 2–5, 1994
75. Jaap R, Zijp J R, ten Bosch J J: Theoretical model for the scattering of light by dentin and comparison with measurements. Appl Optics 32(4) 411–415, 1993
76. Brumer P, Shapiro M: Controlling chemical reactions with lasers. Acc Chemical Research 22(12): 407–413, 1994
77. Zijp J R, ten Bosch J J: Theoretical model for the scattering of light by dentin and comparison with measurements. Appl Optics 32(4), 411–415, 1993
78. ten Bosch J J, Coops J C, Bolt R A: Observing the tooth. The paths of light in visual and instrumental observation. Ned Tijdschr Tandheelkd 100(2): 56–59, 1993
79. Altshuler G B, Grisimov V N: New optical effects in the human hard tooth tissues. Proc. SPIE Lasers and Med 1353: 97–102, 1989
80. Vaarkamp J, ten Bosch J J, Verdonschot E H: Propagation of light through human dental enamel and dentine. Caries Res 29(1): 8–13, 1995
81. Inoyye S, Takeishi K, Lee N, DeMartini M, Hirashima A, Inouye M: Lipoprotein from the outer membrane of *Escherichia coli*: purification, paracrystallization, and some properties of its free form. J Bacteriol 127(1): 555–563, 1976
82. Martini O, Richter D: Eukaryotic ribosomal proteins stimulate *Escherichia coli* stringent factor to synthesize guanosine 5'-diphosphate, 3'-diphosphate (ppGpp) and guanosine 5'-triphosphate, 3'-diphosphate (ppGpp). Mol Gen Genet 9, 166(3): 291–297, 1978
83. Gmeiner J, Schlecht S: Molecular composition of the outer membrane of *Escherichia coli* and the importance of protein-lipopolysaccharide interactions. Arch Microbiol 127(2): 81–86, 1980
84. De Petris S: Ultrastructure of the cell wall of *Escherichia coli* and chemical nature of its constituent layers. J Ultrastruct Res 19(1): 45–83, 1967
85. Klinke T, Klimm W, Gutknecht N: Antibacterial effects of Nd:YAG laser irradiation within root canal dentin. J Clin Laser Med Surg 15(1): 29–31, 1997
86. Odor T M, Watson T F, Pitt Ford T R, McDonald F: Pattern of transmission of laser light in teeth. Int Endod J 29(4): 228–234, 1996
87. Moritz A, Jakolitsch S, Goharkhay K, Schoop U, Kluger W, Mallinger R, Sperr W, Georgopoulos A: Morphologic changes correlating to different sensitivities of *Escherichia coli* and *Enterococcus faecalis* to Nd:YAG laser irradiation through dentin. Lasers Surg Med 26(3): 250–261, 2000
88. Hitchener B J, Egan A F: Outer-membrane damage in sublethally heated *Escherichia coli* K-12. Can J Microbiol 23(3): 311–318, 1977
89. Yatvin M B: Influence of membrane-lipid composition on translocation of nascent proteins in heated *Escherichia coli*. Biochim Biophys Acta 10, 901(1): 147–156, 1987
90. Katsuij N, Tsuchido T, Hiramatsuj R, Fujikawa S, Takano M, Shibasalo I: Heat-induced blebbing and vesiculation of the outer membrane of *E.coli*. J Bacteriol, Dep of Ferm Techn Oska Uni, Inst of Low Temp Sc, Hokkaido Uni, 1523–1531, 1982
91. Tsuchido T, Katsui N, Takeuchi A, Takano M, Shibasaki I: Destruction of the outer membrane permeability barrier of *Escherichia coli* by heat treatment. Appl Environ Microbiol 50(2): 298–303, 1985
92. Braun V, Rotering H, Ohms J P, Hagenmaier H: Conformational studies on murein-lipoprotein from the outer membrane of *Escherichia coli*. Eur J Biochem 15, 70(2): 601–610, 1976
93. Hirota Y, Mordoh J, Jacob F: Related Articles: On the process of cellular division in *Escherichia coli*. 3. Thermosensitive mutants of *Escherichia coli* altered in the process of DNA initiation. J Mol Biol 14, 53(3): 369–387, 1970
94. Yem D W, Wu H C: Physiological characterization of an *Escherichia coli* mutant altered in the structure of murein lipoprotein. J Bacteriol 133(3): 141–142, 1978
95. Sonntag I, Schwarz H, Hirota Y, Henning U: Cell envelope and shape of *Escherichia coli*: multiple mutants missing the outer membrane lipoprotein and other major outer membrane proteins. J Bacteriol 136(1): 280–285, 1978
96. Jung H: A generalized concept for cell killing by heat. Radiat Res 106: 56–72, 1986
97. Moritz A, Schoop U, Jiru E, Goharkhay K, Wernisch J, Sperr W: Morphological Changes of *E. coli* and *E. faecalis* after Er:YAG and Nd:YAG Laser Irradiation through Different Layers of Dentin. Abstract. 2nd Congress of the European Society for Oral Laser Applications, Florence 05/15/2003–05/18/2003
98. Midda M, Renton-Harper P: Lasers in dentistry. Br Dent J 11, 170(9): 343–346, 1991
99. Fegan S E, Steiman H R: Comparative evaluation of the antibacterial effects of intracanal Nd:YAG laser irradiation: an in vitro study. J Endod 21(8): 415–417, 1995
100. Moshonov J, Sion A, Kasirer J, Rotstein I, Stabholz A: Efficacy of argon laser irradiation in removing intracanal debris. Oral Surg Oral Med Oral Pathol Oral Radiol Endod 79(2): 221–225, 1995
101. Gutknecht N, Kaiser F, Hassan A, Lampert F: Long-term clinical evaluation of endodontically treated teeth by Nd:YAG lasers. J Clin Laser Med Surg 14(1): 7–11, 1996
102. Moritz A, Doertbudak O, Gutknecht N, Goharkhay K, Schoop U, Sperr W: Nd:YAG laser irradiation of infected root canals in combination with microbiological examinations. J Am Dent Assoc 128(11): 1525–1530, 1997
103. Ramskold L O, Fong C D, Stromberg T: Thermal effects and antibacterial properties of energy levels required to sterilize stained root canals with an Nd:YAG laser. J Endod 23(2): 96–100, 1997
104. Beriken M, Berkiten R, Oskar I: Comparative evaluation of antibacterial effects of Nd:YAG laser irradiation in root canals and dentinal tubules. J Endod 26(5): 268–270, 2000

105. Piccolomini R, d'Arcangelo C, d'Ercole S, Catamo G, Schiaffino G, Fazio P: Bacteriologic evaluation of the effect of Nd:YAG laser irradiation in experimental infected root canals. J Endod 28(4): 276–278, 2002
106. Folwaczny M, Mehl A, Jordan C, Hickel R: Antibacterial effects of pulsed Nd:YAG laser radiation at different energy settings in root canals. J Endod 28(1): 24–29, 2002
107. Goya C, Yamazaki R, Tomita Y, Kimura Y, Matsumoto K: Effects of pulsed Nd:YAG laser irradiation on smear layer at the apical stop and apical leakage after obturation. Int Endod J 33(3): 266–271, 2000
108. Saunders W P, Whitters C J, Strang R, Moseley H, Payne A P, McGad: The effect of an Nd:YAG pulsed laser on the cleaning of the root canal and the formation of a fused apical plug. Int Endod J 28(4): 213–220, 1995
109. Harashima T, Takeda F H, Kimura Y, Matsumoto K: Effect of Nd:YAG laser irradiation for removal of intracanal debris and smear layer in extracted human teeth. J Clin Laser Med Surg 15(3): 131–135, 1997
110. Goodis H E, White J M, Marshall S J, Marshall G W Jr: Scanning electron microscopic of intracanal walls dentin: hand versus laser treatment. Scanning Microsc 7(3): 979–987, 1993
111. Kaitas V, Signore A, Fonzi L, Benedicenti S, Barone M: Effects of Nd:YAG laser irradiation on the root canal wall dentin of human teeth: a SEM study. Bull Group Int Tech Sci Stomatol Odontol 43(3): 87–92, 2001
112. Zhang C, Kimura Y, Matsumoto K, Harashima T, Zhou H: Effects of pulsed Nd:YAG laser irradiation on root canal wall dentin with different laser initiators. J Endod 24(5): 352–355, 1998
113. Crespi R, Lando G, Covani U: Cleaning of Root Canals with Nd:YAG Laser: An In Vitro Study. J Oral Laser Appl 3(1): 27–31, 2002
114. Altamura C, Majori M, Bedini R, Filippini P: Evaluation of Nd:YAG Laser Effects on Root Canal Walls. J Oral Laser Appl 3(2): 67–72, 2003
115. Blum J Y, Abadie M J: Study of the Nd:YAG laser. Effect on canal cleanliness. J Endod 23(11): 669–675, 1997
116. Barbakow F, Peters O, Havranek L: Effects of Nd:YAG lasers on root canal walls: a light and scanning electron microscopic study. Quintessence Int 30(12): 837–845, 1999
117. Schaller H G, Weihing T, Strub J R: Permeability of dentin after Nd:YAG laser treatment: an in vitro study. J Oral Rehabil 24(4): 274–281, 1997
118. Dederich D N, Zakariasen K L, Tulip J: Scanning electron microscopic analysis of canal wall dentin following neodymium-yttrium-aluminum-garnet laser irradiation. J Endod 10(9): 428–431, 1984
119. Miserendino L J, Levy G C, Rizoiu I M: Effects of Nd:YAG laser on the permeability of root canal wall dentin. J Endod 21(2): 83–87, 1995
120. Moritz A, Gutknecht N, Schoop U, Goharkhay K, Doertbudak O, Sperr W: Irradiation of infected root canals with a diode laser in vivo: results of microbiological examinations. Lasers Surg Med 21(3): 221–226, 1997
121. Moritz A, Gutknecht N, Goharkhay K, Schoop U, Wernisch J, Sperr W: In vitro irradiation of infected root canals with a diode laser: results of microbiologic, infrared spectrometric, and stain penetration examinations. Quintessence Int 28(3): 205–209, 1997
122. Gutknecht N, Moritz A, Conrads C, Lampert F. Der Diodenlaser und seine bakterizide Wirkung im Wurzelkanal: Eine in vitro Studie. Endodontie 3: 217–222, 1997
123. Gutknecht N, Alt T, Slaus G, Bottenberg P, Rosseel P, Lauwers S, Lampert F: A Clinical Comparison of the Bactericidal Effect of the Diode Laser and 5% Sodium Hypochlorite in Necrotic Root Canals. J Oral Laser Appl 2(3): 151–157, 2002
124. Patruta S, Moritz A: In vitro stimulation of the production of tissue inhibitor of matrix metallo proteinases 1 (TIMP-1) in human gingival fibroblasts after diode laser irradiation, JOLA 3/04
125. Moritz A: New Aspects in Laser Supported Endodontics, Abstract. Alpe Adria Kongress, Bled, May 7–8, 2004
126. Paghdiwala A F: Root resection of endodontically treated teeth by erbium:YAG laser radiation. J Endod 19(2): 91–94, 1993
127. Komori T, Yokoyama K, Takato T, Matsumoto K: Clinical application of the erbium:YAG laser for apicoectomy. J Endod 23(12): 748–750, 1997
128. Komori T, Yokoyama K, Matsumoto Y, Matsumoto K: Erbium:YAG and holmium:YAG laser root resection of extracted human teeth. J Clin Laser Med Surg 15(1): 9–13, 1997
129. Moritz A, Schoop U, Goharkhay K, Jakolitsch S, Kluger W, Wernisch J, Sperr W: The bactericidal effect of Nd:YAG, Ho:YAG, and Er:YAG laser irradiation in the root canal: an in vitro comparison. J Clin Laser Med Surg 17(4): 161–164, 1999
130. Jelinkova H, Dostalova T, Duskova J, Kratky M, Miyagi M, Shoji S, Sulc J, Nemec M: Er:YAG and alexandrite laser radiation propagation in root canal and its effect on bacteria. J Clin Laser Med Surg 17(69): 267–272, 1999
131. Schoop U, Moritz A, Kluger W, Patruta S, Goharkhay K, Sperr W, Wernisch J, Gattringer R, Mrass P, Georgopoulos A: The Er:YAG laser in endodontics: results of an in vitro study. Lasers Surg Med 30(5): 360–364, 2002
132. Schoop U, Kluger W, Moritz A, Nedjelik N, Georgopoulos A, Sperr W: Bactericidal Effect of Different Laser Systems in the Deep Layers of Dentin. (in press)
133. Chen W H: Laser root canal therapy. J Indiana Dent Assoc 81(4): 20–23, 2002–2003
134. Matsouka E, Kimura Y, Matsumoto K: Studies on the removal of debris near the apical seats by Er:YAG laser and assessment with a fiberscope. J Clin Laser Med Surg 16(5): 255–261, 1998
135. Takeda F H, Harashima T, Kimura Y, Matsumoto K: A comparative study of the removal of smear layer by three endodontic irrigants and two types of laser. Int Endod J 32(1): 32–39, 1999
136. Shoji S, Hariu H, Horiuchi H: Canal enlargement by Er:YAG laser using a cone-shaped irradiation tip. J Endod 26(8): 454–458, 2000

137. Takeda F H, Harashima T, Kimura Y, Matsumoto K: Efficacy of Er:YAG laser irradiation in removing debris and smear layer on root canal walls. J Endod 24(8): 548–551, 1998
138. Yamazaki R, Goya C, Yu D G, Kimura Y, Matsumoto K: Effects of erbium, chromium:YSGG laser irradiation on root canal walls: a scanning electron microscopic and thermographic study. J Endod 27(1): 9–12, 2001
139. Kesler G, Gal R, Kesler A, Koren R: Histological and scanning electron microscope examination of root canal after preparation with Er:YAG laser microprobe: preliminary in vitro study. J Clin Laser Med Surg 20(5): 269–277, 2002
140. Matsumoto K: Laser in endodontics. Dent Clin North Am 44(49): 889–906, 2000
141. Kimura Y, Yamazaki R, Goya C, Tomita Y, Yokoyama K, Matsumoto K: A comparative study on the effects of three types of laser irradiation at the apical stop and apical leakage after obturation. J Clin Laser Med Surg 17(6): 261–266, 1999
142. Park D S, Lee H J, Yoo H M, Oh T S: Effect of Nd:YAG laser irradiation on the apical leakage of obturated root canals: an electrochemical study. Int Endod J 34(4): 318–321, 2001
143. Gekelman D, Prokopowitsch I, Eduardo C P: In vitro study of the effects of Nd:YAG laser irradiation on the apical sealing of endodontic fillings performed with and without dentin plugs. J Clin Laser Med Surg 20(3): 117–121, 2002
144. Yamazaki R, Goya C, Tomita Y, Kimura Y, Matsumoto K: Study on apical leakage of the teeth after argon laser treatment and obturation. J Clin Laser Med Surg 17(3): 121–125, 1999
145. Kimura Y, Yonaga K, Yokoyama K, Matsuoka E, Sakai K, Matsumoto K: Apical leakage of obturated canals prepared by Er:YAG laser. J Endod 27(9): 567–570, 2001
146. Khan M A, Khan M F, Khan M W, Wakabayashi H, Matsumoto K:. Effect of laser treatment on the root canal of human teeth. Endod Dent Traumatol 13(3): 139–145, 1997
147. Schoop U, Moritz A, Kluger W, Starzengruber P, Goharkhay K., Wernisch J, Sperr W: Laser assisted Apex Scaling: Results of a Pilot Study. J Oral Laser Appl 4(3):175–182, 2004
148. Blankenau R J, Kelsey W P, Powell G L, Cavel W T, Anderson D M: Power density and external temperature of laser-treated root canals. J Clin Laser Med Surg 12(1): 17–19, 1994
149. Anic I, Tachibana H, Matsumoto K, Qi P: Permeability, morphologic and temperature changes of canal dentine walls induced by Nd:YAG, CO_2 and argon lasers. Int Endod J 29(1): 13–22, 1996
150. Cohen B I, Deutsch A S, Musikant B: Effect of power settings on temperature change at the root surface when using a Holmium:YAG laser in enlarging the root canal. J Endod 22(11): 596–599, 1996
151. Cohen B I, Deutsch A S, Musikant B L, Pagnillo M K: Effect of power settings versus temperature change at the root surface when using multiple fiber sizes with a Holmium:YAG laser while enlarging a root canal. J Endod 24(12): 802–806, 1998
152. Machida T, Wilder-Smith P, Arrastia A M, Liaw LH, Berns M W: Root canal preparation using the second harmonic KTP:YAG laser: a thermographic and scanning electron microscopic study. J Endod 21(2): 88–91, 1995
153. Behrens V G, Gutknecht N, Renziehausen R, Lampert F: Die Transmission und Absorption der Temperatur und Energie des Nd:YAG-Lasers im Dentin. ZWR 102(9): 629–634, 1993
154. Farge P, Nahas P, Bonin P: In vitro study of a Nd:YAG laser in endodontic retreatment. J Endod 24(5): 359–363, 1998
155. Lan W H: Temperature elevation on the root surface during Nd:YAG laser irradiation in the root canal. J Endod 25(3): 155–156, 1999
156. Kreisler M, Kohnen W, Beck M, Al Haj H, Christoffers A B, Gotz H, Duschner H, Jansen B, D'Hoedt B: Efficacy of $NaOCl/H_2O_2$ irrigation and GaAlAs laser in decontamination of root canals in vitro. Lasers Surg Med 32(3): 189–196, 2003
157. Kimura Y, Yonaga K, Yokoyama K, Kinoshita J, Ogata Y, Matsumoto K: Root surface temperature increase during Er:YAG laser irradiation of root canals. J Endod 28(2): 76–78, 2002
158. Takashiba S et al.: Perspectives of cytokine regulation for periodontal treatment: fibroblast biology. J Periodontol 74: 103–110, 2003
159. Pitaru et al.: Cellular origins and differentiation control mechanisms during periodontal development and wound healing. J Periodontal Res 29: 81–94, 1994
160. Bliddal H et al.: Soft laser therapy of rheumatoid arthritis. Scand J Rheumatol 16: 225–228, 1987
161. Honmura A et al.: Therapeutic effect of Ga-Al-As diode laser irradiation on experimentally induced inflammation in rats. Lasers Surg Med 12: 441–449, 1992
162. Sakurai Y et al.: Inhibitory effect of low-level laser irradiation on LPS-stimulated prostaglandin E2 production and cyclooxygenase-2 in human gingival fibroblasts. Eur J Oral Sci 108: 29–34, 2000
163. Nomura K et al.: Inhibition of Interleukin-1β Production and Gene Expression in Human Gingival Fibroblasts by Low Laser Irradiation. Lasers Med Sci 16: 218–223, 2001
164. Kreisler M et al.: Low level 809 nm diode laser-induced in vitro stimulation of proliferation of human gingival fibroblasts. Lasers Surg Med 30: 365–369, 2002
165. Feist I S et al.: Adhesion and growth of cultured human gingival fibroblasts and periodontally involved root surfaces treated by Er:YAG laser. J Periodontol 74: 1368–1375, 2003
166. Kreisler M et al.: Effect of diode laser irradiation on survival rate of gingival fibroblast cell cultures. Lasers Surg Med 28: 445–450, 2001

7

Pulp Capping and Pulpotomy in Permanent and Primary Teeth

A. Pescheck, A. Moritz

7.1 Direct Pulp Capping

7.1.1 Introduction

Direct pulp capping is considered as a valid treatment method in today's endodontics, because successful capping can preserve tooth vitality in an exposed cavity. As far back as 1765, Pfaff[1] worked on the problem of treating exposed pulp cavities. From today's standpoint, direct pulp capping is only indicated when the pulp is exposed during removal of healthy dentin. Most importantly, chronic or sub-acute forms of pulpitis, which means an inflammatory alteration of the pulp, must not be present. The major state-of-the-art capping regimens today comprise calcium hydroxide dressing, the total-etch–total-bond technique associated with esthetic composite restorations and as indicated in this chapter here, CO_2 laser irradiation of exposed pulps. Schroeder[2] and Kopel[3] stated that direct capping is indicated only in pulps that have not been affected by inflammation a priori. The pulpal organ itself should have the capacity for tertiary dentin formation, meaning that a plethora of valid cells is present: odontoblasts, fibroblasts and undifferentiated mesenchymal cells must be in the immediate area allowing healing and tight wound closure. Thus, profound caries and subsequent chronic or asymptomatic inflammation of the pulp organ greatly reduces the possibilities of a successful healing process[1]. In addition, the size[4,5] of the wound aperture and the age[6] of the patient influences the therapeutic outcome to a large extent. In general, dentinal wounds smaller than 1 mm^2 exhibit a good chance of pulpal regeneration[4]. The younger the patient, the better the prognosis for dentin bridging and pulpal healing.

In 592 cases followed up to a total of 1429 cases, Reuver[4] found a success rate of 91% in the group of 10–20-year-old patients, which continuously dropped to 58% in the group of 70–80-year-old patients. In a type of opening that the author described as "punctiform", the success rate was ~ 73%. When an area of 1–9 mm^2 was exposed, it was 61%. A total of 68% of the teeth were vital at the last recall examination. However, the timing of the last recall examination varied between 4 months and 24 years in Reuver's study. In 1979, a long-term study by Marti[6] revealed that successful healing depends on the age of the patients. He found a success rate of 84% in 10–25-year-old patients, which dropped to only 44% in 46–70-year-old patients. This may be due to the fact that the pulps of younger subjects are richer in cells and have a higher ability to regenerate.

Further, it was shown that infection and inflammation after treatment occurred also due to a non-sterile procedure or bacterial leakage at the capping site[7]. The use of rubber dam isolation therefore is indispensable[8]. It also appears that capping performed by skilled practitioners is more successful than that performed by students.

Finally, the bleeding occurring after traumatic or iatrogenic exposure of the pulp must not be profuse and has to cease prior to the dressing of the wound. Several studies found that the size of perforation is less important than obtaining hemostasis[9–14]. If bleeding fails to stop after two or three attempts then endodontical treatment should be considered[15,16].

The success rates reported in the literature vary between 44% and 95%[1,4,6,17]. The nature and specificity of the mechanism by which the exposed pulp interface is therapeutically treated determine the properties of the barrier at this site and play a critical role in the outcome of vital pulp therapy.

The healing of the pulp exposures depends on the capacity of the capping material to prevent bacterial microleakage[18]. Pashley[19] stated that to minimize the pulpal response, restorative materials must seal the cavity margins, prevent microleakage and block bacterial substrates from penetrating through dentinal tubules to the pulp. However, if microleakage around various restorations could be measured in vivo, it's likely that all would exhibit some degree of leakage[20].

Therefore, it is desirable to maximize the barrier effect of dentin to provide the best pulpal protection[20].

7.1.2 Conventional Pulp Capping

Long lists of different capping materials have been proposed in recent years with varying success rates.

7.1.2.1 Calcium Hydroxide

Calcium hydroxide has demonstrated its success over a long period of time and is the capping material of choice in most dental schools and private practices.

Several preparations are commercially available[21]. Due to superficial necrosis, resulting from the high alkaline pH of the capping material and the subsequent formation of fiber-rich scar tissue, normal pulp cells are transformed into secondary odontoblasts and tertiary dentin is formed[1].

The conventional treatment regimes are founded on a bacteria-free, tight capping of the pulp wound and a provisional filling with a minimum of microleakage.

The first treatment step is to control the bleeding by washing the area with sterile saline followed by the application of cotton pellets soaked with hydrogen peroxide or 5% sodium hypochlorite. Sometimes it can also be useful to use additionally a hemostatic agent[15]. After the hemostasis, the cavity floor should be treated with a disinfectant[22] such as Consepsis® or Cavity Cleanser®. After air drying, the calcium hydroxide is applied to the site of exposure directly in contact with the pulpal tissue. This has to be done very carefully because it was shown the better the contact of the calcium hydroxide with the pulpal wound, the better the healing chance[15,21]. After the calcium hydroxide dressing, either resin-modified glass ionomer cements or immediate restorative materials are suggested as temporary filling material. Three months later, assuming pulp vitality and no symptoms, a final restoration can be made.

According to numerous investigations, a tight contact between the dressing and the injured pulpal tissue is desirable for the healing process.

The opponents of calcium hydroxide claim that it does not exclusively stimulate sclerotic dentin formation, dentinogenesis, reparative dentin formation or dentin bridge formation[23]. They claim that it disintegrates and is lost after a period of 1 year, that acids will degrade the interface during etching, and that calcium hydroxide will not adhere to bonding resin composite systems. Goracci et al.[24] found that calcium hydroxide placed under composite restorations seemed to pull away from the cavity surface during resin polymerization and a gap between the dentin and the calcium hydroxide occurred. Another study showed multiple tunnel defects (89%) in dentin bridges under the calcium hydroxide. The author of this article suggested that therefore the long-term effect of calcium hydroxide has to be put in serious doubt.

7.1.2.2 Total Etch Technique

The direct pulp capping technique with adhesive systems has recently been advocated with mixed evidence of clinical success from vital pulp therapy performed in animals and human teeth. Recent ISO usage studies have shown a high incidence of dentin bridging with adhesives following proper hemorrhage control and removal of both operative debris and biofilm at the dentin–pulp interface by agents such as NaOCl[5]. Fujitanti[25] compared two different adhesive systems, Clearfil Liner Bond® and Super Bond Liner®, and found that although both of them appear to be effective as pulp capping material, the process and durability of the pulpal healing process was substantially different. Arakawa et al.[26] found in his study slight inflammatory cells in the pulp but the exposed pulp became occluded with dentin bridges within the observation period of 90 days. On the other hand, recent studies performed in human teeth have demonstrated that following the application of different adhesive systems to pulpal wounds, the material delayed pulpal healing, resulting in a lack of dentin bridge formation, even 60 days after the pulp capping procedure[27]. The pulp exposure site showed persistent inflammatory responses evidenced by macrophages and giant cells[28–30]. Finally, Cox et al.[5] stated in his review article that there are important technique-sensitive factors to be considered for pulp healing and dentin bridge formation. Whether the total-etch technique offers an equivalent or superior prognosis will be the subject of many more long-term studies.

7.1.2.3 Mineral Trioxide Aggregate (MTA)

MTA is cement composed of tricalcium silicate, dicalcium silicate, tricalcium aluminate, tetracalcium aluminoferrite, calcium sulfate and bismuth oxide[31]. Mineral trioxide aggregate is very alkaline, and it can be compared to calcium hydroxide when it comes to some of its biological and histological properties. MTA sets in about 3 h in the presence of moisture; working time is 5 min. Histological evaluation demonstrated less inflammation, hyperemia and necrosis, plus thicker dentinal bridge and more frequent odontoblastic layer formation with MTA than with calcium hydroxide[32,33]. Other experiments indicated as well that MTA is an effective pulp-capping material, able to stimulate reparative dentin formation by the stereotypic defensive mechanism of early pulpal wound healing[34]. The material has to be mixed with sterile water to provide a grainy, sandy mixture. The MTA should be placed with the carrier provided or with a large plastic amalgam carrier.

Afterwards the mixture has to be pushed against the exposure site with a moist cotton pellet. The tooth should be temporized with a moist pellet in place because of the long setting time. Pulp status should be evaluated prior to placing a permanent restoration.

7.1.2.4 Bioactive Molecules

Progress in biomedical research has opened new directions for the design of biologically effective pulp therapies. After the application of biocompatible and biodegradable vehicles for local delivery of signaling molecules, pulp capping situations showed induction of fibro dentin/reparative dentin formation[35].

Experimental studies showed that pulpal cells can differentiate directly into odontoblast-like cells in association with specific extracellular matrices (dentinal or fibrodentinal matrix) or TGF β1-containing artificial substrates. Other studies[36,37] investigated the fact that enamel matrix derivate (EMD) used as pulp capping material can cause calcification of dental pulp tissue. Bioactive molecules can be used as the master plan for the achievement of new therapeutic opportunities[38] in the future.

7.1.2.5 Antibiotics

Antibiotics were highlighted as valuable preparations early on. They were suggested for direct pulp capping but have become obsolete in state-of-the-art pulp capping materials. Antibiotics were applied to reduce the bacterial load. But although the bacterial count was proven to be reduced, no growth of tertiary dentin could be found[39].

A study in monkeys[40] investigated that antibacterial drugs added to α-tricalcium phosphate effectively disinfect pulpal lesions, without destroying any of the sound pulp tissue. However, hard tissue barrier formation was not evident or delayed by this mixture as compared with calcium hydroxide.

7.1.2.6. Corticosteroids

Corticosteroids are also of historical interest today in respect to pulpal recovery. They do help to control the pain but no evidence of tertiary dentin formation has been found[41]. Some calcium hydroxide preparations still have corticosteroids added to their formula.

7.1.3 Laser-Assisted Pulp Capping

Lasers have been investigated in dentistry for over two decades, but have come into the forefront as an everyday tool only in the last few years. Refinements in the technology have led to an increasing number of applications. Between 1985 and 1987 Melcer et al.[42-44] suggested that the CO_2 laser could be used for direct pulp capping. They even described successful pulp restoration after direct capping of inflamed pulps with laser[43]. Ebihara et al.[45] used the Nd:YAG laser for exposed pulps of rats and for experimental pulpal capping in dogs[46].

7.1.3.1 Nd:YAG

A retrospective study by Santucci[47] compared the survival rates of a total of 93 permanent teeth in 83 patient; 29 with calcium hydroxide (Dyral®) and 94 with Nd:YAG laser and Vitrebond®. He found that the cumulative proportion of teeth surviving postoperatively in the Dycal group cap was 89.7% at 1 month declining to 79.4% at 3 months, 76% at 6 months and then continued to decline in the final two intervals finishing after 54 months at 43.5%.

For the laser and Vitrebond® direct pulp capping group, the cumulative proportion surviving stood at 98.4% after 1 month, declining to 93.8% at 3 months, 90.3% after 6 months but then held steady in the final two intervals finishing at 90.3% after 54 months. This study showed that the success rates after direct pulp capping with an Nd:YAG laser and Vitrebond® are significantly higher compared to the conventional calcium hydroxide treatment.

7.1.3.2 Er:YAG

The pulpal response to the Er:YAG laser after accidental pulp exposure was evaluated in an vivo study in rats[48]. In comparison to the conventional control group the authors found significantly more dentin formation and a better healing capacity in the laser group. However, further prospective in vivo studies about the YAG lasers with long-term results should be done.

The study by Jayawardena[48] evaluated the pulpal response to the Er:YAG laser after accidental exposure of the pulp. In 76 maxillary first molars of male Wistar rats, cavities were prepared, and pulps were exposed by either Er:YAG laser (150 mJ/ pulse, 10 pulses with a wavelength of $\lambda = 2.94$ μm and a contact tip with a diameter of 600 μm) or conventionally by a slow-speed round bur. The rats were sacrificed immediately, 3 days, 1 week and 2 weeks after the treatment. The histopathological examination found that the Er:YAG laser group showed no bleeding and no dentin chips at the exposure site immediately after pulp exposure. The Er:YAG group showed more reparative dentin formation and formed more frequently dentin bridges at the exposure site than the control group. According to the results of this study, Er:YAG laser-exposed pulp tissue demonstrated good healing capacity with the formation of a dentin bridge and reparative dentin.

7.1.3.3 CO_2 Laser

The CO_2 laser offers new perspectives and possibilities in various medical applications. In addition to being a valuable surgical tool, this wavelength offers also innovative options in the field of conservative dentistry. Furthermore, CO_2 laser irradiation has proven to be a valuable therapy in today's endodontics, primarily as an aid in direct pulp capping. Since the rate of failure for conventional methods is in many cases unsatisfactorily high, the search for an alternative has started to improve the chances of success for direct pulp capping. The question that arose immediately was whether the CO_2-laser would improve these success rates. The most important effects of CO_2 laser irradiation seem to be sterilization and scar formation in the irradiated area due to thermal effects, which may help to preserve the pulp from bacterial invasion. Many authors feel that the absence of pathogenic germs during the pulp capping procedure is associated with a positive treatment outcome. In addition, many authors associate the CO_2 soft tissue surgery with reduced swelling, edema and pain. Thus, laser irradiation should minimize the formation of a hematoma between the pulp tissue and the hydroxide dressing, allowing a tight contact of the dressing to the exposed pulp. Another effect of laser treatment might be the direct stimulation of dentin formation, as indicated by Paschoud and Holz[49].

The CO_2 laser emits at a wavelength of $\lambda = 10.6$ μm, which is readily absorbed in the abundant water of soft tissues. Tissue penetration of the laser beam is minimal (100 μm) and the laser effects remain superficial and limited to the impact area. Since the irradiation of the exposed pulps is undertaken in non-contact mode, iatrogenic bacterial contamination of the treated site can be minimized per se.

Because the CO_2 laser can be operated in a superpulsed mode (as opposed to continuous wave mode – cw mode) thermal stress of the surrounding tissues and thus collateral damage to dental hard tissues are greatly reduced.

Long intervals (1 s) between the pulses (0.1 s), a relatively low power setting of 1 W and the wavelength of $\lambda = 10.6$ μm which is absorbed within ~100 μm by water, seem to be sufficient to avoid any thermal damage of the pulp[50]. Regarding the superpulsed laser, the further reduced thermal stress to the pulp seems to be responsible for higher success rates in comparison to the cw laser.

7.1.3.3.1 Success Rates of CO_2 Laser-Assisted Pulp Capping

According to various long-term studies performed at the Department of Conservative Dentistry of the dental school of the University of Vienna, laser-treated teeth showed only insignificant pulp capping failures whereas pulps dressed with calcium hydroxide alone exhibit a pronounced loss of tooth vitality.

The long-term results of Moritz et al.[51] exhibited a success rate of 93%, 2 years after superpulsed

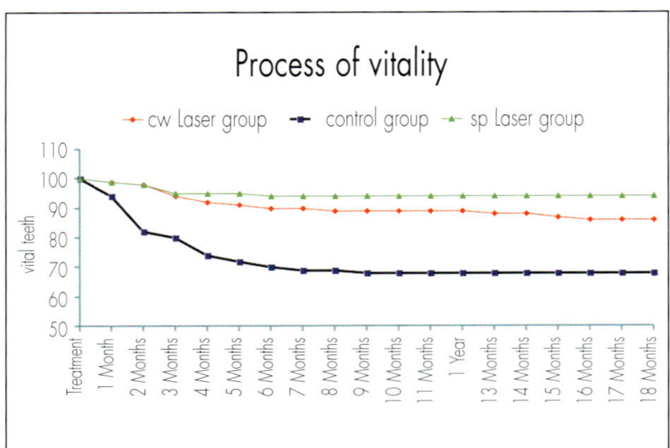

Fig 7-1 Course of vitality of teeth treated with laser-assisted pulp capping either in continuous mode or in the superpulsed mode compared to the conventional method of calcium hydroxide alone. The chance of success improved significantly when the superpulsed laser was applied to the pulps.

CO_2 laser-assisted pulp capping. In a control group, where calcium hydroxide alone had been applied, only 68% of the teeth were vital at the last recall examination. An interesting aspect of this study was the chronological course of vitality. The most noticeable loss of tooth vitality took place within the first 4 months post-treatment. These 4 months seem to be the decisive period[51].

Another study[50] revealed that after 12 months, 89% of the laser-assisted pulp capped teeth remained vital, whereas the success rate of the control group with only calcium hydroxide was considerably lower (68%). In comparing the two studies, it became obvious that the efficiency of laser treatment can be increased by using the superpulsed mode instead of the continuous mode (Fig 7-1).

The randomized study by Moritz et al.[51] determined the effectiveness of the laser application using the superpulsed mode in comparison to a control group with calcium hydroxide. Their study included a total of 260 patients. In 130 patients, pulp capping treatment was carried out with the superpulsed CO_2 laser, whereas the remaining 130 patients were treated with a conventional capping technique with calcium hydroxide. The average age in the laser group was 34.8 years, the youngest patient being 15 years old and the oldest patient 65. The exposure sites had a mean diameter of 0.6 mm, the smallest diameter being 0.2 mm and the largest 1.2 mm. In the control group, the average age was 33.9 years, the youngest patient being 9 years old and the oldest patient being 68. The exposures had a mean diameter of 0.6 mm, the smallest diameter being 0.1 mm and the largest diameter 1.5 mm. The diameters of the exposures were assessed with the help of a calibrated magnifying glass. The exposed pulps were irradiated at a power output of 1 W at several intervals; 0.1-s pulses were followed by 1-s pulse intervals. This procedure was repeated until the exposed pulps were completely scabbed. The treated pulps were then dressed with Kerr Life® and the cavities filled with glass ionomer cement (Ketacfill®). Final filling of the cavities was carried out after 6 months. At the recall examinations 2 years after treatment, 200 patients were still available.

The patients' subjective symptoms and the vitality of the treated teeth were examined; 93% of the teeth in the laser group were vital, they showed a positive reaction to cold and a healthy perfusion index in laser Doppler measurements. Seven teeth were affected by pulpitis and required extirpation. In the control group, 68% remained vital and 32% needed endodontic treatment. None of the groups showed a significant correlation between the size of the exposed pulp region, the patient's age, the type of teeth examined and the success of treatment.

7.1.3.3.2 Procedure of CO_2 Laser-Assisted Pulp Capping

Pulp capping with a CO_2 laser represents an easy, fast and safe method to achieve hemostasis, disinfection and coagulation of exposed pulp areas. The laser beam is applied in a contact-free mode utilizing a He–Ne laser to facilitate targeting. Irradiation commences right after the exposure of the vital pulp. The area is repeatedly irradiated at a power setting of 1 W for 0.1 s with a 1-s interval until hemostasis occurs and the aperture is completely sealed (Figs 7-2 to 7-4). Due to the CO_2 laser's high absorption in water and its superficial mode of action on small blood vessels and capillaries, hemostasis can be achieved usually in 2–3 irradiation cycles.

The lased pulps are dressed with calcium hydroxide and the cavities filled with glass ionomer cement. Final filling of the cavities is recommended after 6 months in order to observe the healing process and the course of vitality. In order to closely supervise the status of tooth vitality, recall examinations should be undertaken monthly for 1 year after treatment.

The same laser parameters can be used for a direct pulp capping in primary teeth (Figs 7-5 to 7-8). For vitality assessment, a conventional cold test can be used. Alternatively, laser Doppler flowmetry can be utilized for direct measurement of the pulpal flow. Typical perfusion curves synchronous with heart beat and vasomotion can be obtained, which allows assessment of the vitality of a tooth.

7.1.4 Laser Doppler Flowmetry

Morikawa et al.[52] developed in 1972 the laser Doppler flowmetry to assess blood flow in microvascular systems such as the retina, the renal cortex or the skin. Gazelius et al.[53] adopted this original method to monitor blood flow in intact teeth. In the laser-Doppler method, laser light in the infrared range, which is delivered to the tissue to be examined, undergoes a Doppler frequency shift. A sensor records the wavelength of the light backscattered by moving particles (erythrocytes).

Conclusions about the blood flow in the capillary region of the pulp can be drawn, by comparing the wavelength of the light transmitted to the tissue under study and the backscattered light. Different wavelengths between λ = 780 and λ = 820 nm have been used for laser Doppler flowmetry. A study by Odor et al.[54] reported a good sensitivity, but poor specificity at a wavelength of λ = 810 nm. Vice versa, he found a

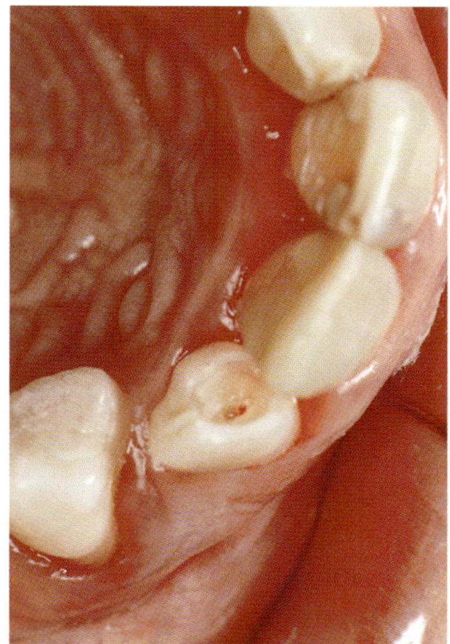

Fig 7-2 Upper secondary incisor with an extensive carious lesion on the mesio-incisal surface. A pinpoint opening of the dental pulp revealed after caries excavation. Before the laser-assisted pulp capping the dentinal wound was covered with a 3% solution of H_2O_2 applied with a sterile gauze in order to prevent contamination of the site.

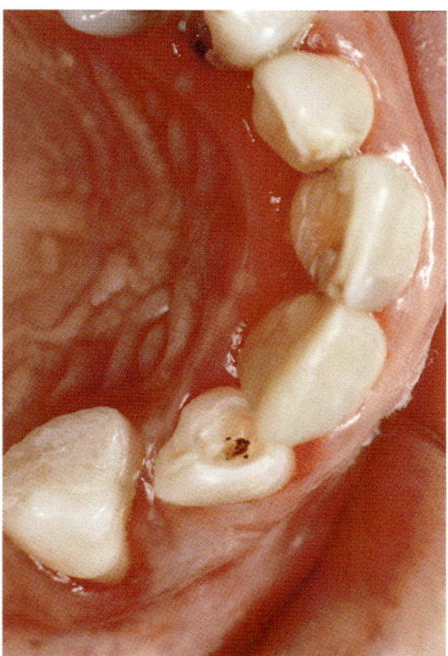

Fig 7-3 The situation after laser application with the coagulated pulp surface. The chosen parameters were 1 W for 0.1 s with 1-s interval until complete hemostasis was achieved.

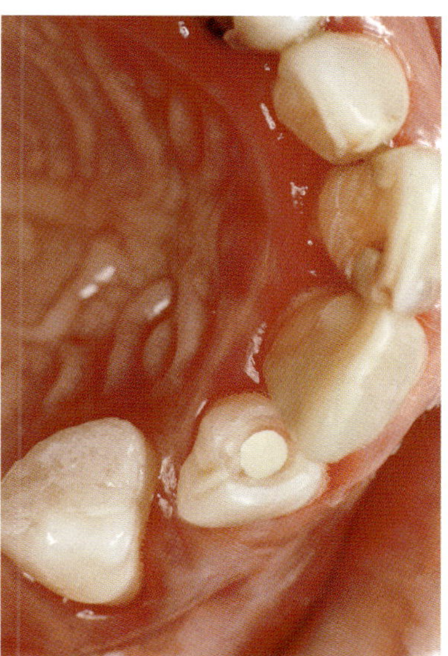

Fig 7-4 The dentinal wound was consequently covered with calcium hydroxide liner (Kerr Life®) as tightly as possible to encourage tertiary dentin formation.

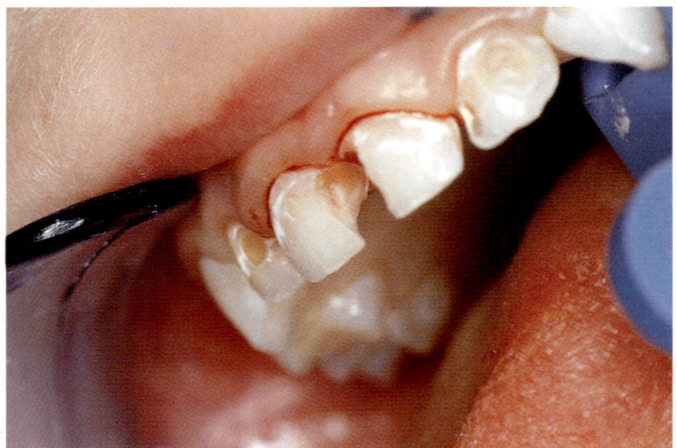

Fig 7-5 Direct pulp capping of exposed pulps of a primary incisor. Situation after caries excavation with a punctiform opening of the pulp.

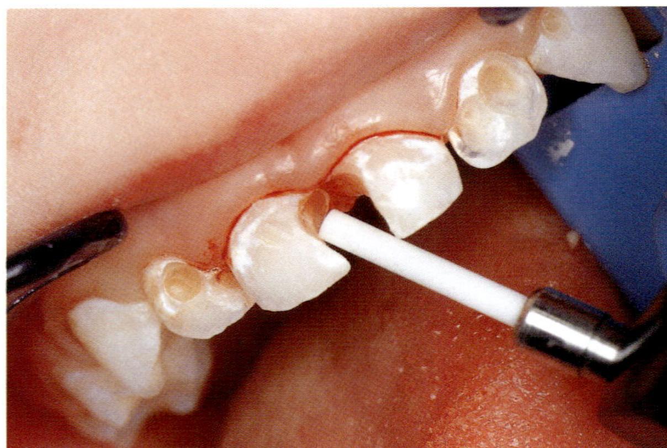

Fig 7-6 Application of the CO_2 laser using a power output of 1 W in a superpulsed mode.

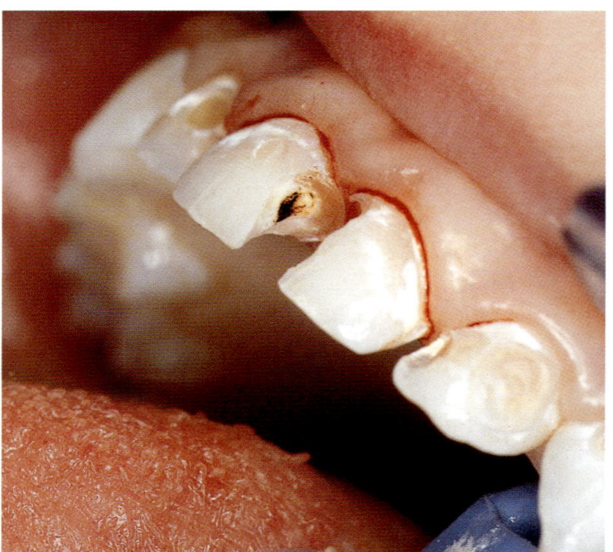

Fig 7-7 The situation after laser application with the sealed pulp.

good specificity and a poor sensitivity at a wavelength of 633 nm. Even non-laser light with a wavelength of 576 nm was suggested for the detection of pulpal perfusion[55]. Vongsavan and Matthews[56] stated that an infrared light between λ = 780 and λ = 810 nm has a better ability to penetrate enamel and dentin than red light with shorter wavelength. The control of vitality with the use of the laser Doppler technique has shown to be very reliable, also in luxated and pre-perfused teeth, as demonstrated by Olgart et al.[57]. In order to avoid motion artifacts, a silicon mask as shown in Fig 7-9 must be used for the application of the laser. Because the measurements are not affected by the function of the sensitive nerve-endings, possible false negative results of an indirect test can be avoided[58].

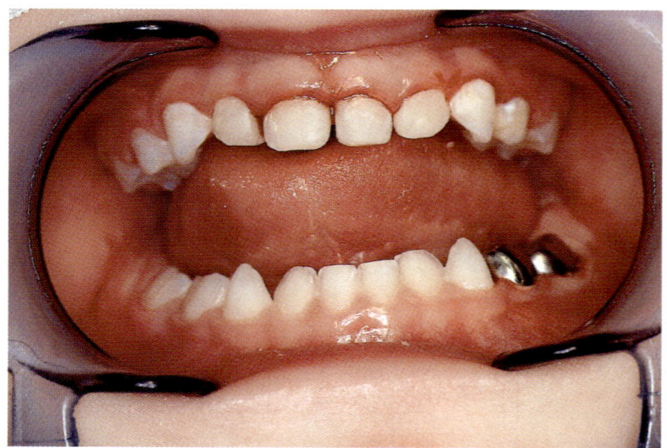

Fig 7-8 At the end of treatment after covering the pulpal wound with calcium hydroxide and the final restoration.

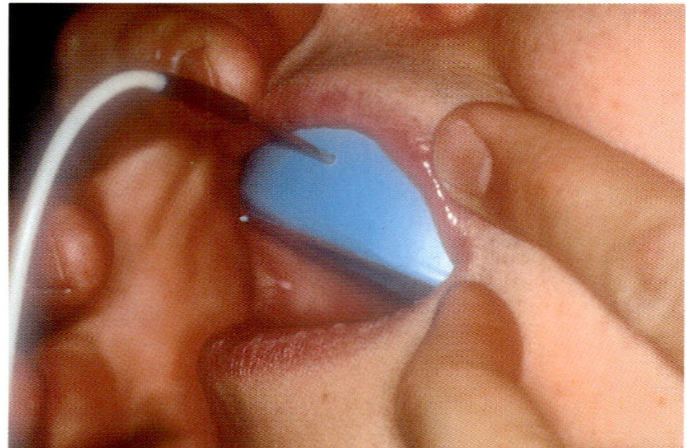

Fig 7-9 Laser Doppler flowmetry. A silicon mask must be applied to stabilize the laser Doppler microprobe to reduce motion artefacts.

7.2 Pulpotomy

7.2.1 Introduction

Pulpotomy is defined as the surgical removal of the coronal pulp in an attempt to maintain the health of the remaining pulp.

The successful treatment of root pulp stumps in vital primary molars after pulpotomy continues to be elusive. In 1904, Sweet[59] introduced the treatment of cariously exposed vital pulp with formocresol solution. Due to its good results[60] the 1:5 dilution of Buckley´s formocresol became a very popular way to treat primary teeth with exposed coronal pulpitis. Because its formaldehyde component has demonstrated mutagenic and carcinogenic potentials[61–65] several biologically more acceptable and effective alternatives have been examined[66]. Several investigations[67] on the use of calcium hydroxide found a clinical and radiological success rate between 19% and 64%. Efforts have been made in pediatric dentistry to find alternatives to formocresol and calcium hydroxide. Options range from eradication by cautery to the possibility of healing with growth factors[68]. However, results indicated that conventional formocresol pulpotomy is histopathologically superior to electrosurgery pulpotomy techniques[69]. Ferric sulfate pulpotomies with a subbase of zinc-oxide-eugenol showed an overall radiographic success rate ranging from 74% to 80%, which is comparable to those reported for 1:5 dilution, 5-min formocresol pulpotomies. The evaluation of the effectiveness of 2% buffered glutaraldehyde with zinc-oxide-eugenol as dressing material, on the radicular pulp showed 75.8% radiographic success rate[70]. Besides the results of the ferric sulfate, glutaraldehyde and iodoform paste, that have a satisfying clinical success rate, other non-pharmacological hemostatic procedures such as Nd:YAG[71,72], Ga-As semiconductor laser[73] and CO_2 laser therapy have been suggested. After the development of the ruby laser by Maiman in 1960[74], the first laser use in endodontics was reported by Weichman and Johnson[75]. Over 30 years ago the CO_2 laser became available and found widespread application in soft tissue surgery. The first laser pulpotomy was performed in 1995 by Shoji et al.[76] using the CO_2 laser in dog's followed by studies of Figueiredo et al.[77], Jukic et al.[78], Wilder-Smith et al.[79] and Dang et al.[80].

The CO_2 laser has the ability to perform precise, bloodless soft tissue surgery with minimal disturbance of the surrounding tissues[81]. Due to these abilities the CO_2 laser is not only an effective tool for direct pulp capping but for the pulpotomy of primary teeth. Wilder-Smith et al.[79] and Dang et al.[80] used the CO_2 laser in dogs and found the laser treatment to be very successful. In both cases they found no damage of the tissues underlying the ablated area produced by the laser irradiation and even demonstrated the presence of secondary dentin and a regular odontoblast layer.

7.2.2 Success Rates

A recent review of Buckley's formocresol used as a primary molar pulpotomy medicament[82] showed the agent to have a long history of clinical success. The use of a 1:5 dilution of formocresol appeared to be equally effective[83]. The long-term clinical results of the one-fifth dilution range between 90% and 98%[84]. However, the use of formocresol became a concern because its formaldehyde component showed carcinogenic and mutagenic potential[61–65]. Therefore other pharmacological agencies have been employed. Several studies using 2% buffered or unbuffered glutaraldehyde attained clinical results ranging between 75% and up to 93%[85,86]. However, toxicological investigations showed that even aqueous solutions of 2% or less are of slight toxicity[87]. In 2000, Tziafas et al.[68] reported a success rate from

74% to 80% for the use of ferric sulfate. In a recent prospective human study on electrosurgical pulpotomy, Fishman et al.[88] found a clinical success rate of 81% and 77% radiographic success.

This indicates that the above mentioned pharmacological agencies did not achieve the good clinical and radiological results of the 1:5 formocresol dilution.

Pescheck et al.[89] found that the CO_2 laser is suitable for primary teeth pulpotomy. They showed after 18 months, clinical and radiological success rates of 98.1% and 91.2%, respectively. The CO_2 laser pulpotomy was comparable to or slightly higher than the formocresol pulpotomy. Preliminary in vivo studies on the pulpotomy of dog teeth have demonstrated good results. The preconditions for successful pulpotomy were atraumatic removal of comprised pulpal tissue[90], hemostasis and minimal dot formation[91] and bacterial elimination[92]. It is also important to place a durable and tight restoration on the treated tooth. In the laser study mentioned above[80] on dogs, only teeth with insufficient fillings failed. Therefore, a restoration with stainless steel crown in primary molars is recommended after pulpotomy.

A clinical success rate of 91.2% was achieved in the superpulsed mode. In comparing the depth of thermal necrosis using the superpulsed CO_2 laser mode or the conventional laser, Fitzpatrick et al.[93] found that the superpulsed mode limited the depth of thermal necrosis by approximately a factor of two. Similarly, the study that used the CO_2 laser for direct capping obtained a markedly higher success rate in the superpulse mode than in the cw mode. A long-term study carried out by Guelmann et al.[94] revealed that the healing success of the pulpal tissue depends on the age of the patient. It is assumed[80] that due to the reduced blood supply through the closed apices of permanent teeth, their capacity for recovery after insult is inferior to that of primary teeth and therefore the laser pulp treatment may well produce better results in primary teeth.

The study by Pescheck et al.[89] treated a total of 212 teeth and observed them over a period of 18 months. The mean age of the 100 children was 4.5 years, the youngest and the oldest being 3 and 8 years old, respectively; 46% were girls and 54% were boys. After 18 months the final study sample consisted of 100 children. The overall clinical success after 18 months was 98.1%. Only 1.9% of the treated molars showed a fistula and therefore had to be extracted.

No teeth were found to exhibit clinical signs of pathologic mobility, any history of pain or early exfoliation. There was no significant difference ($p > 0.05$) between first and second primary molars, the upper or lower jaw, age or sex.

After 18 months, 91.8% of all treated teeth were radiographically unremarkable without any change compared to the baseline radiographs. The most frequently observed pulpal responses were interradicular bone destruction (4.27%) followed by internal resorption (2.52%) and uneven root resorption (1.68%). The success rate was not found to be statistically significantly dependent on the age, gender or treated teeth ($p < 0.05$ level using Fisher's exact test).

7.2.3 Procedure

The excavation of the carious dentin and the removal of the roof of the pulpal chamber, which has to be done with a high-speed hand piece and water spray (Fig 7-10), is done first. The pulp amputation has to be completed with a slow-speed round bur (Fig 7-11). If the child is treated under local anesthesia, a rubber dam should be used. In case that the child is treated in general anesthesia, the use of a rubber dam is not obligatory because of better moisture control and the lack of humidity of the breathing air (Figs 7-12 to 7-18).

Following the amputation the root pulp stumps are lased at the canal orifice (Fig 7-19). This procedure should be repeated for 5 to 10 s until a charred layer is present over the root pulp stumps and there is no evidence of recurrent bleeding.

The hemorrhagic effect can be achieved by a laser power output of 3 W in a superpulsed mode

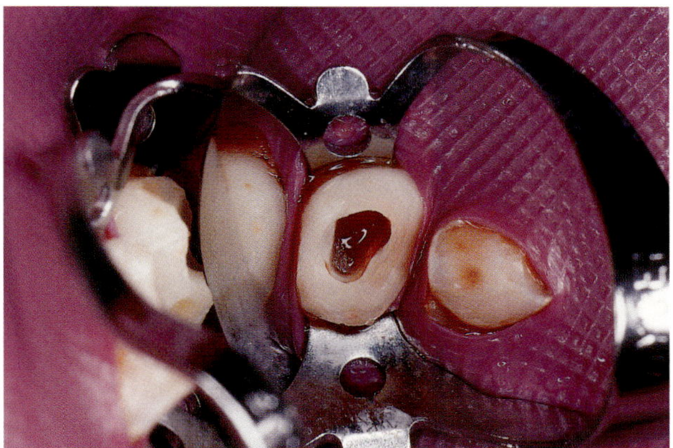

Fig 7-10 First upper left primary molar after excavation and removal of the coronal pulp.

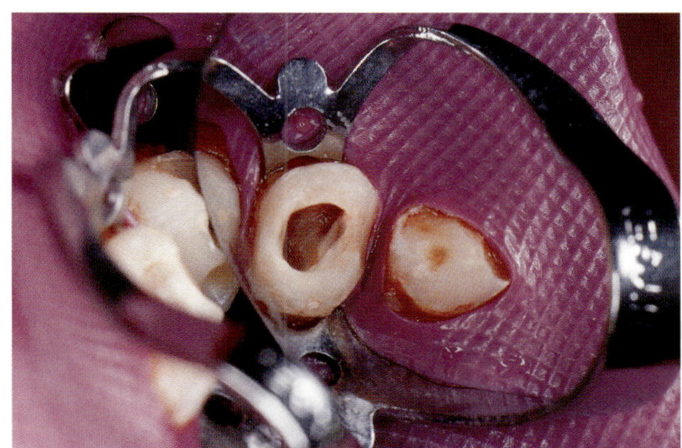

Fig 7-11 Situation after pulp amputation.

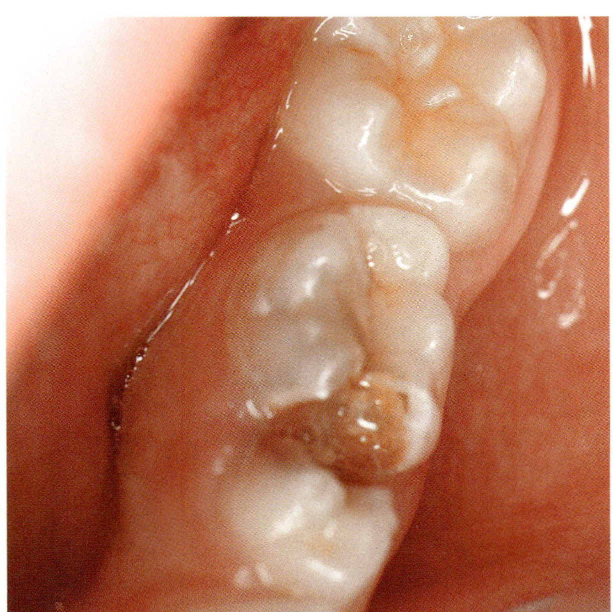

Fig 7-12 Lower left primary molar, situation prior to treatment.

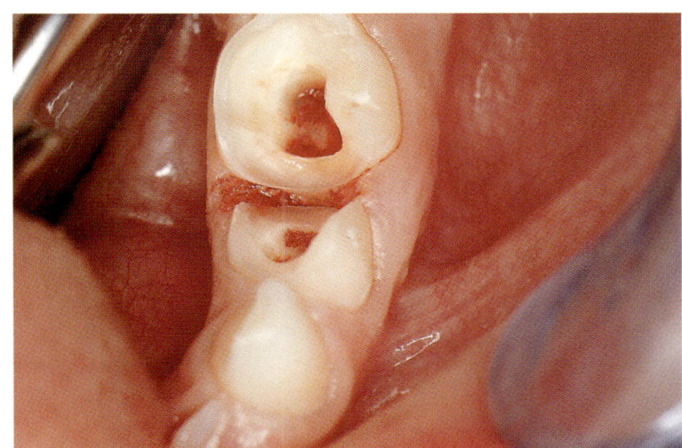

Fig 7-13 Situation after pulp amputation.

defocused (Fig 7-20). If it is not possible to achieve complete hemostasis, the extraction of the primary tooth should be considered and a space holder should be placed (Fig 77-21). For pulpotomies in primary molars it is important to use the shortest tip for the laser hand piece that the manufacturer offers or to shorten it for easy handling in the child's mouth. The ceramic tip is more efficient for hemostasis than a smaller metal tip in which it takes a longer time and more movement of the hand piece to stop the bleeding of the pulp tissue.

After cleaning the cavity with hydrogen peroxide, the treated pulp stumps have to be dressed with zinc-oxide-eugenol and Harvard cement (Fig 7-22) and the tooth should be restored with a stainless steel crown (Fig 7-23).

In some cases it is useful to remove some of the excessive gingiva around the tooth for a better placement of the pediatric steel crown. In those

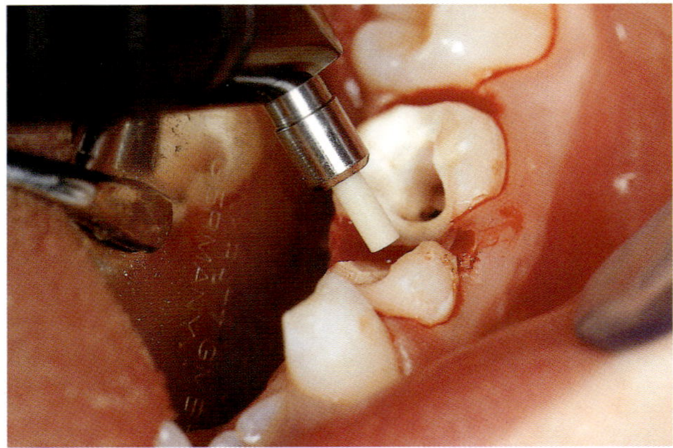

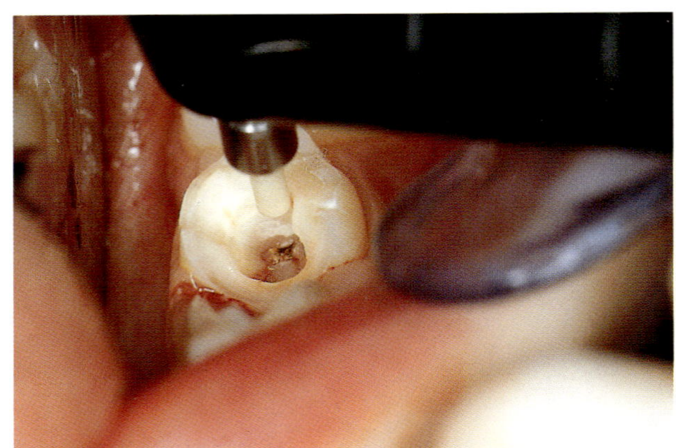

Fig 7-14 and 7-15 CO_2 laser application.

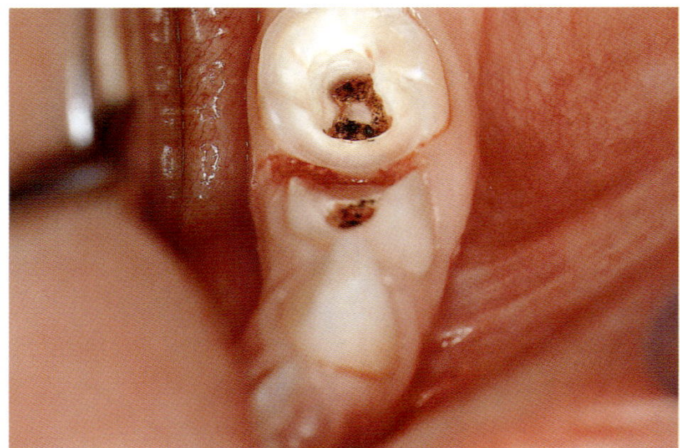

Fig 7-16 After laser irradiation and cleaning, the sealed root pulp stumps.

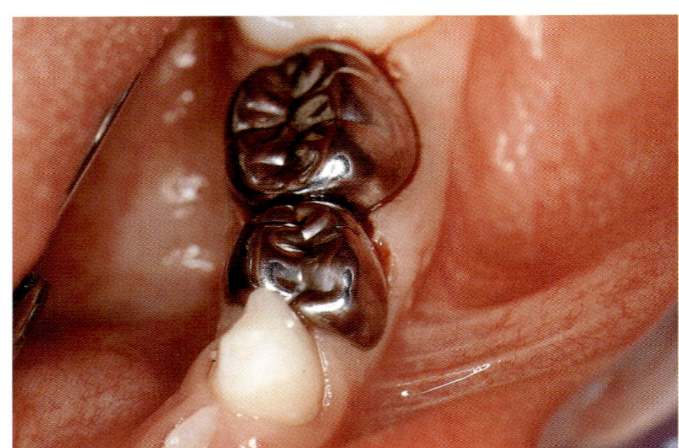

Fig 7-17 After dressing with zinc-oxide-eugenol, the final restoration with a stainless steel crown.

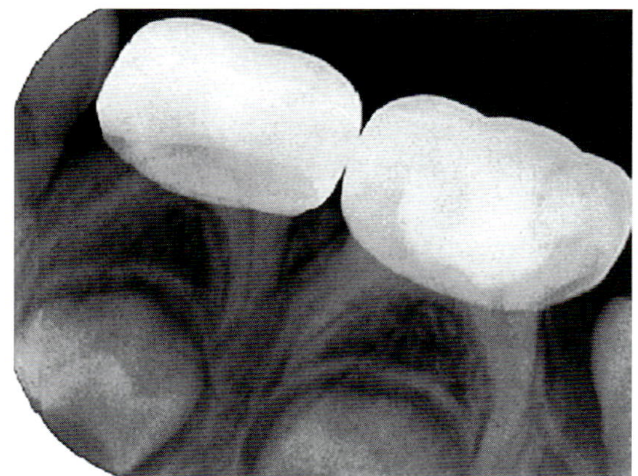

Fig 7-18 Radiograph 18 months after treatment without any signs of inflammation.

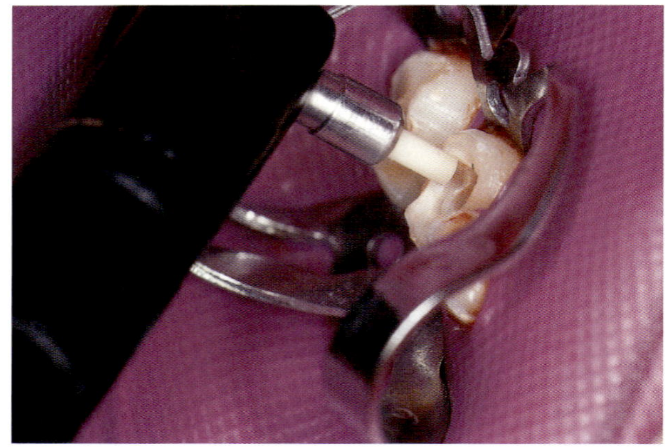

Fig 7-19 CO_2 laser application.

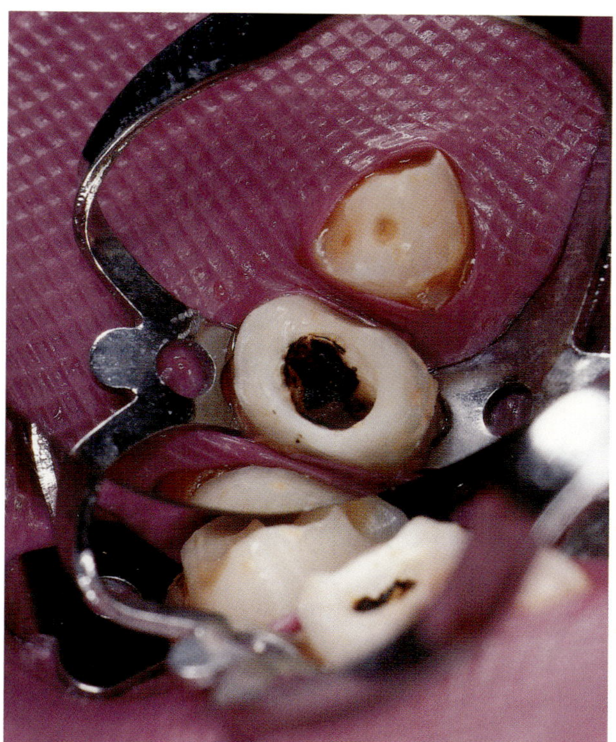

Fig 7-20 After laser irradiation with complete hemostasis.

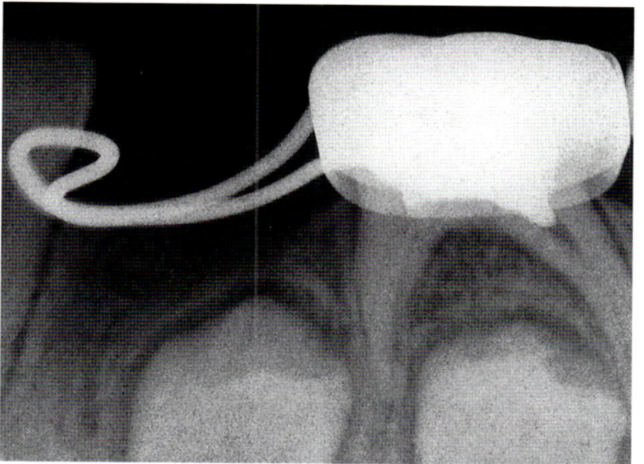

Fig 7-21 Space holder laser-welded to the stainless steel crown.

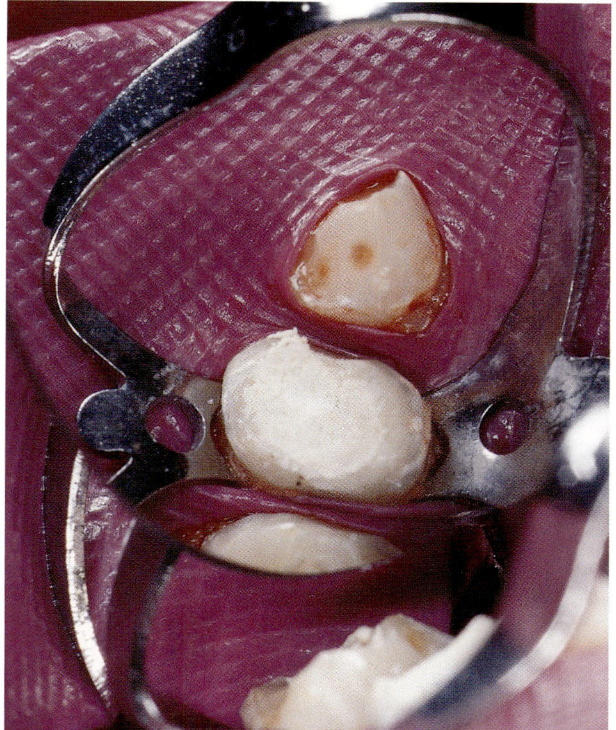

Fig 7-22 After dressing with zinc-oxide-eugenol.

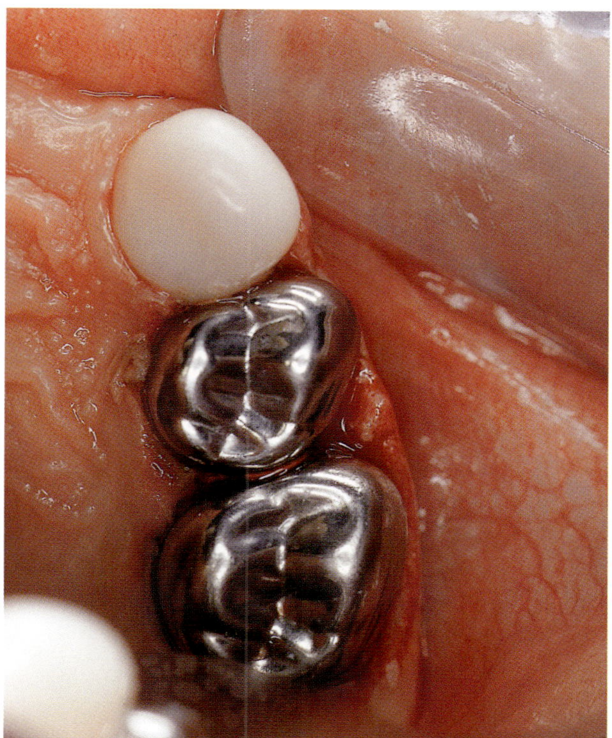

Fig 7-23 The final restoration with a stainless steel crown.

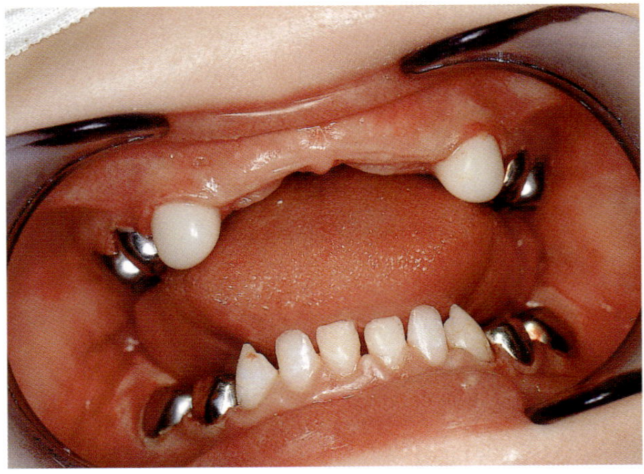

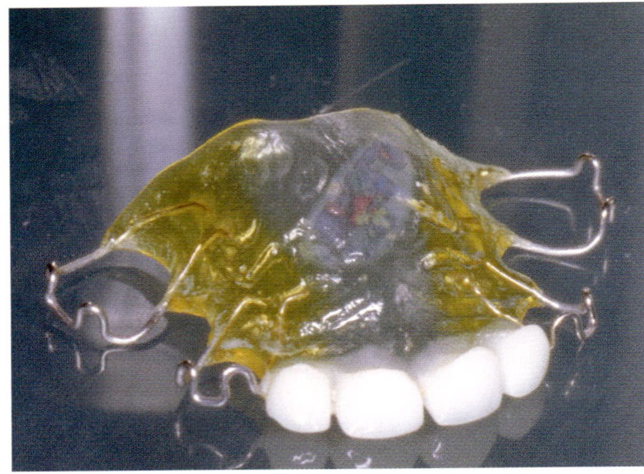

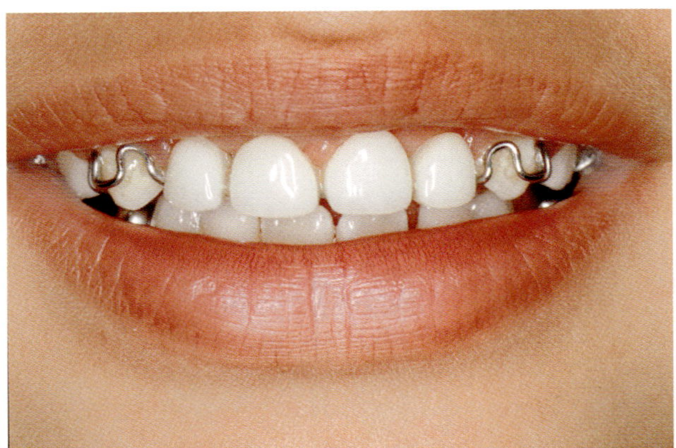

Fig 7-24 to 7-26 In some cases when all primary incisors had to be extracted we offered the patient a pediatric denture.

cases, the CO_2 laser can be used as well. Therefore the power output has to be increased to 4 W and the mode has to be changed from the superpulsed mode into the continuous wave mode. In order to protect the enamel from the laser beam during the removal of the gingiva, a metal instrument should be placed between the enamel and the laser beam. Finally, sufficient suction is important to avoid the inhalation of the removed vaporized material. The same laser parameters can be used to remove the coronal pulp instead of the slow-speed round bur. But, if the coronal pulp is removed and the laser comes closer to the channel orifice, the power output has to be reduced again to 1 W, the continuous wave mode has to be changed back into the superpulsed mode, and the treatment of the amputated pulp stumps follows as described above.

7.3 References

1. Ketterl W: Endodontie. Zahnerhaltung II, Bd. 3 Praxis der Zahnheilkunde. Urban & Schwarzenberg, Wien 1987, 3–81
2. Schroeder A: Endodontie – Ein Leitfaden für Studium und Praxis. Quintessenz Verlag, Berlin 1981, 21–80
3. Kopel H M: Considerations for the direct pulp capping procedure in primary teeth: a review of literature. ASDC J Dent Child 59: 41–49, 1992
4. Reuver J: 592 Pulpaüberkappungen in einer zahnärztlichen Praxis – eine klinische Prüfung (1966–1990). Dtsch Zahnärztl Z 47: 29–32, 1992
5. Cox C F, Tarim B, Kopel H, Gurel G, Hafez A: Technique sensitivity: biological factors contributing to clinical success with various restorative materials. Adv Dent Res 15: 85–90, 2001
6. Marti F: Direkte Pulpaüberkappungen mit Calxyl. Eine Langzeitstudie. Dissertation. Univ. Bern 1979
7. Baume L J, Holz J: Long term clinical assessment of direct pulp capping. Int Dent J 31: 251–260, 1981
8. Hülsmann M: Endodontie. In: Einwag J, Pieper K (Hrsg.): Kinderzahnheikunde. Urban & Schwarzenberg, München, Wien, Baltimore 1997, 301–318
9. Forrester D J, Wagner M L, Fleming J: Pediatric dental medicine. Lea & Febinger, Philadelphia 1981, 436–472
10. Berk H: Vital pulp capping. Presented at the International Association of Dental Research Meeting, Washington DC 1978
11. Masterton J B: Inherent healing potential of the dental pulp. Br Dent J 120: 430–436, 1966
12. Masterton J B: The healing of wounds of the dental pulp. An investigation of the nature of the scar tissue and the phenomena leading to its formation. Dent Pract Dent Rec 16: 325–329, 1966
13. McComb D: Comparison of physical properties of commercial calcium hydroxide lining cements. J Am Dent Assoc 107: 610–613, 1983
14. Torneck C D, Moe H, Howley T P: The effects of calcium hydroxide on porcine pulp fibroblasts in vitro. J Endod 9: 131–136, 1983
15. Stanley H R: Pulp capping: conserving the dental pulp, can it be done? Is it worth it? Oral Surg Oral Med Oral Pathol 68: 628–639, 1989
16. Cox C F, Hafez A A, Akimoto N, Otsuki M, Suzuki S, Tarim B: Biocompatibility of primer, adhesive and resin composite systems on non-exposed and exposed pulps of nonhuman primate teeth. Am J Dent 11: 55–63, 1998
17. Honegger D, Holz J, Baume L J: Controle clinique a long terme du coiffage pulpaire direct (realisé par les etudiants de la SMD, Geneve). Schweiz Monatsschr Zahnheilkd 89: 1020–1041, 1979
18. Cox C F, Keall C L, Keall H J, Ostro E, Bergenholtz G: Biocompatability of surface-sealed dentinal materials against exposed pulp. J Prosthet Dent 57: 1–8, 1987
19. Pashley D H: The effects of acid etching on the pulpodentin complex. Oper Dent 17: 229–242, 1992
20. Pashley D H, Pashley E L: Dentin permeability and restorative dentistry: a status report for the American Journal of Dentistry. Am J Dent 4: 5–9, 1991
21. Foreman P C, Barnes I E: Review of calcium hydroxide. Int Endod J 23: 283–297, 1990
22. Gwinnett A J, Tay F: Early and intermediate time response of the dental pulp to an acid etch technique in vivo. Am J Dent 10: 35–44, 1998
23. Cox C F, Suzuki S: Re-evaluating pulp protection: calcium hydroxide liners vs. cohesive hybridization. J Am Dent Assoc 125: 823–831, 1994
24. Goracci G, Mon G: Scanning electron microscopic evaluation of resin-dentin and calcium hydroxide-dentin interface with resin composite restorations. Quintessence Int 27: 129–135, 1996
25. Fujitani M, Shibata S, Van Meerbeek B, Yoshida Y, Shintani H: Direct adhesive pulp capping: pulpal healing and ultramorphology of the resin-pulp interface. Am J Dent 15(6): 395–402, 2002
26. Arakawa M, Kitasako Y, Otsuki M, Tagami J: Direct pulp capping with an auto-cured sealant resin and a self-etching primer. Am J Dent 16(1): 61–65, 2003
27. Hebling J, Giro E M, Costa C A: Biocompatibility of an adhesive system applied to exposed human dental pulp. J Endod 25(10): 676–682, 1999
28. Costa C A, Hebling J, Teixeira M F: Estudo preliminar da compatibilidade biológica dos adesivos dentinários All Bond 2 e Scotchbond MP. Avaliação histológica de implantes subcutaneos em ratos. Revista de Odontologia da Univ. de Sao Paulo 1996, 11–18
29 Costa C A, Gonzaga H F, Teixeira M F: Avaliação da biocompatibilidade sistema adesivo Prime e Bond 2.0 e do cimento de hidróxido de calcio-Dycal, Análise em microscopia de luz. Revista Odonto 2000-Odontologia. Seculo XXI 1: 8–12, 1997
30. Tziafas D: Experimental bacterial anachoresis in dog dental pulps capped with calcium hydroxide. J Endod 15(12): 591–595, 1989
31. Germain L: Mineral Trioxide Aggregate: A New Material for the New Millennium. Dentistry Today 18: 66–71, 1999
32. Aeinehchi M, Eslami B, Ghanbariha M, Saffar A S: Mineral trioxide aggregate (MTA) and calcium hydroxide as pulp-capping agents in human teeth: a preliminary report. Int Endod J 36(3): 225–231, 2003
33. Pitt Ford T R, Torabinejad M, Abedi H R et al.: Mineral trioxide aggregate as a pulp capping material. J Am Dent Assoc 127: 1491–1494, 1996
34. Tziafas D, Pantelidou O, Alvanou A, Belibasakis G, Papadimitriou S: The dentinogenic effect of mineral trioxide aggregate (MTA) in short-term capping experiments. Int Endod J 35(3): 245–254, 2002
35. Goldberg M, Six N, Decup F, Lasfargues J J, Salih E, Tompkins K, Veis A: Bioactive molecules and the future of pulp therapy. Am J Dent 16(1): 66–76, 2003

36. Tziafas D, Belibasakis G, Veis A, Papadimitriou S: Dentin regeneration in vital pulp therapy: design principles. Adv Dent Res 15: 96–100, 2001
37. Nakamura Y, Hammarstrom L, Matsumoto K, Lyngstadaas S P: The induction of reparative dentine by enamel proteins. Int Endod J 35(5): 407–417, 2002
38. Ishizaki N T, Matsumoto K, Kimura Y, Wang X, Yamashita A: Histopathological study of dental pulp tissue capped with enamel matrix derivative. J Endod 29(3): 176–179, 2003
39. Kirk E E, Meyer M J: Morphology of the mineralizing front and observations of reparative dentine following induction and inhibition of dentinogenesis in the rat incisor. Endod Dent Traumatol 8(5): 195–201, 1992
40. Yoshiba K, Yoshiba N, Iwaku M: Effects of antibacterial capping agents on dental pulps of monkeys mechanically exposed to oral microflora. J Endod 21(1): 16–20, 1995
41. Uitto V J, Antila R, Ranta R: Effects of topical glucocorticoid medication on collagen biosynthesis in the dental pulp. Acta Odontol Scand 33(5): 287–298, 1975
42. Melcer J, Chaumette M T, Melcer F: Experimental research on the preparation of dentin-pulp tissue of teeth exposed to CO_2 laser beams in dogs and macaques (*Macaca mulatta* and *Macaca fascicularis*). C R Soc Biol (Paris) 179: 577–585, 1985
43. Melcer J: Latest treatment in dentistry by means of the CO_2 Laser Beam. Lasers Surg Med 6: 396–398, 1986
44. Melcer J, Chaumette M T, Melcer F: Dental pulp exposed to the CO_2 laser beam. Lasers Surg Med 7: 347–352, 1987
45. Ebihara A, Sawada N, Okuyama M et al.: Histopathological changes of the exposed rat dental pulp irradiated with Nd:YAG laser. J Jap Soc Laser Med 9: 169–172, 1988
46. Ebihara A, Sekine Y, Takeda A, Suda H: Application of Nd:YAG laser irradiation to the experimental direct pulp capping. Jap J Conservat Dent 35: 876–886, 1992
47. Santucci P J: Dycal versus Nd:YAG laser and Vitrebond for direct pulp capping in permanent teeth. J Clin Laser Med Surg 17(2): 69–75, 1999
48. Jayawardena J A, Kato J, Moriya K, Takagi Y: Pulpal response to exposure with Er:YAG laser. Oral Surg Oral Med Oral Pathol Oral Radiol Endod 91(2): 222–229, 2001
49. Paschoud Y, Holz J: Effect of the soft laser on the neoformation of a dentin bridge following direct pulp capping of human teeth with calcium hydroxide. A histological study with the scanning electron microscope. Schweiz Monatsschr Zahnmed 98: 345–356, 1988
50. Moritz A, Schoop U, Goharkhay K, Sperr W: The CO_2 laser as an aid in direct pulp capping. J Endod 24: 248–251, 1998
51. Moritz A, Schoop U, Goharkhay K, Sperr W: Advantages of a pulsed CO_2 laser in direct pulp capping: a long-term in vivo study. Lasers Surg Med 22: 288–293, 1998
52. Morikawa S, Lanz O, Johnson C C: Laser Doppler measurements of localized pulsatile fluid velocity. IEEE Trans Biomed Eng 18(6): 416–420, 1971
53. Gazelius B, Olgart L, Edwall L: Non-invasive recording of blood flow in human dental pulp. Endod Dent Traumatol 2: 219–221, 1986
54. Odor T M, Pitt Ford T R, McDonald F: Effect of wavelength and bandwidth on the clinical reliability of laser Doppler recordings. Endod Dent Traumatol 12(1): 9–15, 1996
55. Diaz-Arnold A M, Wilcox L R, Arnold M A: Optical detection of pulpal blood. J Endod 20(4): 164–168, 1994
56. Vongsavan N, Matthews B: Some aspects of the use of laser Doppler flow meters for recording tissue blood flow. Exp Physiol 78(1): 1–4, 1993
57. Olgart L, Gazelius B, Lindh-Strömberg U: Laser Doppler flowmetry in assessing vitality in luxated permanent teeth. Int Endod J 21: 1–7, 1988
58. Gazelius B, Olgart L, Edwall L: Non-invasive recording of blood flow in human dental pulp. Endod Dent Traumatol 2: 219–221, 1986
59. Sweet C A: Treatment of vital primary teeth with pulpal involvement-therapeutic pulpotomy. J Colorado State Dent Assoc 33: 10–14, 1955
60. Thompson K S, Seal N S, Nunn M E, Huff G: Alternative method in full strength formocresol pulpotomy. Pediat Dent 23: 217–222, 2001
61. Lewis B B, Chestner S B: Formaldehyde in dentistry: a review of mutagenic and carcinogenic potential. J Am Dent Assoc 103: 429–434, 1981
62. Gravenmade E J: Some biochemical considerations of fixation in endodontics. J Endod 1: 233–237, 1973
63. Pashley E L M, Myers D R, Pashley D H, Withford G M: Systemic distribution of ^{14}C-formaldehyde from formocresol-treated pulpotomy sites. J Dent Res 59: 602–607, 1980
64. Nocentini S M, Moreno G, Coppey J: Survival, DNA synthesis and ribosomal RNA transcription in monkey kidney cells treated by formaldehyde. Mutation Res 70: 231–240, 1980
65. Goldmacher V S, Thilley W G: Formaldehyde is mutagenic for cultured human cells. Mutation Res 116: 417–422, 1983
66. Udin R D: Looking at alternatives. CDA J 19: 27–34, 1991
67. Schroeder U: A 2 year follow-up of primary molars, pulpotomized with a gentle technique and capped with calcium hydroxide. Scand J Dent Res 86: 273–278, 1978
68. Tziafas D, Smith A J, Lesot H: Designing new treatment strategies in vital pulp therapy. J Dent 28: 77–92, 2000
69. Oztas N, Ulusu T, Oygur T, Cokpekin F: Comparison of electrosurgery and formocresol as pulpotomy techniques in dog primary teeth. J Clin Pediat Dent 18: 285–289, 1994
70. Shumayrikh N M, Adenubi J O: Clinical evaluation of glutaraldehyde with calcium hydroxide and glutaraldehyde with zinc oxide eugenol in pulpotomy of primary molars. Endod Dent Traumatol 15: 259–264, 1999
71. Ebihara A: Effects of Nd:YAG laser irradiation on the amputated pulp. Jap J of Conservat Dent 32: 1670–684, 1989
72. Kato J, Hashimoto M, Ono H: Pulp reactions of the rat developing molars after pulpotomy with Nd:YAG laser irradiation. J Jap Soc Laser Med 10: 521–524, 1989
73. Kurumada F: A study on the application of Ga-As semiconductor laser to endodontics. The effects of laser irradiation on the activation of inflammatory cells and the vital pulpotomy. Ohu Dent J 17: 233–244, 1990
74. Kimura Y, Wilder-Smith P, Matsumoto K: Lasers in endodontics: a review. Int Endod J 2000; 33: 173–185
75. Weichman J A, Johnson F M: Laser use in endodontics. A preliminary investigation. Oral Surg Oral Med Oral Pathol 31(3): 416–420, 1971

76. Shoji S, Nakamura M, Horiuchi H: Histopathological changes in dental pulps irradiated by CO_2 laser: a preliminary report on laser pulpotomy. J Endod 11(9): 379–384, 1985
77 Figueiredo J A P, Chavantes M C, Gioso M A, Pesce H F, Jatene A D: Pulpotomies with CO_2 laser in dogs. Proceedings of the International Society for Optical Engineering 2394: 15–19, 1995
78. Jukic S, Anic I, Koba K, Najzar-Fleger D, Matsumoto K: The effect of pulpotomy using CO_2 and Nd:YAG lasers on dental pulp tissue. Int Endod J 30(3): 175–180, 1997
79. Wilder-Smith P, Peavy G M, Nielsen D, Arrastia-Jitosho A M: CO_2 laser treatment of traumatic pulpal exposures in dogs. Lasers Surg Med 21(5): 432–437, 1997
80. Dang J, Wilder-Smith P, Peavy G M: Clinical Preconditions and treatment modality: effects on pulp surgery outcome. Lasers Surg Med 22: 25–29, 1998
81. Shaw D W, Sheller B, Barnes B D: Electrosurgical pulpotomy: a 6 month study in primates. J Endod 10: 500–505, 1987
82. Waterhouse P J: Formocresol and alternative primary molar pulpotomy medicaments: a review. Endod Dent Traumat 11: 157–162, 1995
83. Morawa A P S, Straffon L H, Han S S, Corpron R E: Clinical evaluation of pulpotomies using dilute formocresol. ASDC J Dent Child 42: 360–363, 1975
84. Garcia-Godoy F: Direct pulp capping and partial pulpotomy with diluted formocresol in primary molars. Acta Odontol Pediat 5: 57–62, 1984
85. Aranjo F B, Ely L B, Pergo A M, Pesce H F: A clinical evaluation of 2% buffered glutaraldehyde in pulpotomies of human deciduous teeth: a 24-month study. Braz Dent J 6: 41–44, 1995
86. Tsai T P, Su H L, Tseng L H: Glutaraldehyde preparations and pulpotomy in primary molars. Oral Surg Oral Med Oral Pathol 76: 346–350, 1993
87. Ballantyne B, Jordan S L: Toxicological, medical and industrial hygiene aspects of glutaraldehyde with particular reference to its biocidal use in cold sterilization procedures. J Appl Toxicol 21: 131–151, 2001
88. Fishman S, Udin R D, Good D L, Rodef F: Success of electrofulguration pulpotomies covered by zinc oxide and eugenol or calcium hydroxide: a clinical study. Pediat Dent 18: 385–390, 1996
89. Pescheck A, Pescheck B, Moritz A: Pulpotomy of Primary Molars with the Use of a Carbon Dioxide Laser: Results of a Long-term In Vivo Study. J Oral Laser Appl 2: 165–169, 2002
90. Granath L, Hagman G: Experimental pulpotomy in human bicuspids with reference to cutting techniques. Acta Odontol Scad 29: 155–163, 1971
91. Shalman E R, Mc Iver F, Burkes E J: Comparison of electrosurgery and formocresol as pulpotomy techniques in monkey primary teeth. Pediat Dent 9: 189–194, 1987
92. Weine F S: Alternatives to routine endodontic therapy. In: Weine F S (ed.): Endodontic Therapy, 4th ed. Mosby, St. Louis 1989, 616–653
93. Fitzpatrick R E, Goldman M P, Ruiz-Esparza J: Clinical advantages of the CO_2 laser superpulsed mode. J Dermatol Surg Oncol 20: 449–456, 1994
94. Guelmann M, Fair J, Turner C, Courts F J: The success of emergency pulpotomies in primary molars. Pediat Dent 24: 217–220, 2002

8

Laser-Assisted Periodontal Therapy

U. Schoop

with contributions from A. Moritz, R. Blum, G. Romanos, F. Schwarz

8.1 Introduction

8.1.1 General

If some decades ago, the treatment of carious lesions and their consequences was at the center of dental treatment, nowadays, periodontal diseases and their consequences are considered as the main danger for tooth- and bone-loss worldwide in the group of over 35-year-old people. For this reason, the development of suitable diagnostic and therapy procedures represents, within periodontal treatments, one of the greatest challenges of modern dentistry. With the introduction of lasers in this area, very interesting and elegant perspectives have emerged, which should be integrated into the normal treatment means of each practitioner. Through a certain paradigm shift in periodontal therapy over the past years, the non-surgical treatment of pockets with a medium depth (4–5 mm) has come to the fore. These cases certainly represent a major part of the patients suffering from periodontal disease and the laser hereby preferably shows its strengths in conjunction with scaling and root planing. The following contribution aims to show the additional advantages of laser-assisted periodontal treatment, but also the limits of periodontal laser therapy, and to present, in this way, a guideline for a successful treatment concept.

8.1.2 Specific Problems of the Indication

8.1.2.1 Etiology, Definitions and Pathogenesis: Gingivitis – Periodontitis – Gingival Recession

Generally, periodontal disease means bacterially-caused inflammatory as well as non-inflammatory damage, and thus recessive changes of the gingival and/or periodontal tissue. The term **gingivitis** means that the inflammation procedure stays

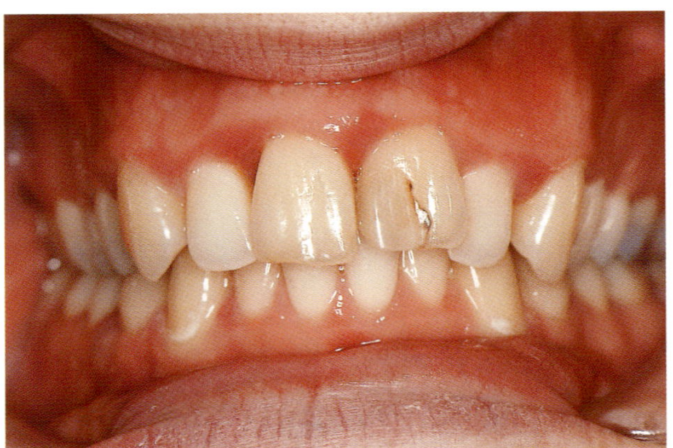

Fig 8-1 Gingivitis: redness and swelling of the gingiva.

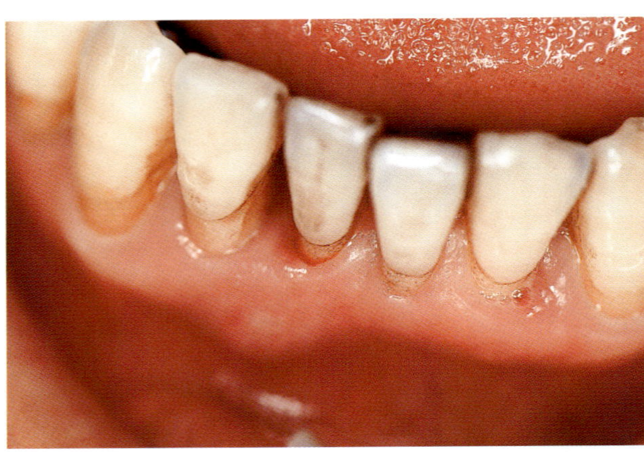

Fig 8-2 Periodontitis. The gingiva is swollen, the symptoms of gingivitis can be seen. In addition, a strong shrinkage of the periodontal tissues with attachment loss imposes.

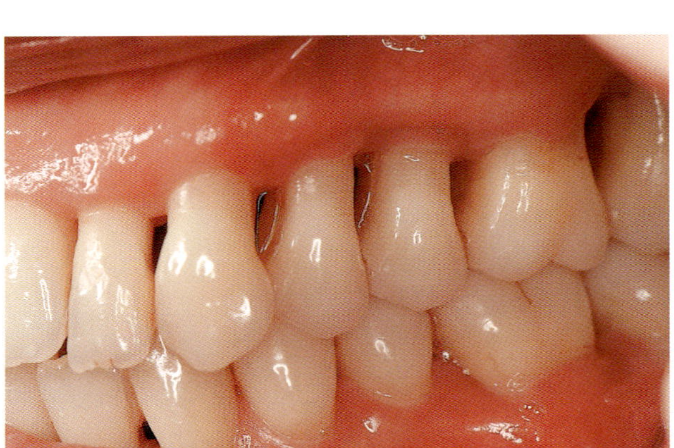

Fig 8-3 Periodontitis. Through the recession of the periodontal tissues the gingival neck areas are exposed.

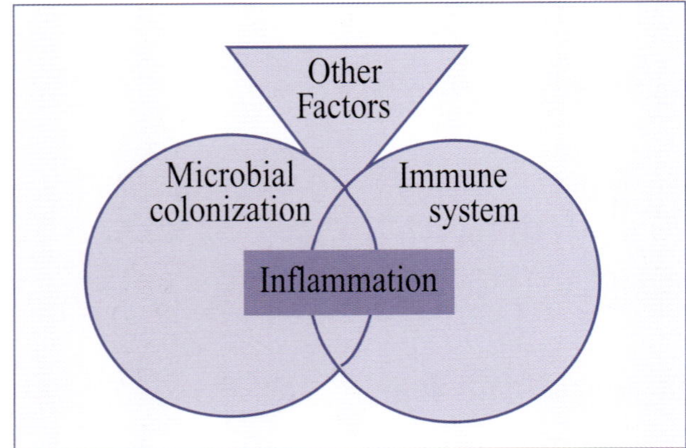

Fig 8-4 Diagram of etiology – through an interaction of several key factors, periodontitis is induced.

limited to the gingival area and that there is no loss of attachment present.

It is possible that gingivitis can exist for many years, without developing into **periodontitis**. Furthermore, in principle, gingivitis is reversible by good oral hygiene and consistent plaque control and scaling. Normally gingivitis results from bacterial plaque due to a lack of mouth hygiene. In addition, changes of the gingiva are possible with metabolic disturbances, general illnesses and in the context of the side effects of medicine (e.g., pregnancy, Cyclosporin A-hyperplasia, Hydantoin-hyperplasia etc.).

If the inflammation process does not remain limited to the gingiva, and if also periodontal supporting tissues are touched, then a loss of attachment is present and we speak of periodontitis.

In opposition to these inflammatory-decrease forms stand the clinically inflammation-free decrease of gingiva and bone, which is called **recession**.

The etiology of periodontitis has not been completely clarified to date. As described by Listgarten[1,2] in 1986 and 1987, several factors seem to interact in its emergence, where the crucial criteria seem to be dependent on the pathogenicity of the microorganisms, their ability to penetrate into the tissue and the individually different response of the host, depending on his immune status and his resistance. Even with treatment, periodontitis

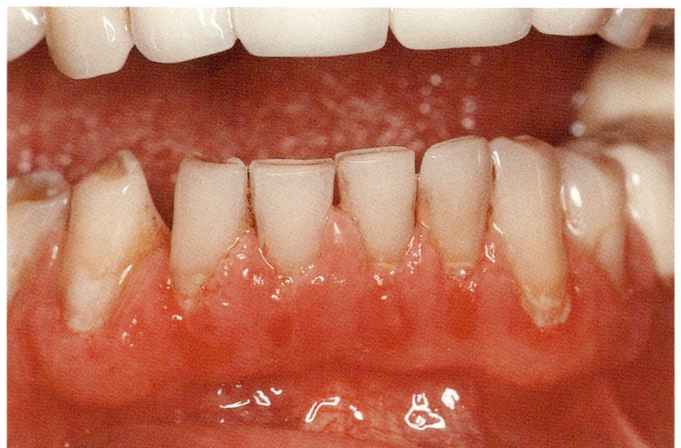

Fig 8-5 Plaque. The accumulations on the gingival margin are discernible. The gingiva appears reddened and swollen. Ulcerations can additionally be seen.

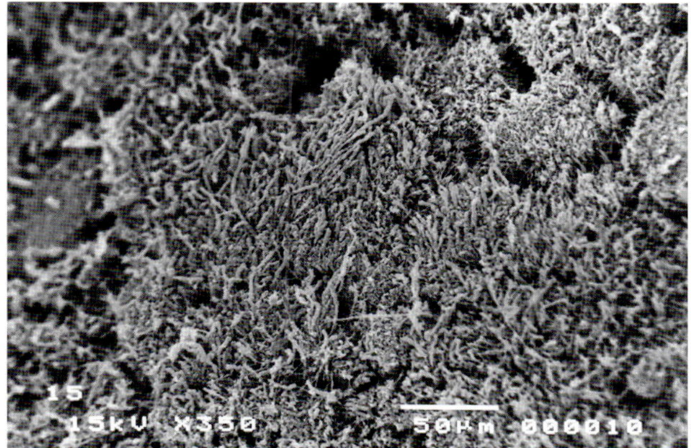

Fig 8-6 Tooth surface after 48 h. A dense bacterial culture develops.

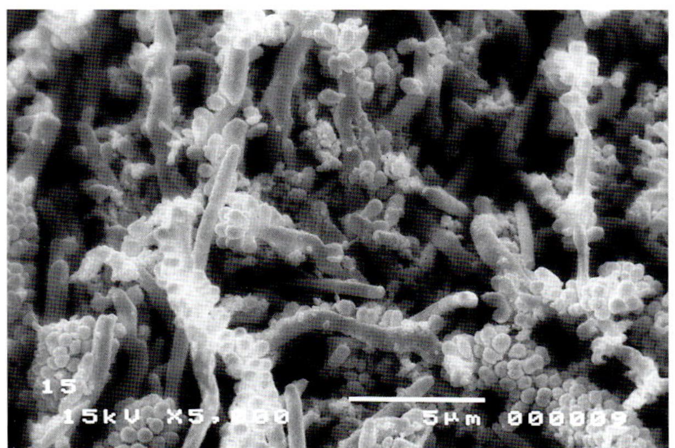

Fig 8-7 48-h-old plaque, high magnification.

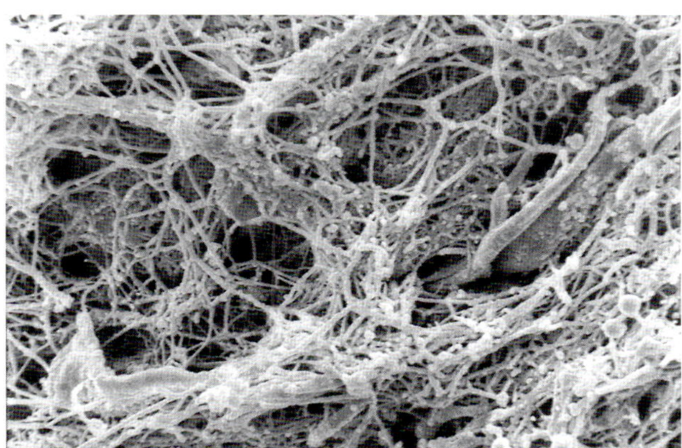

Fig 8-8 After 72 h. The dense web formation of the biofilm is discernible.

is only partially reversible and the starting situation found in a healthy person can never be achieved.

Plaque is considered as the main cause of the emergence of periodontitis and its persistence. However, periodontitis does not necessarily occur in the presence of plaque; a healthy status of gingiva and periodontium is possible when lesser amounts of plaque and less virulent microorganisms come together with a positive host-defense. A thin adherent plaque layer, often only a few cell layers thick, can be compatible with a clinically healthy gingiva.

Plaque, which ranks among the primary causes of inflammatory periodontal disease, is a structured, yellowish-gray calculus, which cannot be rinsed off, but must be removed mechanically with a toothbrush or other suitable instruments. It consists of bacteria, which stick together firmly, one with another, through the glycoproteins of the saliva and polysaccharides produced by the bacteria themselves.

Even on an absolutely clean tooth, a 0.1–0.8-µm-thick dental cuticle consisting of saliva-glycoproteins settles within a few minutes to hours, whereupon mainly gram-positive, colony-building bacteria settle within the first 24 h (streptococci, actinomycetes). With further growth of the plaque, gram-negative cocci as well as gram-positive and -negative small rods and filaments appear within the next few days. After ~3 weeks, particularly at

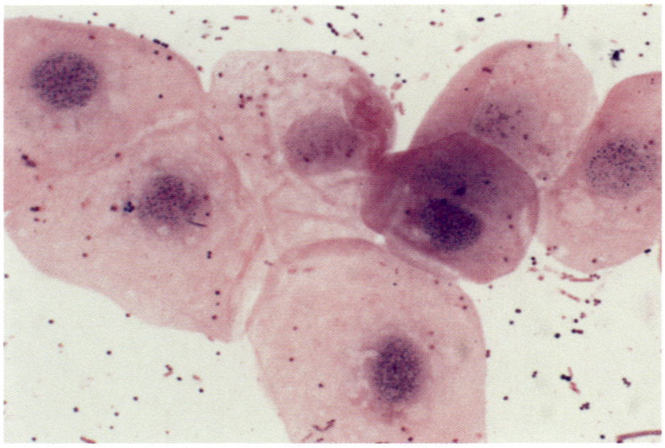

Fig 8-9 Bacterial flora, epithelial cells, smear.

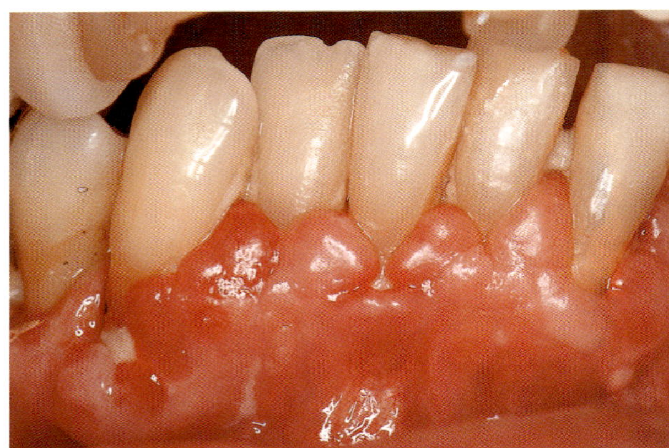

Fig 8-10 Plaque. The accumulations on the gingival margin are discernible. The gingiva shows a hyperplasia.

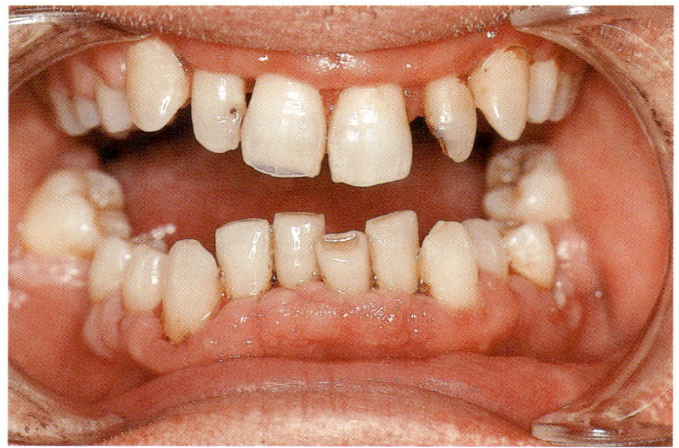

Fig 8-11 Interlocked position: the position of the teeth impedes the removal of plaque and therefore promotes gingivitis.

the gingival border, there is a significant increase of filaments, as described by Listgarten et al.[3,4] in 1975 and 1976.

The bacterial flora leads the tissue to an intensified immigration of polymorphonuclear leucocytes and exudation into the gingival sulcus. The junctional epithelium is now loosened up in the presence of the developing gingivitis and bacteria can penetrate between tooth and epithelium into the subgingival area, thus creating a **gingival pocket**.

Supra-gingival plaque is the main factor in the emergence of gingivitis. The development of plaque is promoted by so-called natural and iatrogenic plaque-promoting factors.

Among the natural factors rank:
- confining and interlocked position of the teeth
- the enamel–cementum border, which likewise shows roughness
- indentations of root surfaces
- mouth respiration, because the saliva is more viscous
- badly accessible pits and fissures

Among the iatrogenic causative factors rank:
- over-hanging edges of fillings
- edges of crowns
- prosthodontic clips and saddles.

If now this supra-gingival plaque is mineralized by the components of the saliva, calculus occurs, especially at weak points, such as the neighborhood of the exit of the major salivary glands. Particularly concerned are the lingual parts of the lower maxillary front teeth (Glandula sublingualis) and the vestibular surfaces of the upper molars (Glandula Parotis). Already in the early phases of plaque formation, transformation of soft, still-cleanable linings begins into hard, mineralized tartar. Already after 1–2 days, the first core of mineralization develops, which consolidates itself to centers of mineralization. After an average of 10–20 days, firm mineralized tartar develops from the soft plaque.

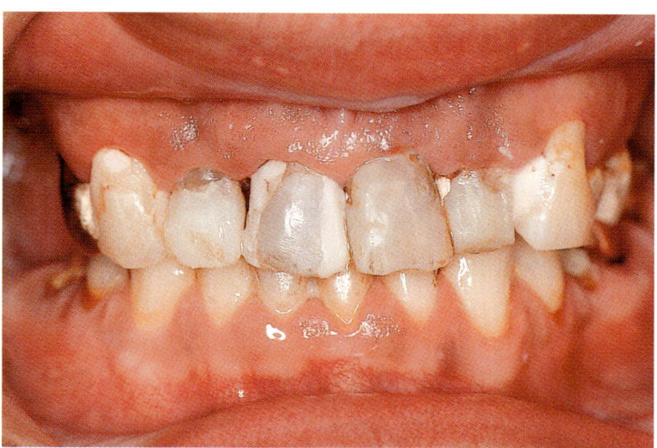

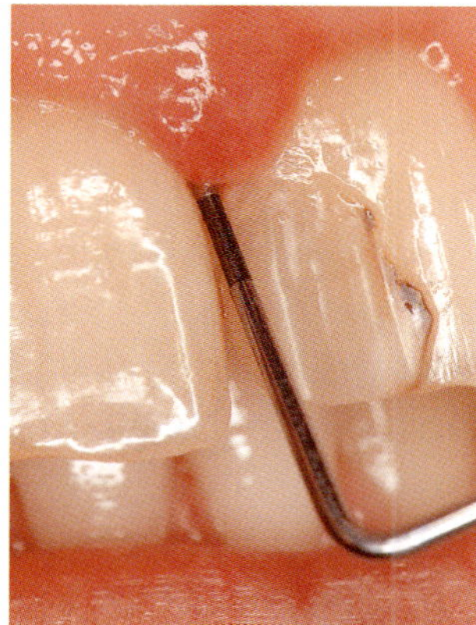

Fig 8-12a and b Overhanging edges of fillings. The persisting irritation favors the development of gingivitis.

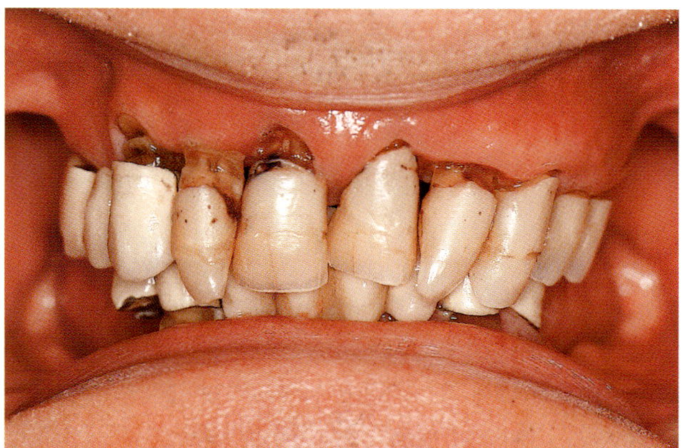

Fig 8-13 Overhanging edges of crowns.

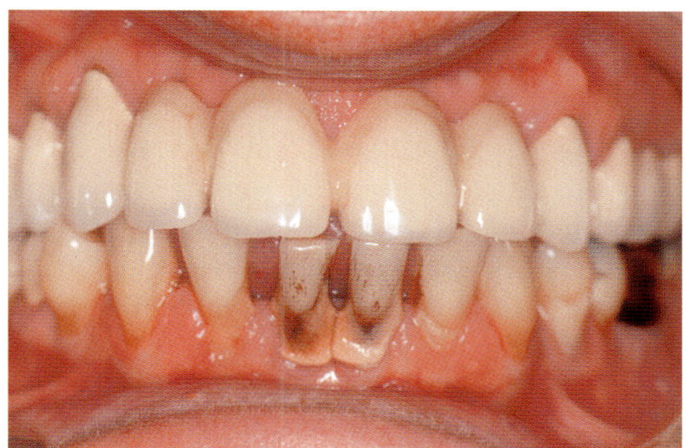

Fig 8-14 Calculus. In teeth 31 and 41 the accumulations can be clearly discerned.

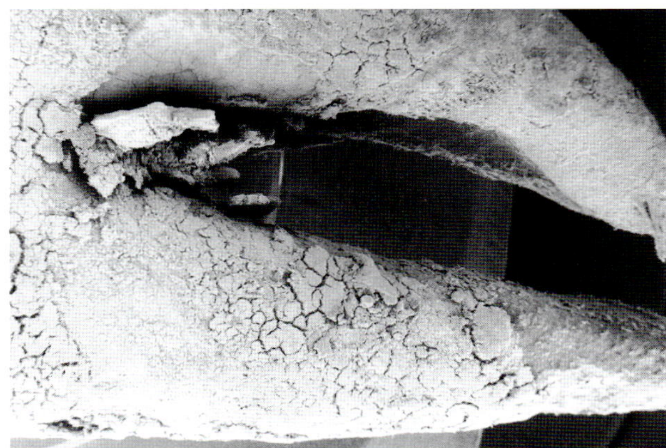

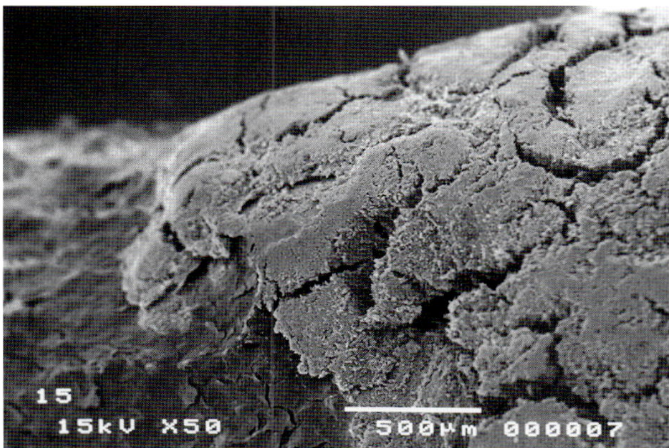

Fig 8-15 and 8-16 SEM pictures of concrements.

8.1.2.2 Subgingival Plaque, Subgingival Calculus – Concrements

Subgingival plaque is now the main factor in the emergence of periodontitis. The supra-gingival plaque and the following gingivitis loosen the junctional epithelium. The so-weakened epithelial adhesion at the tooth makes it now possible for the bacteria of the plaque to push themselves in a thin layer in the apical direction between the tooth and the junctional epithelium. It results in the formation of a gingival pocket.

One can differentiate between adherent and non-adherent plaque. The adherent layer is on the tooth's root surface, and it is a different type of thick layer, similar to the plaque of gingivitis, consisting particularly of filaments and gram-positive cocci. The adherent layer can now calcify giving subgingival tartar. This subgingival tartar is also called **concrement**. Neither subgingival nor supra-gingival tartar cause inflammatory procedures in the periodontium, despite the rough surface. Tartar does, however, have an important role as a retention place for settling microorganisms. The difference between tartar and concrement exists in the origin of the components and the color. The origin of the concrement components is not saliva, but blood serum and the components of the liquid of the pocket. The storage of blood coloring material in the mineralized plaque explains the brownish-black color. The concrement stays in the periodontal pockets and contributes substantially to the maintenance of periodontitis. In comparison with supra-gingival tartar, the mineralization clearly takes longer; furthermore, there are no favorite localizations, concrement can occur in any place on the root surface. Therefore, diagnosis and therapy are very difficult.

Non-adherent plaque, consisting of amounts of loose bacteria accumulations, also called "swimmers", are found on the side of the soft tissue of the pockets and consist almost exclusively of gram-negative anaerobic bacteria. They increase substantially in acute phases and seem to play a major part in the progress of periodontitis[5,6].

8.1.2.3 Periodontopathogenic Bacteria, Endotoxin, Exotoxin

The pathogenic capacity of the plaque is determined primarily by the kind of available microorganisms and their metabolism products. The **periodontopathogenic plaque bacteria** have certain characteristics, which can accelerate the destruction of the periodontium. The enzymes, among them enzymes like collagenases, hyaluronidases, chondroitinsulfatases, neuramidases and different proteases, produced by them, dissolve collagen structure facilitating thus the penetration of the microorganisms into the tissue. Furthermore, metabolism products of the bacteria, such as ammonia, indole and hydrogen sulfide, attack the tissue directly. Different bacteria produce specific toxins, whereby **endotoxins** and **exotoxins** are differentiated.

Among the endotoxins rank lipopolysaccharides from the wall of gram-negative bacteria, which cause an increased inflammatory defense reaction. Exotoxins are antigens, which are produced by the microorganisms, such as the leucotoxin produced by *Actinobacillus actinomycetemcomitans*, which leads to the decay of polymorphonuclear granulocytes.

The inflammatory periodontopathologies have been regarded for a long time as a consequence of a non-specific plaque settling. It was assumed that only the quantity of the plaque was responsible for the inflammatory procedures in the periodontium. Since the discovery of specific types of bacteria in connection with certain forms of the inflammatory diseases of the periodontium, it is assumed, however, that the quality of the plaque has a crucial influence on the kind of illness. Among the assumed pathogenic bacteria rank: *Actinobacillus actinomycetemcomitans, Bacteroides forsythus, Eikenella corrodens, Fusobacterium nucleatum, Peptostreptococcus micros, Porphyromonas gingivalis* and spirochetes.

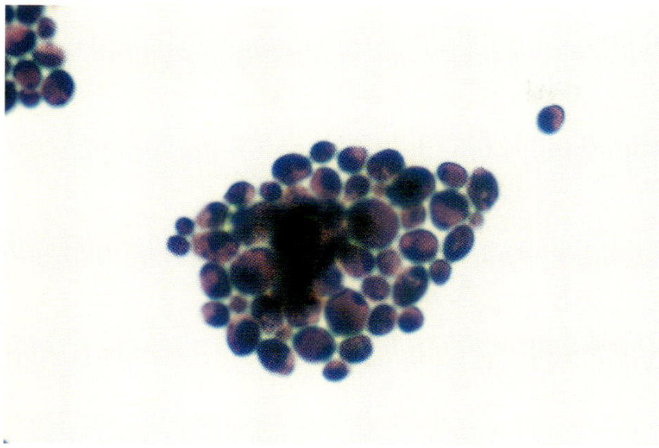

Fig 8-17 *Candida albicans.*

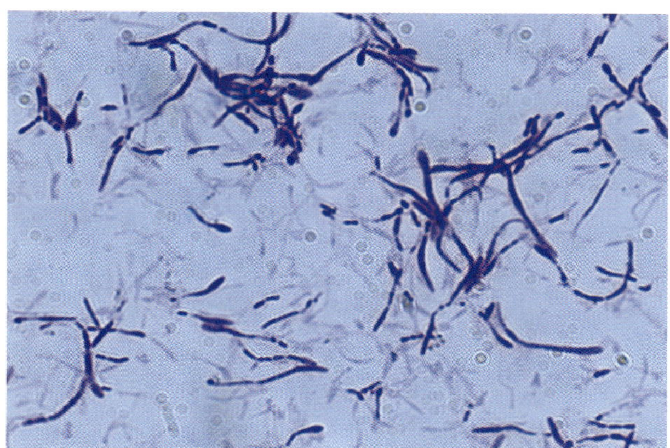

Fig 8-18 *Actinobacillus actinomycetemcomitans.*

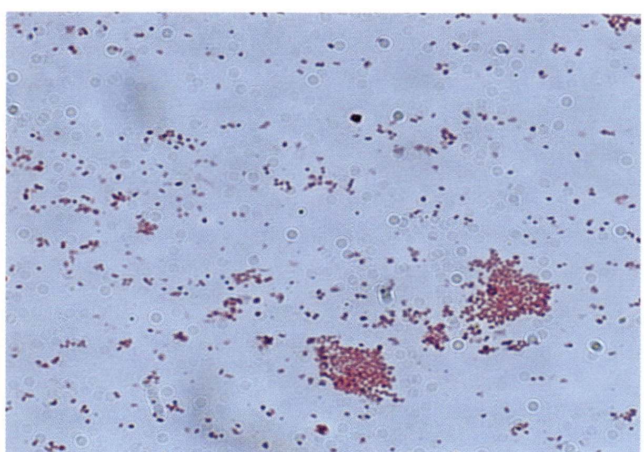

Fig 8-19 *Porphyromonas gingivalis.*

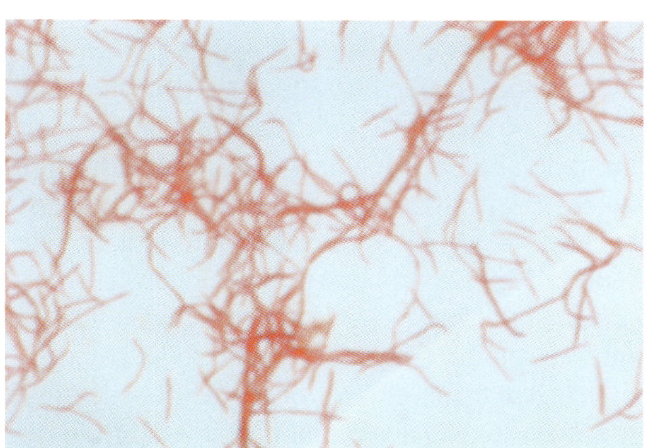

Fig 8-20 *Fusobacterium nucleatum.*

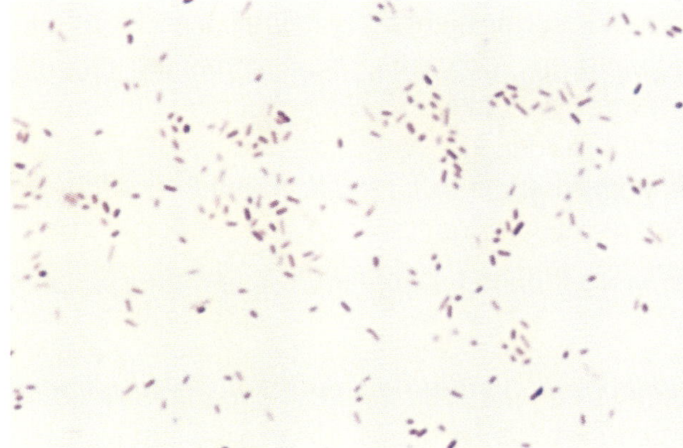

Fig 8-21 *Prevotella intermedia.*

8.1.2.4 Secondary Causes

The secondary cause of periodontal illnesses contains factors that cannot release inflammatory reactions alone. There is differentiation between local and systemic factors. Among the **local factors** rank tartar, tooth anatomy (enamel-pearls, enamel-cementum border), tooth positions (tilting, interlocked position) and incorrect preserving and prosthetic restorations, since they strengthen **plaque retention**. Further factors are open carious lesions, which represent a bacteria reservoir, mouth respiration, which obstructs normal salivation, non-physiological occlusive forces, which cause **occlusal trauma** and lead to changes in the desmodontium and thus to an increased tooth mobility, existing niches like gingival and periodontal pockets, the consistency, composition and quantity of the saliva and finally the most important individual risk factor, **tobacco consumption**, which has a restraining influence on fibroblasts and leads to decreased salivation and reduced function of the polymorphonuclear granulocytes.

Among the systemic factors are ranked general illnesses, during which there can also be pathogenic changes to the gingiva or in the periodontium. These changes must be differentiated from the plaque-caused forms of gingivitis and periodontitis, which usually come about as a second step to inflammatory changes due to plaque, since during these illnesses, mouth hygiene is also often impaired. Among these illnesses, metabolic illnesses rank, such as **diabetes** type I (the increase of glucose in the cervicular fluid promotes bacteria growth); avitaminoses such as scurvy with impairment of collagen synthesis; malfunctions in the immune defense such as with Chediak Higashi syndrome, and syndromes where there is a lack of antibodies; illnesses with dermatological problems such as Pemphigus vulgaris and Lichen ruber planus; viral illnesses such as Gingivistomatitis herpetica and HIV infection, and finally, genetically-caused syndromes, which accompany gingivo-periodontal features, like Papillon Lefèvre syndrome or Down syndrome.

8.1.2.5 Histology

Inflammation of the periodontium, due to plaque, is divided histologically into four steps, as described by Page and Schroeder[7]:

- the initial lesion
- the early lesion
- the established lesion
- the advanced lesion

The initial lesion develops after new plaque formation from a clinically healthy gingiva and develops within 2–4 days. This condition is completely reversible. From the marginal edematous swelling results a subgingival space, into which the supra-gingival plaque can penetrate. Already at this stage, there is dismantling of the perivascular collagen.

The early lesion develops from an uninfluenced initial lesion within 14 days. The characteristics of this stage are the intensified accumulation of defense-cells in the gingival connective tissue, the further loss of collagen and tearing of the junctional epithelium at the bottom of the sulcus.

Both the initial and the early lesion describe the condition of a clinically clearly-defined gingivitis.

The established lesion develops in a few weeks from the early lesion and seems, like the two specified above, to be still completely reversible with optimal mouth hygiene. Clinically it appears as chronic gingivitis, which is bound always to the presence of a subgingival plaque. It now reaches an almost complete dissolution of the gingival supporting tissue and apical proliferation of the junctional epithelium, which begins to be converted into a pocket epithelium. The exact mechanisms that lead to the detachment of the junctional epithelium of the tooth are not yet sufficiently clarified. A pocket of 2–3 mm appears, which however remains limited to the gingiva only.

The advanced lesion, however, describes a destructive process in the periodontium. A complete healing cannot be achieved despite optimal mouth hygiene. With the existing periodontal inflammation, phases of exacerbation (acute) alternate with phases of stagnation (chronic). The lesion begins to expand itself now to alveolar bone and desmodontium, where the interdental bone is affected more frequently by dismantling than the vestibular, lingual or interradicular bones. The consequence is the formation of a periodontal pocket.

The inflammatory defense reaction released by the pathogenic bacteria and their toxins, contributes, likewise, to the destruction of the periodontium.

The polymorphonuclear granulocytes of the non-specific defense have the ability to phagocyte and kill microorganisms, and to digest and/or destroy cell rubble. In the case of this digestion by lysosomal enzymes, enzymatic substances (e.g., collagenases) are released into the surrounding tissue, whereby dissolution of tissue structures can occur.

The T-lymphocytes of the specific defense release lymphokines, which lead among other factors to an activation of osteoclasts.

Furthermore, certain factors of the inflammation reaction, like prostaglandins and interleukins, promote the activity of osteoclasts.

8.1.2.6 Classification of Periodontal Diseases

In 1999, an international workshop[8] for the classification of periodontal diseases took place in Oak Brook, Illinois. Based on a comprehensive literature review, a new classification of periodontal diseases was defined, which is arranged as follows.

8.1.2.6.1 Gingivitis

The clinical picture of gingivitis is characterized by a reddening, swelling and by a possible ulceration. An increased flow-rate of the sulcus fluid, a bleeding after sounding of the sulcus and an increased probing depth without loss of attachment are present. It is necessary to differentiate here between essentially plaque- and non-plaque-induced forms of the illness.

Pure plaque-induced gingivitis is caused by microorganisms of the plaque. In the subgingival plaque gram-positive rods and cocci prevail. The facultative anaerobic microorganisms outweigh the strictly anaerobic bacteria. Local factors, such as, for instance, supernatant edges of fillings, aggravate the case. The typical inflammation characters like bleeding and swelling remain limited on the gingiva; bone destruction is not observed. The sulcus can be deepened to a gingival pocket. The prognosis of plaque-induced gingivitis is dependent only on the mouth hygiene of the patient; with good cooperation it is possible to have a complete reorganization of the gingiva.

If systemic factors are in addition to the presence of dental plaque, then this is systemically modified gingival disease. To this group belong puberty-gingivitis, pregnancy-gingivitis and diabetes-gingivitis, as well as the medicament-caused forms of the illness, for instance the Cyclosporin-associated gingiva-hyperplasia.

The second main group of gingival illnesses is determined by the non-plaque-induced forms of gingivitis. These are specific infections, for instance those caused by *Neisseria gonorrhea* or *Treponema pallidum*, and all forms caused by viruses or fungi. Further, genetically caused, as well as allergic appearances of gingival illnesses and gingivitis, in the context of systemic illnesses (lichen planus, pemphigoid, lupus erythemathodes, etc.) are also included. The last subgroup of the plaque-independent gingival diseases is finally formed by the injury-conditioned ones (chemically, mechanically, thermally).

8.1.2.6.2 Chronic Periodontitis

Chronic periodontitis is the most frequent form of periodontitis. It is an infectious, inflammatory illness of the tooth-retaining apparatus with progressive loss of attachment and dismantling of the alveolar bone, the main symptoms being pocket formation and also recession. This form of periodontitis is most frequent in adults starting from the 4th decade, but it can occur in children and young people. The etiological factors are usually subgingival tartar and a differently associated microflora. Depending upon the extent of the illness it can be differentiated into a **localized form**, with less than 30% of the surfaces involved, and a **generalized form**, with more than 30% of the surfaces concerned. The degree of the illness is called "light", if 1–2 mm of loss of attachment is present, "moderate" with 3–4 mm and "severe" with more than 5 mm loss of attachment. Some cases of chronic periodontitis do not respond to therapeutic measures, and are regarded as therapy-refractory periodontitis.

8.1.2.6.3 Aggressive Periodontitis

Aggressive periodontitis, a familial illness, is likewise an infectious, inflammatory illness of the tooth-retaining apparatus with rapid loss of attachment. Frequently present characteristics are the discrepancy between the periodontal destruction and the quantity of the etiological factors, an increased proportion of *Actinobacillus actinomycetemcomitans* in the subgingival flora and increased tissue level of prostaglandin-E2 and interleukin-1β. There is a **localized form**, which starts around puberty and concerns the 1st molar and the incisors, and a **generalized form** starting from around 30 years and which concerns at least three teeth which are not the 1st molar nor the incisors. The underlying pathogens cause an increased serum anti-body titer within the localized form, whereas in the generalized form, no increased serum anti-body titer is determined.

8.1.2.6.4 Periodontitis as a Manifestation of Systemic Diseases

To this group belong the periodontal diseases caused by blood diseases (Neutropenia, Leukemia) or genetically caused sickness (Down syndrome, Papillon–Lefèvre syndrome, Chediak–Higashi syndrome, etc.).

8.1.2.6.5 Necrotizing Periodontal Diseases

To this group belong **necrotizing ulcerative gingivitis (NUG)** and **necrotizing ulcerative periodontitis (NUP)**. While the first form remains limited to the gingiva and is characterized by the occurrence of ulcerations and pseudo-membranes, the latter is an acute periodontal infection, whereby the necroses spread on the periodontal ligament and the alveolar bone. It appears frequently as a manifestation of severe systemic defense weakness, e.g., during immunosuppression or lack of nutrition, and there exists a close relationship with HIV infection. It leads to a rapid attachment loss, frequently without the formation of deep pockets, and the formation of sequesters is possible.

8.1.2.6.6 Abscesses of the Periodontium

Gingival, periodontal and pericoronal abscesses are classified in this group.

8.1.2.6.7 Periodontitis in Combination with Endodontic Lesions

As the periodontium and the endodontium can be considered to have a certain relationship as a functional unit, diseases from one can influence directly the state of health of the other.

8.1.2.6.8 Developmental or Acquired Deformities and Conditions

In this range we count factors like tooth anatomy, tooth restorations, abnormal position of the frenulum and muscle beginnings, abnormal pigmentation, occlusal traumata and a multiplicity of other influences on the gingival and periodontal health.

8.2 Laser Versus Conventional Therapy

8.2.1 Conventional Therapy

The aim of the therapy of inflammatory periodontal diseases is mostly complete recovery of the tissue and the re-establishment of anatomical and physiological conditions in as much as is possible. An existing gingivitis is reversible with consistent oral hygiene. With periodontitis, constant controls, the motivation of the patient and treatments like root planing, surgery procedures and antibiotics are at the center of attention. A valuable addition, both in conventional and surgical therapy, is the employment of different laser systems.

The course of treatment of systematic periodontal therapy is divided into three large sections:

- the initial therapy
- the corrective phase (possibly by surgery)
- the supporting periodontal therapy (recall)

The goal of the **initial therapy** is the removal of gingivitic changes, stopping the existing illness and the obtention of plaque- and tartar-free oral conditions.

In the context of the initial phase, the oral hygiene measures are accomplished by the patient, whereby the patient must be instructed precisely and gradually about correct mouth hygiene with appropriate help (e.g., dental floss, interdental brushes, superfloss). Furthermore, the motivation and control of the patient cooperation are central to this. The task of the dentist consists in eliminating possible bacterial hiding-places, supernatant fillings and, in the sense of a professional tooth cleaning, removing the existing supra- and subgingival calculus.

The supra-gingival tartar clings relatively loosely to the smooth surface of the enamel and can be removed easily with scraping hand instruments such as scalers and chisels. Beside these hand instruments, ultrasonic scalers are used during the scaling.

The subgingival concrements are intimately bound with the roughness of the root cementum and thus difficult to remove. For the removal of the subgingival concrements, the infected root cement, the granulation tissue and pocket epithelium curettes are used in the sense of "deep scaling". There is differentiation between universal curettes (e.g., Columbia) and special curettes (e.g., Gracey). They are used similar to sharply cutting scalpels at the root cement. Every one of the differently-formed curettes has a tooth-surface-specific range of application. With this classical closed curettage results a cleaning and a smoothing of the root cement. The disadvantage of this closed curettage is that the root cleaning must be accomplished without direct view. The advantage is that the gingival recessions are smaller than with curettage with flap-surgery (open curettage).

The final polishing of the tooth surface and complete removal of discolorations is accomplished by machine-driven rotary soft brushes or rubber cups in combination with a few abrasive polishing pastes. In this way the tooth surfaces are smoothed and thus the possibility of plaque retention is minimized.

Surgical corrective measures are used, if the goals of the initial phase are reached to a large extent but, nevertheless, active remaining pockets are still present. Active pockets are characterized by bleeding on careful probing. Particularly with pocket depths that exceed 5 mm, a surgical procedure is in most cases indicated. With flap-surgery the gingiva is mobilized by a sulcular incision and a flap is formed. Then, under direct view, the root surface is cleaned and the infected pocket epithelium is removed. The advantage of the open curettage versus the closed curettage is the production of good visibility and the "sharp curettage" of the infected soft tissue with a scalpel. The disadvantage of this procedure is the occurrence of tissue contractions, which can lead to exposed dental necks after healing.

Supporting periodontal therapy is an essential component of the periodontal therapy. Periodontal patients must be considered as chronically sick patients, who require constant control and remotivation. Therefore, only a conscientiously accomplished aftercare, with repeated supra- and subgingival plaque controls, makes possible the durable success of the treatment result obtained in the initial and the surgical corrective phase.

8.2.2 Laser

Different laser systems have gained more and more significance in the therapy of periodontitis. It is important for the surgeon to be always conscious of the possibilities and limits of the laser. Always, laser application has to be regarded as additional to conventional methodology, even if sometimes the range of non-surgical therapy can be extended by laser application.

Before lasers can be applied, the patient must be prepared in the sense of a complete initial therapy. With recent developments in the area of laser technology, it appears conceivable that the removal of concrements may also be possible with the help of the laser; primarily ,however, one takes advantage of the bactericidal effect of certain wavelengths. Numerous studies from diverse fields of dental medicine have proven that lasers within the infrared range exhibit excellent antibacterial effect and also are able to deactivate bacterial toxins[9–11]. This effect unfolds at a power output that lies clearly underneath a threshold for thermal damage to soft and hard tissues. Also, a direct stimulation of periodontal regeneration in the sense of soft-laser-effects is being discussed.

Thin, flexible light-conductor systems lead the laser beam to almost any desired location. It seems normal to use these advantages also in the area of periodontal therapy. The bibliography at the end of this chapter offers an overview of current studies in this area and a detailed argument pro and contra the different wavelengths.

8.2.2.1 Applied Lasers

Besides the CO_2 laser (λ = 10,600 nm), which is used in periodontal surgery, the most important wavelengths in this area are those of the Nd:YAG laser (λ = 1,064 nm) and those of the diode laser (λ = 810 or λ = 980 nm). Both lasers work with flexible light conductors, which make application possible in periodontal pockets.

With the development of special applicators, the employment of lasers, whose indications were limited to the preparation of tooth hard substances, was made possible in the area of periodontics. In particular, this applies to the Er:YAG laser (λ = 2,960 nm), and in addition, with an Er,Cr:YSGG (λ = 2,780 nm) and a frequency-

Fig 8-22 (left) Example of an Nd:YAG laser system.

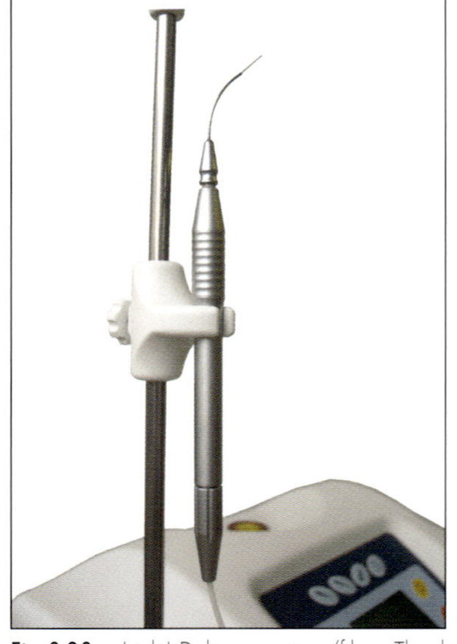

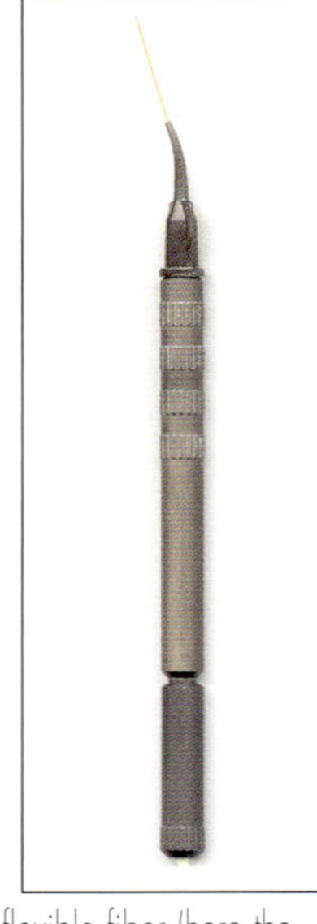

Fig 8-23 (right) Delivery system/fiber. The thin flexible fiber (here the one of an Nd:YAG laser is depicted) can be introduced easily into the periodontal pocket and grants complete coverage of the root surface.

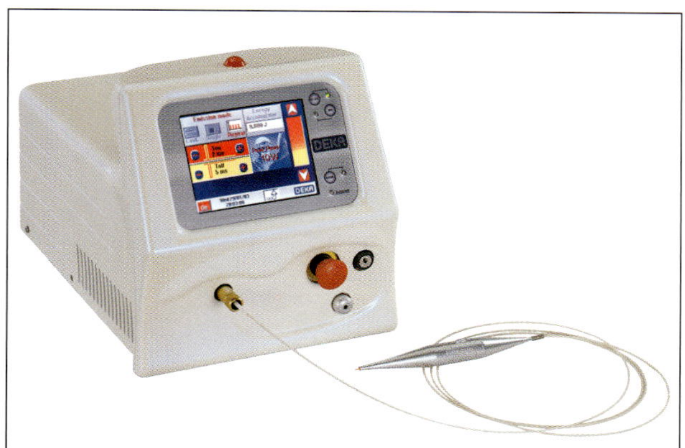

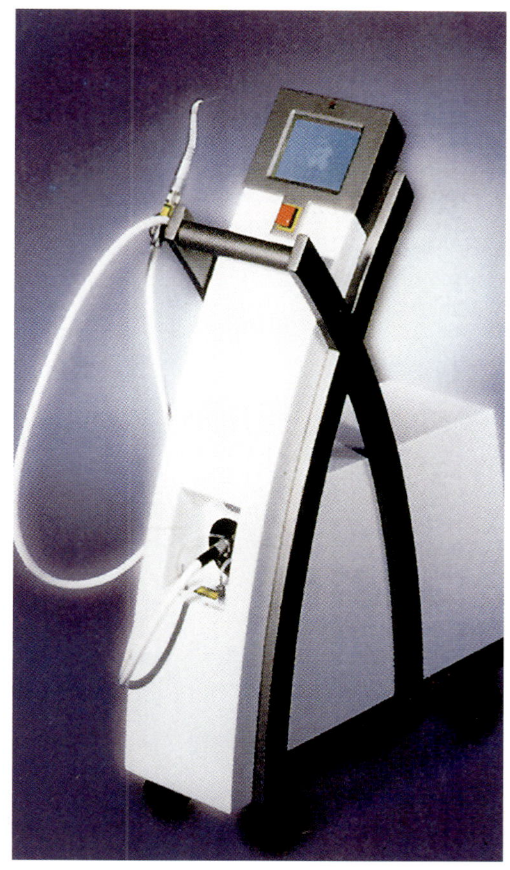

Fig 8-24 and 8-25 Examples of diode laser systems.

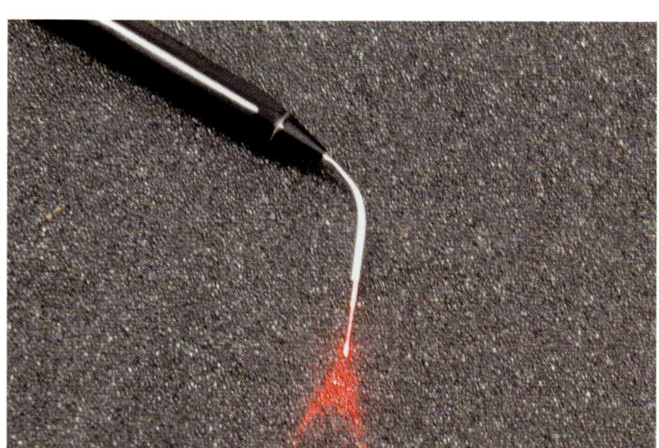

Fig 8-26 Delivery system (bare fiber) of a diode laser.

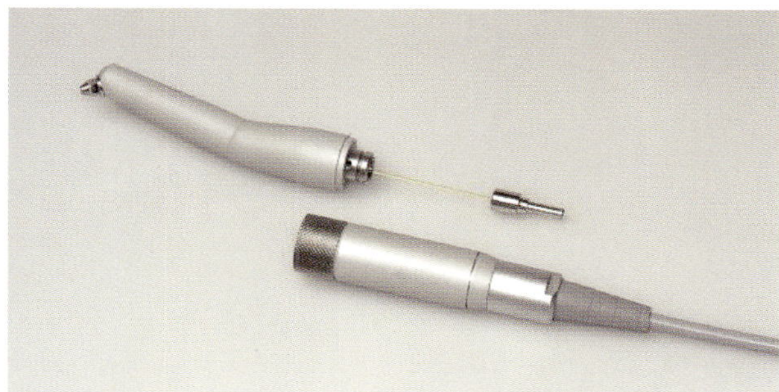

Fig 8-27 Hand piece of a diode laser with exchangeable fiber tips. The part of the delivery system that comes in contact with the patient can be exchanged or sterilized, respectively — a major advantage in periodontics.

doubled alexandrite laser (λ = 377 nm), it was possible to achieve good success in this field. The following figures 8-28 to 8-31 give an overview in the context of the wavelengths used in periodontal therapy.

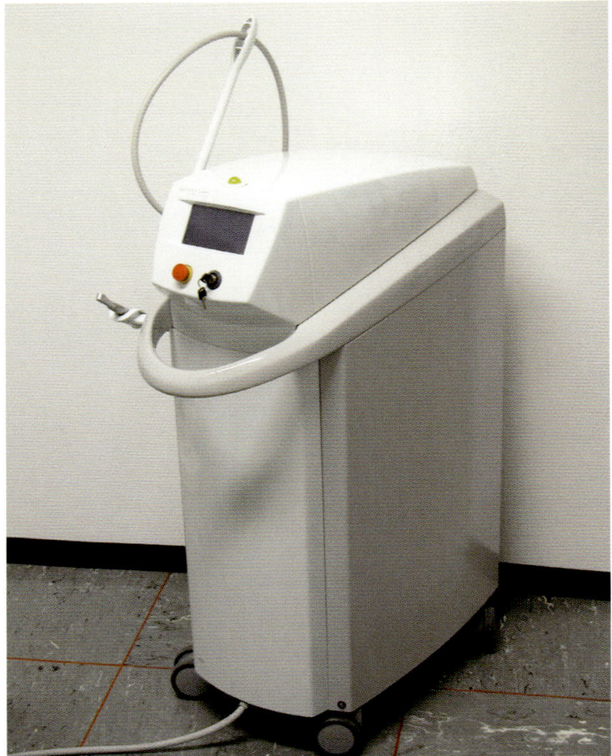

Fig 8-28 Example of an Er:YAG laser system.

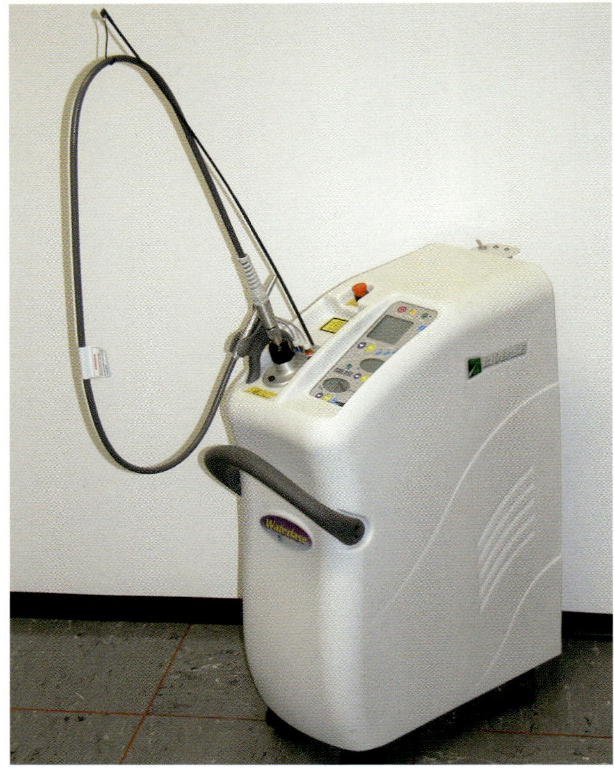

Fig 8-30 Er,Cr:YSGG laser system.

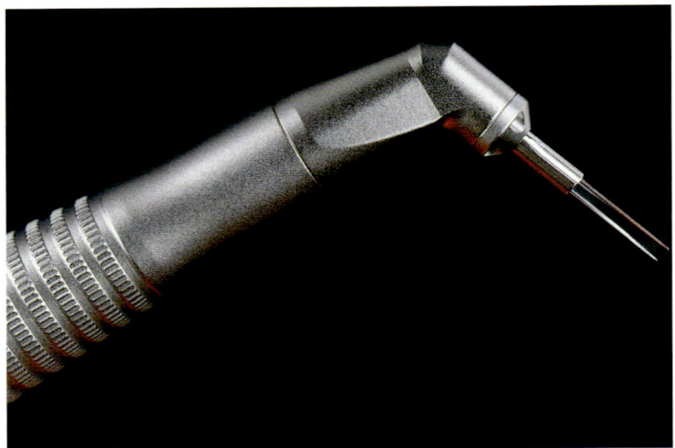

Fig 8-29 Delivery system of an Er:YAG laser: because of ots size, the chisel-shaped fiber tip can be introduced only to limited extent in periodontal pockets. The cooling water necessary for this wavelength is conducted along the chisel tip.

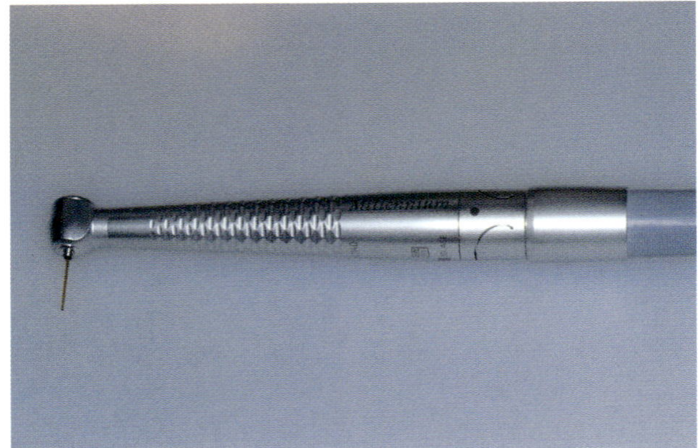

Fig 8-31 Hand piece of an Er,Cr:YSGG laser with a thin flexible fiber.

8.2.3 Impact of the Different Lasers on Tissues

The most important effect of all lasers in the context of periodontal therapy is their antibacterial effect. With low power settings, extremely satisfying results can be obtained. In the case of "preparation wavelengths", particularly the one of the Er:YAG laser, this laser is capable of removing concrements from the root surface. Feedback systems even allow for the selective removal of concrements in connection with protection of the sound root surface. New developments, like the frequency-doubled alexandrite laser will provide similar benefits.

If the output power is increased, also the pocket epithelium, in the sense of a closed curettage, can be removed with the Nd:YAG or the diode laser. In contrast to conventional methods, the laser facilitates a complete deepithelization.[12,13] Still higher settings finally extend the indication field to the range of periodontal surgery, where lasers can be used in the context of flap surgery. Here advantage is taken of the favorable characteristics of the Nd:YAG and the diode wavelengths, which permit efficient cutting and coagulating. A more rapid and complication-free healing comes as a further advantage. The laser also provides interesting aspects in the treatment of peri-implantitis (see section 11.9.7).

Last but not least, the soft-laser effects, which are present with each hard-laser application, should be mentioned. Depending on the power setting and penetration depth, the laser light becomes attenuated when passing through the irradiated tissue down to energy densities that correspond to the irradiation of a soft laser. Its effects, like cell stimulation and probably pain inhibition, have to be taken into account. For a more detailed overview and literature about this topic, see the chapter 13 in the present book.

8.2.4 Pro and Contra the Respective Lasers – Literature Discussion

As already suggested, the antibacterial effect of laser radiation in the infrared range is an advantage, which is common to all lasers mentioned and which offers large advantages to the user in relation to conventional treatment. In addition, the effect of the lasers on the root surface and the surrounding soft tissue is of great importance. The respective effects depend strongly on the wavelength used and their absorption in the different tissues. The following section gives a detailed and scientifically well-founded overview of the lasers applied in periodontal therapy and their specific interactions with the targeted tissues.

8.2.4.1 Diode Laser

Studies concerning the diode laser ($\lambda = 810$ nm) show that the bactericidal effect of this laser is excellent. If one compares conventionally treated control groups with patients who benefited from laser irradiation, this becomes clear. Neither with mechanical removal of concrement alone, nor in combination with antibacterial rinsing solutions could similarly good results be reached. Overall, scientists point out the outstanding effect of the diode laser on the periodontal "problem bacillus", *Actinobacillus actinomycetemcomitans*.

The reduction of bacteria in periodontal pockets by irradiation with a diode laser.

The goal of this pilot study by Moritz et al.[9], was to examine the effect of a diode laser, with a wavelength of 810 nm, on the microorganisms in periodontal pockets.

Fifty patients with pockets of at least 4 mm and different important periodontal indices were evaluated, in order to have reference values for the study. With sterile paper-points, microbiological samples were taken out of the pockets of the patients. Further, they were treated with scaling and 1 week later laser treatment was applied. After 1 more week, samples were taken again by means of paper points and the patients were treated again by scaling, but without laser treatment afterwards. Two weeks later, again samples with paper points were taken. All of the samples taken were analyzed in order to evaluate whether a reduction of the bacterial flora in the pockets had taken place. The comparison of the samples taken at the beginning and at the end of the treatment showed that irradiation with the diode laser offers the possibility of the elimination of the bacteria in periodontal pockets, especially those of *Actinobacillus actinomycetemcomitans*.

The conclusion was drawn that the diode laser is an effective and useful addition to the conventional instrumental treatment. Even if concrement removal with hand instruments may appear sufficient, the laser is a good alternative to chemical rinsing solutions in order to reduce further the bacterial load. The great advantage of the laser is in the special effect on the germ *Actinobacillus actinomycetemcomitans*, known for playing an important part in the destruction of the periodontal retaining apparatus and its destruction is highly important for the success of the therapy.

The goal of another study by Moritz et al.[10] was to examine the long-term effects of the diode laser in periodontal therapy, with regards to its possibilities in reduction of bacteria and periodontal regeneration.

Fifty patients were divided into a laser group and a control group. Microbiological samples were taken. Six treatments per month were done according to an accurate pattern. Periodontal indices as well as the pocket depths were measured, the patients were well-instructed in oral hygiene and a scaling therapy was accomplished. Afterwards, the deepest pocket of each quadrant in the group of lasers was microbiologically examined. Subsequently, all teeth were treated with the diode laser. The control group was submitted to the same procedure; instead of the laser treatment the pockets were rinsed with hydrogen peroxide. At each treatment date, the hygiene of the patient was controlled. After 6 months a renewed determination of the values of the periodontal indices and a recent investigation of the microbiological samples from the pockets took place. The number of bacteria such as *Actinobacillus actinomycetemcomitans, Prevotella intermedia* and *Porphyromonas gingivalis* was measured.

The bacteria reduction in the group treated with lasers was significantly higher in comparison to the control group, the bleeding index in the laser group amounted to 96.9%, in the control group 66.7%. The pocket-depth in the laser group was reduced significantly compared to the control group.

The diode laser has a bactericidal effect according to this study and is able to reduce, in combination with a scaling therapy, the inflammation of the tissue.

Concerning the effect of the wavelength on the root surface itself, no clearly positive effects can be proven, such as for instance the improvement of the attachment.

The effect of diode laser irradiation on the attachment rate of the cells of the periodontal ligament. This in vitro study by Kreisler et al.[14] examined the effect of a diode laser of wavelength 810 nm on periodontium affected by periodontal disease. The goal of the study was to evaluate the effect of the laser treatment on the root surface with regards to the attachments.

Cells of the periodontal ligaments of diseased periodontia of molars were taken and cultivated. A total of 150 of these roots were smoothed with scalers and curettes, and treated afterwards with abrasive air flow devices; 75 of these roots were then lased, the other 75 not. The irradiation time was 20 s with 1 W. The roots were then covered with the cultivated periodontal ligament cells and incubated for a duration of 72 h. Then they were washed with phosphate buffer solution and the cells, which remained on the roots, were marked with methylene blue. The cell density per mm^2 was examined by microscope.

There was no significant difference between the two groups; the cell density on the roots that had been treated with the diode laser was only slightly higher than that on the roots that had not been illuminated with laser. The average values were 66 cells/mm^2 in the group of lasers and 63.7 cells/mm^2 in the other group.

This in vitro study proved that the diode laser does not have a significantly positive effect on the reattachment of periodontally damaged teeth. Whether this investigation translates also into vivo conditions is, however, questionable.

The effect of the diode laser on root surfaces in vitro. A goal of another in vitro study by Kreisler et al.[15] was to examine possible morphologic changes in root surfaces after irradiation with a GaAlAs diode laser of wavelength 809 nm.

Teeth extracted for periodontal reasons were treated with curettes and sandblasting devices. The thus-prepared root surfaces were illuminated with 0.5–2.5 W for 10–30 s per sample with the laser. Additionally, a part of the root surfaces was covered either with saline solution or a thin blood film before the laser treatment. The roots were examined with the optical microscope and additionally photographs were compared, which had been taken before and after the treatment.

The evaluation of the results showed that those samples that were dry or had been covered with saline solution did not exhibit visible surface changes caused by the laser irradiation. On the surfaces covered by a blood film, dependent on the energy parameters, small to serious damage could be observed and with 2.5 W a partial to total carbonization was visible.

According to the authors, the diode laser can thus lead to a strong impairment of the periodontal hard tissue, if the parameters of irradiation are not adequate.

Comparable results were observed by Schwarz et al.[16] when using a GaAlAs diode laser in vivo. Periodontally compromised, not preservable teeth, were irradiated directly prior to their extraction with an energy setting of 1.8 W (pulse/pause relation 1:10). The histological evaluation revealed carbonizations and crater-shaped destruction of the root surface, and the majority extended into the dentin. In contrast, an irradiation after the extraction and rinsing of the root surface with sterile saline solution did not cause any morphological modifications. No removal of concrements could be observed, under in-vivo as well as under in-vitro conditions. According to the authors, the diode laser should only be applied as adjuvant therapy subsidiary to hand-instrumented or ultrasonic-supported cleaning of the root surface. In this connection it should be taken into account that bleeding periodontal pockets produce a blood layer on the root surface and thus lead to destruction and carbonization of the dental hard tissue due to the high absorption of the diode laser's wavelength in hemoglobin. For this reason, the periodontal pocket should be sufficiently rinsed with sterile saline solution or further treatment should be postponed by 1 day.

If the employment of the diode laser does not seem to lead directly to an improvement of the reattachment, however, the success in reduction of the bacteria in deep periodontal pockets speaks for itself. Particularly the bacteria that lead to periodontitis seem to respond strongly to the diode laser. Thus the diode laser is certainly superior to chemical rinsing solutions for reduction of bacteria; its wavelength can be regarded as a valuable tool in the field of periodontal therapy. It allows for an efficient treatment, which is well accepted by the patients. As with any instrument used by a dentist, all the safety precautions and correct handling have to be obeyed. It is particularly important to keep the fiber in motion and never stationary to exclude thermal side-effects. If we pay attention to this, the diode laser does not produce damage to periodontal hard and soft tissues, but leads to the desired therapeutical modifications.

8.2.4.2 Nd:YAG Laser

Something similar applies to the Nd:YAG laser with its wavelength of 1,064 nm. Here also, the antibacterial effect stands in the foreground, while the attachment rate might not be affected directly. As wavelengths within the short-wave infrared range do not show a considerable absorption in hard tissues, this is obvious. Only with high laser energies outside the therapeutic range in vitro, can melting and cracks in the root cement be observed; with clinical application such side effects are not to be feared while working with the correct laser parameters. In addition to its excellent antibacterial effect, the possibility of laser-supported removal of pocket epithelium is another indication.

Nd:YAG laser versus scaling and root planing in periodontal therapy. The goal of the clinical study by Liu et al.[17] was to show the effectiveness of periodontal therapy with this laser and to compare the Nd:YAG laser with scaling and root planing. In eight patients with periodontitis, the content of interleukin-1β in the gingival sulcus fluid was measured, since this represents a strong stimulant for the absorption of bone and stands at the same time for the progression of periodontitis.

Two periodontal damaged teeth with pocket depths from 4 to 6 mm and a horizontal bone loss of 3 mm per quadrant were selected. Each quadrant was then assigned to one of the following groups: a group that was treated only with the laser, a group treated with scaling and root planing only, a third group, treated first with laser and 6 weeks later with hand instruments, and finally a group that was treated first by hand instruments and 6 weeks after with the laser.

Samples of the gingival sulcus fluids were taken and examined by means of an ELISA test for the quantity of existing interleukin-1β. One test at the beginning and another 12 weeks later evaluated the clinical parameters and the results of the investigations of the sulcus fluids after the therapy.

In all four groups a reduction of interleukin-1β and an improvement of the clinical parameters were found. In a comparison of the group that was only mechanically cleaned, with the laser group, a clearly smaller quantity of interleukin-1β was found in the former. A still further reduction of the interleukins could be obtained in the combined laser/scaling group, this significant reduction could not be reached in either the laser group or the scaling-laser group.

The largest effect could be achieved thus in the group that was treated first with the laser and cleaned afterwards mechanically. In the group that first had mechanical cleaning and afterwards laser treatment, this result could not be obtained. The worst result obtained was with exclusive laser therapy: it was clearly less effective in this study than a purely instrumental treatment.

The clinical efficiency of the Nd:YAG laser in combined periodontal therapy. In the double-blind study by Neill and Mellonig[18], 10 patients with periodontitis were submitted to one of the three following treatments:

(1) exclusive scaling and root planing,
(2) laser treatment combined with scaling and root planing
(3) control group

Agreeing with the study mentioned above, that the best possible treatment is that in which lasers and mechanical cleaning could be used together, the applied pulsed Nd:YAG laser with low energy led to an elimination of those bacteria that are in close relationship with the development and the progression of periodontitis.

The effects of a pulsed Nd:YAG laser on the subgingival bacterial flora and on the root cement. The purpose of this in vivo study by Ben Hatit et al.[11] was the comparison of laser combined with instrumental treatment with just-instrumental treatment in reference to the effect on the periodontopathogenic bacteria *Actinobacillus actinomycetemcomitans, Bacteroides forsythus, Porphyromonas gingivalis* and *Treponema denticola*.

Fourteen patients aged 30–75 years with pocket depths of at least 5 mm were examined, with a total of 150 periodontally involved sites. In the first group a conventional mechanical cleaning was accomplished and afterwards a laser treatment, which took 60 s per pocket. The second group served as a control group and was treated exclusively with hand instruments. Samples (DNA probes) were taken in the first group before the instrumental treatment, after the instrumental treatment, after the laser treatment and finally 2, 6 and 10 weeks after. In the second group the samples were taken before and after the instrumental treatment and likewise 2, 6 and 10 weeks later.

In both groups reduction of pathogens and total bacterial load occurred. The microbiological analysis of the reductions of the first group showed a clear reduction of all four bacteria after the treatment in comparison with the condition before. In the control group a clearly weaker result was obtained.

The best results were obtained with low energy (1 W). At these energy settings no cementum damage was seen, however, higher energies led to melting and cracks on the hard tissues.

Evaluation of Nd:YAG laser in the therapy of periodontal pockets. The goal of this study by Radvar et al.[19] was to find out whether the Nd:YAG laser, with an energy of 50 mJ and/or 80 mJ and 10 pulses per second, could influence positively the clinical parameters in the case of periodontal disease. These energy settings were selected, because in other publications higher energy settings had, on the one hand, described surface-damaging and, on the other hand, a bactericidal effect had been proven in vitro with 80 mJ.

Eighty periodontally damaged teeth, scheduled for extraction, in 11 patients were examined; the patients were divided into the following four groups:

(1) laser treatment with 50 mJ and 10 pps for a duration of 3 min
(2) laser treatment with 80 mJ and 10 pps for a duration of 3 min
(3) curettage
(4) untreated control group

At the beginning and after the therapy, the pocket depths, the bleeding index, the plaque index, the gingival index and the volume of gingival sulcus fluid were measured. Samples were taken before and after therapy as well as 6 weeks after, in order to evaluate the colony forming units (CFU) of the strict anaerobes.

An improvement of the clinical parameters was found only in the curettage group. A reduction of the CFUs occurred in the curettage group as well as in the laser-group, treated with energy of 80 mJ, but only the group that had been treated with curettes could maintain the low value until 6 weeks after the therapy. The desired goal of improvement of the clinical and micro-biological parameters in periodontitis patients, by treatment with an Nd:YAG laser with energies of 50 and 80 mJ, could not be achieved in this study.

Effects of Nd:YAG laser irradiation and root planing on the root surface: structural and thermal effects. The purpose of the study by Wilder-Smith et al.[20] was to clarify the question whether the radiation of an Nd:YAG laser could have a cleaning effect on the root surface, without damaging the microstructures.

Sixty extracted teeth were not treated, or only illuminated with laser, only instrumentally cleaned or treated with both laser and mechanical means. The intra-pulpal and the surface temperature during the laser treatment were measured and the surface changes were examined by means of a scanning electron microscope.

The intra-pulpal temperature rose from 9° to 22° C and the surface temperature from 18° to 36° C. Additionally, small changes in the root surfaces were determined. Although the laser was very effective in removing the smear layer, the authors did not recommend the application of an Nd:YAG laser to support periodontitis therapy because of the substantial rise of temperature in this study.

The effect of a pulsed laser beam on the gingiva. In the study by Gold and Vilardi[21], the effectiveness of the removal of the pocket epithelium in patients with moderate periodontitis by a pulsed Nd:YAG laser with low energy settings was examined.

Gingival tissue samples from six patients were taken after application of pulsed Nd:YAG and were microscopically examined. The energy settings were 1.25 and 1.75 W and the frequency 20 Hz. The duration of treatment lay between 2 and 3 min.

The samples were fixed and processed in the usual way. Four representative ranges were examined with 25× and 100× magnification of each tooth using an optical microscope. Most samples (83%) showed up traces of vital basal cell rests at the coronar sulcus edge (17%), a complete epithelium removal. The underlying connective tissue did not show signs of necrosis or carbonization. The morphology exhibited only minimum modifications compared with the controlled areas, concerning the removal of the pocket epithelium. During an output of 1.25–1.75 W, a pulsed Nd:YAG laser is suitable to remove the pocket epithelium of moderately deep pockets.

The effect of the Nd:YAG laser on root surfaces and the subgingival bacterial flora. The goal of this in vivo study by Cobb et al.[22] was to evaluate the effects of a pulsed Nd:YAG laser alone and in combination with mechanical cleaning. Eighteen teeth with periodontal pockets of eight different patients were treated as follows: five teeth were cleaned with curettes and afterwards treated for 3 min with laser at an energy of 3.0 W. Two teeth were cleaned mechanically and then illuminated for 3 min with laser of energy 2.25 W. Four teeth were treated with laser of energy 1.75 W for 1 min and then cleaned with curettes, four teeth treated with laser of energy 1.75 W only. The remaining three teeth served as a control group and remained untreated. Before and after the respective treatments, microbiological samples were taken from the pockets and examined for *Actinobacillus actinomycetemcomitans, Porphyromonas gingivalis* and *Prevotella intermedia*. All teeth, with the exception of two teeth extracted 7 days after treatment, were extracted immediately after the treatment and examined with the scanning electron microscope.

All teeth, regardless of the course of treatment, showed certain laser-induced changes of the root surfaces. The remarkable fact was that the laser-treated concrement was free of its usual plaque-covered surfaces. The investigation of the microbiological samples of the pockets showed a significantly lower level of the examined pathogens after the treatment. Nevertheless, certain concrement and plaque remnants were visible in all groups of treatments.

The effect of Nd:YAG laser used in combination with root planing on root surfaces. A goal of the in vitro study of Morlock et al.[23] was to examine the effect of an Nd:YAG laser on root surfaces, where the laser was used either alone or in combination with mechanical cleaning.

Non-erupted third molars were used which were divided and treated as follows:

(1) untreated control group
(2) root planing
(3) laser treatment with an energy of 1.25 W
(4) laser treatment with an energy of 1.50 W
(5) laser treatment with 1.25 W followed by root planing
(6) laser treatment with 1.50 W and then root planing

All treated teeth were prepared and subsequently examined with the scanning electron microscope.

One could determine, with the exception of the control group, damage to the root cement in all groups, particularly in the laser-treated samples, crater-like defects and carbonization were found frequently; furthermore, exposed dentin tubules were observed, which resulted from the "peeling" of the root cement. According to the authors of this study, every application of the Nd:YAG laser, even with low energy, leads to changes in the root surface.

The effect of Nd:YAG laser and combined treatment on the attachment of fibroblasts at root surfaces. This in vitro study by Thomas et al.[24] had as its goal to examine the attachment rate of fibroblasts on healthy root surfaces which had been treated either only with an Nd:YAG laser or by means of root planing and abrasive powder jet devices in combination with the laser.

Twenty-eight included 3rd molars were used, which were divided into the following four treatment groups:

(1) control group
(2) exclusive laser treatment group
(3) treatment with laser followed by root planing
(4) laser treatment combined with application of airflow

The roots treated with laser were irradiated for 1 min with an energy of 75 mJ and 20 pps, where the root surfaces were kept wet with distilled water. After the four groups had been treated as mentioned, the roots were incubated with fibroblast cultures and prepared for the scanning electron microscope.

The root surfaces of the control group exhibited the highest number of fibroblasts, followed by the group that had been treated first with laser and afterwards with powder jet devices. A substantially smaller number of fibroblasts were yielded in the combined lasers/scaling group and the worst result was obtained in the exclusive laser group.

The removal of the smear layer from root surfaces after root planing with an Nd:YAG laser. This study of Ito et al.[25] compared, by means of a scanning electron microscope, the effectiveness of removing the smear layer by an Nd:YAG laser followed by root planing on one hand and by the use of citric acid on the other. Fifteen periodontally damaged teeth with a loss of attachment of at least 5 mm, which had been extracted due to the prognosis offering no prospects, were examined. The existing concrement was removed with the ultrasonic scaler and the root surfaces were smoothed afterwards with Gracey-curettes. Thirty samples were assigned to one of the two following groups: group A (25 teeth) was irradiated with an Nd:YAG laser at 20 W during 0.3, 0.5, 1.0, 2.0 or 3.0 s, the corresponding energy levels amounted to 84.93, 141.54, 283.09, 566.17 and 849.26 J/cm^2. In group B, five teeth were dipped for 3 min in saturated citric acid (pH 1). The peripheral surfaces, thus untreated areas, in both groups served as control groups. Finally, all teeth were fixed and examined under the scanning electron microscope.

The root surfaces of both control groups exhibited an irregular morphology, corresponding to the amounts of smear layer still existing. The surfaces treated with laser and citric acid showed a smooth morphology, thus the removal of the smear layer was totally possible.

The irradiation with Nd:YAG laser made possible a complete removal of the smear layer; it thus can be used alternatively to other methods for this purpose.

Concrement removal with Nd:YAG laser using low energies. This study of Arcoria and Vitasek-Arcoria[26] examined the possibility of concrement removal using an Nd:YAG laser with 1.09 and 2.19 W. The power densities amounted to 49.2 and 98.4 J/cm^2. Extracted molars with solid deposits of subgingival tartar at the root surfaces were irradiated with an Nd:YAG laser of the described energy. An additional group of teeth was treated with Gracey-curettes and another part of the teeth served as an untreated control group. All teeth were then examined with the scanning electron microscope.

The Nd:YAG laser applied with 1.09 W could not affect the integrity of the concrement at the root surfaces, with 2.19 W concrement removal could be achieved, in such a way that treated surfaces were similar to those on which the Gracey-curettes had been applied. In both cases no considerable damage could be determined on the root surfaces.

The effect of the Nd:YAG laser on concrement, dentin and cement. The goal of this in vitro study by Radvar et al.[27] was to evaluate the effect of an Nd:YAG laser with different energy levels on dentin, cement and the removal of subgingival tartar deposits.

In the first part of the study, 32 extracted teeth were submitted to a laser treatment. In the second part of the study, the root cement of three extracted teeth and the exposed dentin (after mechanical cleaning) of three more extracted teeth were irradiated with the laser. Then all 38 teeth were examined with the scanning electron microscope.

The treatment with the laser had generally larger effects on the removal of the concrement than on the cement or the dentin. Higher energy levels affected more effectively the removal of subgingival deposits. The root cement and the exposed dentin were not affected by the laser treatment with settings of 50 mJ.

Structural and functional changes of the cement surface after irradiation with the Nd:YAG laser. Tewfik et al.[28] studied the effects of the Nd:YAG laser regarding the topography of the root cement and on a possible fibroblast attachment. Fifteen extracted teeth were scaled with curettes and divided into four groups: group 1 represented the untreated control group, groups 2, 3 and 4 were irradiated with 4 W for 1 s, where the distance from the fiber to the tooth surface consisted in group 2 of 1 mm, in group 3 of 3 mm and in group 4 of 5 mm. The 4th group was thus irradiated with the lowest energy, since the energy decreases with the distance. A part of the roots treated in such a way was prepared and examined with the scanning electron microscope. The remaining part of the roots was covered with fibroblast cultures and the attachment rate of the fibroblasts was evaluated.

The investigation with the scanning electron microscope showed that the changes in the root surfaces increased with the rising energy; with 1 mm distance, cracks and fissures in the cement were observed. On the other hand, a larger number of fibroblasts could be determined in the areas irradiated with high energy than with the control group and the root surfaces irradiated with lower energy.

Advantages of the Nd:YAG laser application. Sjostrom and Friskopp[29] came to the conclusion that the application of the Nd:YAG laser in the fields of periodontal therapy provides distinct advantages. Among others, pain reduction, the improvement in concrement removal and the hemostatic effect of the laser irradiation are described.

The studies mentioned above showed both positive and negative results. The best results obtained by Nd:YAG laser are the elimination of periodontopathogenic germs such as *Actinobacillus actinomycetemcomitans, Bacteroides forsythus, Prevotella intermedia* and *Treponema denticola*. Good success could be achieved with the removal of the pocket epithelium and the reduction of interleukin-1β, which has a stimulating effect on the bone resorption. A problem with the application of this laser, according to the opinion of some authors, could be the temperature rise and thus a possible damage to the pulp and the root cement. This raises the question, as to how far certain in-vitro studies can be compared with the situation in vivo, particularly because different parameters have been applied. In vivo studies and numerous reports of successful use clearly depict the Nd:YAG laser as a very valuable tool in periodontal treatment.

The diode and the Nd:YAG lasers have in common that both wavelengths can be delivered directly to the application place with the help of extremely thin, flexible light conductors. Practically all areas of the root surface can be easily reached. Thermal side effects can be excluded when the right parameters and procedures are obeyed.

8.2.4.3 CO_2 Laser

Even if the main indication for the application of the CO_2 laser, with its wavelength of 10,600 nm, in the fields of dentistry is oral surgery, several authors have proven the positive effects of this wavelength with regard to its bactericidal impact, and the ability to remove pocket epithelium and to condition the root surface.

In an in-vivo study, Israel et al.[30] showed that the application of the CO_2 laser in open flap surgery could impede the growth of pocket epithelium to a large extent, in comparison with a control group.

Crespi et al.[31] investigated the attachment rate of fibroblasts on CO_2 laser-irradiated root surfaces in an in-vitro study. They found that the CO_2 laser applied with low power settings is very capable of conditioning the root surface.

The morphology of root surfaces irradiated with a CO_2 laser was investigated by Barone et al.[32]. If the laser was used in defocused mode, the formation of cracks and craters on the root surface could be prevented. The so-conditioned surface was smooth, and open dentinal tubules were sealed.

8.2.4.4 Er:YAG Laser

The Er:YAG laser exhibits an excellent antibacterial effect. Already at low energies, problem bacteria are reliably eliminated with this wavelength. Furthermore, the Er:YAG laser also opens the possibility of removing concrement and plaque from the root surface. This possibility of removal of the concrement by the Er:YAG laser, however, means also roughening of the root surface, since ablation does not take place selectively. The development of special feedback systems could offer a possible way out here. The Er:YAG laser's own delivery system, with a comparatively large chisel-like tip, limits the employment of this wavelength to accessible regions. Further improvements will be necessary in order to extend the range of application of this very-promising wavelength.

Great attention must also be given to a sufficient water cooling with the application of the Er:YAG laser in order to exclude thermal damage of the irradiated surfaces.

The effect of an Er:YAG laser on periodontal damaged root surfaces. In the study by Schwarz et al.[33], 160 roots were treated with the Er:YAG laser, 80 in vivo and 80 immediately after the extraction. The energy settings varied from 120 to 180 mJ. The treated root surfaces were electron microscopically examined.

The in-vitro-treated surfaces showed crater-like defects, which, with higher energy levels, reached into the dentin. In comparison, in-vivo-treated root surfaces showed a homogeneous and smooth morphology, the surface changes did not correlate with the height of the energy level.

The authors conclude a clinical applicability of the Er:YAG laser even with higher energy settings and a modified ablation mechanism under in vivo conditions. The efficacy of the Er:YAG laser in the removal of concrements is comparable with hand instrumentation[16,34] (Fig 8-33). In addition, periodontally compromised Er:YAG laser-irradiated root surfaces showed a significantly higher biocompatibility in cultures of human PDL fibroblasts in comparison to those which have been only hand- or ultrasonic-instrumented. This could be explained by the lack of a smear layer after laser therapy[35].

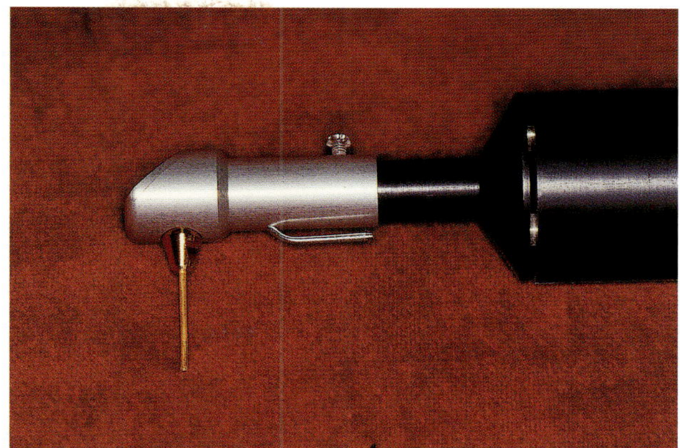

Fig 8-32 Delivery system of a CO_2 laser (hollow waveguide).

Laser scaling with the Er:YAG laser. In this in vitro study Aoki et al.[36] studied the effectiveness of the Er:YAG laser in concrement removal. Fifty-three extracted periodontally damaged teeth were used, that exhibited large quantities of concrement. On the one hand a laser with water spray, an energy from 10 to 120 mJ per pulse and a frequency of 10 cycles per second was used, and on the other hand a laser without water spray and an energy of 30 mJ per pulse and the same frequency. The morphologic changes, the temperature development and the effectiveness were evaluated.

The best result was obtained with the Er:YAG laser with water irrigation, an energy of 30 mJ per pulse and a frequency of 10 cycles per second. The concrement could be removed efficiently from the roots; a small temperature rise during the laser treatment was observed at the same time.

In this study it was shown that the Er:YAG laser represents a suitable aid to the removal of concrement.

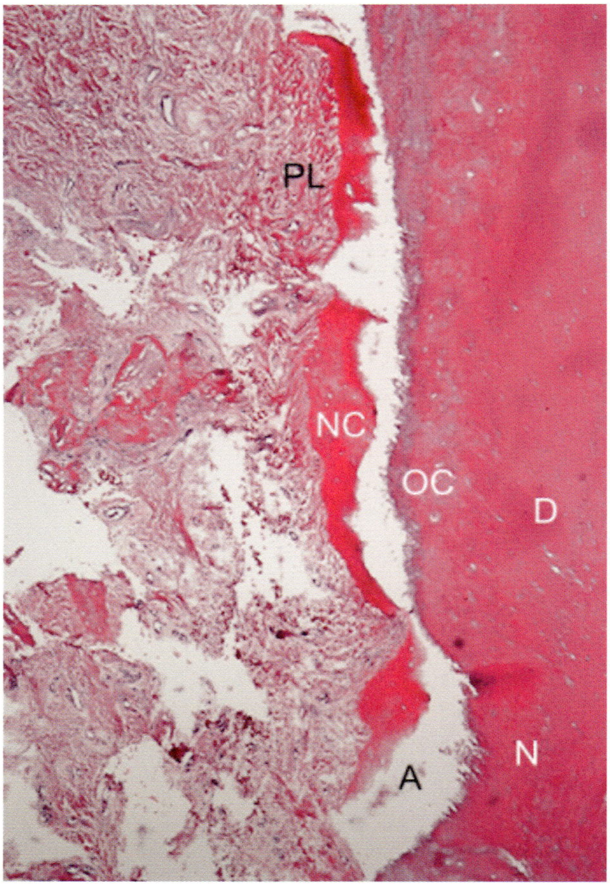

Fig 8-33 Human histological sample 6 months after flap surgery and instrumentation of the root surface and removal of the granulation tissue with an Er:YAG laser. The healing is characterized by the formation of a long junctional epithelium. A, artifact; D, dentin; LJE, long junctional epithelium; N, notch; OC, old cementum (hematoxylin–eosin stain; original magnification x25).

The effect of the Er:YAG laser on root surfaces and the pulpal temperature. In this in vitro study by Schoop et al.[37] an Er:YAG laser with a wavelength of $\lambda = 2.94$ µm and a maximum radiation energy of 400 mJ was used in order to examine its effects on root surfaces, the pulpal temperature and the periodontal connective tissue.

In the first part of the study 20 extracted human teeth were divided in four groups. The specimens of the first group were each irradiated five times during 5 s with 100 mJ. The second group was treated manually, while the third group was treated manually and with laser. The fourth group served as untreated control group. After the different treatments, the result was evaluated by means of a scanning electron microscope.

In the second part of the study 10 teeth, which had been treated with different laser settings, were examined for a possible increase of the temperature in the pulp.

In the third part of the study, teeth of sheep were treated with different laser settings, in order to evaluate the effect on the root surfaces and the adjacent connective tissue, where one group was treated only manually and a second group served as control group.

During the evaluation of the results it was observed that a satisfying removal of the subgingival concrement from the root surfaces with the Er:YAG laser was possible; the root surfaces, however, exhibited a clearly rougher morphology than those that had been treated either only manually or combined.

The temperature in the pulp increased by maximally 4.5°C when the laser was set to 100 mJ. With this setting, no damage of the hard and soft tissue could be found, whereas with higher energy settings rough root surfaces and damage to the remaining parts of the periodontium could be determined.

The Er:YAG laser is thus able to remove concrements when a setting of 100 mJ is applied, where the roughness at the root surface, developed thereby, is comparable with that caused by manual scaling. The temperature rise in the pulp can be called tolerable, if appropriate water cooling is present and an interval of 15 s is respected. One can consider the damage caused on hard and soft tissues as negligible.

The Er:YAG laser seems to be a very promising instrument for the removal of subgingival plaque and concrement.

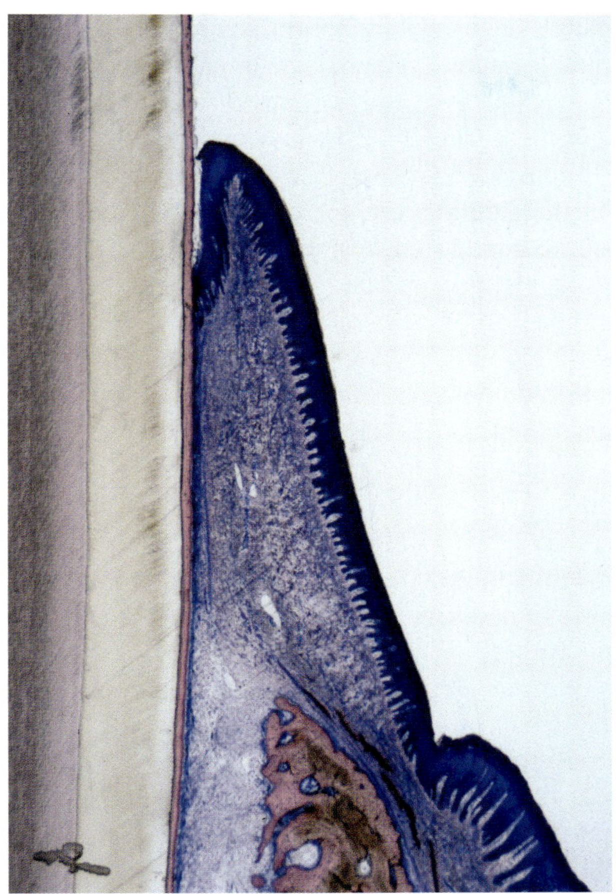

Fig 8-34 Section through a sheep's molar, buccal/lingual. Control group. The unimpaired anatomical situation is discernible.

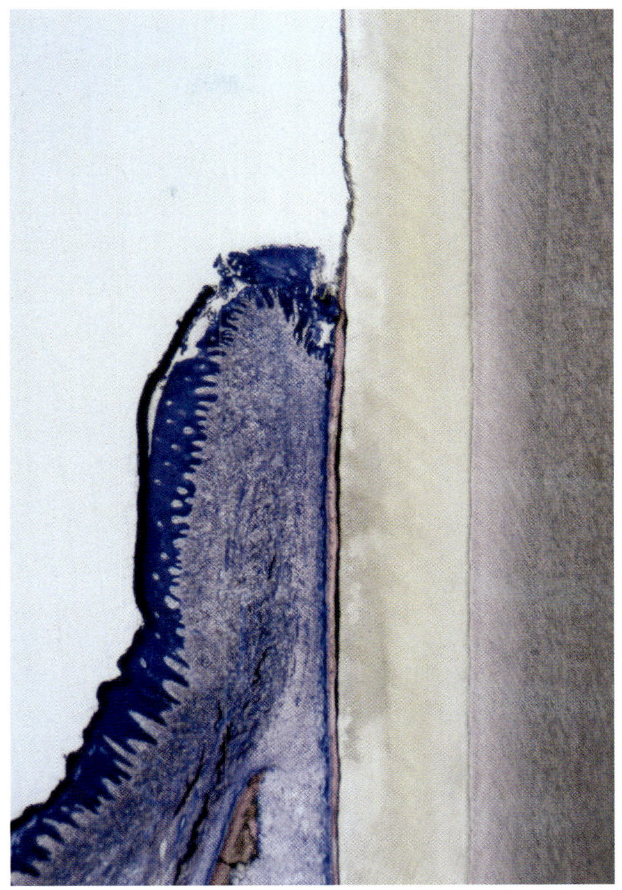

Fig 8-35 Section through a sheep's molar, buccal/lingual. Lased side. The roughening of the root surface and a discrete damage of the soft tissue can be seen.

The impacts of Er:YAG laser irradiation on root surfaces and the adjacent tissues. Folwaczny et al.[38] assessed the impact of Er:YAG laser irradiation on the root surface and adjacent tissues using histological samples obtained from the respective structures, after teeth of human bodies had been irradiated in situ. In contrast to the preceding scanning electron studies, certain apparently thermally-caused alterations of the ultrastructure of the root cementum and the underlying dentin could be observed.

These alterations were observed up to a depth of 611 µm and were independent of the irradiation energy.

Removing concrement with the Er:YAG laser and a new delivery system using different parameters. In this in vitro study Folwaczny et al.[39] tried to justify the employment of an Er:YAG laser in combination with a delivery system specifically developed for removing concrement. Fifty extracted teeth were divided in two groups: 25 teeth with existing concrement and 25 teeth with no concrement. The radiation source was an Er:YAG laser with a wavelength of $\lambda = 2.94$ µm, a pulse duration of 250 µs and a pulse frequency of 15 per second. Each group was divided into four sub-groups, which were irradiated with, in each case, 300 laser pulses up to 60, 80, 100 and 150 mJ. The evaluation of the concrement removal was assessed with a three-dimensional laser scanning system (100 points on the surface per specimen and an accuracy of 5 μm) and special software. In order to evaluate the surface changes caused by the laser, a scanning electron microscope was used.

The statistical results showed that in the group with existing concrement, far better results could be obtained. In the group without existing concrement, no thermal damage could be determined with the electron microscope.

Due to this study it could be shown that the Er:YAG laser with a lower energy setting is quite comparable with the conventional instrumentation with regards to concrement removal.

The impact of Er:YAG laser irradiation on the root surface structure. In another study, Folwaczny et al.[40] evaluated the influence of Er:YAG laser irradiation on the roughness of root surfaces. Untreated, lased and conventionally scaled root surfaces, were compared in vitro. The roughness values were obtained using a profilometer; the results were submitted to a statistical evaluation. The authors came to the conclusion that there were no significant differences regarding the roughness, regardless of whether the samples were laser-irradiated or conventionally scaled. In addition, there was no dependency observed on the laser parameters used or the angulation of the hand piece.

Regarding the absolute amount of hard substance removed, there are clear dependencies on the energy used and the ablation of the hand piece (Folwaczny et al.[41]). The more material is ablated, the higher the power setting and the more obtuse the angle between the fiber and the root surface.

Frentzen et al.[42] compared the ablation rates of conventional scaling with a laser-supported curettage and came to the conclusion that the laser produces a higher surface roughness and more dental hard substance is ablated.

In contrast, Eberhard et al.[43] illustrated in an in-situ study that conventional scaling is slightly superior to the Er:YAG laser regarding concrement removal, but also invokes a higher loss of root cementum. The teeth used in the study were treated in vivo, and for further procedures they were subsequently extracted.

Israel et al.[44] compared the impacts of CO_2-, Nd:YAG- and Er:YAG-laser irradiation on root surfaces in vitro. Depending on the energy setting used, the Nd:YAG and the CO_2 lasers produced melting and cracks on the root surface. In contrast, the Er:YAG laser irradiation led to a roughening of the surface and the exposure of collagenous fibers. The authors therefore contribute great potential to the wavelength of the Er:YAG laser in the field of periodontology.

An in vitro study by Yamaguchi et al.[45] examined the effects of the Er:YAG laser on subgingival deposits by means of a scanning electron microscope.

Fifteen premolars were used, which had been extracted for orthodontic reasons. The teeth were divided in three different groups:

- five teeth without any treatment,
- five teeth partially treated without damage of the root cement
- five teeth whose root-dentin was partly exposed after the treatment.

The success rate of cleaning the subgingival deposits with Er:YAG laser was about 83.1%, and the areas treated by laser showed only small morphologic changes. Despite these good results, the authors suggest that further clinical investigations are necessary to establish the Er:YAG laser in periodontics.

With an in vitro study, Aoki et al.[46] examined the effectiveness of Er:YAG laser scaling and the morphologic and histological changes of root surfaces in direct comparison to subgingival ultrasonic scaling.

Fifty-three extracted teeth with concrement deposits were used. The laser was used with an energy level of 40 mJ/pulse and 10 pulses/min under water cooling. The ultrasonic device was used with the clinically usual standard energy levels. The changes in the root surfaces were examined by means of a light and a scanning electron microscope. The Er:YAG laser achieved just as good a concrement removal rate as the ultrasonic scaler, without causing a considerable rise in temperature. The surfaces treated with the laser were macroscopic, somewhat rougher than those treated with the ultrasonic scaler; small micro structural and thermal changes could be determined. The effectiveness of the laser scaling was hardly less than that of the ultrasonic.

Treatment with laser offers, thus, a good alternative to instrumental treatment, however, with the same effectiveness; the ultrasonic device, however, better respects the integrity of the hard tissue.

Changes to root surfaces and the influence on fibroblast adhesion by irradiation with the Er:YAG laser. This combined in vitro study of Schoop et al.[47] examined the effects of the Er:YAG laser with a wavelength of $\lambda = 2.94$ µm on the root surface morphology, the possibility of concrement removal and a possibly better fibroblast adhesion by laser irradiation.

In the first part of the study, 15 extracted teeth with concrement were examined, five specimens were irradiated, five times in each case during 5 s with an energy of 100 mJ (group 1). A further five teeth were cleaned only manually (group 2), the remaining five (group 3) were cleaned manually and with the laser (same conditions as in group 1).

In the second part of the study, 32 extracted teeth were used, from which 26 samples exhibited concrement at the root surfaces. The remaining six were free from concrement and served as a control group (group 4). With a diamond band saw, a 2-mm-thick layer was cleared away consisting of radicular dentin, root cement and concrement from each of the 26 teeth. Then, nine teeth were irradiated five times for 5 s with the Er:YAG laser with an energy of 100 mJ (group 1). A further nine teeth were cleaned with Gracey-curettes (group 2). The remaining eight specimens were treated in a combined way, first with the laser as in group 1 and afterwards manually as in group 2 (group 3). Mouse fibroblasts, which had been cultivated before, were applied on the thus-prepared root surfaces.

The results were examined and evaluated using a scanning electron microscope.

Concerning the first part of the study, in group 1 there was a rough root surface, caused by the laser. A better result was obtained in group 3, and in group 2 relatively smooth surfaces were found.

The evaluation of the second part of the study showed that the best results concerning the adhesion of fibroblasts were obtained in group 3. The lowest number of fibroblasts was found in group 2.

The Er:YAG laser thus facilitates the concrement removal and offers better conditions for the adhesion of fibroblasts than pure manual cleaning.

Feist et al.[48] also asked the question, whether the Er:YAG laser irradiation of root surfaces could possibly improve the adherence rate of fibroblasts. The utilized teeth were divided into three groups and either treated with conventional scaling or laser irradiation at 60 mJ/10 Hz or 100 mJ/10 Hz, respectively. The thus-prepared surfaces were cultivated with human gingival fibroblasts. An evaluation using a scanning electron microscope took place 1, 2 and 3 days after the cell culture was initiated. It could be shown that an irradiation with a power setting of 60 mJ at 10 Hz was more beneficial to the establishment of fibroblasts than scaling or laser irradiation with higher energies.

The bactericidal effect of the Er:YAG laser on periodontopathogenic bacteria. In an in vitro study, Ando et al.[49] assessed the effect of the Er:YAG laser on periodontopathogenic bacteria. A bacterial suspension was spread on agar plates and subsequently irradiated. Through Er:YAG laser irradiation, a high bactericidal effect was obtained, even if a comparison with other studies is not easy to accomplish because of the methods used (agar plates instead of root surfaces).

The bactericidal effect of the Er:YAG laser on the periodontopathogenic microbial flora also was the subject of an in-vitro study by Folwaczny et al.[50]. The root surfaces of 125 extracted teeth were inoculated with a suspension of *E. coli, Staphylococcus aureus, Actinobacillus actinomycetemcomitans, Eikenella corrodens* and *Peptostreptococcus micros*. This was followed by a laser irradiation at different power settings and a bacteriological evaluation which proved a high bactericidal effect of the Er:YAG laser on the investigated microorganisms.

Clinical evaluation of the Er:YAG laser concerning soft tissue surgery and scaling. Thirty-one patients with soft tissue lesions and 60 patients with subgingival tartar deposits were treated with the Er:YAG laser in this study by Watanabe et al.[51] The criteria for the evaluation of the clinical applicability were: pain, redness, swelling of the gingiva and subjective criteria of the patients, such as noise and vibrations during the laser treatment.

Additionally, bleeding and wound healing were evaluated during and after surgical application as well as the effectiveness of the laser-scaling and/or the roughness of the root surface after the scaling.

With the surgical application of the laser, less bleeding and better results of wound healing were observed compared with conventional surgical methods.

In 95% of the cases the removal of the subgingival calculus deposits of the root surfaces was easy, and although the surfaces showed light irregularities, these were clinically not significant in 98% of the cases. The subjective evaluation of the patients was likewise positive; only a few complained about unpleasant noises or vibrations.

Because of the absence of complications and side effects during this clinical study the application of the Er:YAG laser can be judged meaningful in soft tissue surgery and an alternative to instrumental scaling as well.

Non-surgical periodontal therapy with the Er:YAG Laser. Fifteen patients with progressed marginal periodontitis were treated by Schwarz et al.[52] with an Er:YAG laser after a hygiene phase of 4 weeks. In none of the participants were postoperative complications like impaired wound healing, wound infections or abscess formation observed. In the beginning of the study 59% of the tooth surfaces showed bleeding on probing, which was reduced to 19% after 6 months ($P \leq 0.001$). During the study, the mean initial probing depths of 4.7 ± 0.7 mm were reduced to 3.1 ± 0.6 mm after 6 months ($P \leq 0.001$). The gingival recessions slightly increased from 1.4 ± 0.8 mm in the beginning to 1.5 ± 0.7 mm after 6 months ($P \geq 0.05$). The mean clinical attachment level was reduced from 6.1 ± 1.1 mm in the beginning to 4.6 ± 1.0 mm after 6 months ($P \leq 0.001$). The changes of the clinical parameters were statistically highly significant in comparison to the initial values ($P \leq 0.001$).

A first clinical comparison with conventional scaling and root planing showed heterogeneous results. In a study accomplished by Jepsen et al.[53] a mean attachment gain of 0.3 ± 0.2 mm in the laser group and 0.4 ± 0.3 mm in the control group was observed in 10 patients after 3 months. The differences were not statistically significant ($P \geq 0.05$).

The goal of another clinical study by Schwarz et al.[54] was to compare the effectiveness of the Er:YAG laser with classical scaling and root planing.

Twenty patients with average periodontal destruction were treated by quadrants, either with an Er:YAG laser (energy of 160 mJ/pulse and frequency of 10 Hz) or with conventional hand instruments. During the treatment, then 3 and 6 months after, the plaque index, the gingiva index, the bleeding index, the pocket depths, the gingival recession and the clinical loss of attachment were measured. Subgingival plaque was sampled and examined by means of a dark field microscope for cocci, mobile and immobile rods and spirochetes.

The plaque index remained almost unchanged, while the gingival index in both groups could be significantly reduced after 6 months. The bleeding index decreased in the laser group from 56% at the beginning to 13% after 6 months. In the group that had been treated with hand instruments, the bleeding index sank from 52% to 23%. The pocket depths in the laser group dropped from 4.9 mm to 2.9 mm, whereas in the non-laser-treated group, a pocket reduction from 5.0 mm to 3.4 mm was obtained. The clinical attachment loss had sunk in the group of lasers from 6.3 mm to 4.4 mm, in the other group from 6.5 mm to 5.5 mm. In both groups a strong increase of cocci and immobile rods took place, but a significant reduction of the spirochetes and mobile rods was registered. The treatment time in the laser group was 5 minutes for teeth with one root and 10 minutes for teeth with more than one root. In the control group, the treatment time amounted to 9 minutes for single-rooted teeth and 15 minutes for teeth with more than one root.

Due to the significant reduction of the bleeding index and the clinical attachment loss in the group treated with lasers, the Er:YAG laser can be considered as a meaningful alternative to hand instruments in the treatment of periodontitis.

The results of a recently published study show that the clinical parameters could be maintained in both treatment groups over a period of 24 months[55]. The attachment loss after 24 months accounted for 4.9 ± 0.4 mm in the laser group ($P \leq 0.001$), and 5.8 ± 0.4 mm in the control group ($P \leq 0.001$).

In addition, it could be shown that supplementary hand instrumentation after the Er:YAG laser irradiation did not invoke an improvement of the clinical parameters[56]. The mean probing depth was reduced from 5.2 ± 0.8 mm in the beginning to 3.2 ± 0.8 mm after 12 months ($P \leq 0.001$) in the laser + SRP group and from 5.0 ± 0.7 mm in the beginning to 3.3 ± 0.7 mm after 12 months ($P \leq 0.001$) in the control group. The mean attachment loss was reduced from 6.9 ± 1.0 mm in the beginning to 5.3 ± 1.0 mm after 12 months ($P \leq 0.05$) in the laser group and from 6.6 ± 1.1 mm in the beginning to 5.0 ± 0.7 mm after 12 months ($P \leq 0.05$) in the control group. Nevertheless, the differences between the two groups were not statistically significant ($P \geq 0.05$).

The first clinical data proved also that the attachment gain after non-surgical periodontal therapy with an Er:YAG laser is comparable to the one achieved by ultrasonic scaling[57].

Surgical and regenerative periodontal therapy with the Er:YAG laser. To date, only two controlled clinical studies exist which permit discussion of the application of the Er:YAG laser in surgical and regenerative periodontal therapy. Sculean et al.[58] assessed the cleaning of the root surfaces and the removal of granulation tissue with energy settings of 160 mJ/10 Hz in the field of open periodontal therapy. In relation to the hand-instrumented cleaning of root surfaces and defects, a clinically comparable attachment gain could be observed 6 months post-operation. The differences between the two groups were not statistically significant ($P \geq 0.05$).

Schwarz et al.[59] combined the use of the Er:YAG laser with the application of an enamel-matrix protein (EMD) in the field of regenerative periodontal therapy. The control group was treated by hand-instrumented root surface- and defect-cleaning, followed by a conditioning of the root surfaces with EDTA and the application of EMD. The mean probing depth in the laser group decreased from 8.6 ± 1.2 mm in the beginning to 4.6 ± 0.8 mm after 6 months ($P \leq 0.001$) and in the control group from 8.1 ± 0.8 mm in the beginning to 4.0 ± 0.5 mm after 6 months ($P \leq 0.001$). The mean attachment loss decreased from 10.7 ± 1.3 mm in the beginning to 7.5 ± 1.4 mm after 6 months ($P \leq 0.05$) in the laser group and in the control group from 10.4 ± 1.1 mm in the beginning to 7.1 ± 1.2 mm after 6 months ($P \leq 0.05$). The differences between the two groups were statistically not significant ($P \geq 0.05$).

The treatment of hypersensitive dental necks with the Er:YAG laser. In a clinical study it was additionally proven that the Er:YAG laser facilitates an effective treatment of hypersensitive dental necks[60]. A group of 30 patients with, in total, 104 contralateral hypersensitive, caries-free pairs of teeth were treated either with an Er:YAG laser at 80 mJ/3 Hz or with Dentin Protector (polyurethane-Iisocyanate 22.5%, methylene chloride 77.5%, Vivadent, Germany) using the "split-mouth" study design. An additional untreated pair of teeth served as a control in each patient. The qualitative assessment of the hypersensitivity (grade 1–4) was accomplished by applying an air spray to the mouth of the blindfolded patient for 3 s at a distance of 2 mm to the root surface immediately after the therapy and 1 week, 2 and 6 months after the therapy. Both treatment measures led to a significant reduction in comparison to the untreated control group. The Er:YAG laser, however, yielded a significantly higher reduction after 2 and 6 months in comparison to Dentin Protector®. The actual impact mechanism of the Er:YAG laser in the treatment of hypersensitive dental necks is still unknown and subject to current investigations.

Feedback system. If a system for the measurement of laser fluorescence is coupled to an Er:YAG laser, as in the case of the KeYIII laser made by KaVo, selective concrement removal should be facilitated. The control unit only releases the laser beam as long as the laser fluorescence measurement gives evidence of the existence of concrements. If the root surface is free from deposits, the laser is stopped and no more sound tissue is ablated.

Laser light of a diode laser with a wavelength of $\lambda = 655$ nm was assessed in a study by Krause et al.[61] with regard to its ability to detect concrements on root surfaces using laser fluorescence. Root surfaces loaded with concrement were submitted to laser fluorescence measurements in vitro; the Diagnodent System, normally used for the diagnosis of caries, was applied. After a mechanical removal of the concrements, the investigation was repeated. Significant differences were found regarding the laser fluorescence in comparison with the concrement-loaded samples. The authors came to the conclusion that laser fluorescence at a wavelength of $\lambda = 655$ nm is suitable for the detection of subgingival concrements.

To assess the impacts of a feedback system coupled to an Er:YAG laser, an in-vitro study has been accomplished at the University Clinic of Vienna. The buccal root surfaces of concrement-loaded extracted teeth were treated with the Er:YAG laser in conjunction with the activated feedback system. For control purposes, the lingual sides were treated with the laser and the feedback system remained deactivated. The thus-treated root surfaces were assessed by means of a scanning electron microscope. It could be shown that the root surfaces, which were irradiated with the help of the feedback system, were clearly smoother, but still showed signs of slight ablation.

The Er:YAG laser facilitates the removal of concrements and offers a better environment for the adhesion of fibroblasts than mechanical cleaning.

The critical view of the studies mentioned above leads to the conclusion that the Er:YAG laser is only at the beginning of its success in periodontal therapy. The advantages seem to outweigh the disadvantages by far. From the view of the patient, the laser is surely the best alternative to conventional instrumental treatment, since the laser provides nearly painless and rapid treatment. From the medical view, the disadvantage of the laser treatment is that it leaves micro-roughness, but that cannot be excluded with other working methods either, which simply means that every technique has some disadvantage. The indication for concrement removal, which the Er:YAG laser achieves with high effectiveness, is confirmed by these studies; also, we can conclude that by treatment with the Er:YAG laser, an improvement of the reattachment can be achieved. The rise in pulpal temperature induced by the laser can be neglected when using appropriate parameters and water cooling.

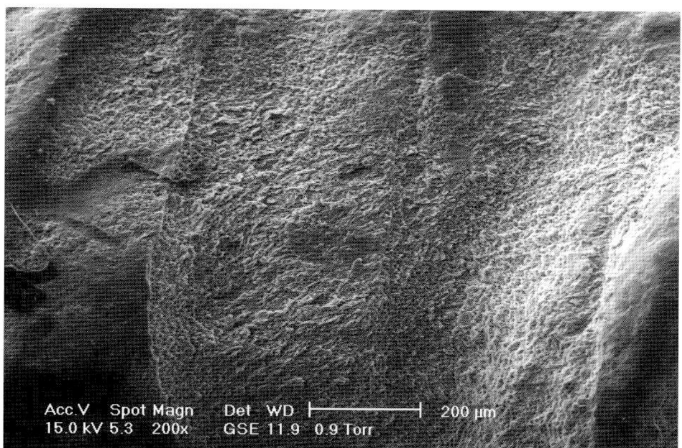

Fig 8-36 Root surface lingual, irradiated with the feedback system deactivated (×200); the areas roughened by the laser are clearly discernible.

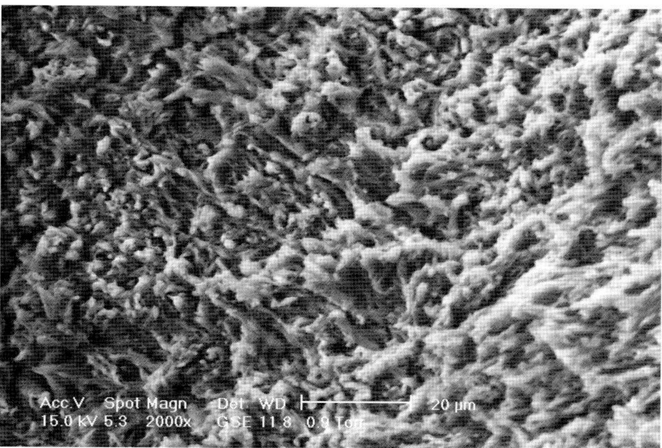

Fig 8-37 Root surface lingual, irradiated with the feedback system deactivated (×2000); the areas roughened by the laser are clearly discernible.

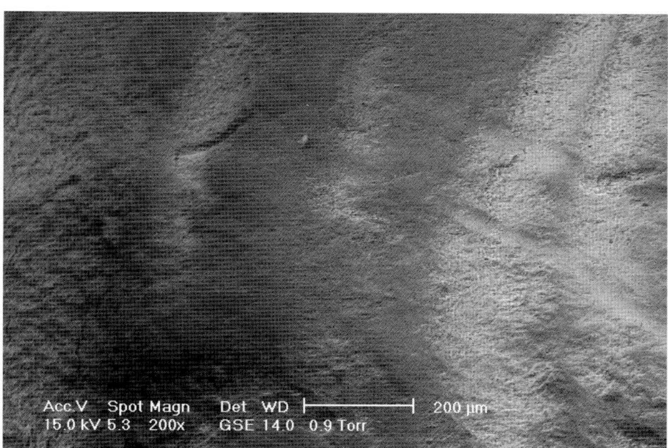

Fig 8-38 Root surface buccal, irradiated with the feedback system activated (×200); the surface appears clearly smoother; the ablation took place in single spots.

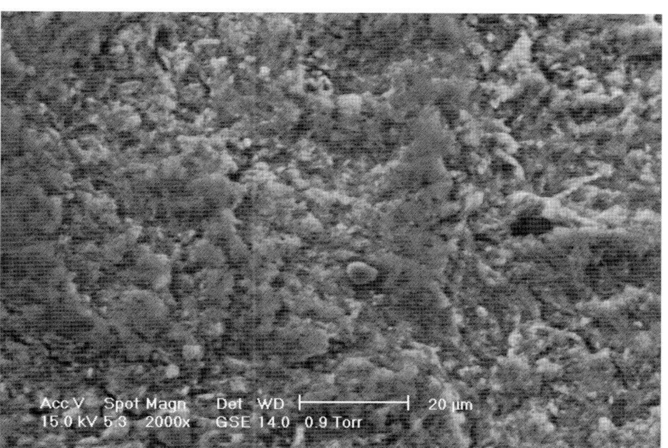

Fig 8-39 Also in this picture (high magnification, ×2000) a rough surface can be seen, although in a lower amount in comparison to Fig 8-37.

8.2.4.5 The Er,Cr:YSGG Laser

For the Er,Cr:YSGG laser, the statements about the Er:YAG laser largely apply, even if only a few investigations on the application of this laser in periodontics are available to date. A good bactericidal effect is known for this wavelength, and the removal of subgingival concrements seems to be possible, althrough, not selectively. Sufficient water cooling is indispensable when using this laser.

Investigations by Kimura et al.[62] showed that the effect of this laser on root surfaces might be comparable to those of the Er:YAG laser: concrement can be removed from the root surface – this, however, is again at the price of a roughening of the cement surface.

8.2.4.6 The Frequency-Doubled Alexandrite Laser

The introduction of this "new" wavelength into the field of periodontal therapy could open up highly interesting aspects: with the use of the frequency-doubled alexandrite laser, it should be possible in future to remove plaque and concrements selectively, under maximized preservation of the root surface.

After this laser, with a wavelength of $\lambda = 377$ nm, proved its ability of selective caries removal, in the studies of Henning et al. and Rechmann et al.[63,64], Rechmann et al. began an investigation on the application of this laser in the context of periodontal therapy[65]. At repetition rates of up to 110 cycles per second and pulse duration between 100 and 200 ns they succeeded in clearing away plaque and concrement selectively from enamel and root surfaces. The treated hard tissues remained completely intact, proven by light and scanning electron microscopy. A bactericidal effect of the wavelength of $\lambda = 377$ nm was proven in a study of Henning et al.; also, a good applicability and efficient water cooling of the treated area are attributed to the delivery system[66].

The frequency-doubled alexandrite laser could revolutionize the entire range of laser-based periodontal therapy. Selective concrement removal with a good antibacterial effect and an easy applicability make this laser appear to be ideal tool in this field.

8.3 Practical Procedure

8.3.1 Anamnesis

In principle, the procedures described here are similar to those that are recommended in the context of any periodontal therapy. It begins with the collection of a general-medical and dental anamnesis, in order to evaluate periodontal pathogenic-relevant basic illnesses and to evaluate the general condition of the denture. Special attention in the context of the dental anamnesis must be focused on the recognition of occlusal disturbances and periodontally unfavorably arranged restorations.

The periodontal anamnesis serves to evaluate and document all relevant parameters. Only on the basis of these data can further therapy be planned. Of particular importance here is the assessment of

- pocket depth
- mobility of the teeth
- plaque accumulations
- severity of the inflammation
- radiographic findings
- restorations/periodontal compatibility

For the measurement of pocket depths, periodontal probes are used, which permit by means of their mm-marks an estimation, not only of the actual pocket depth, but also of the general attachment loss.

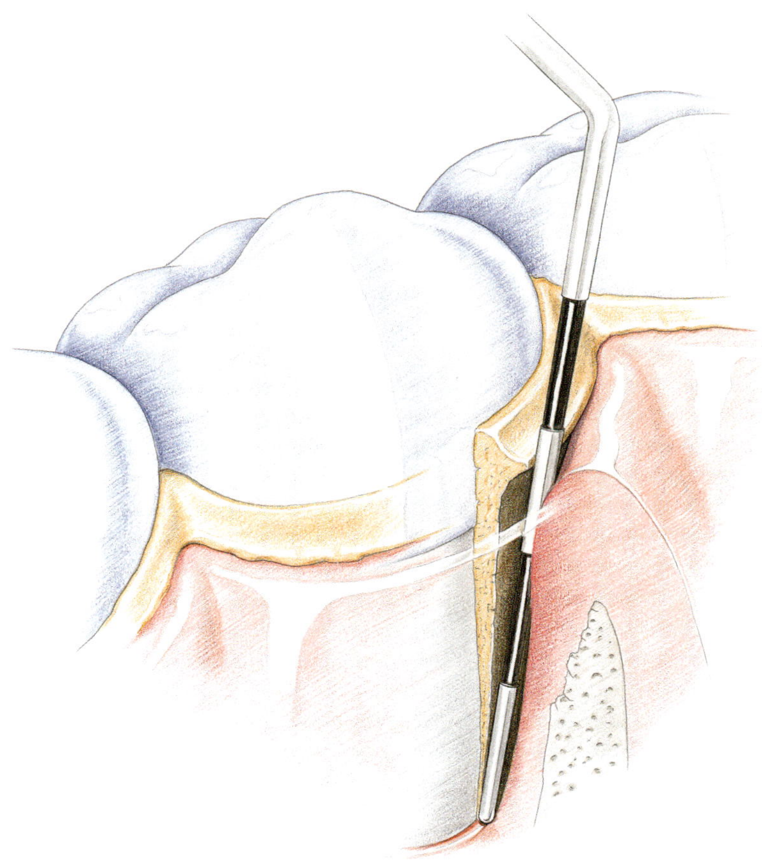

Fig 8-40 Measuring of pocket depths.

Fig 8-41 Measuring of pocket depths.

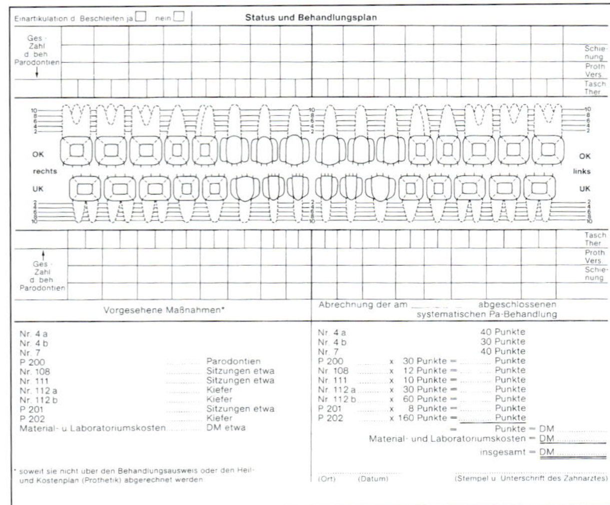

Einartikulation d. Beschleifen ja ☐ nein ☐

Status und Behandlungsplan

Ges.-Zahl d. beh. Parodontien

Schienung
Proth. Vers.
Tasch. Ther.

OK rechts | OK links
UK | UK

Tasch. Ther.
Proth. Vers.
Schienung

Ges.-Zahl d. beh. Parodontien

Vorgesehene Maßnahmen*

Nr. 4 a		
Nr. 4 b		
Nr. 7		
P 200	....	Parodontien
Nr. 108	....	Sitzungen etwa
Nr. 111	....	Sitzungen etwa
Nr. 112 a	....	Kiefer
Nr. 112 b	....	Kiefer
P 201	....	Sitzungen etwa
P 202	....	Kiefer
Material- u. Laboratoriumskosten	....	DM etwa

* soweit sie nicht über den Behandlungsausweis oder den Heil- und Kostenplan (Prothetik) abgerechnet werden

Abrechnung der am ________ abgeschlossenen systematischen Pa-Behandlung

Nr. 4 a				40 Punkte
Nr. 4 b				30 Punkte
Nr. 7				40 Punkte
P 200	....	x 30 Punkte =	....	Punkte
Nr. 108	....	x 12 Punkte =	....	Punkte
Nr. 111	....	x 10 Punkte =	....	Punkte
Nr. 112 a	....	x 30 Punkte =	....	Punkte
Nr. 112 b	....	x 60 Punkte =	....	Punkte
P 201	....	x 8 Punkte =	....	Punkte
P 202	....	x 160 Punkte =	....	Punkte

= Punkte = DM ....
Material- und Laboratoriumskosten = DM ....
insgesamt = DM ....

(Ort) (Datum) (Stempel u. Unterschrift des Zahnarztes)

Fig 8-42 Anamnesis sheet.

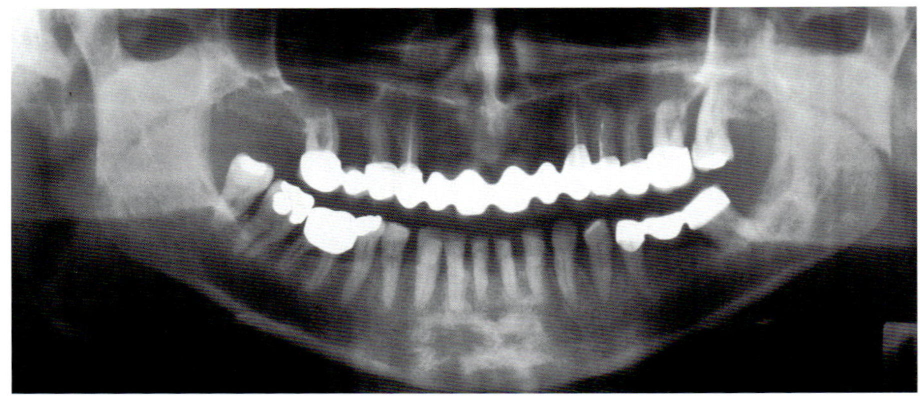

Fig 8-43 Panoramic X-ray. The generalized bone loss is clearly discernible.

The collected data are noted on a suitable anamnesis sheet (Fig 8-42).

The grade of tooth mobility is also recorded on this sheet and is noted following a scale from 0 (normally stable) to 4 (extremely high mobility).

In order to assess the plaque formation quantitatively, several indices are used, like the Plaque-Index (PI) according to Silness and Löe or the Hygiene Index (HI) according to O'Leary et al. and Lindhe.

The PI covers the thickness of plaque along the gingival margin using a scale from 0 to 3, where a value of 0 stands for "no plaque" and a value of 3 represents a large quantity of plaque along the gingival margin and interdental spaces filled with plaque.

A more accurate evaluation of the individual plaque load is facilitated by the HI. The plaque is stained at first, and then the presence of plaque is recorded in all four quadrants of a tooth. This measurement is done in all teeth. If the number of plaque-free locations is divided by the total number of measuring sites and the result is multiplied by 100, the percentage portion of clean sites is obtained. A HI of 100% would mean a set of teeth free from plaque.

The severity of an inflammation can be described by so-called gingival indices. The Gingiva-Index (GI) according to Löe and Silness evaluates the grade of inflammation and bleeding following a scale from 0 (no discoloration, no bleeding) to 3 (severe inflammation and swelling,

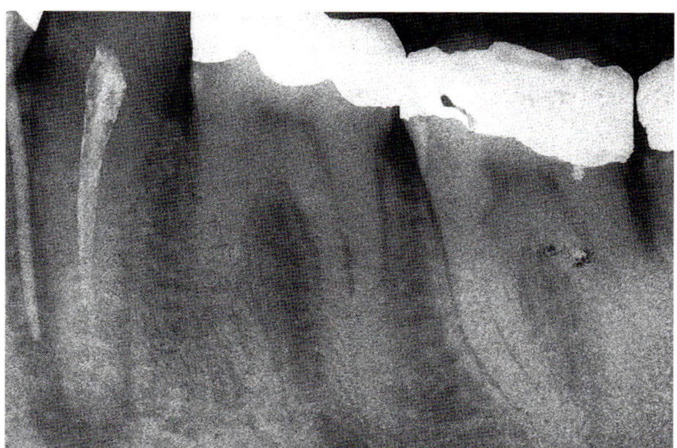

Fig 8-44 X-ray, small picture. Endo/periodontal problem.

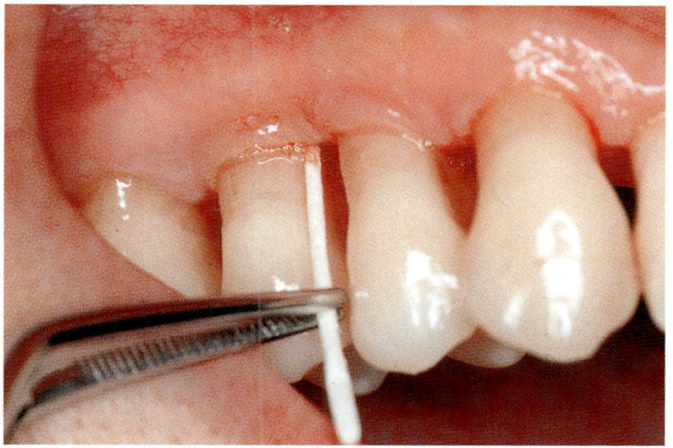

Fig 8-45 Bacteriological sampling with a sterile paper point.

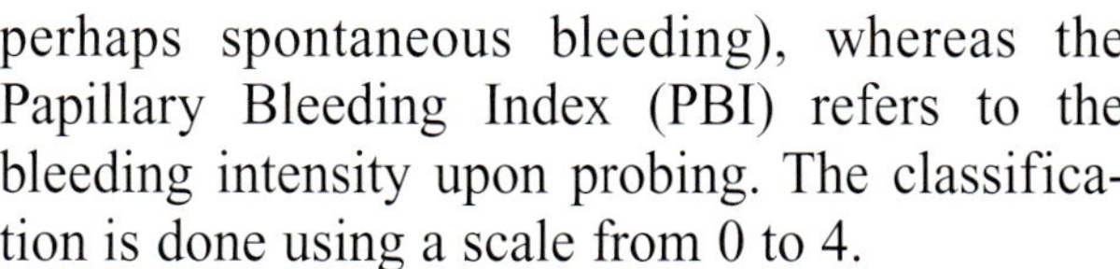

perhaps spontaneous bleeding), whereas the Papillary Bleeding Index (PBI) refers to the bleeding intensity upon probing. The classification is done using a scale from 0 to 4.

In order to assess the severity of periodontitis with an index, it must comprise the attachment loss besides the grade of inflammation (like GI or PBI). This task is fulfilled by indices like the Periodontal Disease Index (PDI) or the Community Periodontal Index of Treatment Needs which has been developed by the WHO. These indices have a measurement of the attachment loss and the inflammation indicators in common, whereas the latter also describes the treatment needs in coarse grades.

Great importance is also attributed to the radiological examination. Whereas the orthopantomography gives a good overview of the general situation, in particular a right angle status provides a good status of osseous conditions. Bitewings can be a good diagnostic complement.

In addition, also a bacteriological probe should be taken, in order to get information about the microbiologic spectrum and the total bacterial load and to evaluate the eventual accompanying treatment with antibiotics.

8.3.2 Clinical Preparation

Again the same procedure should be applied as in the context of a conventional initial therapy.

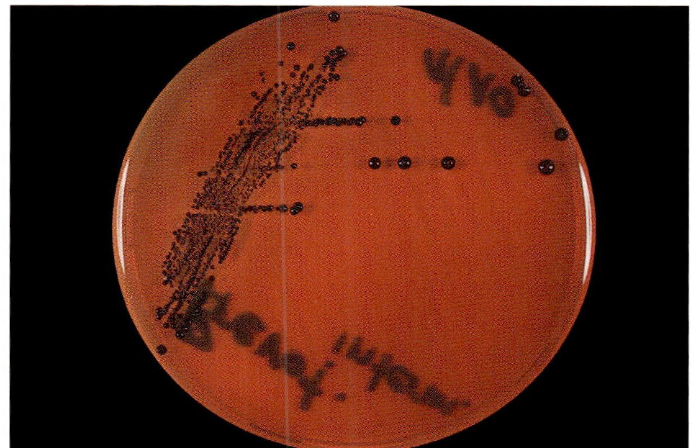

Fig 8-46 Bacterial culture. Here: *Prevotella* sp.

Plaque and concrements are removed by tooth cleaning and curettage, overhanging edges of fillings are eliminated and the patient is informed about the right measures concerning oral hygiene.

8.3.3 Modus Operandi

Since in the context of the pretreatment, the patient was freed to a large extent from tartar and concrement, laser radiation can exert its optimal effect at the target destination. In principle, and for all lasers, the following procedure is selected (see Figs 8-49 to 8-51):

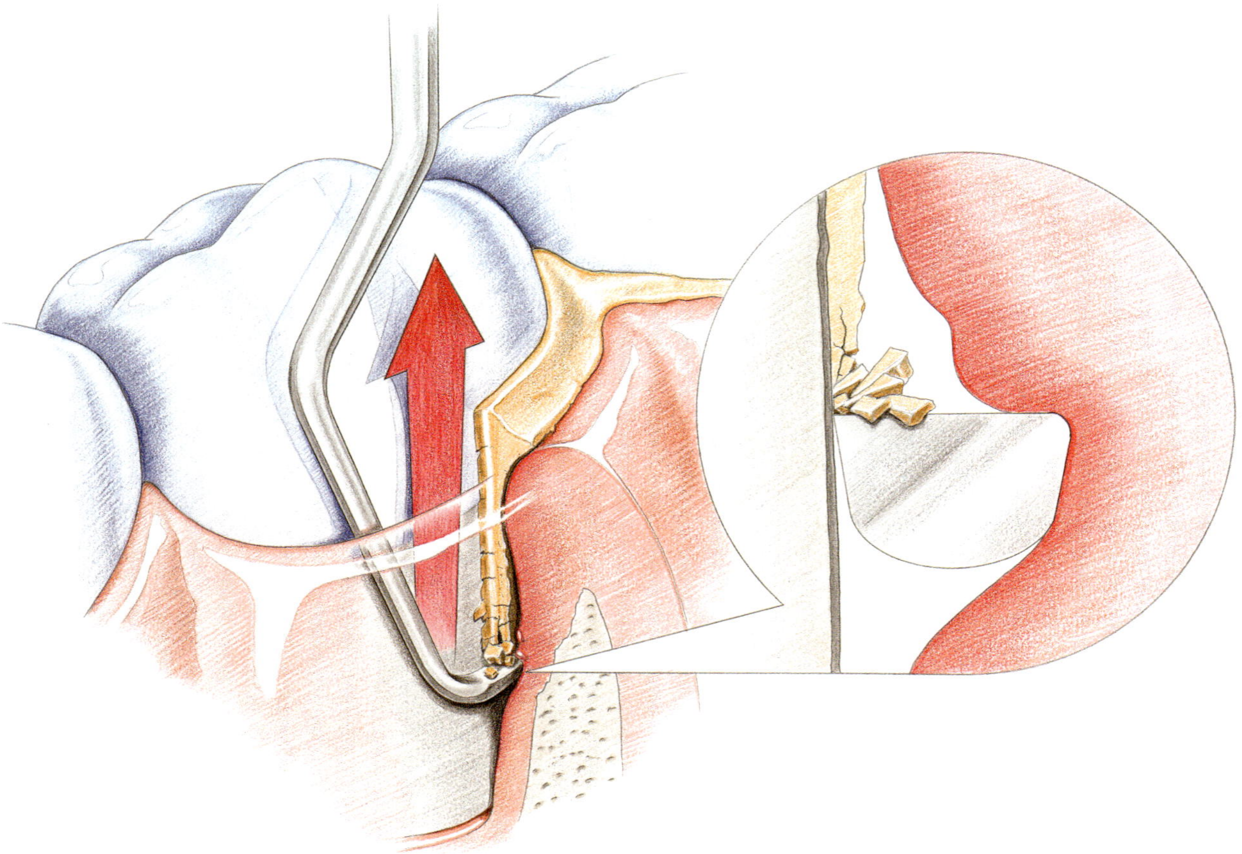

Fig 8-47 Scaling.

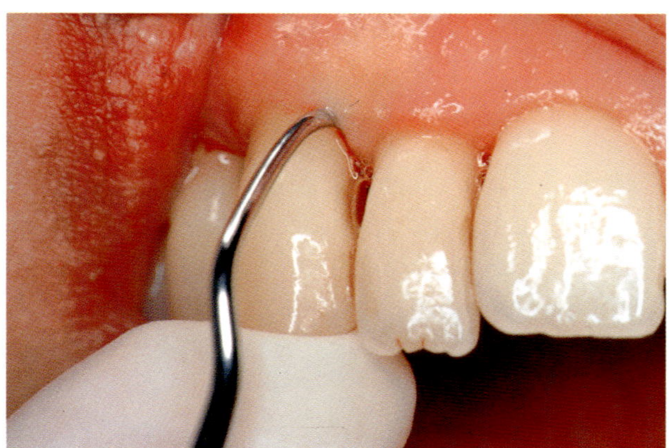

Fig 8-48 Scaling.

The light conductor (a fiber with a diameter between 200 and 400 μm) is introduced without use of force, like a probe, step by step into the periodontal pocket. After the activation of the laser the fiber is removed from the bottom of the pocket by sinusoidal movements to the outside of the pocket within 5 s. This is necessary in order to irradiate, on the one hand, as much of the root surface as possible and, on the other hand, to avoid localized overheating. The choice of the correct laser parameters is also of great importance. For pocket disinfection, the Nd:YAG laser is used with a setting of maximally 1.5 W with 15 Hz, with the diode laser, maximally 2.5 W is selected with 15 Hz. These values ensure a high-grade antibacterial effect with, at the same time, small thermal side effects. To accomplish a gingivectomy, higher settings can be chosen advisedly up to ~3 W for both wavelengths. In the case of the Er:YAG laser, a setting of 100 mJ at 15 Hz should not be exceeded, because this setting ensures

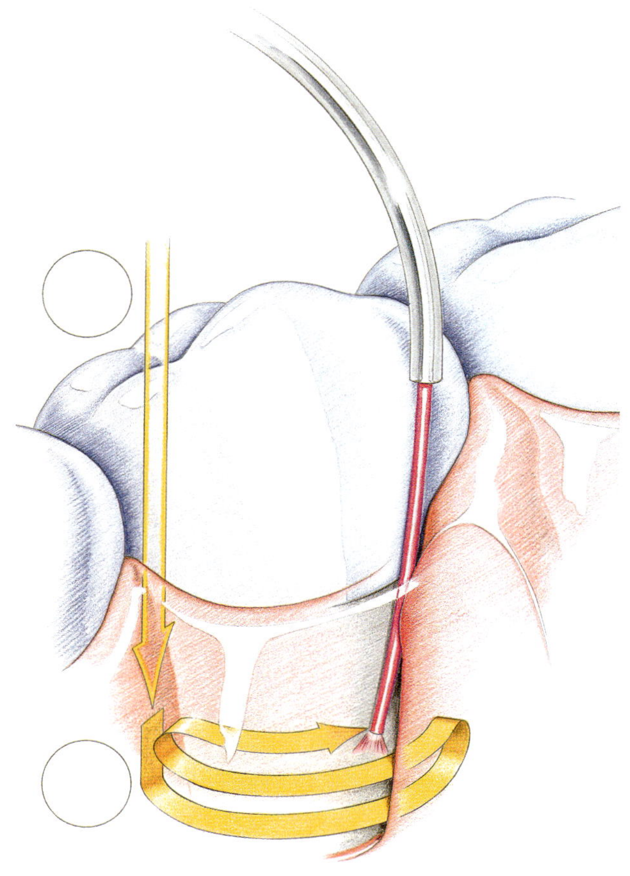

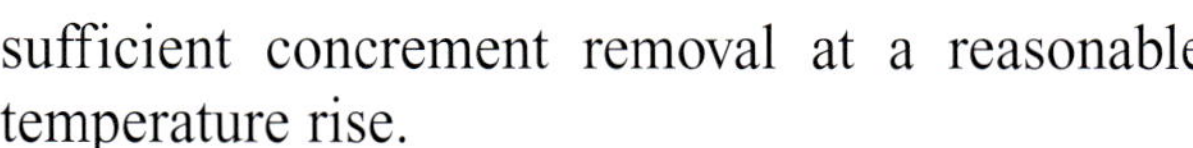

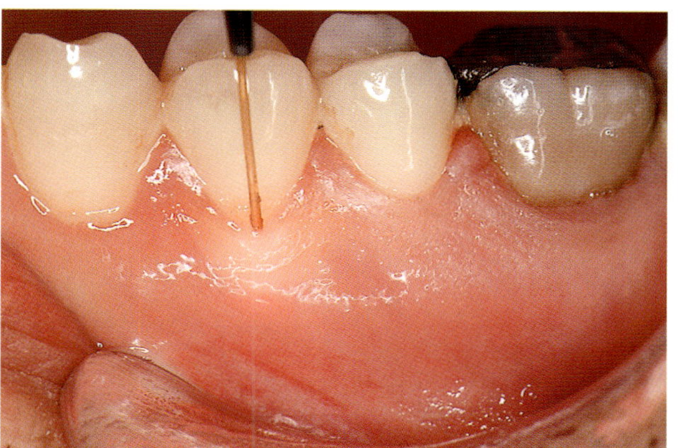

Fig 8-49 and 8-50 Irradiation of a periodontal pocket with a Nd:YAG laser.

sufficient concrement removal at a reasonable temperature rise.

To provide the correct settings for each laser system available would go far beyond the scope of this chapter. In particular, all the possibilities for adjustment are not available in each individual system. The parameters mentioned above could be regarded as a coarse guideline, beyond which the user must consult the manufacturers' recommendations and work out suitable parameters.

Now, if all four sides of a tooth were irradiated, one begins again with the first quadrant and repeats the entire procedure until each side has been treated five times for 5 s.

In most cases, the treatment is perceived as not uncomfortable or painful by the patient, and local anesthesia is very rarely necessary.

Table 8-1 Treatment scheme.

Appointment 1		– Evaluation of the medical history – Information and oral hygiene instructions – Removal of superficial concrements and plaque
Appointment 2	after 1 week	– Periodontological evaluation, indices (pocket depths, bleeding, mobility, PBI...) – X-ray status – Again oral hygiene instructions – Photodocumentation – Therapy planning – Bacteriology – Conventional scaling – Laser (probably at a separate appointment) – Eventually antibiotics
Appointment 3	after 1 $^1/_2$ weeks	– laser (to prevent the regrowth of pocket epithelium)
Appointment 4	after 2 weeks	– Hygienic check-up (Microbiology)
Appointment 5	after 2 months	– Hygienic check-up (Microbiology) – Re-evaluation – Perhaps supplementary treatment (surgery, if the patient is free from inflammation, pocket depths more than 5 (6–7) mm, API, PBI below 20%, otherwise again initial therapy) – Laser irradiation
Appointment 6	after 4 months	– Hygienic check-up – Laser irradiation
Appointment 7	after 6 months	– Re-evaluation (Microbiology) – Evaluation of the periodontal indices – Hygienic check-up – Regular recall

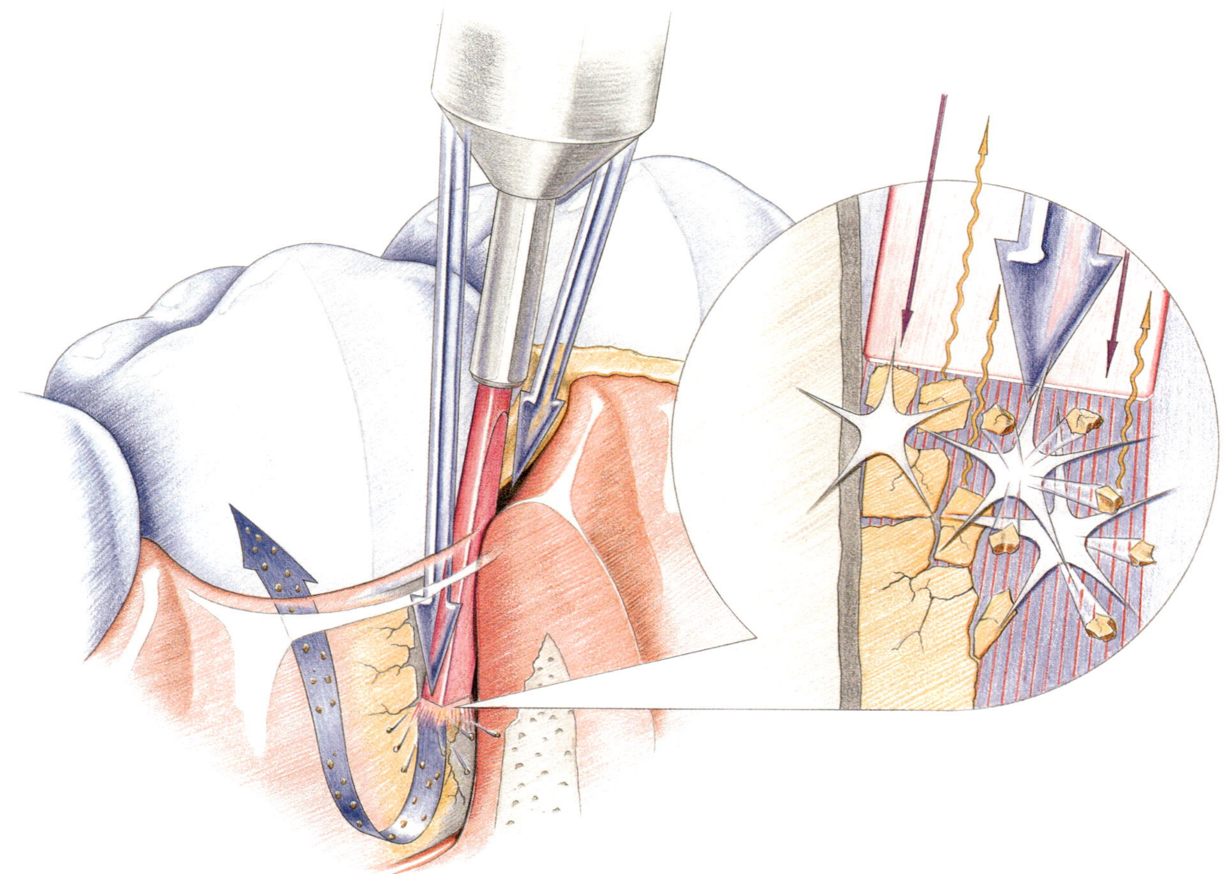

Fig 8-51 Irradiation of a periodontal pocket with an Er:YAG laser (chisel-shaped tip). Inset: diagrammatic representation of feedback mechanism.

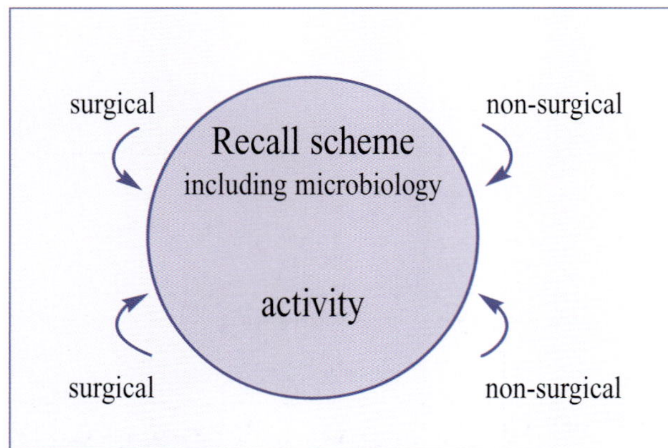

Fig 8-52 The figure points out the importance of a repeated evaluation of the achieved treatment success.

In order to ensure and perpetuate therapy success within the context of the laser-supported periodontal treatment, a regular recall, and monitoring of the mouth hygiene in the sense of maintenance therapy, is absolutely necessary. Also, a periodic repetition of the laser irradiation after 3 to 6 months can sometimes be useful. Table 8-1 (see page 369) gives an overview of a possible treatment plan.

The aim of recall appointments is not only a check-up of the oral hygiene, but facilitates a re-evaluation of the treatment applied so far and its success. If a conventional therapy in conjunction with a laser therapy should not yield the desired success, a surgical procedure (perhaps in combination with laser therapy) could be necessary. Fig 8-52 illustrates this.

8.4 Case Reports

8.4.1 Clinical Case Report[67]

8.4.1.1 Medical History

General medical history. There were no special findings to be recorded.

Special medical history. A 36-year-old female patient attended the Poliklinik für Zahnärztliche Chirurgie und Aufnahme of the Westdeutschen Kieferklinik, Heinrich Heine Universität Düsseldorf with a painful swelling in the area of the right upper jaw existing for 4 days. Through the medical history it was discovered that tooth 16 had been trepanated and left open by an emergency dentist 2 days ago. Despite antibiotic therapy (penicillin V) and endodontic pretreatment, the swelling and the patient's discomfort further increased in intensity.

8.4.1.2 Findings

Extraoral findings. Only normal structures were found.

Intraoral findings. The clinical inspection revealed a distinct vestibular and palatinal swelling of the marginal gingiva in the area of teeth 15–18 (Fig 8-53). Mobility was grade I for 15, 17 and 18, and grade I–II for tooth 16, with a distinct sensitivity to horizontal percussion. All teeth, with the exception of 16 showed a normal reaction on cold. The highest probing depths were found at the teeth 16 with 9 mm (mb, db), 17 with 8 mm (dp) and 18 with 7 mm (mp). In addition, furcation affection grade I on the buccal side of tooth 16 could be found. During the measurement of pocket depth, purulent secretion was expressed in the region of the swelling. The bleeding on probing showed a value of 100%.

Microbiological findings. As a further diagnostic tool, a molecular genetic test system for the combined determination of five periodontopathogenic marker organisms was applied (microDent®, Hain Diagnostika, Nehren, Germany). The evaluation showed a high prevalence of the aggressive marker bacterium *Actinobacillus actinomycetemcomitans* (Table 8-2).

Table 8-2 DNA- assessment of periodontopathogenic marker organisms before and after Er:YAG laser therapy (microDent®, Hain Lifescience, Nehren). Tooth 16, location: disto-buccal.

Periodontopathogenic marker organisms	Bacterial counts pre op	Bacterial counts post op (4 weeks)
Actinobacillus actinomycetemcomitans	$< 10^5$ (++)	$< 10^3$ (-)
Porphyromonas gingivalis	$< 10^5$ (+)	$< 10^4$ (-)
Prevotella intermedia	$< 10^4$ (-)	$< 10^4$ (-)
Bacteroides forsythus	$< 10^5$ (+)	$< 10^4$ (-)
Treponema denticola	$< 10^5$ (+)	$< 10^4$ (-)

– = bacterial count below the cut-off
\+ = high bacterial count*
++ = very high bacterial count*
* Evaluated bacterial counts (Aa: $>10^3$; Pg, Pi, Bf and Td: $> 10^4$) normally represent treatment needs.

Radiographic findings. The orthopantomography revealed a generalized horizontal bone resorption in the upper and lower jaw with vertical bone destructions distally at tooth 26 and mesially at tooth 36 and a non-erupted tooth 48. On the intraoral X-ray picture, a peri- and interradicular lightening in the region of the mesio–buccal root could be determined. On both pictures, lucency mesial on tooth 17 represents approximal caries.

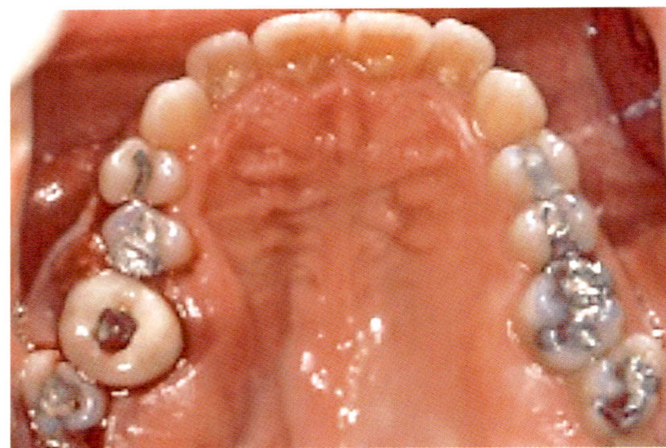

Fig 8-53 Periodontal abscess in the region of the teeth 15 to 18 beginning from a periodontal-endodontal lesion on tooth 16.

8.4.1.3 Diagnosis

A periodontal abscess was present in the teeth 15–18, which has developed from a periodontal–endodontic lesion on tooth 16. Further findings were a periodontitis marginalis superficialis et profunda, tooth 18 without antagonist, a non-erupted tooth 48 and approximal caries on tooth 17.

8.4.1.4 Therapy

As a therapy of choice, the root canals of tooth 16 were further instrumented and rinsed (Chlorhexidine 0.2%). In addition, scaling and root planing was accomplished on teeth 15–18 with hand instruments (Gracey curettes, Hu-Friedy, Chicago, Illinois) and subsequent subgingival rinsing with Chlorhexidine (0.2%). In the periodontal pocket of tooth 16 an iodoform strip was placed. The antibiotic therapy with Clindamycin was halted.

The next day, the patient returned with an increase of swelling and pain. The whole area of the marginal gingiva at the teeth 14–18 was dark red and showed clear signs of spontaneous bleeding. After local anesthesia vestibular and in the area of the right nervus palatinus major, a laser treatment of the teeth 14–18 was accomplished. An Er:YAG laser (KEYIII®, KaVo, Biberach, Germany) with a wavelength of $\lambda = 2.94$ µm and a pulse duration of 250 µs was used.

The treatment was carried out with the hand piece P 2061 (KEY III®, KaVo, Biberach, Germany) and a chisel tip of dimension 0.5 × 1.65 mm and a setting of 160 mJ/pulse and a frequency of 10 Hz. The guidance of the fiber was accomplished from coronal to apical in parallel tracks with an angulation of about 15–20° in relation to the tooth's axis (Figs 8-54 to 8-56).

As soon as the next day, a distinct decrease of the swelling could be observed. In addition, no purulent secretion could be expressed. Within 5 days, the swelling disappeared completely (Fig 8-57). The marginal gingiva showed a physiologic texture with pinkish color and bleeding on probing of 23%.

The probing depths were 5 mm in the locations mentioned above after 4 weeks while the gingival recessions increased only minimally. The molecular genetic test system revealed a reduction of the aggressive periodontopathogenic marker germ *Actinobacillus actinomycetemcomitans* below the detection limit (microDent®, Hain Diagnostika, Nehren, Deutschland) (see Table 8-2). The peri- and interradicular osteolysis clearly decreased after a medical dressing ($CaOH_2$). In further treatment, the endodontic therapy of tooth 16, a systematic periodontal therapy, and the extraction of tooth 18 without antagonist and the filling therapy of tooth 17 were accomplished.

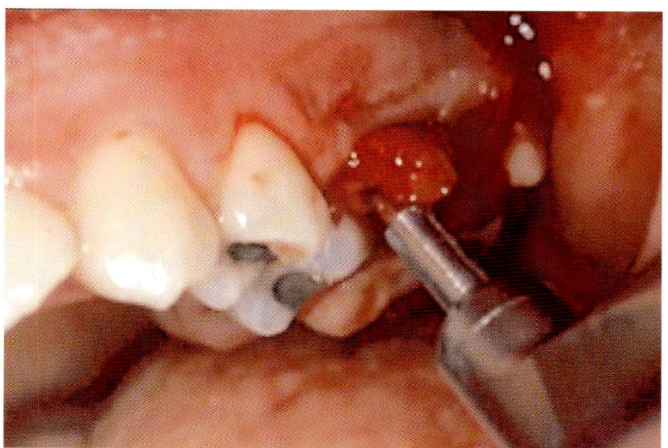

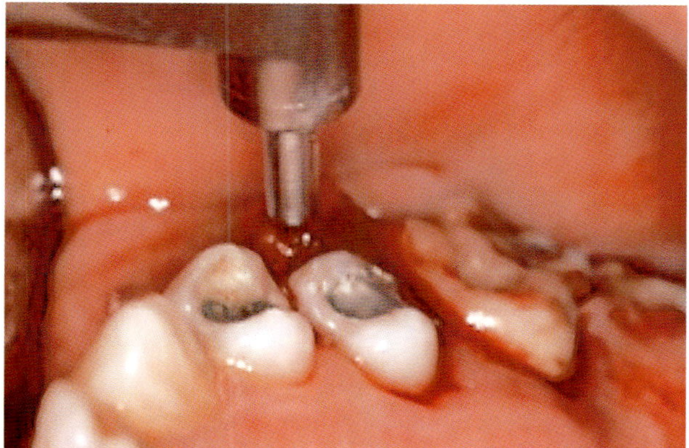

Fig 8-54 and 8-55 The angulation of the fiber tip should be 15° to 20° in relation to the tooth axis.

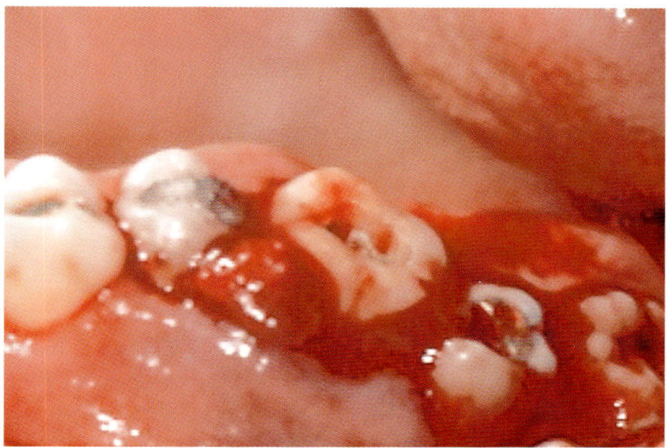

Fig 8-56 Situation immediately after the Er:YAG laser irradiation.

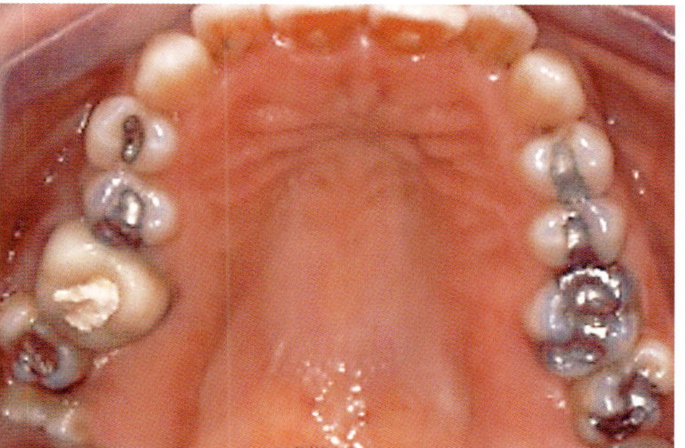

Fig 8-57 Situation 5 days after laser therapy. The marginal gingiva shows a physiologic texture with pinkish color and only a slight increase of the gingival recessions.

8.4.1.5 Conclusions

Clinical cases always rank as the lowest "level of evidence" and should therefore not be used for therapy recommendations. Nevertheless, they are suitable for the confirmation of the results from randomized, prospective controlled clinical studies, which account for the highest level of evidence-based medicine. Consequently, the case study could indicate the superiority of the Er:YAG laser to conventional instrumentation of the root surface mainly in initially high probing depths and the presence of aggressive periodontopathogenic bacteria. Nevertheless, it must be pointed out that the long-term stability of periodontal–endodontical lesions is first of all dependent on the successful endodontic therapy.

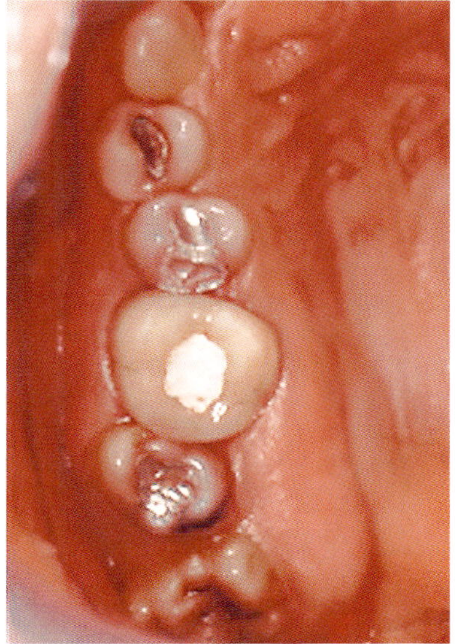

Fig 8-58 The situation 4 weeks postoperative shows stable conditions.

8.5 References

1. Listgarten M A: Pathogenesis of periodontitis. J Clin Periodontol 13: 418–425, 1986
2. Listgarten M A: Nature of periodontal diseases: Pathogenic mechanism. J Periodont Res 22: 172–178, 1987
3. Listgarten M A, Mayo H E, Tremblay R: Development of dental plaque on epoxy resin crowns in man. A light and electron microscopic study. J Periodontol 46: 10–26, 1975
4. Listgarten M A: Structure of the microbial flora associated with periodontal health and desease in man. A light and electron microscopic study. J Periodontol 47: 1–8, 1976
5. Slots J: Subgingival microflora and periodontal disease. J Clin Periodontol 6: 351–382, 1979
6. Lindhe J: Textbook of Clinical Periodontology. Munksgaard, Copenhagen 1983
7. Page R C, Schroeder H E: Pathogenesis of inflammatory periodontal disease. A summary of current work. Lab Invest 33: 235–249, 1976
8. International Workshop for a Classification of Periodontal Diseases and Conditions October 30–November 2, 1999, Oak Brook, IL
9. Moritz A, Gutknecht N, Doertbudak O, Goharkhay K, Schoop U, Schauer P, Sperr W: Bacterial reduction in periodontal pockets through irradiation with a diode laser: a pilot study. J Clin Laser Med Surg 15(1): 33–37, 1997
10. Moritz A, Schoop U, Goharkhay K, Schauer P, Doertbudak O, Wernisch J, Sperr W: Treatment of periodontal pockets with a diode laser. Lasers Surg Med 22(5): 302–311, 1998
11. Ben Hatit Y, Blum R, Severin C, Maquin M, Jabro M H: The effects of a pulsed Nd:YAG laser on subgingival bacterial flora and on cementum: an in vivo study. J Clin Laser Med Surg 14(3): 137–143, 1996
12. Romanos GE, Renner PJ, Everts H, Nentwig GH: Veränderungen an der Wurzeloberfläche frisch extrahierter Zähne nach Anwendung eines Nd:YAG-Lasers. Eine in vitro REM-Untersuchung. Die Quintessenz 49: 497–500 (1998)
13. Romanos GE, Purucker P, Renner PJ: Laseranwendung in der Parodontologie. Aktueller Stand. Parodontologie 9: 299–312 (1998)
14. Kreisler M, Meyer C, Stender E, Danblader M, Willershausen-Zonnchen B, d`Hoedt B: Effect of diode laser irradiation on the attachment rate of periodontal ligament cells: an in vitro study. J Periodontol 72(10): 1312–1317, 2001
15. Kreisler M, Al Haj H, Daublander M, Gotz H, Duschner H, Willershausen B, D`Hoedt B: Effect of diode laser irradiation on root surfaces in vitro. J Clin Laser Med Surg 20(2): 63–69, 2002
16. Schwarz F, Sculean A, Berakdar M, Szathmari L, Georg T, Becker J: In vivo and in vitro effects of an Er:YAG laser, a GaAlAs diode laser, and scaling and root planing on periodontally diseased root surfaces: a comparative histologic study. Lasers Surg Med 32: 359–366, 2003
17. Liu C M, Hou L T, Wong M Y, Lan W H: Comparison of Nd:YAG laser versus scaling and root planing in periodontal therapy. J Periodontol 70(11): 1276–1282, 1999
18. Neill M E, Mellonig J T: Clinical efficacy of the Nd:YAG Laser for combination periodontitis therapy. Pract Periodont Aesthet Dent 9(6 Suppl.): 1–5, 1997
19. Radvar M, MacFarlane T W, MacKenzie D, Whitters C J, Payne A P, Kinane D F: An evaluation of the Nd:YAG laser in periodontal pocket therapy. Br Dent J 20, 180(2): 57–62, 1996
20. Wilder-Smith P, Arrastia A M, Schell M J, Liaw L H, Grill G, Berns M W: Effect of Nd:YAG laser irradiation and root planing on the root surface: structural and thermal effects. J Periodontol 66(12): 1032–1039, 1995
21. Gold S I, Vilardi M A: Pulsed laser beam effects on gingiva. J Clin Periodontol 21(6): 391–396, 1994
22. Cobb C M, McCawley T K, Killoy W J: A preliminary study on the effects of the Nd:YAG laser on root surfaces and subgingival microflora in vivo. J Periodontol 63(8): 701–707, 1992
23. Morlock B J, Pippin D J, Cobb C M, Killoy W J, Rapley J W: The effect of Nd:YAG laser exposure on root surfaces when used as an adjunct to root planing: an in vitro study. J Periodontol 63(7): 637–641, 1992
24. Thomas D, Rapley J, Cobb C, Spencer P, Killoy W: Effects of the Nd:YAG laser and combined treatments on in vitro fibroblast attachment to root surfaces. J Clin Periodontol 21(1): 38–44, 1994
25. Ito K, Nishikata J, Murai S: Effects of Nd:YAG laser radiation on removal of a root surface smear layer after root planing: a scanning electron microscopic study. J Periodontol 64(6): 547–552, 1993
26. Arcoria C J, Vitasek-Arcoria B A: The effects of low-level energy density Nd:YAG irradiation on calculus removal. J Clin Laser Surg 10(5): 343–347, 1992
27. Radvar M, Creanor S L, Gilmour W H, Payne A P, McGadey J, Foye R H, Whitters C J, Kinane D F: An evaluation of the effects of an Nd:YAG laser on subgingival calculus, dentine and cementum. An in vitro study. J Clin Periodontol 22(1) 71–77, 1995
28. Tewfik H M, Garnick J J, Schuster G S, Sharawy M M: Structural and functional changes of cementum surface following exposure to a modified Nd:YAG laser. J Periodontol 65(4): 297–302, 1994
29. Sjostrom L, Friskopp J: Laser treatment as an adjunct to debridement of periodontal pockets. Swed Dent J 26(2): 51–57, 2002
30. Israel M, Rossmann J A, Froum S J: Use of carbon dioxide laser in retarding epithelial migration: a pilot histological human study utilizing case reports. J Periodontol 66(3): 197–204, 1995
31. Crespi R, Barone A, Covani U, Ciaglia R N, Romanos G E: Effects of CO_2 laser treatment on fibroblast attachment to root surfaces. A scanning electron microscopy analysis. J Periodontol 73(11): 1308–1312, 2002
32. Barone A, Covani U, Crespi R, Romanos G E: Root surface morphological changes after focused versus defocused CO_2 laser irradiation: a scanning electron microscopy analysis. J Periodontol 73(4): 370–373, 2002

33. Schwarz F, Putz N, Georg T, Reich E: Effect of an Er:YAG laser on periodontally involved root surfaces: an in vitro and in vivo SEM comparison. Lasers Surg Med 29(4): 328–335, 2001
34. Sculean A, Schwarz F, Windisch P, Keglevich T, Gerharz D, Becker J: Clinical and histologic evaluation of human intrabony defects treated with an Er:YAG laser. Periodontal Practice Today (Perio) 2004 (in press)
35. Schwarz F, Aoki A, Sculean A, Georg T, Scherbaum W, Becker J: In vivo effects of an Er:YAG laser, an ultrasonic system and scaling and root planing on the biocompatibility of periodontally diseased root surfaces in cultures of human PDL fibroblasts. Lasers Surg Med 33: 140–147, 2003
36. Aoki A, Ando Y, Watanabe H, Ishikawa I: In vitro studies on laser scaling of subgingival calculus with an erbium:YAG laser. J Periodontol 65(12): 1097–1106, 1994
37. Schoop U, Moritz A, Maleschitz P, Goharkhay K, Kluger W, Wernisch J, Sperr W: The impact of Er:YAG laser irradiation on root surfaces: an in vitro evaluation. J Oral Laser Appl 1(1), 2001
38. Folwaczny M, Benner KU, Flasskamp B, Mehl A, Hickel R: Effects of 2.94 micron Er:YAG laser radiation on root surfaces treated in situ: a histological study. J Periodontol 74(3): 360–365, 2003
39. Folwaczny M, Mehl A, Haffner C, Benz C, Hickel R: Root substance removal with Er:YAG laser radiation at different parameters using a new delivery system. J Periodontol 71(2): 147–155, 2000
40. Folwaczny M, George G, Thiele L, Mehl A, Hickel R: Root surface roughness following Er:YAG laser irradiation at different radiation energies and working tip angulations. J Clin Periodontol 29(7): 598–603, 2002
41. Folwaczny M, Thiele L, Mehl A, Hickel R: The effect of working tip angulation on root substance removal using Er:YAG laser radiation: an in vitro study. J Clin Periodontol 28(3): 220–226, 2001
42. Frentzen M, Braun A, Aniol D: Er:YAG laser scaling of diseased root surfaces. J Periodontol 73(5): 524–530, 2002
43. Eberhard J, Ehlers H, Falk W, Acil Y, Albers H K, Jepsen: Efficacy of subgingival calculus removal with Er:YAG laser compared to mechanical debridement: an in situ study. J Clin Periodontol 30(6): 511–518, 2003
44. Israel M, Cobb C M, Rossmann J A, Spencer P: The effects of CO_2, Nd:YAG and Er:YAG lasers with and without surface coolant on tooth root surfaces. An in vitro study. J Clin Periodontol 24(9 Pt 1): 595–602, 1997
45. Yamaguchi H, Kobayashi K, Osada R, Sakuraha E, Nomura T, Arai T, Nakamura J: Effects of irradiation of an Er:YAG laser on root surfaces. J Periodontol 68(12): 1151–1155, 1997
46. Aoki A, Miura M, Akiyama F, Nakagawa N, Tanaka J, Oda S, Watanabe H, Ishikawa I: In vitro evaluation of Er:YAG laser scaling of subgingival calculus in comparison with ultrasonic scaling. J Periodontol Res 35(5): 266–277, 2000
47. Schoop U, Moritz A, Kluger W, Frei U, Maleschitz P, Goharkhay K, Schöfer C, Wernisch J, Sperr W: Changes in root surface morphology and fibroblast adherence after Er:YAG laser irradiation. J Oral Laser Appl 2: 83–93, 2002
48. Feist I S, De Micheli G, Carneiro S R, Eduardo C P, Miyagi S, Marques M M: Adhesion and growth of cultured human gingival fibroblasts on periodontally involved root surfaces treated by Er:YAG laser. J Periodontol 74(9): 1368–1375, 2003
49. Ando Y, Aoki A, Watanabe H, Ishikawa I: Bactericidal effect of erbium YAG laser on periodontopathic bacteria. Lasers Surg Med 19(2): 190–200, 1996
50. Folwaczny M, Mehl A, Aggstaller H, Hickel R: Antimicrobial effects of 2.4 micron Er:YAG laser radiation on root surfaces: an in vitro study. J Clin Periodontol 29(1): 73–78, 2003
51. Watanabe H, Ishikawa I, Suzuki M, Hasegawa K: Clinical assessments of the erbium:YAG laser for soft tissue surgery and scaling. J Clin Laser Med Surg 14(2): 67–75, 1996
52. Schwarz F, Sculean A, Arweiler N, Reich E: Nicht-chirurgische Parodontalbehandlung mit einem Er:YAG Laser. Parodontologie 4: 329–336, 2000
53. Jepsen S, Rühling A, König J, Dietzel K, Keller U, Albers H K: Treatment of periodontitis with a novel Er:YAG laser system. J Dent Res Abstract No. 2281, 2000
54. Schwarz F, Sculean A, Georg T, Reich E: Periodontal treatment with an Er:YAG laser compared to scaling and root planing. A controlled clinical study. J Periodontol 72(3): 361–367, 2001
55. Schwarz F, Sculean A, Berakdar M, Georg T, Reich E, Becker J: Periodontal treatment with an Er:YAG laser or scaling and root planing. A 2-year follow-up split-mouth study. J Periodontol 74: 590–596, 2003
56. Schwarz F, Sculean A, Berakdar M, Georg T, Reich E, Becker J: Clinical evaluation of an Er:YAG laser combined with scaling and root planing for non-surgical periodontal treatment. A controlled, prospective clinical study. J Clin Periodontol 30: 26–34, 2003
57. Sculean A, Schwarz F, Berakdar M, Arweiler N, Becker J: Periodontal treatment with an Er:YAG laser compared to ultrasonic instrumentation. J Periodontol 2004 (in press)
58. Sculean A, Schwarz F, Berakdar M, Windisch P, Arweiler N, Romanos G E: Healing of intrabony defects following surgical treatment with or without an Er:YAG laser. A pilot study. J Clin Periodontol 2004 (in press)
59. Schwarz F, Sculean A, Georg T, Becker J: Clinical evaluation of the Er:YAG laser in combination with an enamel matrix protein derivative for the treatment of intrabony periodontal defects: a pilot study. J Clin Periodontol 30: 975–981, 2003
60. Schwarz F, Arweiler N, Georg T, Reich E: Desensitizing effects of an Er:YAG laser on hypersensitive dentine. J Clin Periodontol 29: 211–215, 2002
61. Krause F, Braun A, Frentzen M: The possibility of detecting subgingival calculus by laser-fluorescence in vitro. Lasers Med Sci 18(1): 32–35, 2003
62. Kimura Y, Yu D G, Kinoshita J, Hossain M, Yokoyama K, Murakam Y, Nomura K, Takamura R, Matsumoto K: Effects of erbium, chromium: YSGG laser irradiation on root surface: morphological and anatomic analytical studies. J Clin Laser Med Surg 19(2): 69–72, 2001
63. Henning T, Rechmann P, Pilgrim C, Schwarzmaier H J, Kaufmann R: Caries Selective Ablation by Pulsed Lasers. SPIE Proceedings of Lasers in Orthopedics, Dent Vet Med 1424: 99–105, 1991

64. Rechmann P, Henning T, von den Hoff U, Kaufmann R: Caries Selective Ablation Using a 2nd Harmonic Alexandrite-Laser. Proceedings of the Third International Congress on Lasers in Dentistry 1992, Salt Lake City, UT, 123–124
65. Rechmann P, Henning T: Lasers in Periodontology – New Trends. J Oral Laser Appl 2: 7–14, 2002
66. Henning T, Rechmann P, Heinz H, Hadding U: Influence of Second Harmonic Alexandrite-Laser Radiation on Bacterial Growth. SPIE Proceedings of Lasers in Dentistry II 2672: 40–45, 1996
67. Schwarz F, Rothamel D, Becker J: Behandlung eines parodontalen Abszesses mit dem Er:YAG Laser. Parodontologie 14: 67–75, 2003

9

Dentin Hypersensitivity

K. Goharkhay, J. Wernisch, A. Moritz

9.1 Introduction

If the dentin surface has been exposed, the dentinal tubules, which are open to both the oral cavity and the pulp cavity, provide a connection between the oral environment and the sensitive nerve endings of the tooth pulp. The dentinal tubules are filled with long odontoblastic processes, also referred to as Tomes' fibers, and with an interstitial hard tissue fluid, also termed dentinal liquor.

Several stimuli can cause unpleasant sensations on exposed dentinal surfaces. Dentin hypersensitivity is characterized by short, sharp pain arising from exposed dentin in response to stimuli typically thermal, evaporative, tactile, osmotic or chemical and which cannot be ascribed to any other form of dental defect or pathology (Chapter 9.1.1 Theories of dentin hypersensitivity).[1,2] Essentially, exposure of the dentin results from one of two processes, either removal of the enamel covering the crown of the tooth, or denudation of the root surface by loss of cement and overlying periodontal tissues. Removal of the enamel may

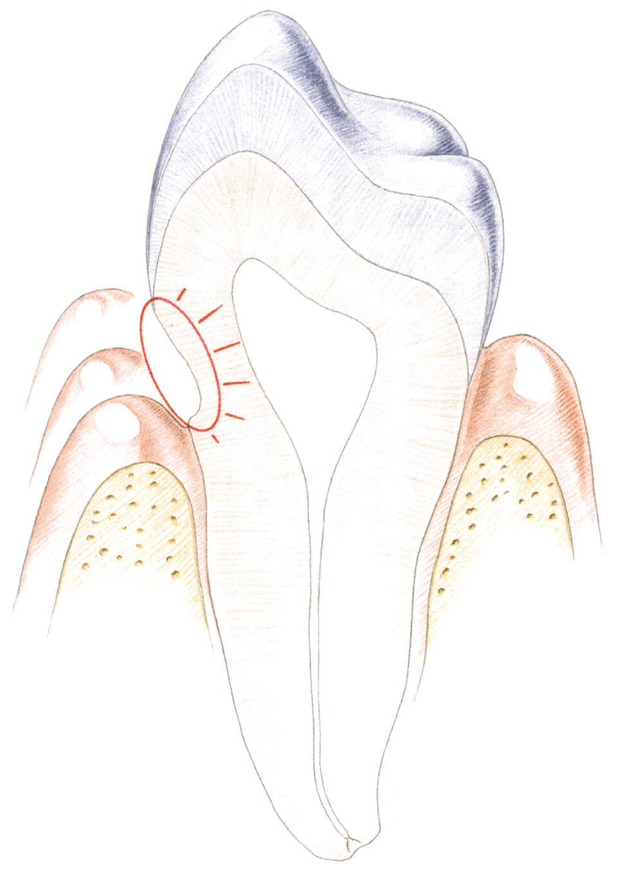

Fig 9-1 Exposed cervical dentin area.

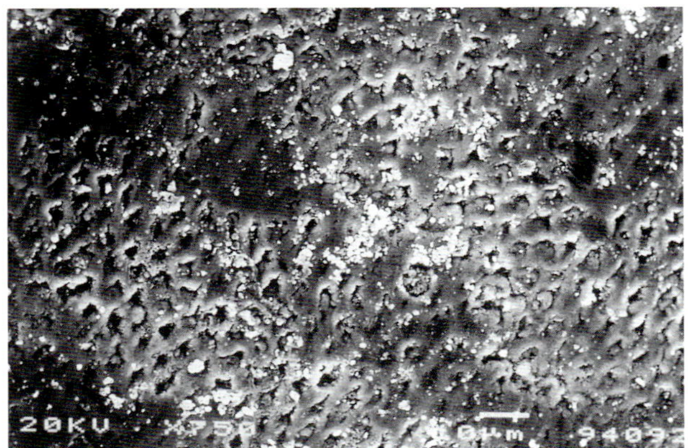

Fig 9-2 SEM 750x, open dentinal tubules of the cervical dental neck area.

result from attrition relating to occlusal abnormalities, toothbrush abrasion, dietary erosion, habits, or a combination of these factors. Aetiologically important are also the increased incidence of gingival recessions with advancing age, chronic periodontal disease and certain forms of periodontal surgery.[3–6] Sensitivities can also be seen after scaling and root planing.

Areas of sensitive cervical dentin display patent dentin tubules.[7] Hypersensitive teeth demonstrate tubular diameters that are significantly wider (2 times) than those of non sensitive teeth, so it would appear that treatment focused at decreasing the radius is a prerequisite for effective desensitization.[8] Thus, in those individuals where no symptoms arise from dentin exposure, occlusion of tubules may have resulted from the formation of dead tracts, or the laying down of irregular secondary dentin, or the development of sclerosed dentin.[9,10] (Chapter 9.1.2 Natural pulpal defense mechanisms).

However, blockage of the tubules at the dentin surface by other means may occur and may include dentifrice ingredients and oral debris.[11]

The prevalence of this discomfort causing symptomatic conditions ranges between 8.9% and 15% in the adult western population.[12–14]

The severity of the pain, or the patient's interpretation of this, appears to determine whether treatment is sought.[15–17] In our present state of knowledge we must agree with the conclusion of Tyldesley and Mumford[18] that since pain on stimulation may arise where the pulp[19–21] is normal, inflamed or necrotic, the patient's experience of pain, or lack of it, is not a satisfactory indication of the pulp condition. The very subjective measurement of pain arising from exposed dentin, which may be further modified by psychological factors, makes an accurate assessment of the extent of the problem difficult.[22] Nevertheless, dentin hypersensitivity, besides directly causing patient discomfort, may indirectly pose other problems, in particular those associated with reduced oral hygiene.[11] The failure to practise satisfactory plaque control has well established consequences with respect to gingival health. Furthermore, in those patients where dentin surfaces are exposed as a result of gingival surgery, the success of treatment in the long term may be compromised.[24,25]

9.1.1 Theories of Dentin Hypersensitivity[26]

9.1.1.1 Hydrodynamic Mechanism

The most widely accepted theory for the transmission of stimuli to the pulp is by a hydrodynamic mechanism[27,28], with a rapid movement of fluid within the dentinal tubules. The idea of a fluid in dentinal tubules was presented by Fish[29]. Analysis of human dentinal fluid suggested that the fluid is extracellular[30]. The wall of the dentinal tubule was found to be considerably more mineralized than the rest of the dentin[31]. Brännström theorized that the contained fluid would obey the same physical laws as liquids in glass capillaries[28]. Scanning electron microscopic investigations of human dentinal tubules demonstrated ~ 45,000/mm^2 at the pulp, 29,500/mm^2 in the middle dentin and 20,000/mm^2 peripherally, with the diameter of tubules decreasing from 2.5 µm at the pulp to 0.9 µm peripherally[32]. Interestingly, odontoblast processes were seen only in the tubules near the pulp.

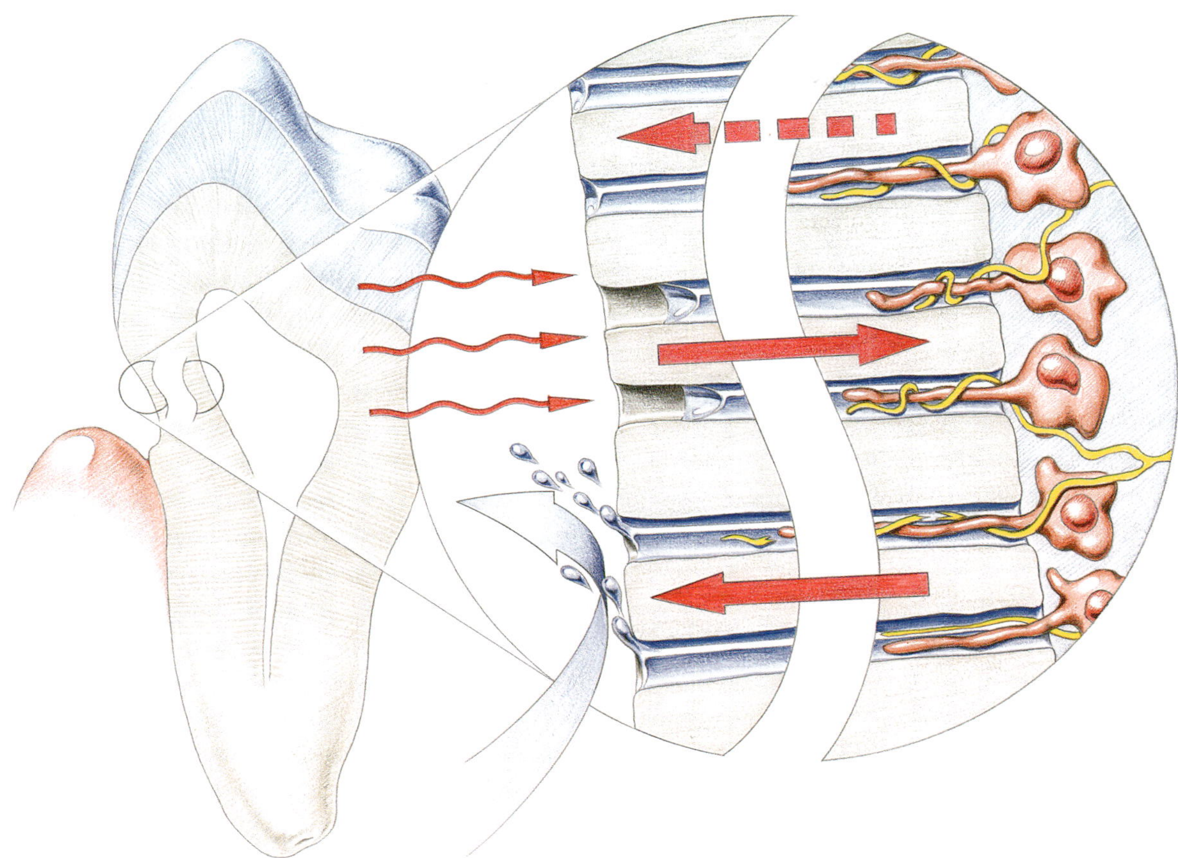

Fig 9-3 Hydrodynamic theory: dentinal fluid flow.

Pain would appear to be produced by the rapid displacement of the tubular contents at the pulp dentin-border as opposed to the slow outward fluid flow, which seems to occur normally[28]. In vitro, the application of a physiological pulpal pressure of 30 mm Hg for 24 h produced a fluid flow of 0.6 μl/mm^2 of exposed fractured dentin[33,34]. This gradient would empty an open tubule 10 times during 24 h. In vivo, this pressure was sufficient to displace cells into the tubules[35]; however, cell "aspiration" is common beneath "leaky" fillings or unprotected dentin but does not correlate with the occurrence of pain[36]. Nevertheless, with the application of stimuli such as cold water[37], hypertonic solutions such as sugar, calcium chloride, absorbent material[35,38,39], probing or air blasts, there is a rapid outward flow of the tubular contents accompanied by the sensation of pain. It was estimated that pain-producing stimuli created an outward fluid flow in tubules of 2–4 mm/s[40,41].

Brännström and Johnson[42] summarized that rapid flow in the pulpal part of the dentinal tubule can be expected to result in deformation, not only of the cellular processes but also of nerve fibers which might be present in the dentinal tubules or adjacent pulp. Consistent with the hydrodynamic theory, studies in the cat have shown that pain receptors of the tooth are not chemoreceptors but very likely mechanoreceptors[43]. This hypothesis is further supported by the recording of physical stimuli known to cause fluid movement including air blasts, cold and reduced pressure[44]. The application of heat, however, produces an inward movement of the tubular contents at the pulp dentinal border[39]. This shift would not be expected

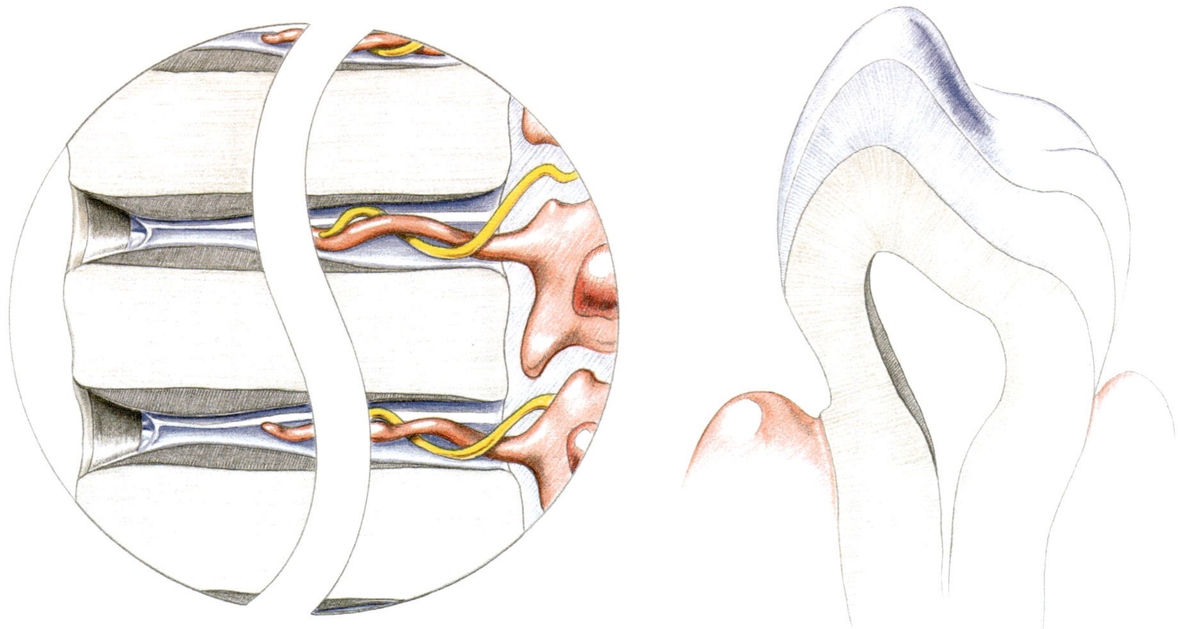

Fig 9-4 Calcification and sclerosis of dentinal tubules.

to activate nerve fibers in the same manner. In experiments in vivo it was observed that an elevation in temperature by 30°C above ambient did not produce pain, whereas an equivalent reduction in temperature almost invariably did so[39]. Interestingly, the pain produced by the prolonged application of heat is of a dull nature, totally different from the sharp pain elicited by cold or an air blast[45].

Horiuchi and Matthews[46], whilst in agreement, observed that dentin did not behave as a normal semi-permeable membrane, and fluid movement could not always be predicted by osmotic pressures of applied stimuli. These investigators concluded that not all stimuli producing pain did so by this mechanism.

9.1.1.2 Dentinal Receptor Mechanism

The postulation of the dentinal receptor mechanism carries the implication that the odontoblast has a special sensory function and that the functional complex with the nerve ending in or near the odontoblastic layer acts as an excitatory synapse. The odontoblast and its process has been perceived as a transducer mechanism[47–51].

9.1.1.3 Modulation of Nerve Impulses by Polypeptides

A number of polypeptides have been implicated as regulators of neural transmission. Of these, plasma kinins (kallikinins or bradykinins) and substance P have been postulated as modulators of nerve impulses in the pulp[52]. These substances may selectively alter the permeability of the odontoblastic cell membrane (hyperpolarisation), so that pulp neurons are more prone to discharge upon receipt of subsequent stimuli.

9.1.2 Natural Pulpal Defense Mechanisms[53]

The pulp has several natural defenses to protect itself from irritating stimuli.

9.1.2.1 Calcification

Pulpal calcification and the formation of secondary dentin, peritubular dentin, and dentinal sclerosis have been demonstrated[54,55]. This natural occlusion of the peritubular dentin by calcium crystals is the tooth's physiologic response to dentinal sensitivity. The tooth may naturally desensitize itself with a peritubular dentin mineralization.

9.1.2.2 Bacterial Plaque

Another defense mechanism that may decrease dentinal sensitivity is the formation of plaque in the acquired salivary pellicle material, coupled with salivary occlusion. A dog study showed that plaque decreased sensitivity[56].

9.1.2.3 Sclerosis

Electron microscopic studies on teeth with incisor attrition revealed partially or completely obliterated dentinal tubules. The sclerotic zones beneath the region of attrition were occluded by peritubular, dentin-like material.[10]

9.2 Conventional Treatment Methods

9.2.1 Therapy Requirements[25]

In 1935, Grossman[57] suggested the following requirements for a satisfactory material for the treatment of dentin hypersensitivity, which would appear to still hold good today[26]:

1. non-irritant to the pulp
2. relatively painless on application
3. easily applied
4. rapid in action
5. effective for a long time
6. without staining effects
7. consistently effective

9.2.2 Historic Treatment Methods[53]

Opium therapy, the earliest recorded treatment method, dates from 400 BC and was still advocated as late as 1000 AD[58]. A wide variety of treatments such as henbane plant and crushed beetles were recommended until the late 1800s.

Cocaine was introduced in 1859 and other medicaments such as creosote and tannic acid and arsenic were used at the turn of the century. In the 1920s, aqueous solutions of iodine with silver nitrate were recommended.

Silver iodide was reported to be effective for relieving dentinal sensitivity and did not blacken the tooth surface as did silver nitrate alone. Fat-soluble vitamins A and D were suggested by Franken as part of a nutritional theory of hypersensitivity[57].

In 1935, Grossman refined the treatment of sensitive teeth by specifying where specific modes of therapy should be used. Silver nitrate was most effective on the cement dentinal surfaces of the posterior teeth and on the lingual surfaces of the anterior teeth[59]. Because it did not stain, formalin was most used on the labial surface of the anterior teeth. Sodium potassium carbonate was suggested in areas of attrition and erosion[57].

Hot olive oil, formaldehyde, silver nitrate, zinc chloride, sodium carbonate, and sodium fluoride were used in the 1950s[57]. Many of these materials are obtunding agents. Some are used to stimulate the formation of secondary dentin, and some are adhesive and used for covering the sensitive areas. Most dentists agree that an agent may be effective (1) in one individual but not in another, (2) on one tooth but not others, and (3) against one stimulus but not others.

9.2.3 Common Agents[53,60]

Therapies employed to relieve this condition have relied upon the astringent or coagulating effects of various agents, the occluding properties of others, or the ability to render calcium less soluble[61]. Amongst the most common agents now being used, the literature contains references to the efficacy of the following.

9.2.3.1 Strontium

A 10% strontium chloride hexahydrate dentifrice was evaluated for more than a decade[62–68]. In vitro studies report that strontium chloride only slightly reduces dentinal fluid flow. This slight reduction is thought to occur when the abrasive filler occludes the tubules[69]. Some studies have shown improvement in more than 80% of patients. However, it is noteworthy that all investigations demonstrated a strong placebo effect (25% to 45%) on control patients[70]. This placebo effect may be caused by a natural desensitizing process, irritational or abrasive effects from the ingredients in the paste, or a psychological component.

Strontium has been shown to penetrate all calcified tissues, including dentin[71]. It therefore affects dentin hypersensitivity by blocking the outer organic matrix of the root surface. In vivo[72] and in vitro[73] studies demonstrate significant penetration of strontium ions into the dentin. When deposits in tubules are observed, the permeability of dentin is reduced, which may explain the positive effect on dentin hypersensitivity.

Calcium remineralization is higher when calcium and strontium are administered together compared with calcium administered alone. The strontium ions may have some value in accelerating the calcification and eventual obturation of the dentinal tubules[74]. Possible detrimental side effects on the pulp have also been suggested.

9.2.3.2 Sodium Monofluorophosphate (MFP)

Caries research is well documented as to the anticaries effectiveness of commercially available dentifrices containing 0.76% MFP[66,75–77]. Several groups have also suggested its effectiveness in the treatment of hypersensitive teeth[66,78]. From a chemical point of view, MFP-enamel interaction shows that the formation of fluoride hydroxyapatite occurs without calcium. It was concluded that MFP is hydrolyzed in the presence of hydroxyapatite and this hydrolysis occurs at the surface of the apatite crystals[79]. The fluoride ion is evidence for the interaction of MFP with hydroxyapatite. In vitro or in the presence of saliva, MFP produced no visual changes on the surface of the dentin as assessed by scanning electron microscopy, and the tubules remained patent[80].

9.2.3.3 Sodium Fluoride

Various forms of fluoride are used for treatment of dentinal hypersensitivity. Many studies have shown its effectiveness clinically as well as in evaluation in vitro of fluid flow decrease[81–91].

Topical fluoride most likely results in the formation of a fluoride-hydroxyapatite. The addition of fluoride ions decreases the diameter of the dentinal tubules, which effectively reduces the potential to stimulate the pulp via the hydrodynamic mechanism. It also encourages formation of a harder, more insoluble dentin that makes it more durable and protective.

Greenhill and Pashley[69], in their in vitro study on hydraulic conduction, showed that acidulated sodium fluoride solution reduced hydraulic conduction to 24.5%. Two percent neutral sodium fluoride reduced this conduction to 17.7% and sodium fluoride applied through iontophoretic techniques reduced it to 33%. Thus, fluoride-containing medicaments do alter fluid flow and could provide a benefit in the treatment of hypersensitivity[85].

9.2.3.4 Calcium Hydroxide[10,92–95]

Calcium hydroxide ($Ca(OH)_2$) is thought to promote a hypermineralized cement that insulates the dentin. It has been used widely beneath restorations[92,95]. It has little or no direct effect on dentin sensory activity and its long-term effectiveness is attributed to the ability to cause increased peritubular dentin mineralization. Greenhill and Pashley[69] noted a 21% decrease in dentinal fluid movement in vitro when calcium hydroxide was used.

9.2.3.5 Potassium Nitrate[92]

Physiologic experiments, using isotonic KCl, show no effect on producing or relieving dentin sensitivity unless applied directly to the pulp. In vitro tests revealed that 30% potassium nitrate was ineffective in decreasing dentinal fluid flow even though clinicians have found effectiveness at 5% levels[96]. In a double-blind clinical study comparing 5% potassium nitrate, 10% strontium chloride, 2% sodium citrate in pluronic gel, and 1.4% formalin paste, the 5% potassium nitrate paste was found to be superior overall[97].

9.2.3.6 Formaldehyde[98–101]

Several reports in the 1950s and 1960s described considerable reduction in sensitivity when formalin was incorporated into a dentifrice. The in vitro studies of Addy and Morgan[102] demonstrated that a commercially available toothpaste containing formaldehyde was one of the few pastes that appeared to have little or no effect on the dentin surface. Formaldehyde works as a protein precipitant, but the exact mode of action in reducing hypersensitivity is unclear.

9.2.3.7 Sodium Citrate-Pluronic Gel[103,104]

The action of sodium citrate and pluronic gel is thought to be derived from the polyglycol's ability to precipitate dentinal or salivary proteins. Direct dentinal occlusion with the filler has been shown to reduce dentinal fluid flow in vitro by about 19%[69]. Early marketing acclaimed its good flavour, but reported little on its desensitizing properties.

9.2.3.8 Stannous Fluoride[89]

It has been demonstrated that low concentrations of aqueous solutions of stannous fluoride will effectively control dentin hypersensitivity. As with sodium fluoride, the formation of a barrier blocking tubule openings is the speculated mode of action. Blunder et al.[80] demonstrated that in vitro stannous fluoride, as well as sodium fluoride, may precipitate on the dentinal surface and occlude the tubules. Penney and Karlsson[77] showed that tin diffuses less readily than fluoride into the dentin. Fluoride is of similar molecular size to the hydroxyl group. Tin undergoes ionic exchange and its chemical role in the reduction of hypersensitivity appears negligible.

9.2.3.9 Glucocorticoids

The anti-inflammatory effect of glucocorticoids is well known and many believe that their topical application to cavity preparation and surgically exposed dentin decreases dentinal sensitivity. Using topical prednisone in an uncontrolled study of gold restoration, it was found that the steroid was successful in reducing thermal sensitivity; however, it did not reduce pulp inflammation histologically[105]. Steroid application to dentin increased peritubular dentin mineralization[94]. The dentinal tubule lumen was reduced, resulting in less dentinal tubule fluid movement. The exact mechanism of steroid-induced mineralization has yet to be ascertained.

9.2.3.10 Resins and Adhesives

Dayton et al.[106] and Brännström et al.[107] demonstrated an immediate and long-lasting blockage of sensation after sealing the tubules or impregnating them with unfilled resin or dentin bonding material.

Olgart et al.[108] reviewed the root surface condition before resin impregnation. Dentin softened by acidic foods or bacterial plaque must be removed. Prophylactic removal tends to clog the tubules, whereas acid conditioning before resin placement has been controversial. Brännström et al.[107] recommended acid placement before resin-adhesive placement, but Doering and Jensen[109] do not advocate acid contact with the dentin.

Light-cured dentin bonding agents adhere better to the tubular wall and the dentin surface. After 18 months, a lasting effectiveness of 89%–90% is found. Doering and Jensen's results[109] revealed that 74% had no pain 3 months after placement of a light-cured dentin bonding agent. Preliminary data on postperiodontal surgical patients reveals that only one of 26 patients needed more than two coats of resin to relieve hypersensitivity. All others achieved immediate relief with one or two applications.

9.2.3.11 Glass Ionomer Cement[110]

Wycoff[111] believes that the glass-ionomer cements are kindest to the pulp and do not require etching.

There is excellent adhesion to the tooth structure so that it can be placed without mechanical tooth preparation. The material is hydrophilic and has good mechanical strength and adhesion. In addition, it is esthetic and appears to be non-irritating to the pulp.

9.2.3.12 Bioactive and Biocompatible Glasses[112]

Bioactive and biocompatible glasses have been developed as bone replacement materials and previous studies have demonstrated that these glasses can induce or aid osteogenesis in physiological systems[113]. Furthermore, particulate Bioglass® has been used for periodontal osseous repair[114]. It is evident from these reports that bioactive glass has the capacity to bond with bone tissue and, according to Schepers and Ducheyne, bone tissue repair and growth is enhanced by its osteoconductive properties[115].

The bonding of bioactive glass particles to bone begins with the exposure of the glass to aqueous solutions. Sodium ions in the glass exchange with hydrogen ions from the body fluids causing the pH to increase. Calcium and phosphate ions subsequently migrate from the glass forming a calcium-phosphate-rich surface layer under which is a layer that becomes increasingly silica-rich because of the loss of the sodium, calcium and phosphate ions[113–115]. It is this observation with regard to the silica-rich layer together with the small size of bioactive glass particles which enabled the investigators to consider using bioactive glass particles as a possible desensitizing agent for the reduction of dentin sensitivity.

9.2.3.13 Oxalate-Containing Products[116]

Oxalate-containing products have been tested both in vitro[117] and in vivo[118–120]. Studies have suggested that oxalate-containing products may interact with the dentin surface, producing precipitates of calcium and phosphate with the potential to aid tubule occlusion[121,122]. This type of desensitizing mechanism would require the preservation of the original oxalate within the product in order for such specific surface reactions to take place. Gillam et al.[123] have provided some useful observations concerning the deposition of oxalate-containing products onto the exposed dentin surface, particularly with respect to the possible mode of tubule occlusion. All oxalate-containing products covered the dentin surface as well as occluding the tubules to varying degrees.

Table 9-1 Treatment options (modification of Jacobsen 2001[230])

1. Desensitization of the nerve	a. potassium nitrate b. low level laser therapy c. Nd:YAG Laser d. neural therapy (infiltrations with local anesthetics) e. laser acupuncture	
2.Coverage of dentinal tubules	a. periodontal surgery/grafting b. composite/GIC restoration c. crown placement d. plugging (sclerosis) of dentinal tubules	1. ions/salts a. stannous fluoride b. Na fluoride/stannous fluoride combination c. potassium oxalate d. ferrous oxide e. strontium chloride f. in combination with an adhesive 2. precipitates – proteins/amino acids a. glutaraldehyde 3. resins a. dentin sealers b. methyl methacrylate 4. Laser treatment
3. Endodontics		

9.3 Laser Application for Dentin Hypersensitivity Treatment

Conventional treatment methods as described before (Chapter 9.2) have the great disadvantage that they have to be repeated regularly, to achieve a continuous relief from pain[124–126]. Because acids contained in food or aggressive tooth brushing cause gradual removal of precipitations and superficial coatings[127], the treatment agent must be applied repeatedly. The use of lasers might open up new dimensions in the treatment of dentin hypersensitivity.

The lasers used for the treatment of dentin hypersensitivity are divided into two groups: low output power (low-level) lasers (He-Ne and GaAlAs (= diode) lasers), and middle output power lasers (Nd:YAG, Er:YAG and CO_2 lasers)[128–131].

The possibility of a placebo effect must be taken into consideration, especially as patient reports were positive immediately after laser treatment, whereas normally one would expect the cumulative effect of any therapy to provide a gradual improvement from visit to visit. A strong placebo effect is commonly described in clinical dentin hypersensitivity trials. This effect consists of a complex mixture of physiologic and psychological interactions, depending considerably on the doctor–patient relationship, with both parties needing to believe that the treatment is valuable and desiring to obtain relief of symptoms. Investigators have described patients obtaining relief without any treatment due to the placebo effect. This is thought to vary from 20% to 60% in dentin hypersensitivity clinical trials.[132]

Recurrence of hypersensitivity varied with each laser and treatment protocol and depended on the irradiation methods and time after treatment. The recurrence rate of hypersensitivity after He-Ne laser treatment has been reported to range from 7.4% to 66%; that of the GaA1As laser (830 nm wavelength) from 6.0% to 75%, that of the Nd:YAG laser measured up to 34%, and that of the CO_2 laser measured up to 50%. The mechanism of recurrence is unknown. Laser effects are considered to be due to the effects of sealing of dentinal tubules, nerve analgesia or placebo effect. The sealing effect is considered to be lasting, whereas nerve analgesia or a placebo effect are not.[6]

9.3.1 Low Output Power (Low-level) Lasers[6]

Low output power laser therapy has been utilized in humans since the early 1970s. Initially, this form of energy delivery was used to support wound healing[133–135]. Subsequently, in the 1980s, the benefit of low output-delivery systems as an anti-inflammatory tool was delineated[136,137]. Then, it was demonstrated that low output power laser therapy stimulates nerve cells in a clinical environment[134–140].

9.3.1.1 He-Ne Laser (Helium-Neon)

The He-Ne laser (wavelength 633 nm) was used for the treatment of dentin hypersensitivity by several investigators at an output power of 6 mW for 0.5–5 min[141–145]. Irradiation modes were of two types: pulsed (5 Hz only) and continuous wave (cw) mode. Treatment effectiveness rate ranged from 55% to 100%. Wilder-Smith et al. achieved a treatment effectiveness of only 5.2–17.5%[146].

The mechanism involved is mostly unknown. According to physiological experiments, He–Ne laser irradiation does not affect peripheral Aδ- or C-fiber nociceptors[147], but does affect electric activity (action potential), which in the healthy nerve increased by 33% following a single transcutaneous irradiation[138,139]. This was found to be a long-lasting effect, inducing an increase in the size of the nerve's action potential for more than 8 months after cessation of irradiation[138]. He-Ne laser irradiation at 6 mW does not affect the enamel or dentin surface morphologically, but a small fraction of the laser energy is transmitted through enamel or dentin to reach the pulp tissue[148]. With low output power lasers, there is no danger of causing skin burns, or damaging cells[149].

9.3.1.2 GaAlAs Laser (Gallium, Aluminum, Arsenide)

GaAlAs (diode) lasers were initially restricted to GaAs systems. In their early stages of development, GaAs systems were difficult to run for long periods in a cw mode because of the propensity of the chip to overheat. However, by 1979, experiments using a new diode were looking very promising. This new chip, which used wafer-thin crystals of GaAlAs, could produce a variety of wavelengths from 720 to 904 nm, all within the infrared spectrum. It could also generate a continuous wave with no likelihood of overheating. Three wavelengths (780, 830 and 900 nm) of GaAlAs have been used for the treatment of dentin hypersensitivity.

A GaAlAs laser at 780 nm was used for the treatment of dentin hypersensitivity by Matsumoto et al.[150,151], Ebihara et al.[152] and Kawakami et al.[153] at an output power of 30 mW in cw mode. Irradiation time ranged from 0.5 to 3 min. Treatment effectiveness ranged from 85% to 100%.

A GaAlAs laser at 830 nm was used by Matsumoto et al.[154], Setoguchi et al.[155], Hamachi et al.[156], Wakabayashi et al.[157], Mezawa et al.[158], Tachibana et al.[159], Gerschman et al.[160] and Liu and Lan[161]. An output power of 20 to 60 mW was used for the treatment. Irradiation mode was cw and irradiation time ranged from 0.5 to 3 min. Treatment effectiveness rate was dependent on the output power, and ranged from 30% to 100%.

Use of a GaAlAs laser at 900 nm at 2.4 mW, 1.2 kHz for 2.5 min had a treatment effectiveness ranging from 73.3% to 100%[162].

It is postulated that this type of low output power laser mediates an analgesic effect related to depressed nerve transmission. According to physiological experiments using the GaAlAs laser at 830 nm, this effect is caused by blocking the depolarization of C-fiber afferents[163,164]. GaAlAs laser emissions at 904 nm have an analgesic effect on the cat tongue although the mechanism remains unclear[165]. GaAlAs laser irradiation at a maximum power of 60 mW does not affect the enamel or dentin surface morphologically, but a small fraction of the laser energy at 830-nm wavelength is transmitted through enamel or dentin to reach the pulp tissue[166].

9.3.1.3 Laser Acupuncture

Other areas of laser irradiation for cervical dentin hypersensitivity treatment induce the nerve fibers related to the symptomatic region and acupuncture of sites such as M. adductor pollicis and M. lobulus auriculae.[167] Treatment effectiveness is dependent on the area irradiated.

9.3.2 Middle Output Power Lasers

9.3.2.1 Nd:YAG, Ho:YAG, Diode Laser

Several authors used Nd:YAG laser at 1,064 nm for the treatment of dentin hypersensitivity.[168–176] The output power was varied and ranged from 0.3 to 10 W, but 1 or 2 W output was most common. Irradiation methods were dependent on the laser powers and varied from 0.3 W for 90 s out of contact to 2 W for 0.5 s on black ink in contact mode. One investigator applied even 10 W for 0.1 s Treatment effectiveness ranged from 52% to 100%. When using Nd:YAG laser irradiation, the use of black ink as an absorption enhancer can prevent deep penetration of the Nd:YAG laser beam through the enamel and dentin and exces-

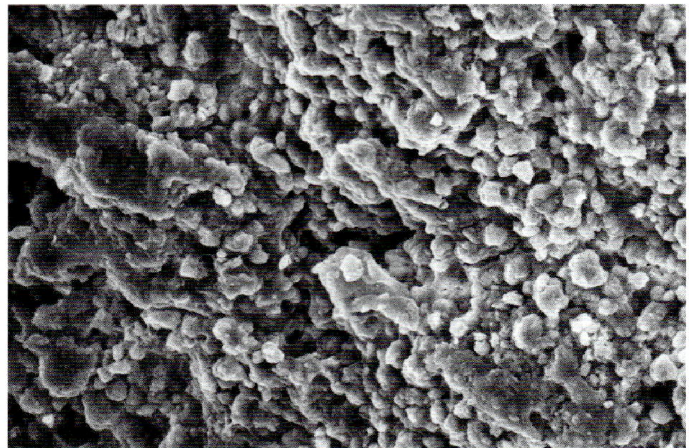

Fig 9-5 SEM 1000X, Nd:YAG laser irradiation at 0.5 W, 10 Hz, incomplete closure of dentinal tubules with an inhomogeneous dentin surface.

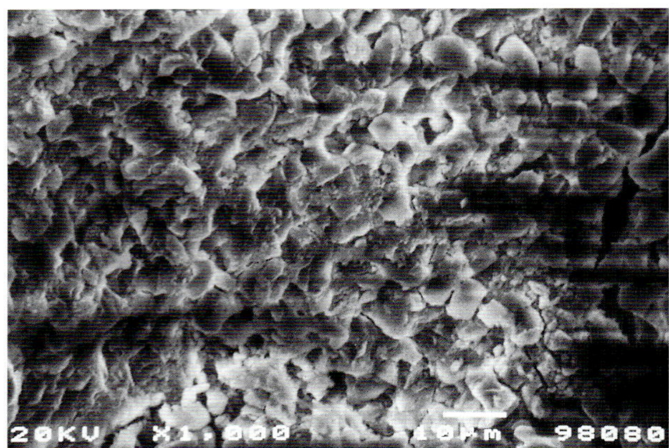

Fig 9-6 SEM 1000X, fluoride gel and Nd:YAG laser irradiation at 0.5 W, 10 Hz, inhomogeneous dentin surface with some dentinal tubules open.

sive effects in the pulp.[177] The use of black ink for enhancing the effects of Nd:YAG laser irradiation to treat dentin hypersensitivity has been reported to be more effective than without.[170,173,174,178]

The mechanism of Nd:YAG laser effects on dentin hypersensitivity is thought to be the laser-induced occlusion or narrowing of dentinal tubules,[171,173,179] as well as direct nerve analgesia. Laser energy at 1064 nm is transmitted through dentin,[180] producing thermally mediated effects on microcirculation,[181] and pulpal analgesia via its nerve system.[182] A variety of theories have been put forward as to how the laser produces its analgesic effect. It has been hypothesized that the laser energy interferes with the sodium pump mechanism, changes the cell membrane permeability and/or temporarily alters the endings of the sensory axons.[183] Irradiation by semiconductor laser has a suppressive effect by blocking the depolarization of very slowly conducting C-fiber afferents only, but it was reported that the blocking of not only C-fibers, but also rapidly conducting Aβ-fibers is performed by Nd:YAG laser irradiation.[184] The mechanism of desensitization can also be regarded as a denaturation of the odontoblastic processes or as an "overcooking" of the dentinal liquor.[175,176]

As mentioned, there is a significantly high correlation between the morphology[185] and the number[186,187] of open dentinal tubules and dentin hypersensitivity. During the irradiation of root dentin, a fusing of the dentinal tubules has been described, along with a vitrification of the dentinal surfaces.[128,188] Otherwise, no complete closure of the dentinal tubules can be observed in the dental neck region. In contrast, even adverse effects like an increase in colour penetration have been reported.[189] The absence of a smear layer can be regarded as the reason for this effect.[188]

Liu et al.[190] found that the sealing depth achieved by Nd:YAG laser irradiation at 30 mJ/pulse and 10 pps on dentinal tubules was less than 4 mm. However, in an in vitro study by Goharkhay et al.[191] scanning electron microscopic and stain penetration tests revealed topographically only incomplete closure of dentinal tubules with an inhomogeneous dentin surface when irradiated with the Nd:YAG laser at 0.2 or 0.5 W, 10 Hz, with and without prior application of a stannous fluoride gel. Higher energy resulted in a greater number of closed tubules with an increased removal of dentin.

In the use of the laser in vivo, thermal effects on pulpal tissues are of concern. Compared to other lasers, the Nd:YAG laser beam penetrates deeply through dentin,[180] bone, and non-pigmented soft tissues.[192] Irradiation causing temperature rises exceeding the threshold of pulpal tolerance will cause thermal injury to the pulp. Previous studies have demonstrated that healthy pulp tissue is not injured thermally if the laser equipment is used at the correct specifications and the temperature increase to the pulp remains under 5.5° C.[193] Pulpal disruption did occur in laser-treated rat specimens with remaining dentin thickness of less than 1 mm, while pulps of intact and prepared teeth with remaining dentin thickness exceeding 1 mm were the same as controls, and observed after laser exposures up to 240 J (2 W, 20 Hz for 2 min) using the Nd:YAG laser. No histologically measurable response was observed using a power of 50mJ/pulse at 10 Hz for 30 s (total energy: 15 J) using rats.[194] However, treatment effects must be well controlled when using black ink as absorption enhancer. It was reported that irradiation at 2 W and 20 Hz for 10 sec induced pulpal temperature rises of 13.4°C through 2 mm thickness of remaining dentin.[195]

Lier et al.[196] concluded, that the effect of treatment of hypersensitive teeth with Nd:YAG laser did not, after 16 weeks, differ from those of a placebo.

In contrast to favourable congress contributions, no scientific publications proving the efficiency of the diode- and Ho:YAG lasers are available. The diode laser application in combination with a fluoride gel could be advantageous due to the continuous wave or chopped working mode of this device. Irradiation with a diode laser (810 nm) at 0.2 or 0.5 W, 10 Hz, shows no closure in the cervical neck region. Ho:YAG laser (2940 nm) treatment partial can lead to sealing of the dentinal tubules at a lower power setting (0.2 W), but not at a higher setting (0.5 W). The dentin surface has a non homogeneous surface structure. Pulpal effects of semiconductor laser devices have been investigated previously. The GaA1As laser at a wavelength of 780 nm, and an output power of 30 mW for 3 min caused no thermal or other damage to pulp tissues in monkeys.[168] According to an in vitro thermometric study, GaA1As laser irradiation at the parameters of 30 mW (cw) at 780 nm wavelength, 60 mW (cw) at 830 nm wavelength, and 10 W (pulsed) at 900 nm wavelength do not cause significant intrapulpal temperature rises.[197]

Furthermore, bacteria also seem to play an important role in sensitivity of teeth. The pain threshold of the nerve fibers seems to be lowered in presence of inflammation mediators.[198] In this context it is important to point to the results of previous studies which have shown the high bactericidal potential of middle output power lasers.[199–207]

9.3.2.2 Er:YAG Laser (Erbium-Doped: Yttrium, Aluminum and Garnet)

Desensitizing effects of an Er:YAG laser (wavelength 2940 nm) are reported by Schwarz et al.[208] Irradiation occurred at an energy level of 80 mJ/pulse, 3 Hz with water irrigation in a defocused manner for 2 min/tooth by scanning in an overlapping pattern. Significant improvement immediately after treatment remained at the same level for the follow-up at 6 months.

The energy setting used is lower than the ablation thresholds of dental hard tissues. The high absorption of the Er:YAG laser emission wavelength in water may result in an evaporation of the dentinal fluid and the smear layer. In a comparative study the Er:YAG laser was the most effective tool in removing the smear layer from root canal walls[209]. Thus, it could be suggested that a deposition of insoluble salts in the exposed tubules is responsible for an obturation of the dentin tubules.

Investigations at the University of Vienna resulted in the splitting off of dentinal hard tissue without sealing of the dentinal tubules, when irradiated with two different Er:YAG lasers even at the lowest possible power settings of 0.2 and 0.5 W, with and without prior application of a stannous fluoride gel. The treated surfaces, however, did not show any melted area[191].

The Er:YAG laser shows the lowest limitation due to thermal side effects because of its thermomechanical ablation mechanism and the high absorption of its wavelength by water[210–213.] An Er:YAG laser has a water absorption characteristic ~15 times greater than that of the CO_2 and even 20000 times greater than the Nd:YAG laser[214,215]. The resulting penetration depth of the Er:YAG laser is in the µm range.

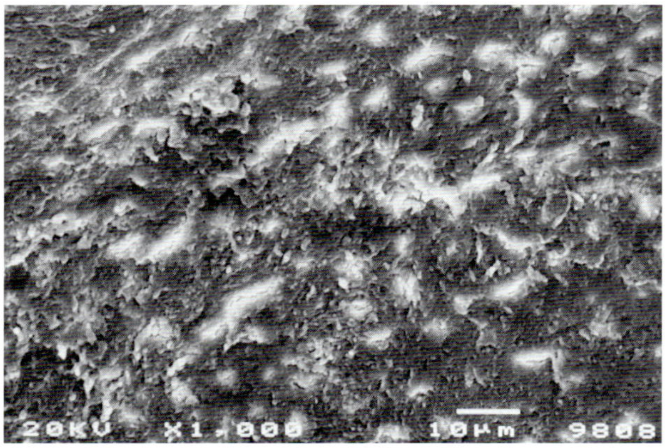

Fig 9-7 SEM 1000X, Er:YAG laser irradiation at 0.2 W, open dentinal tubules.

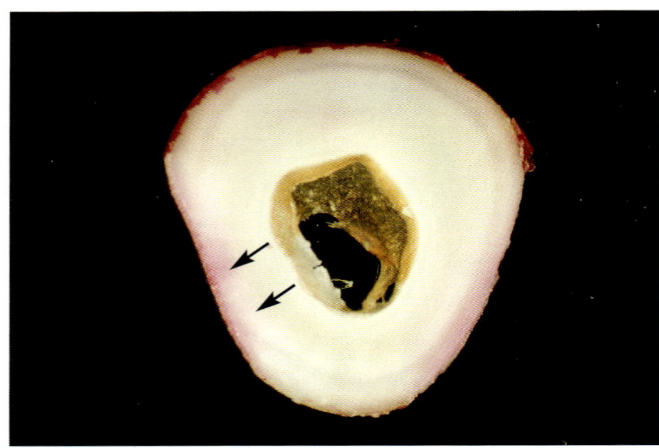

Fig 9-8 1000X, fluoride gel and Er:YAG laser irradiation at 0.2 W, stain penetration into open dentinal tubules.

9.3.2.3 CO_2 Laser (Carbon Dioxide)

The CO_2 Laser (10.6 µm) is the most frequently discussed laser for the treatment of dentin hypersensitivity. The impact of this laser is based on a closure or stricture of the dentinal tubules.

In principle, there are two possibilities to utilize the CO_2 laser. Either a sole CO_2 laser application, that means the exposed dentin is directly irradiated (direct method) or as first described by Moritz et al.[216–219] in combination with a fluoride gel (indirect method). In this case, stannous fluoride gel is first applied to the cleaned dental neck area and the actual laser irradition is carried out through the gel layer. Output powers described in the literature of 0.5 and 1 W, and the cw mode were used for both methods. Irradiation time ranged from 0.5 to 5 s, and irradiation was repeated 5-10 times. There have been no reports on nerve analgesia by CO_2 laser irradiation.[220]

9.3.3 Direct Method

Using the CO_2 laser at moderate energy densities, mainly sealing of dentinal tubules is achieved, as a reduction of permeability due to the occlusion or narrowing of dentinal tubules. CO_2 laser irradiation, may like other wavelengths, also cause dentinal desiccation, yielding temporary clinical relief of dentinal hypersensitivity.[221] The sealing depth achieved by CO_2 laser irradiation at 0.3 W for 0.1 s on dentinal tubules is usually measured to be 2–8 µm.[222] Using the CO_2 laser, no damage was reported after pulpal exposure to 3 W of power for 2 s in the cw mode using monkeys and dogs.[223] The long-time success rate of the sole laser application seems to be questionable: A treatment success of only 50% was reported.[224]

9.3.4 Indirect Method

The indirect method, the CO_2 laser irradiation through a thin layer of stannous fluoride, was first described by Moritz et al. This procedure was developed based on the consideration to combine the advantages of laser- and fluoride therapy and thereby to achieve a durable treatment success. Combined use of laser irradiation with the chemical agent stannous fluoride[218,219] which is incorporated into the dentinal surface for several years, guarantees freedom of pain for a long period of time. Before using the procedure in patients in vivo, comprehensive studies were carried out in vitro to document the safety and efficiency of the treatment method.

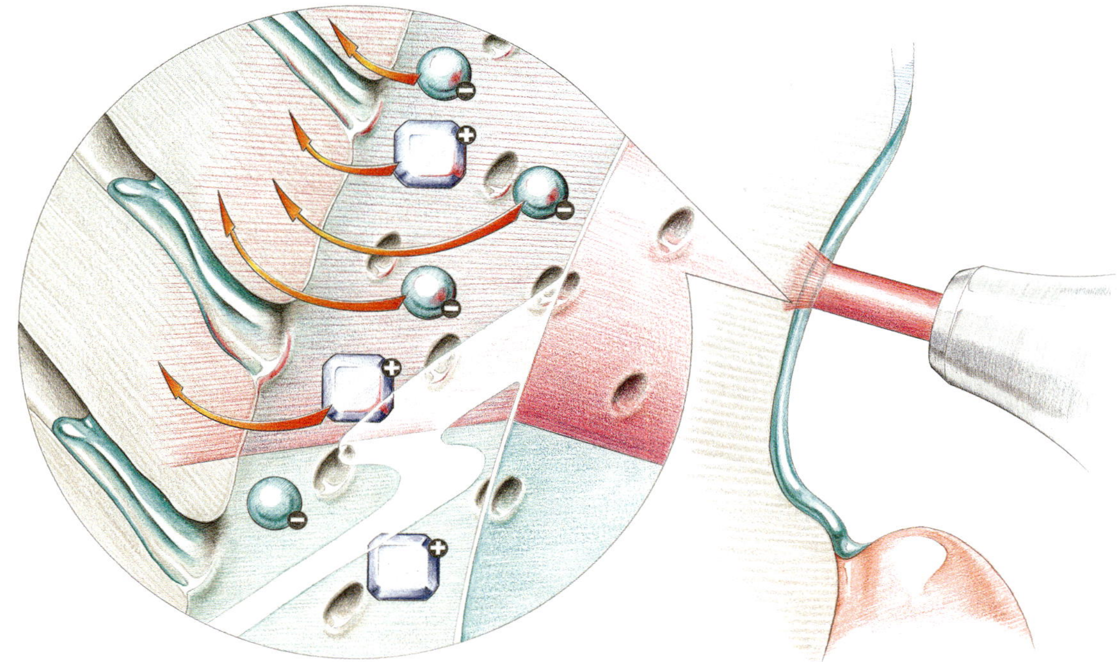

Fig 9-9 Irradiation of the dentinal surface through a thin layer of fluoride gel.

9.3.4.1 Stain penetration and SEM

The fusing ability of common middle-output-power lasers examined in a stain penetration and SEM (scanning electron microscopy) study revealed that at present the continuous wave CO_2 laser at a output power of 0.5 W in combination with prior application of a thin layer of stannous fluoride gel is the only laser to achieve optimum closure of dentin surfaces with a very homogenous surface structure in the scanning electron microscope.[191]

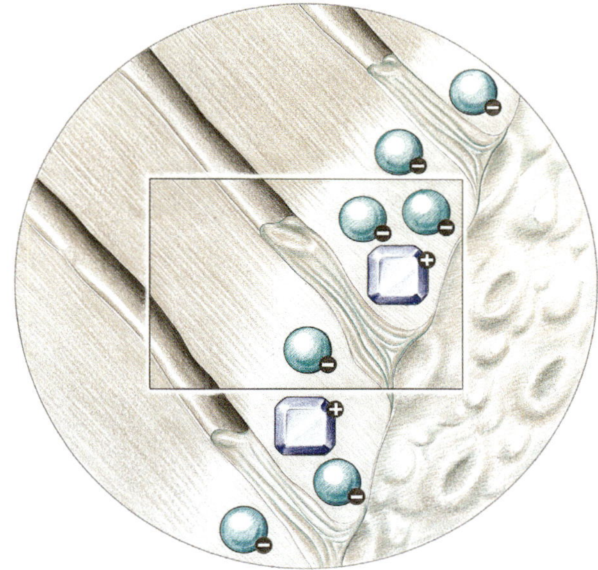

Fig 9-10 Incorporation of fluoride into the dentinal surface.

9.3.4.2 Temperature measurements

To exclude thermal damage of the dental pulp after CO_2 laser irradiation, temperature measurements were performed. With the CO_2 laser, the enamel and dentin surfaces reach very high temperatures, but only low temperatures are measured in the pulp chambers.[177] At parameters of 0.5 to 1 W an intrapulpal temperature rise below 1°C was measured. This is related to the very high absorption and low penetration of light in hard

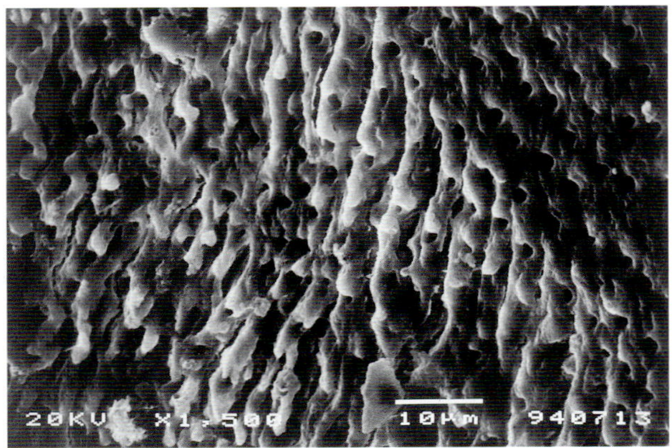

Fig 9-11 SEM 1500X, open dentinal tubules of the cervical dental neck area.

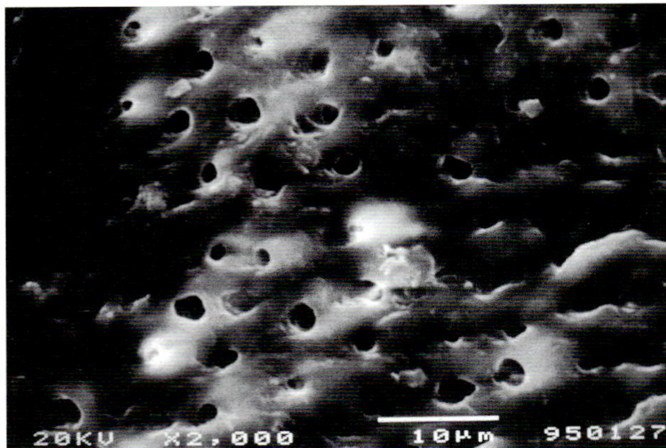

Fig 9-12 SEM 2000X, CO_2 laser irradiation at 0.5 W, no fluoridation, open tubuli.

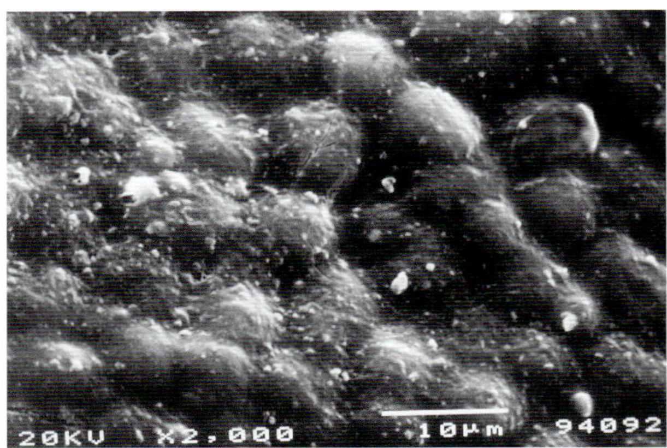

Fig 9-13 SEM 2000X, fluoride gel and CO_2 laser irradiation at 0.5 W.

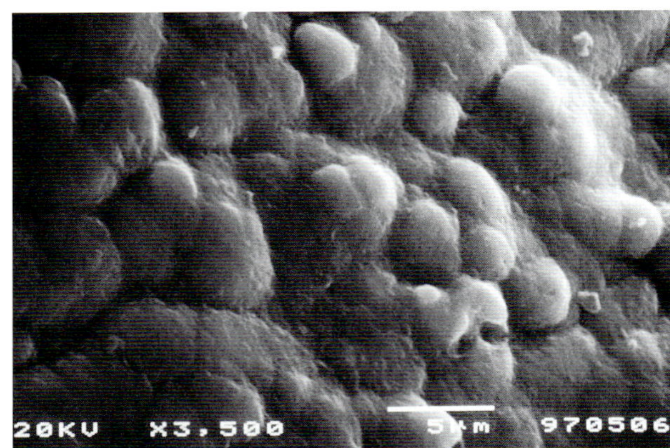

Fig 9-14 SEM 3500X, fluoride gel and CO_2 laser irradiation at 0.5 W, extraction 18 months after in vivo treatment.

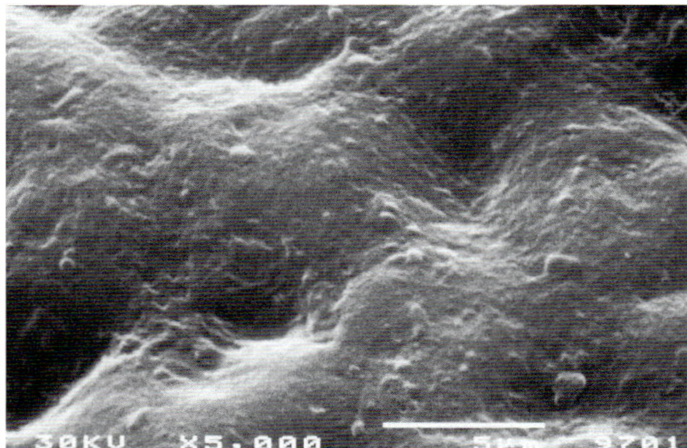

Fig 9-15 SEM 5000X, fluoride gel and CO_2 laser irradiation at 0.5 W, extraction 18 month after in vivo treatment.

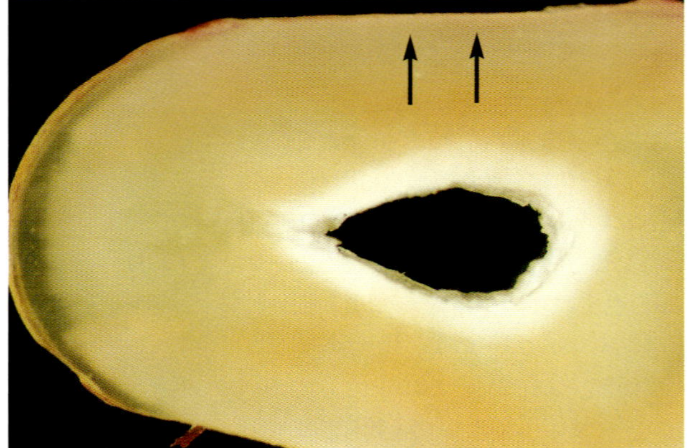

Fig 9-16 Fluoride gel and CO_2 laser irradiation at 0.5 W, no stain penetration into dentinal tubules.

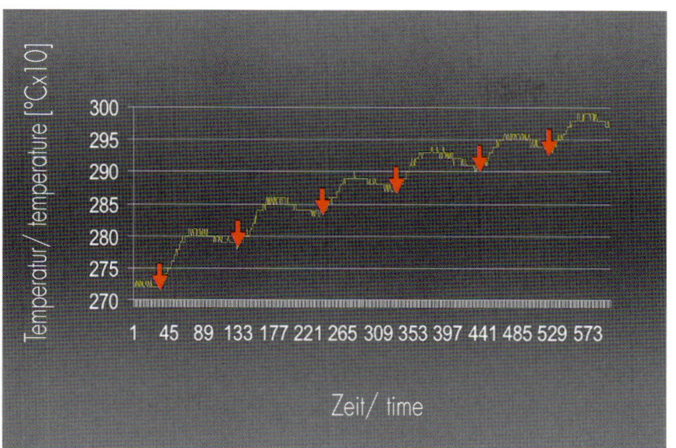

Fig 9-17 CO_2 laser irradiation at 0.5 W, max. temperature increase < 2.5°C.

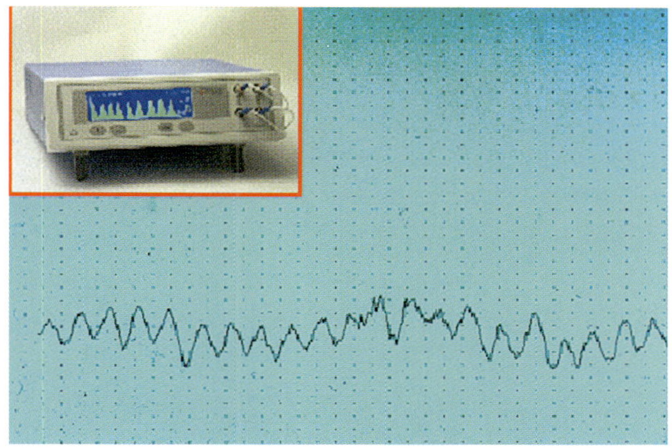

Fig 9-18 Laser Doppler flowmetry: no change in pulpal blood flow after laser treatment.

dental tissues at this wavelength. Intermittent lasing of 6 times for 5 seconds with 20-second breaks excludes thermal damage to the pulp because the maximum temperature rise at 0.5 W does not exceed 2.5°C.[216,217] The safety of the CO_2 Laser therapy is confirmed by this finding to a large extent.

9.3.4.3 Clinical Adoption

Comprehensive clinical studies were carried out to ensure the efficiency of the treatment method. Although there are many methods of clinically assessing dentin hypersensitivity, most investigators use either a sharp explorer or a blast of cold air to measure sensitivity. These are the oldest.[127] The evaluation of treatments for dentin hypersensitivity is extremely difficult regardless of the methods or materials employed. In estimating treatment effects in hypersensitive teeth, investigations are handicapped by an inability to observe patient response objectively and are dependent upon the patient's interpretation, which has been useful and popular in the fields of internal medicine and psychology, is considered to be good for objective judgment.[226] And this is effective for evaluation of human dental pain.[227]

Moritz et al. decided to use the patients' subjective freedom from symptoms after application of specific stimuli (touch, cold, heat, sweet, sour) as the only criterion for the success of treatment.[217]

Prior to treatment, the patients were asked to subjectively evaluate the pain caused by hypersensitive dental necks on a scale ranging from 0 (free from pain) to 4 (unbearable). This evaluation was carried out for each of the following pain-producing stimuli: touch, heat, cold, sweet and sour.

The sensitivity to touch was assessed by exerting pressure on the respective region with an ASH Brodontic 25 G-probe. The sensitivity to heat and cold was evaluated by rinsing the hypersensitive area with water at a temperature of 55°C and 10°C, respectively. The sensitivity to the pain-producing stimuli "sweet" and "sour" was assessed by applying sugar and citric acid solution, respectively.

In this in vivo study by Moritz et al. the efficacy of laser treatment was examined in 72 patients with dentin hypersensitivity and 72 control patients.

When success was defined as complete freedom from pain, the success rate in the laser group was 94.5%; when marked pain relief was included in the definition of treatment success, 98.6% of the patients were treated successfully. Treatment of the control group with conventional dental neck fluoridation resulted no marked improvement.

All patients showed no effect on perfusion indices immediately before and after CO_2 laser treatment at 0.5 W in the cw mode for 5 s with 20 s interval as well as 1 week after treatment.[217] Other Laser

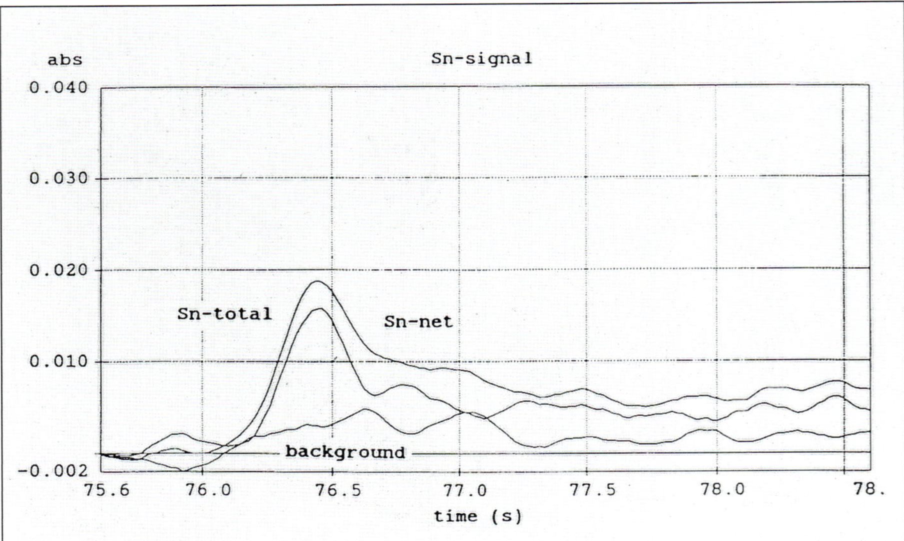

Fig 9-19 AAS: traces of tin 18 months after treatment

Doppler examination revealed also no change in pulpal blood flow due to laser treatment.[228]

9.3.4.4 Physical Basics

To assess the treatment method's exact mode of action, detailed physical examinations (AAS, XPS, EPMA, X-ray diffraction) were carried out at the Institute of Solid State Physics at the Technical University of Vienna. Teeth, that had been irradiated with the CO_2 laser and stannous fluoride in vivo after a written consent from the patients, served as a basis for these investigations. The teeth had been extracted 18 months after the treatment for orthodontic reasons.

AAS

AAS (atomic absorption spectroscopy examinations) revealed traces of tin in very small dentin samples (in the µg range) from dental neck regions at 18 months indicating that stannous fluoride had been integrated into the dentinal surface and that it had remained there for the observed duration.[217] AAS allows quantitative evaluation of minimal amounts of an element (in the ng range) in samples whose components are known.

XPS

X-ray photoelectron spectroscopy (XPS) allows statements about the bonding characteristics. The information depth is several atomic layers, the detection limit around 1%. The spectra revealed a shift in the binding energy: The stannous fluoride peak was missing, actually being integrated into the calcium fluoride peak and leveling off to the baseline. The elements fluorine, phosphorus, calcium, and tin were examined for a possible chemical shift (that allows a conclusion about bonding characteristics). The carbon peak (Cls) was used as reference line. The statistical data evaluation revealed no shifts in phosphorus, calcium, or tin within the samples, while a marked difference in the bonding energy of fluorine was observed between treated samples (C) and untreated samples (A). These findings indicate that irradiation with the CO_2 laser results in a change in the bonding characteristics of fluorine. Bonding of fluorine to dentin at the outermost surface (approximately 1 nm) of the tooth is obviously improved when CO_2 laser treatment is combined with the application of SnF_2 gel. Therefore a chemical bond between the stannous fluoride gel and the dental neck surface can be assumed.

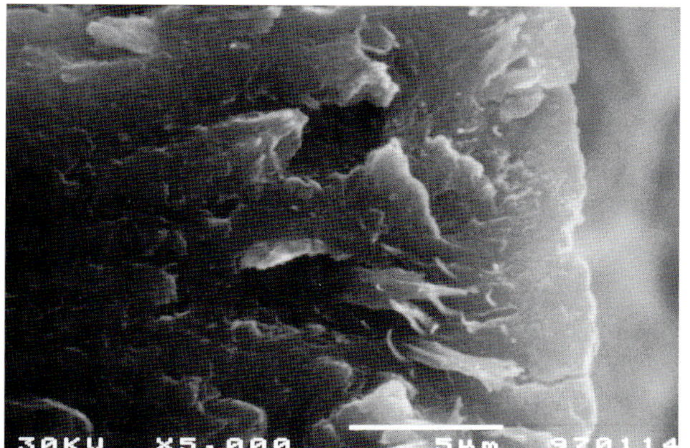

Fig 9-20 SEM 2000X, image of the fracture in a homogeneous site (no layer discernible on topogram; clean fracture).

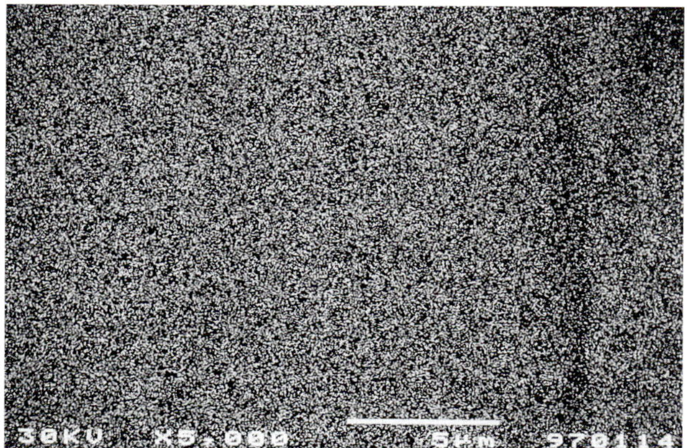

Fig 9-21 X-ray energy disperse image of the same site with an ~2–3-µm-thick layer deficient of calcium, deficient in phosphorus and a zone enriched with tin, 2000X.

Fig 9-22 X-ray diffraction, no structural change after fluoride gel application and CO_2 laser irradiation at 0.5 W.

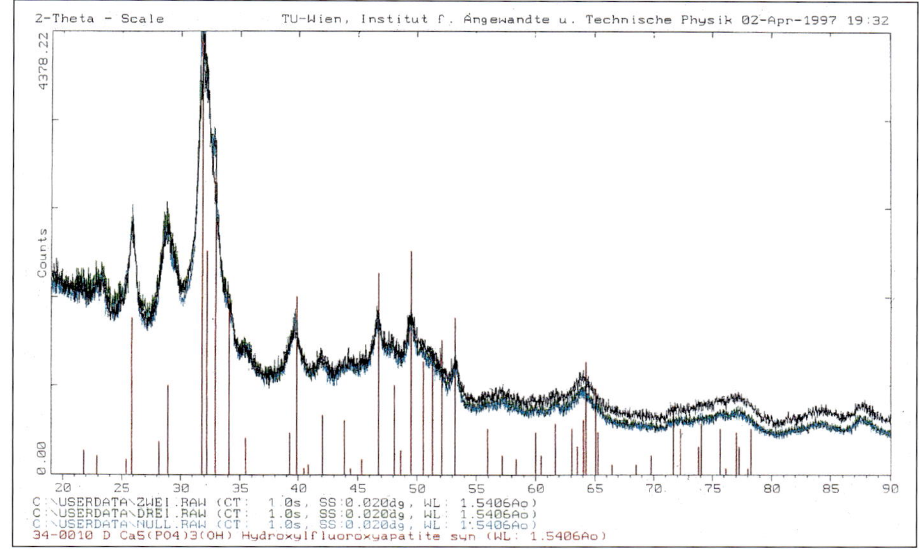

EPMA

Electron probe microanalysis (EPMA) allows evaluation of the distribution of certain elements of surfaces in combination with SEM. X-ray energy dispersive images of the cross sections of lased teeth showed a 2 to 3 µm thick layer deficient in calcium (Ca K α) and phosphorus (Phosphor K α) and enriched with tin (tin L α). Fluorine in very low concentrations can also be detected with this method. Normally, the EPMA is carried out using a wavelength-dispersive detector system – in this case no detection of fluorine is possible. In the actual case, the measurements were accomplished with an energy-dispersive detector system (EDS). Scanning electron microscopic pictures revealed no structural change.

EPMA examinations of tin are rather difficult (the limit of detection is around 0.1%). The depth information of dentin is around 3 µm (at 20 kV accelerating voltage). According to the tin signal, the mean tin concentration near the surface was around 1%. Because background noise could not be suppressed, the tin signal (SnLα) was not very significant. However, in long-term spot measure-

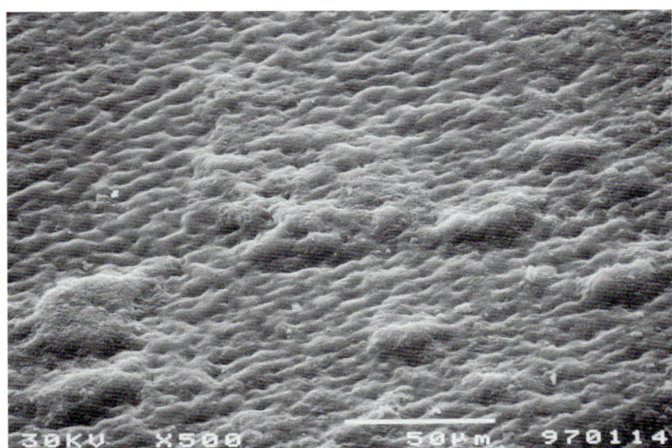

Fig 9-23 SEM 500X, nearly complete closure of dentinal tubules 6 months after fluoride gel and CO_2 laser irradiation at 0.5 W in vivo.

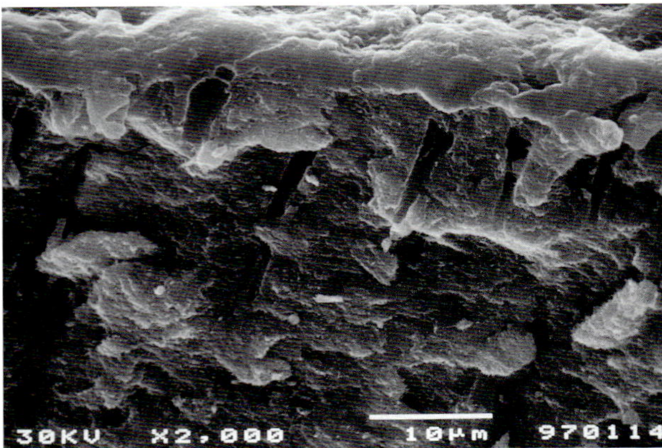

Fig 9-24 2000X, SEM image of the fracture site with gel residues after fluoride gel and CO_2 laser irradiation at 0.5 W.

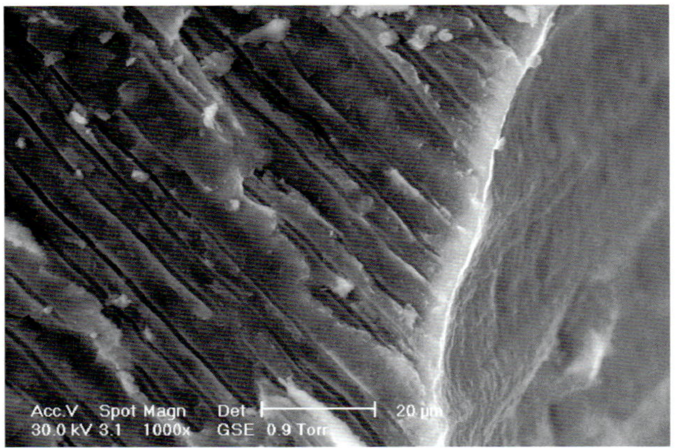

Fig 9-25 1000X, SEM image of the fracture site with gel residues after fluoride gel and CO_2 laser irradiation at 0.5 W.

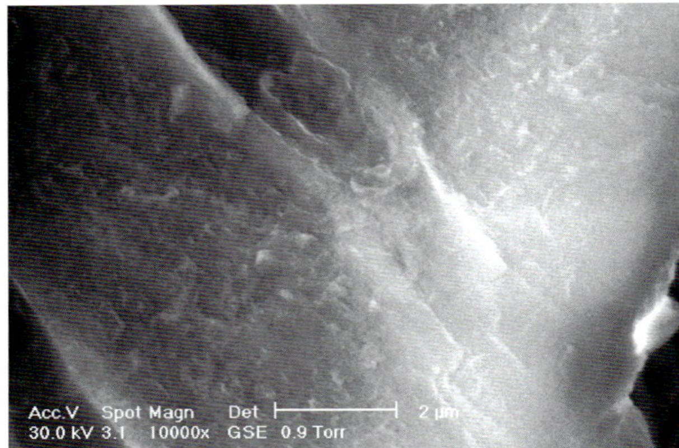

Fig 9-26 SEM, 10000X, magnification of Fig 9-25, detail of a closed dentinal tubule.

ments, there was a clear difference in tin concentration between the tooth region near the surface and the inner tooth region.

The results of XPS and EPMA indicate that there are physical and chemical bonds between stannous fluoride gel and the treated dental neck surface following irradiation with the CO_2 laser. The amazingly swift improvement of the clinical situation as well as the encouraging long-term effect and the high rate of acceptance achievable by the combined treatment emphasize the usefulness of the CO_2 laser in the field of hypersensitive dental necks. Due to the above-mentioned physical properties and the specific wavelength of the CO_2 laser a highly resistant protective layer on sensitized dentin can be generated. This layer induced by physical and chemical bonding mechanisms provides a superior defense against external stimuli.[219]

9.4 Clinical Procedure in Treatment of Hypersensitive Dentin

1. Appointment:

1. initial examination to eliminate any possible reason that may mimic dentin hypersensitivity (e.g., fracture, cracked tooth or irreversible pulpitis)
2. identification and if possible elimination of the etiology or process causing the hypersensitivity, e.g.,
   a. exposure to acids (e.g., sodas, fruit juice, wine, bulimia)
   b. incorrect oral hygiene technique (e.g., toothbrush abrasion)
   c. poor plaque control (acidic bacterial byproducts)
   d. excessive (home-) bleaching
   e. cervical erosion
   f. gingival retraction
   g. malocclusion
   h. iatrogenic (e.g., concrement removal, scaling, root planing)
3. patients information of treatment steps and written confirmation
4. if necessary, professional oral hygiene
5. evaluation of pain on a scale ranging from 0 (free from pain) to 4 (unbearable pain) before treatment, by stimulating with an air blast or alternative different stimuli (e.g., touch, cold, heat, sweet, sour)
6. rinsing and drying of the cervical area (application of rubber dam)
7. eye protection for every person in the room
8. application of a thin layer of stannous fluoride gel prior to irradiation
9. operation mode of the CO_2 laser is continuous wave at an output power of 0.5 W
10. five seconds of contact-free lasing of the hypersensitive dental neck region (around 5 mm^2) under continuous movement of the hand piece (at a distance of 1 cm – focal spot 1 mm^2)
11. 20 s break
12. six times repetition of the procedure for an overall exposure time of 30 s/region
13. evaluation of pain

2. Appointment: after 1 week
Like steps 5–13 of Appointment 1

3. Appointment: after 2 weeks
Like steps 5–13 of Appointment 1 if necessary

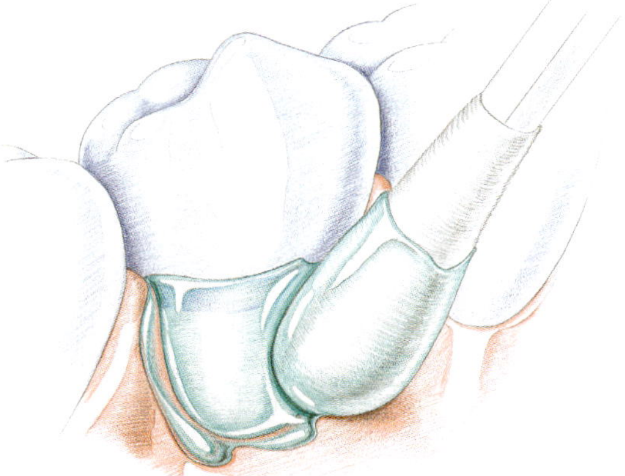

Fig 9-27 Application of a thin layer of stannous fluoride gel.

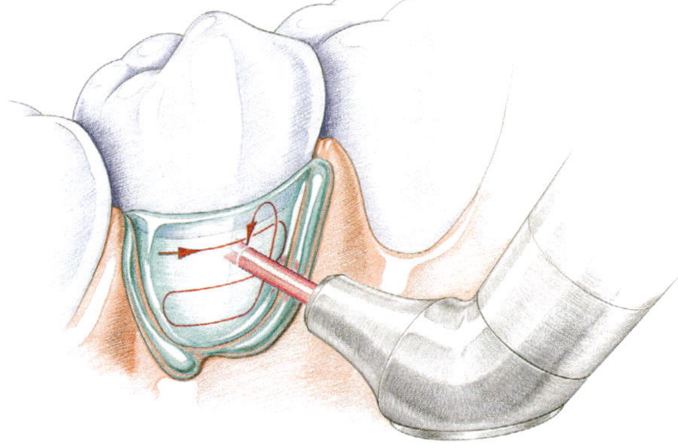

Fig 9-28 Laser treatment of the hypersensitive dental neck under continuous movement.

9.5 Case

Sensitive cervical region of tooth 45 of a 32 year old patient, first appointment.

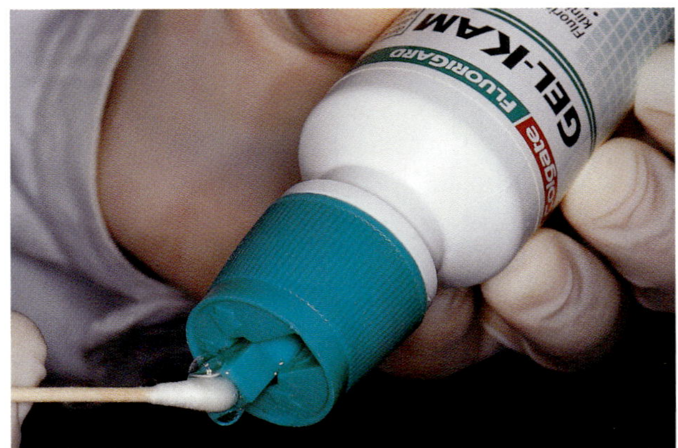

Fig 9-29 Commercial stannous fluoride gel.

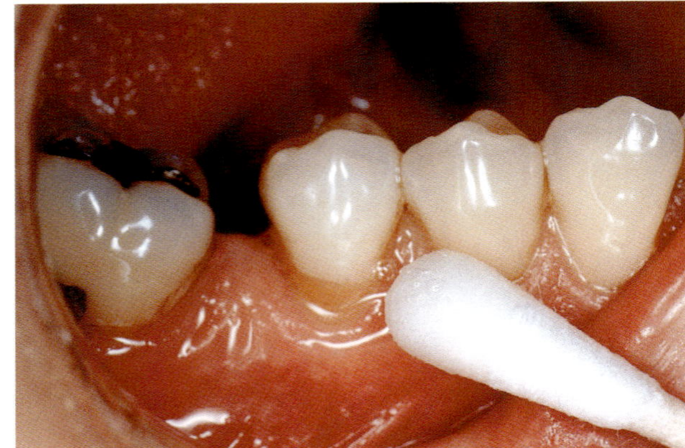

Fig 9-30 Application of a thin layer of stannous fluoride gel in region 45.

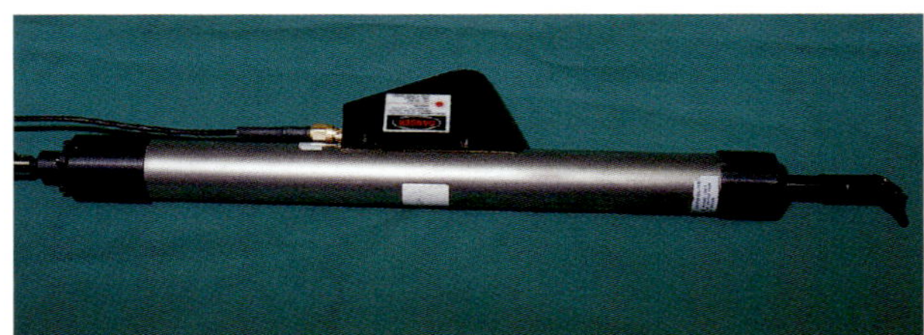

Fig 9-31 Continuous wave CO_2 laser with a minimal output power of 0.5 W.

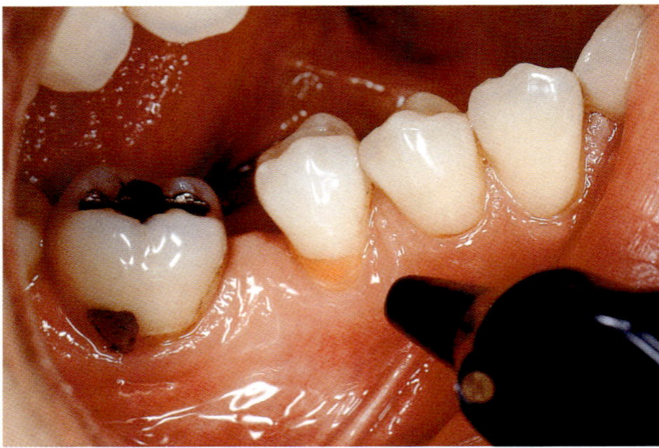

Fig 9-32 Laser treatment of the hypersensitive dental neck under continuous movement with a 0.5 W cw CO_2 laser.

9.6 References

1. Holland G R, Narhi M N, Addy M, Gangarosa L, Orhardson S (1997) Guidelines for the design and conduct of clinical trials on dentine hypersensitivity. Journal of Clinical Periodontology 24: 808–813
2. Seltzer S, Bender I, Ziontz M (1963) The dynamics of pulp inflammation: Correlation between diagnostic data and actual histologic findings in the pulp. Oral Surgery, Oral Medicine & Oral Pathology 16: 846–871
3. Woofter C (1969) The prevalence and aetiology of gingival recession. Periodontal Abstract 17: 45–50
4. Schluger S, Yuodelis R A Page R C (1978) Periodontal Disease. Philadelphia: Lea & Febinger
5. Glickman I (1979) Glickman´s Clinical Periodontology, ed. Garranza W B, pp. 103–104. Philadelphia: Saunders & Co
6. Kimura Y, Wilder-Smith P, Matsumoto K (2000) Lasers in endodontics: a review. International Endodontic Journal 33:173–185
7. Ishikawa S (1969) A clinico-histological study on the hypersensitivity of dentine. Journal of the Japanese Stomatological Society 36: 68-88
8. Rimondini L, Baroni C, Carrassi A (1995) Ultrastructure of hypersensitive and non-sensitive dentine. Journal of Clindical Periodontology 22: 899 – 902
9. Johanson G, Brännström M (1971) Pain reacting to pain stimulus in teeth with experimental fillings. Acta Odontologica Scandinavica 29: 639–647
10. Brännström M, Garberoglio R (1980) Occlusion of tubules under superficially atritted dentine. Swedish Dental Journal 4: 87-91
11. Hiatt W H, Johansen E (1972) Root preparation. I. Obturation of dentinal tubules in treatment of root hypersensitivity. Journal of Periodontology 43: 373–380
12. Graf G, Galasse R (1977) Morbidity, prevalence and intraoral distribution of hypersensitive teeth. Journal of Dental Research 56, Special Issue, 162, abstr. 479
13. Flynn J, Galloway R, Orchardson R (1985): The incidence of 'hypersensitive' teeth in the West of Scotland. J Dent 13(3):230–6
14. Scherman A, Jacobsen PL (1992): Managing dentin hypersensitivity: what treatment to recommend to patients. J Am Dent Assoc 123(4):57–61
15. Anderson D J, Ronning G A (1966) Osmotic excitants of pain in human dentine. Archives of Oral Biology 7: 513–523
16. Anderson D J, Curven M P, Howard L V (1958) The sensitivity of human dentine. Journal of Dental Research 37: 669–677
17. Stephan R M (1937) Correlation of clinical tests with microscopic pathology of the dental pulp. Journal of Dental Research 16, 267–278
18. Tyldesley W R, Mumford J M (1970) Dental pain and the histological condition of the pulp. Dental Practitioner 20: 333–336
19. Dachi S F (1965) The relationship of pulpitis and hyperaemia to thermal sensitivity. Oral Surgery, Oral Medicine & Oral Pathology19: 776–785
20. Lundy T, Stanley H R (1969) Correlation of pulpal histopathology and clinical symptoms in human teeth subjected to experimental irritation. Oral Surgery, Oral Medicine & Oral Pathology 27: 187–201
21. Brännström M (1962a) Observations on exposed dentine and the corresponding pulp tissue. A preliminary study with replica and routine histology. Odontologisk Revy 13: 235–245
22. Everett F G, Hall W B, Phatak N M (1966) Treatment of hypersensitive dentine. Journal of Oral Therapeutics and Pharmacology 2: 300-310
23. Löe H, Theilade E, Jensen S B (1965) Experimental gingivitis in man. Journal of Periodontology 36: 177–187
24. Grant D A, Stern I, Everett F (1972) Orban´s Periodontics. 4th ed., pp 414–416. St. Louis: C. V. Mosby
25. Uchiada A, Wakano Y, Fukuyama O, Miki T, Iwayama Y, Okady H (1980) Controlled clinical evaluation of a 10% strontium chloride dentrifice in the treatment of dentine hypersensitivity following periodontal surgery. Journal of Periodontology 51, 578–581
26. Dowell P, Addy M (1983) Dentine hypersensitivity. A Review. Journal of Clinical Periodontology 10: 341–350
27. Brännström M (1962c) A hydrodynamic mechanism in the transmission of pain producing stimuli through the dentine. In Sensory Mechanisms in Dentine, ed. Anderson D J, 73–79, Oxford: Pergamon Press
28. Brännström M (1966) Sensitivity of dentine. Oral Surgery, Oral Medicine & Oral Pathology 21: 517–526
29. Fish E W (1927) The circulation of lymph in dentine and enamel. Journal of the American Dental Association 14: 804–817
30. Coffey C T, Ingram M J, Bjorndal A M (1970) Analysis of human dentinal fluid. Oral Surgery 30: 835–837
31. Johansen E, Parks H F (1962) Electron microscopic observations on sound human dentine. Archives of Oral Biology 7: 185–194
32. Garberoglio R, Brännström M (1976) A scanning electron microscopic investigation of human dentinal tubules. Archives of Oral Biology 21: 355–362
33. Beveridge E E, Brown A C (1956) The measurement of human dentinal intrapulpal pressure and its response to clinical variables. Oral Surgery 19: 655–688
34. Johnson G, Olgart L, Brännström M (1973) Outward fluid flow in dentine under a physiologic pressure gradient: Experiments in vitro. Oral Surgery, Oral Medicine & Oral Pathology 35:238–248
35. Brännström M, Aström A (1964) A study in the mechanism of pain elicited from the dentine. Journal of Dental Research 43: 619–625
36. Kramer I R H (1955) The relationship between dentine sensitivity and movements in the contents of the dentinal tubules. British Dental Journal 98: 391–392

37. Brännström M, Johnson G (1970) Movements of the dentine and pulp liquids on application of thermal stimuli – an in vitro study. Acta Odontologica Scandinavica 28: 59–70
38. Brännström M (1962b) The elicitation of pain in human dentine and pulp by chemical stimuli. Archives of Oral Biology 7: 59–62
39. Brännström M, Aström A (1972) The hydrodynamics of the dentine, its possible relationship to dentinal pain. International Dental Journal 22: 219–227
40. Brännström M, Linden L A, Aström A (1967) The hydrodynamics of the dental tubule and pulp fluid. Caries Research 1: 310–317
41. Berggren G, Brännström M (1965) The rate of flow in dentinal tubules due to capillary attraction. Journal of Dental Research 44: 408–415
42. Brännström M, Johnson G (1978) The sensory mechanism in human dentine as revealed by evaporation and mechanical removal of dentine, Journal of Dental Research 57: 49–53
43. Hagerstam G, Olgart L, Edwall L (1975) The Excitatory action of acetylcholine on intradental sensory units. Acta Physiologica Scandinavica 93: 113–118
44. Hagerstam G (1976) The effect of Veratrine and Actonitrine on the excitability of sensory units in the tooth of the cat. Acta Physiologica Scandinavica 98: 1–7
45. Brännström M, Johnson G, Linden L A (1969) Fluid flow and pain response in the dentine produced by hydrostatic pressure. Odontologisk Revy 20: 15–30
46. Horiuchi M, Matthews M (1973) In vitro observations of fluid flow through human dentine caused by pain producing stimuli. Archives of Oral Biology 18: 275–294
47. Scott, D, Stewart, G G (1965) Excitation of the dentinal receptor of the cat by heat and chemical agents. Oral surgery 20:784–794
48. Yamada M (1969) Recording of nerve potential. International Dental Journal 19: 239–249
49. Scott D, Temple T R (1965) Neurophysiological response of single receptor units in the tooth of the cat. Journal of Dental Research 44: 20–27
50. Matthews B (1970) Nerve impulses recorded from dentine in the cat. Archives of Oral Biology 15: 523–530
51. Ten Cate A R, Shelton I (1966) Cholinesterase activity in human teeth. Archives of Oral Biology 11: 423–428
52. Kroeger D C (1968) Possible role of neurohumoral substances in the pulp. In Biology of the Dental Pulp Organ: A Symposium, ed. Finn S B, pp. 334–346. Birmingham University: Alabama Press
53. Krauser J T (1986) Hypersensitive teeth. Part II: Treatment. The Journal of Prosthetic Dentistry 56: 307–311
54. Hall DC (1968) Pulpal calcifications – A pathologic process. In Symons NB, editor: Dentin and Pulp: Their structure and Reaction. Dundee, Scotland, DC Thomas and Co, 269–273
55. Bernick S (1967) Age changes to the bloody supply to human teeth. Journal of Dental Research 54: 544
56. Karlson UL, Penny D A (1975) Natural Desensitization of exposed tooth roots in dogs. Journal of Dental Research 54:982
57. Grossmann LE (1935) The treatment of hypersensitive dentine. JADA 22: 592–6
58. Emling R C (1982) Historical overview of causes and treatment of dental hypersensitivity. Compendium of Continuing Education in Dentistry. Suppl No. 3, 92–94
59. Anderson D J, Mathews B (1966) An investigation into the reputed desensitising effect of applying silver nitrate and strontium chloride to human dentine. Archives of Oral Biology 11: 1129–1135
60. Zappa U (1994) Self-applied treatments in the managenent of dentine hypersensitivity. Arch oral Biology 39: 107–112
61. Blitzer B (1967) A consideraton of the possible causes of dentine hypersensitivity. Treatment by strontium-ion dentifrice. Periodontics 5: 318–321
62. Cohen A (1961) Preliminary study of the effects of strontium chloride dentifrice for the control of hypersensitive teeth. Oral Surgery, Oral Medicine & Oral Pathology 14: 1046–1052
63. Skurnik H (1963) Preliminary report on a strontium containing dentifrice. Journal of Periodontology 34: 183–185
64. Meffert R M, Hoskins S W (1964) Effect of strontium chloride dentifrice in relieving dental hypersensitivity. Journal of Periodontology 35: 232–235
65. Shapiro W B, Kaslick R S, Chasens A I (1970) The effect of a strontium chloride toothpaste on root hypersensitivity in a controlled clinical study. Journal of Periodontology 41: 702–703
66. Shapiro W B, Kaslick R S, Chasens A I, Weinstein D (1970) Controlled clinical comparison between a strontium chloride and sodium monofluorophosphate toothpaste in diminishing root hypersensitivity. Journal of Periodontology 41: 523–525
67. Carrasco H P (1971) Strontium chloride toothpaste – effectiveness as related to duration of use. Pharmacology Therapeutics in Dentistry 1: 209–215
68. Hernandez, Mohammed C, Shannon I, Volpe A, King W (1972) Clinical study evaluating the desensitising effect and duration of 2 commercially available dentifrices. Journal of Peridontology 43: 367–372
69. Greenhill J D, Pashley D H (1981) The effects of desensitising agents on the hydraulic conductance of human dentine in vitro. Journal of Dental Research 60: 686–698
70. Yankell S L (1982) At-home treatment. Compendium of Continuing Education in Dentistry, Suppl. No. 3
71. Hodge H C, Gawett E, Thomas E (1946) The adsorption of strontium at 40 degrees by enamel, dentine, bone and hydroxyapatite as shown by radioactive isotope. Journal of Biology and Chemistry 163: 1–6
72. Ross M R (1961) Hypersensitive teeth: Effect of strontium chloride in a compatible dentifrice. Journal of Periodontology 32: 49–52
73. Kun L (1976) Biophysical study of the modification in dental tissues induced by the topical application of strontium. Schweiz Monatsschr. Zahnheil. 86: 611–615
74. Shorr E, Carter A (1952) The usefulness of strontium as an adjunct to calcium in remineralization Bull. Hosp. Jt. Dis. 86: 103–106

75. Bolden T E, Volpe A R, King W J (1968) The desensitising effect of a sodium monofluorophosphate dentifrice. Periodontics 6: 112–114
76. Hazen S P, Volpe A R, King W J (1968) Comparative desensitising effect of dentifrices containing sodium monofluorophosphate, stannous fluoride and formalin. Periodontics 6:230–232
77. Kanause M C, Ash M M (1969) The effectiveness of sodium monofluorophosphate dentifrice on dental hypersensitivity. Journal of Periodontology 40: 38–40
78. Hernandez F, Mohammed C, Shannon I, Volpe A, King W (1972) Comparative desensitizing effect of dentifrices containing sodium monofluorophosphate, stannous fluoride and formalin. Periodontics 6: 230–233
79. Gron P, Caslavska V (1981) Fluoride deposition in enamel from monofluorophosphate application. Caries Research 15: 90–95
80. Blunder R et al. (1981) The effects of compounds used clinically in the management of dentine hypersensitivity on some physical properties of dentine. Int Assoc Dent Res, Br. Div., Abstr. No. 130
81. Carlo G T, Ciancio S G, Seyrek S K (1982) An evaluation of iontophoretic application of fluoride for tooth desensitization. Journal of American Dental Association 105: 452–455
82. Ehrlich J, Hochman N, Gedalia I et al. (1975) Residual fluoride concentrations and scanning electron microscopic examimation of root surfaces of human teeth after topical application of fluoride in vivo. Journal of Dental Research 54: 897
83. Gangarosa L P, Park N (1978) Practical consideration in iontophoresis of fluoride for desensitization of dentin. Journal of Prosthetic Dentistry 39: 173–177
84. Gangarosa L P (1981) Iontophoretic application of fluoride by tray techniques for desensitisation of multiple teeth. Journal of the American Dental Association 102: 50
85. Hoyt W H, Bibby B G (1943) Use of sodium fluoride for desensitising dentine. Journal of the American Dental Association 68: 216–225
86. Tal M, Oron M, Gedalia I et al. (1976) X-ray defraction and scanning electron microscope investigation of fluoride-treated dentin in man. Arch. Oral Biology 21: 285–290
87. Minkov B, Marmari I, Gedalia I, Garfunkel A (1975) The effectiveness of sodium fluoride treatment with and without iontophoresis on the reduction of hypersensitive dentine. Journal of Periodontology 46: 246–249
88. Murthy K S, Talim S T, Singh I (1973) A comparative evaluation of topical application and iontophoresis of sodium fluoride for desensitization of hypersensitive dentin. Oral Surgery 36: 448
89. Miller J T, Shannon I L, Kilgore W G et al. (1969) The use of water-free stannous fluoride-containing gel in the control of dentinal hypersensitivity. Journal of Periodontology 40: 490–495
90. Penney D A, Karlsson U L (1976) Fast desensitization of tooth roots by topically applied stannous fluoride and strontium chloride in dogs. Arch. Oral Biology 21: 339
91. Schaeffer M L, Bixler D, Pao-L Y (1971) The effectiveness of iontophoresis in reducing cervical hypersensitivity. Journal of Periodontology 42: 695–699
92. Green B L, Green M, Mc Fall J (1977) Calcium hydroxide and potassium nitrate as desensitising agents for hypersensitive root surfaces. Journal of Periodontology 48: 667–672
93. Jorkjend L, Tronstad L (1972) Treatment of hypersensitive root surfaces by calcium hydroxide. Scand J Res 80: 264
94. Mjor I A (1967) Histologic studies of human coronal dentine following the insertion of various materials in experimentally prepared cavities. Arch. Oral Biology 12: 441
95. Levin M P, Yearwood L L, Carpenter W N (1973) The desensitising effect of calcium hydroxide and magnesium hydroxide on hypersensitive dentine. Oral Surgery 35: 741–746
96. Berman L H (1985) Dentinal Sensation and hypersensitivity. Journal of Periodotology 56: 216–219
97. Tarbet W J, Silverman G, Stolman J M, Fratarcangelo P A (1980) Clinical evaluation of a new treatment for dentinal hypersensitivity. Journal of Periodontology 51: 535–540
98. Fitzgerald G (1956) A clinical evaluation of a new agent for the relief of hypersensitive dentin. Dental Diagnostics 62: 492–500
99. Abel I (1958) Study of hypersensitive teeth in a new therapeutic aid (formalin). Oral Surgery 11:67–70
100. Forrest J D (1963) A clinical assessment of 3 desensitising toothpastes containing formalin. British Dental Journal 114: 103–106
101. Smith B A, Ash M M (1964) Evaluation of a desensitising dentifrice (formaldehyde). Journal of the American Dental Association 68: 639–647
102. Addy M, Morgan T (1982) The effect of toothpaste on the electrical appearances of dentine. International Association of Dental Research, Br. div., Abstract No. 102
103. Zinner D D, Duany L F, Lutz H J (1977) A new desensitising dentifrice: preliminary report. Journal of the American Dental Association 95: 982–985
104. Wie S H, Lainson P A, Henderson W et al. (1980) Evaluation of dentifrices for the relief of hypersensitive tooth surfaces. Quintessence International 11: 67–71
105. Mosteller J H (1962) The use of prednisolone in the elimination of postoperative thermal sensitivity. Journal of Prosthetic Dentistry 12: 1176–1180
106. Dayton R E, de Marco T J, Swedlow D (1974) Treatment of hypersensitive root surfaces with dental adhesive materials. Journal of Perodontology 45: 873–878
107. Brännström M, Johnson G, Nordenvall K J (1979) Transmission and control of dentinal pain: resin impregnation for the desensitisation of dentine. Journal of the Americal Dental Association 99: 612–618
108. Olgart L, Brännström M, Johnson G (1974) Invasion of Bacteria into dentinal tubules – experiments in vivo and in vitro. Acta Odontologica Scandinavica 32: 61–70
109. Doering J, Jensen M E (1985) A new photo-curing dentin bonding material. AIDR abstracts
110. Gillam DG, Bulman J S, Eijkman M A J, Newman H N (2002) Dentists perceptions of dentine hypersensitivity and knowledge of its treatment. J of Oral Rehabilitation 29: 219–225
111. Wycoff S J (1982) Current treatment for dentinal hypersensitivity. Compendium for Continuing Education in Dentistry, Suppl. No. 3.

112. Gillam DG, Mordan NJ, Sinodinou AD, Tang JY, Knowels JC, Gibson (2001): The effects of oxalate-containing products on the exposed dentine surface: an SEM investigation. J Oral Rehabil. 28(11):1037–44
113. Hench LL, Splinter RJ, Allen WC, Greenlee TK (1971) Bonding mechanisms at the interface of ceramic prosthetic materials. Journal of Biomedical Materials Research 2: 117–121
114. Zamet JS, Darbar U, Griffiths GS, Bulman JS, Bragger U, Burgin W, Newman HN (1997) Particulate bioglass as a grafting material in the treatment of periodontal intrabony defects. Journal of Clinical Periodontology 24:410–417
115. Litkowski LJ, Hack GD, Sheaffer HB, Greenspan DC (1997) Occlusion of dentine tubules by 45S5 Bioglass®, Bioceramics 10: 411–416
116. Ling T Y Y, Gillam D G, Barber P M, Morgan N J, Critchell J (1997) An investigation of potential desensitizing agents in the dentine disc model. A SEM study. Journal of Oral Rehabilitation 24:191–197
117. Zhang Y, Agee K, Pashley D H, Pashley E L (1998) The effects of Pain-Free® on dentine permeability and tubule occlusion over time, in vitro. Journal of Dental Research 69:168–175
118. Suggs A K, Cox C F, Cox L K, Suzuki S, Suzuki S H (1996) Colloidal MSE for differential diagnostics and treatment of dentin hypersensitivity. In: Proceedings of International Conference on Dentin/Pulp Complex (ed. Shimono M, Meada T, Suda H, Takahashi K) p. 245. Quintessence Publishing Co. Ltd, Tokyo
119. Gillam D G, Coventry H F, Manning R H, Newman H N, Bulman J S (1997) Comparison of two desensitizing agents for the treatment of cervical dentine sensitivity. Endodontics and Dental Traumatology 13: 36–40
120. Morris M F, Davis R D, Richardson B W (1999) Clinical efficacy of two dentin desensitizing agents. American Journal of Dentistry 12: 72–80
121. Sena F J (1990) Dentinal permeability in assessing therapeutics agents. Dental Clinics of North America 34: 474–480
122. Dragolich W E, Pashley D H, Brennan W A, Robert B O, Horner J A & Van Dyke T E (1993) An in vitro study of dentinal tubules occlusion by ferric oxalate. Journal of Periodontology 64: 1045–1050
123. Gillam D G, Morgan N J, Sinodinou A D, Tang J Y, Knowles J C, Gibson I R (2001) The effects of oxalate-containing products on the exposed dentine surface: an SEM investigation. Journal of Oral Rehabilitation 28: 1037–1044
124. Gillam D G, Newman H N, Bulman J S, Davies E H (1992) Dentifrice abrasivity and cervical dentinal hypersensitivity. Journal of Periodontology 63(1): 7–12
125. Cuenin M F, Scheidt M J, O´Neal R B et al. (1991) An in vivo study of dentine sensitivity: The relation of dentine sensitivity and the patency of dentine tubules. Journal of Periodontology 62(11): 668– 673
126. Rost A (1963) Die Behandlung sensibler Zahnhälse mit Infiltrationsanästhesie. Zahnärztliche Praxis 26: 71–74
127. Addy M, Dowell P (1983) Dentine hypersensitivity – A review. II. Clinical and in vitro evaluation of treatment agents. Journal of Clinical Periodontology 10: 351–363
128. Dederich D N, Zakariasen K L, Tulip J (1984) Scanning electron microscopic analysis on canal wall dentin following neodymium-yttrium-aluminum-garnet laser irradiation. J. Endod.10: 428–431
129. Melcer J, Chaumette M T, Melcer F, Dejardin J, Hasson R, Merard R, Pinaudeau Y (1984) Treatment of dental decay by CO_2 Laser beam: Preliminary results. Lasers Surg Med 4: 311–321
130. Keller U (1993) Laser in der Zahnmedizin – Indikationen und klinische Perspektiven. Zahnärztliche Praxis 2: 38–43
131. Featherstone JDB, Nelson DGA (1987) Laser effects on dental hard tissue. Adv Dent Res 1(1): 21–26
132. West N X, Addy M, Jackson R J, Ridge D B (1997) Dentine hypersensitivity and the placebo response. A comparison of the effect of strontium acetate, potassium nitrate and fluoride toothpastes. Journal of Clinical Periodontology 24: 209–215
133. Kimura Y, Takebayashi H, Iwase T, Nara Y, Marioka T (1991) Effect of helium-neon laser irradiation on wound healing in rats. Surgical and Medical Lasers 4: 14–16
134. Kimura Y, Takebayashi H, Iwase T, Nara Y, Marioka T (1993) The enhancement of transforming growth factor-β activity by helium-neon laser on wound healing in rats. Lasers in the Life Sciences 5: 209–217
135. Kimura Y, Iwase T, Marioka T, Wilder-Smith P (1997) Possible platelet-derived growth factor involvement on helium-neon laser stimulated wound healing in rats. Lasers in the Life Sciences 7: 267–284
136. Karu T I (1988) Molecular mechanism of the therapeutic effect of low-intensity laser radiation. Lasers in the Life Sciences 2: 53–74
137. Karu T (1989) Photobiology of low-power laser effects. Health Physics 56: 691–704
138. Rochkind S, Nissan M, Razon N, Schwartz M, Bartal A (1986) Electrophysiological effect of HeNe laser on normal and injured sciatic nerve in the rat. Acta Neurochirurgica 83: 125–130
139. Rochkind S, Nissan M, Barr-Nea L, Razon M, Schwartz M, Bartal A (1987) Response of peripheral nerve to He-Ne laser: experimental studies. Lasers in Surgery and Medicine 7: 441–443
140. Jarvis D, Bruce MacIver M, Tanelian D L (1990) Electrophysiologic recording and thermodynamic modeling demonstrate that helium-neon laser irradiation does not affect peripheral Aδ- or C-fiber nociceptors. Pain 43: 235–242
141. Senda A, Gomi A, Tani T, Yoshino H, Hara G, Yamaguchi M, Matsumoto T, Narita T, Hasegewa J (1985) A clinical study on "Soft Laser 632", a He-Ne low energy medical laser. Aichi-Gakuin Journal of Dental Science 23: 773–780
142. Matsumoto K, Nakamura G, Tomonara H (1986) Study on the treatment of hypersensitive dentine by HeNe laser irradiation. Japanese Journal of Conservative Dentistry 29: 312–317
143. Gomi A, Kamiya K, Yamashita H, Ban Y, Senda A, Hara G, Yamaguchi M, Narita T, Hasegawa J (1986) A clinical study on "Soft laser632", a HeNe low energy medical laser. Aichi Gakuin Journal of Dental Science 24: 390–399

144. Matsumoto K, Nishihama R, Onodera A, Wakabayashi H (1988) Study on treatment of hypersensitive dentine by HeNe laser. Journal of Showa University Dental Society 8: 180–184
145. Mezawa S, Shiono M, Sato K, Mikami T, Hayashi M, Maeda K, Ogawa M, Saito T (1992) The effect of low power laser irradiation on hypersensitive dentine: differing effect on the irradiated area. Journal of Japanese Society for Laser Dentistry 3: 87–91
146. Wilder-Smith P (1988) The soft laser: Therapeutic tool or popular placebo? Oral Surg OralMed Oral Path 66: 654–658
147. Jarvis D, Bruce MacIver M, Tanelian DL (1990) Electrophysiologic recording and thermodynamic modeling demonstrate that helium-neon laser irradiation does not affect peripheral Aδ- or C-fiber nociceptors
148. Watanabe H (1993) A study of He-Ne laser transmission through the enamel and dentine. Journal of Japanese Society for Laser Dentistry 4: 53–62
149. Strang R, Moseley H, Carmichael A (1988) Soft lasers – Have they a place in dentistry? British Dental Journal 165: 221–225
150. Matsumoto K, Funai H, Wakabayashi H, Oyama T (1985) Study on the treatment of hypersensitive dentine by GaAlAs laser diode. Japanese Journal of Conservative Dentistry 28: 766–771
151. Matsumoto K, Tomonari H, Wakabayashi H (1985) Study on the treatment of hypersensitive dentine by laser. Place of laser irradiation. Japanese Journal of Conservative Dentistry 28: 1366–1371
152. Ebihara A, Takeda A, Araki K, Suda H, Sunada I (1988) Clinical evaluation of GaAlAs-semiconductor laser in the treatment of hypersensitive dentine. Japanese Journal of Conservative Dentistry 31: 1782–1787
153. Kawakami T, Ibaraki Y, Haraguchi K, Odachi H, Kawamura H, Kubota M, Mijata T, Watanabe T, Iioka A, Nittono M, Odachi T, Ohnuma S, Sekiguchi N, Yokouchi A, Matsuda K (1989) The effectiveness of GaAlAs semiconductor laser treatment to pain decrease after irradiation. Higashi Nippon Dental Journal 8: 57–62
154. Matsumoto K, Nakamura Y, Wakabayashi H (1990) A clinical study on the hypersensitive dentine by 60 mW GaAlAs semiconductor laser. Journal of Showa University Dental Society 10: 446–449
155. Setoguchi T, Mastunaga M, Chinjyu N, Yokata N, Sueda T (1990) The effects of soft laser irradiation and strontium chloride application on dentine hypersensitivity induced by periodontal treatment. Japanese Journal of Conservative Dentistry 33: 620–627
156. Hamachi T, Iwamoto Y, Hirofuji T, Kabashima H, Maeda K (1992) Clinical evaluation of GaAlAs-semiconductor laser in the treatment of cervical hypersensitive dentine. Japanese Journal of Conservative Dentistry 35: 12–17
157. Wakabayashi H, Tachibana H, Matsumoto K (1992) A clinical study on the hypersensitive dentine by 40 mW GaAlAs semiconductor laser. Journal of Showa University Dental Society 12: 10–16
158. Mezawa S, Shino M, Maeda K, Ogawa M, Saito T (1992) The effect of low power laser irradiation on hypersensitive dentine: differing effect according to the irradiated area. Journal of Japanese Society for Laser Dentistry 3: 87–91
159. Tashibana H, Wakabayashi H, Matsumoto K (1992) A clinical study on the hypersensitive dentine by 20 and 40 mW GaAlAs semiconductor laser. Journal of Showa University Dental Society 12: 343–347
160. Gerschman A, Ruben J, Gebart-Eaglemont (1994) Low level laser therapy for dentinal tooth hypersensitivity. Australian Dental Journal 39: 353–357
161. Liu H-C, Lan W-H (1994) The combined effectiveness of the semiconductor laser with Duraphat in the treatment of dentine hypersensitivity. J Clin Laser Med Surg 12: 315–319
162. Iida M, Ando Y, Watanabe H, Ishikawa I (1993) Effect of GaAlAs-semiconductor laser irradiation on dentin hypersensitivity of exposed root surface and influence to microflora in dento-gingival region. Journal of Japanese Society for Laser Dentistry 4: 3–7
163. Wakabayashi H, Hamba M, Matsumoto K, Nakayama T (1992) Electrophysiological study of irradiaton of semiconductor laser on the activity of the trigeminal subnucleues caudal neurons. Journal of Japanese Society for Laser Dentistry 3: 65–74
164. Wakabayashi H, Hamba M, Matsumoto K, Tachibana H (1993) Effect of irradiation by semiconductor laser on responses evoked in trigeminal caudal neuron by tooth pulp stimulation. Lasers in Surgery and Medicine 13: 605–610
165. Mezawa S, Iwata K, Naito K, Kamogawa G (1988) The possible analgesic effect of soft-laser irradiation on heat nociceptors in the cat tongue. Archives of Oral Biology 33: 693–694
166. Watanabe H, Nakamura Y, Wakabayashi H, Matsumoto K (1991) Study on laser transmission through tooth structures by 40 mW Ga-AlAs semiconductor laser. Journal of Japanese Society for Laser Dentistry 4: 53–62
167. Matsumoto K, Wakabayashi H,Funato A, Shirasuka T (1985) Histopathological findings of dental pulp irradiated by GaAlAs laser diode. Japanese Journal of Conservative Dentistry 28: 1361–1365
168. Matsumoto K, Funai H, Shrasuka T, Wakabayashi H (1985) Effects of Nd:YAG laser in Treatment of cervical hypersensitive dentine. Japanese Journal of Conservative Dentistry 28: 760–765
169. Renton-Harper P, Midda M (1992) Nd:YAG laser treatment of dentin hypersensibility. British Dental Journal 172: 13–16
170. Gelskey S C, White J M, Pruthi V K (1993) The effectiveness of the Nd:YAG laser in the treatment of dental hypersensitivity. Journal of Canadian Dental Association 59: 377–386
171. Lan WH, Liu H-C (1996) Treatment of dentine hypersensitivity by Nd:YAG laser. J Clin Laser Med Surg 14(2): 89–92
172. Gutknecht N, Moritz A., Dercks H W, Lampert F (1997) Treatment of hypersensitive teeth using neodymium:yttrium-aluminium-garnet lasers: A comparison of the Use of Various Settings in an in Vivo Study. J Clin Laser Med Surg 15 (4): 171–174
173. Yonaga K, Kimura Y, Matsumoto K (1999) Treatment of cervical dentin hypersensitivity by various methods using pulsed Nd:YAG laser. Journal of clinical Laser Medicine & Surgery 17: 205–210

174. Kobayashi K, Yamaguchi H, Kumai A, Tanaka M, Sakuraba E, Nomura T, Nakamura J, Arai T (1999) Pain relief effects of Nd:YAG laser irradiation on dentin hypersensitivity during periodontal treatment. Journal of Japanese Society of Periodontology 41: 180–187
175. White J M, Goodis H E (1990) Effect of Nd:YAG laser treatments on hydraulic conductance of dentin (Abstract 481). Journal of Dental Research 69: 169–173
176. Goodis H E, White J M, Rose C M et al. (1989) Dentin surface modification by the Nd:YAG laser. Trans Acad Dent Materials 2: 246–252
177. Launay Y, Mordon S, Cornil A, Brunetaud J M, Moschetto Y (1987) Thermal effects of lasers on dental tissues. Lasers in Surgery and Medicine 7: 473–477
178. Morioka T, Suzuki K, Tagomori S (1984) Effect of beam absorptive mediators on acid resistance of surface enamel by Nd:YAG laser irradiation. Journal of Dental Health 34: 40–44
179. Lan WH, Liu H-C (1995) Sealing of human dentinal tubules by Nd:YAG laser. Journal of Clinical Laser Medicine & Surgery 13: 329–333
180. Zennyu K, Inoue M, Konishi M, Minami M, Kumazaki M, Fujii B, Lee C S (1996) Transmission of Nd:YAG laser through human dentin. Journal of Japanese Society for Laser Dentistry 7: 37–45
181. Funato A, Nakamura Y, Matsumoto K (1991) Effects of Nd:YAG laser irradiation on microcirculation. Journal of Clinical Laser Medicine and Surgery 9: 467–474
182. Whitters C J, Hall A, Creanor S L, Moseley H, Gilmour W H, Strang R, Saunders W P, Orchardson R (1995) A clinical study of pulsed Nd:YAG laser-induced pulpal analgesia. Journal of Dentistry 23: 145–150
183. Myers T D, McDaniel J D (1991) The pulsed Nd:YAG dental laser: review of clinical applications. Journal of California Dental Association 19: 25–30
184. Orchardson R, Peacock J M, Whitters C J (1997) Effect of pulsed Nd:YAG laser radiation on action potential conduction in isolated mammalian spinal nerves. Lasers in Surgery and Medicine 21: 142–148
185. Oyama T, Matsumoto K (1991) A clinical and morphological study of cervical hypersensitivity. Journal of Endodontics 17: 500
186. Matsumoto K, Izumi M, Nagasawa H (1980) Scanning electron microscopic study on the hypersensitivity of dentin. Japanese Journal of Conservative Dentistry 23: 247–251
187. Matsumoto K, Nakamura G, Morita Y, Oti K, Suzuki K (1982) Scanning electron microscopic study on the hypersensitivity of the exposed root surface. Japanese Journal of Conservative Dentistry 25: 142–147
188. Gutknecht N, BehrensVG: Die Bearbeitung der Wurzelkanalwände mit dem Nd:YAG Laser. Zahnärztl Welt 100: 748–755, 1991
189. Gutknecht N, Ermert M, Lampert F: Farbpenetrationsversuche am Dentin nach Behandlung mit einem Nd:YAG Laser. Dtsch Zahnärztl. Z. 49, 157, 1994
190. Liu H-C, Lin C-P, Lan W-H (1997) Sealing depth of Nd:YAG laser on human dentinal tubules. Journal of Endodontics 23: 691–693
191. Goharkhay K, Moritz A, Wernisch J, Schoop U, Pattera C, Rumetzhofer A und Sperr W (2000) Oberflächeneffekte unterschiedlicher Laserwellenlängen im Zahnhalsdentin in vitro. Stomatologie 97/2: 47–52
192. Dederich DN (1993) Laser\tissue interaction: What happens to laser light when it strikes tissue? Journal of American Dental Association 124: 57–61
193. Zach L, Cohen G (1965) Pulp response to externally applied heat. Oral Surgery, Oral Medicine, and Oral Pathology 19: 515–530
194. White JM, Goodis H E, Kudler J (1995) Laser thresholds in pulp exposure: a rat animal model. Proceedings of the International Society for Optical Engineering 2394: 160–169
195. White J M, Fagan M C, Goodis H D (1994) Intrapulpal temperatures during pulsed Nd:YAG laser treatment of dentin, in vitro. Journal of Periodontology 65: 255–259
196. Lier BB, Rosing CK, Aass AM, Gjermo P (2002): Treatment of dentin hypersensitivity by Nd:YAG laser. J Clin Periodontol. 29(6):501–506
197. Arrastia A M A, Machida T, Wilder-Smith P, Matsumoto K (1994) Comparative study of the thermal effects of 4 semiconductor lasers on the enamel and pulp chamber of a human tooth. Lasers in Surgery and Medicine 15: 116–118
198. Olgart L, Brannström M, Johnson G (1974) Invasion of bacteria into dentinal tubules – experiment in vivo and in vitro. Acta Odontologica Scandinavica 32: 61–70
199. Ando Y, Aoki A, Watanabe H, Ishikawa I (1996) Bactericidal effect of the Er:YAG laser on periodontopathic bacteria. Lasers in Surgery and Medicine 19: 190–200
200. Hibst R, Stock K, Gall R, Keller U (1996) Controlled tooth surface heating and sterilization by Er:YAG laser radiation. Lasers in Surgery and Medicine 2922: 119–126
201. Moritz A, Gutknecht N, Schoop U, Goharkhay K, Doertbudak O, Sperr W: Rapid Report: Irradiation of Infected Root Canals with a Diode Laser In Vivo: Results of Microbiological Examinations. Journal of Lasers in Surgery and Medicine 21: 221–226, 1997
202. Moritz A, Doertbudak O, Gutknecht N, Goharkhay K, Schoop U, Sperr W (1997): Nd:YAG Laser Irradiation of Infected Root Canals in Combination with Microbiologic Examinations. JADA 128: 1525–1530
203. Moritz A, Gutknecht N, Goharkhay K, Schoop U, Wernisch J, Sperr W (1997): In Vitro Irradiation of Infected Root Canals with a Diode Laser: Results of Microbiologic, Infrared Spectrometric, and Stain Penetration Examinations. Quintessence International 28/3: 205–209
204. Moritz A, Gutknecht N, Doertbudak O, Goharkhay K, Schoop U, Schauer P, Sperr W (1997): Bacterial Reduction in Periodontal Pockets Through Irradiation with a Diode Laser: A Pilot Study. Journal of Clinical Laser Medicine and Surgery 15/1: 33–37
205. Moritz A, Schoop U, Goharkhay K, Schauer P, Doertbudak O, Wernisch J, Sperr W (1998): Treatment of Periodontal Pockets With a Diode Laser. Journal of Lasers in Surgery and Medicine. 22: 302–311

206. Moritz A, Schoop U, Goharkhay K, Jakolitsch S, Kluger W, Wernisch J, Sperr W (1999): The Bactericidal Effect of Nd:YAG-, Ho:YAG- and Er:YAG - Laser Irradiation in the Root Canal: An in Vitro Comparison. Journal of Clinical Laser Medicine and Surgery 17/4: 161–164
207. Moritz A, Jakolitsch S, Goharkhay K, Schoop U, Kluger W, Mallinger R, Sperr W, Georgopoulos A (2000): Morphologic Changes Correlating to Different Sensivities of *Escherichia coli* and *Enterococcus faecalis* to Nd:YAG Laser Irradiation Through Dentin. Journal of Lasers in Surgery and Medicine 26: 250–261
208. Schwarz F, Arweiler N, Georg T, Reich E (2002) Desensitizing effects of an Er:YAG Laser on hypersensitive dentine. J Clin Periodontol 29: 211–215
209. Takeda FH, Harashima T, Kimura Y, Matsumoto K (1999) A comparative study of the removal of smear layer by three endodontic irrigants and two types of of laser. International Endodontic Journal 32, 32–39
210. Pick R M ; Pecaro, B C , Silberman, C J (1985) The laser gingivectomy: The use of CO_2 laser for removal of phenytoin hyperplasia. Journal of Peridontology 56: 492–496
211. White J M, Goodis H E, Rose C L (1987) Use of the pulsed Nd:YAG laser for intraoral soft tissue surgery. Lasers in Surgery and Medicine 7: 207–213
212. Midda M (1992) The use of lasers in periodontology. Current Opinion in Dentistry 2: 104–108
213. Aoki A, Ando A, Watanabe H, Ishikawa I (1996) Bacterial effect of the Er:YAG laser on periodontopathic bacteria. Lasers in Surgery and Medicine 19: 190–200
214. Walsh J T, Flotte T J, Deutsch T F (1989) Er:YAG laser ablation of tissue; Effects of pulse duration and tissue type on thermal damage. Lasers in Surgery and Medicine 9: 314–326
215. Walsh J T, Cummings J P (1994) Effect of the dynamic optical properties of water on mid-infrared laser ablation. Lasers in Surgery and Medicine 15: 295–305
216. Moritz A, Gutknecht N, Schoop U, Wernisch J, Lampert F. Sperr W (1995) Effects of CO_2 laser irradiation on treatment of hypersensitive dental necks: results of an in vitro study. J Clin Laser Med Surg 13(6): 397–400
217. Moritz A, Gutknecht N, Schoop U, Goharkhay K, Ebrahim D, Wernisch J und Sperr W (1996) The Advantage of CO_2 Treated Dental Necks in Comparison with a Standard Method: Results of an in Vivo Study. Journal of Clinical Laser Medicine and Surgery 14: 27–32
218. Moritz A, Gutknecht N, Schoop U, Goharkhay K, Ebrahim D, Wernisch J und Sperr W (1997) Die Wirkung des CO_2 Lasers bei der Behandlung von empfindlichen Zahnhälsen. Ergebnisse einer In-vivo-Studie. Stomatologie 7/1:27–32
219. Moritz A, Schoop U, Goharkhay K, Aoid M, Teichenbach P, Lothaller M A, Wernisch J, Sperr W (1998) Long term effects of CO_2 laser irradiation on treatment of hypersensitive dental necks: Results of an in vivo study. Journal of Clinical Laser Medicine and Surgery 16: 211–215
220. Zhang C, Matsumoto K, Kimura Y, Harashima T, Takeda F H, Zhou H (1988) Effects of CO_2 laser in treatment of cervical dentin hypersensitivity. J of Endodontics 24: 595–597
221. Bonin P, Boivin R, Poulard J (1991) Dentinal permeability of the dog canine after exposure of a cervical cavity to the beam of a CO_2 laser. Journal of Endodontics 17: 116–118
222. Fayad M I, Carter J M, Liebow C (1996) Transient effects of low-energy CO_2 laser irradiation on dentinal impedance: Implications for treatment of hypersensitive teeth. Journal of Endodontics 22: 526–531
223. Kimura Y, Wilder-Smith P, Krasieva T B, Liaw L-H L, Matsumoto K (1998) Effects of CO_2 laser on human dentin: a confocal laser scanning microscopic study. Lasers in the Life Sciences 8: 1–12
224. Melcer J, Chaumette M T, Melcer F, Zeboulon S, Hasson R, Merard R, Pinaudeau Y, Dejardin J, Weill R (1985) Preliminary report on the effect of the CO_2 laser beam on the dental pulp of the *Macaca mulatta* primate and the beagle dog. Journal of Endodontics 11: 1–5
225. Zhang C, Matsumoto K, Kimura Y, Harashima T, Takeda F H, Zhou H (1988) Effects of CO_2 laser in treatment of cervical dentin hypersensitivity. J of Endodontics 24: 595–597
226. Miserendino L J, Neiburger E J, Walia H, Luebke N, Brantley W (1989) Thermal effects of continuous wave CO_2 laser exposure on human teeth: an in vitro study. Journal of Endodontics 15: 302-305
227. Ohnhaus E E, Adler R (1975) Methodological problems in the measurement of pain: A comparison between the verbal rating scale and the visual analogue scale. Pain 1, 379–384
228. Kuriwada-Satoh S, Shoji N, Sasano T, Sanjo D (1996) The quantitative measurement of dental pain. Japanese Journal of Conservative Dentistry 39: 1587–1592
229. Wilder-Smith P (1988) A new method for the non-invasive measurement of pulpal blood flow. Int Endod J 21:307–312
230. Jacobsen P L (2001) Clinical Dentin Hypersensitivity: Understanding the Causes and Prescribing a Treatment. Journal of Contemporary Dental Practice 2: 1–8

10

Laser-Assisted Bleaching

P. Verheyen, L. J. Walsh, J. Wernisch, U.Schoop and A. Moritz

10.1 Introduction

The search for beauty can be traced to the earliest civilizations. Dental art has been part of this quest to enhance the esthetics of the teeth and mouth. Esthetic improvement by chemical means of well-shaped but discolored teeth is highly desirable because of its conservative nature. A professional response to the unrelenting quest for whiter teeth dates back at least 2000 years. First-century Roman physicians maintained that brushing teeth with urine, in particular Portuguese urine, whitened teeth. In the 1300s, the most requested dental service, other than extractions, was tooth whitening. Barber surgeons, after abrading the enamel with coarse metal files, would apply "aquafortis", a solution of nitric acid, to whiten the teeth. This common practice continued into the 18th century. In the late 1800s, the combination of hydrogen peroxide, ether and electricity was reported to be an effective method of lightening teeth. Circa 1916, hydrochloric acid was used to successfully treat "Colorado brown stain", endemic fluorosis. In 1937, the combination of five parts 100% hydrogen peroxide with one part ether and heat was reported as a treatment for this same type of discoloration. Two years later, successful bleaching of fluorosis staining using 30% hydrogen peroxide, ether and heat was used. In 1966, the use of hydrochloric acid combined with hydrogen peroxide was advocated. It was not until 1970 that hydrogen peroxide was demonstrated to be effective for the treatment of dentinal discoloration as well. Nowadays, the chemical agents and specific procedures that are used depend on a number of factors, including the type, intensity, and location of the discoloration.

10.2 In General

Tooth discoloration can be defined as a changing of the color of a tooth in a way that it differs markedly from the adjacent teeth; and in most cases it is a deviation to the darker hues. Genetic malformations and development disorders can affect several teeth of the dentition or may cause a general discoloration. Discoloration is then defined as a general tooth color, which differs from the average color across a population. Average tooth color varies from white-yellow to yellow with grey, brown, green and pink shades. Tooth discoloration interferes with normal esthetics. Tooth shape and tooth color are the main factors of influence in the esthetics of a dentition. Nowadays, poor esthetics is one of the most important reasons for people to ask for dental care. The vastly improved bleaching techniques of today have eliminated the need for invasive treatments with irreversible damage to the teeth and periodontal tissues, e.g., fixed crowns. Teeth bleaching is a simple, effective and relatively cheap method of treating tooth discolorations[1] and must be the treatment of choice before more invasive techniques are used, such as direct- or indirect-veneering[2]. The indications for bleaching and the outcome of a treatment are highly dependent on the etiology of the discoloration. It is crucial to know in advance what has caused the discoloration[1,3].

10.2.1 Causes of Tooth Discoloration

Tooth discolorations are classified as extrinsic and intrinsic discolorations. Extrinsic discolorations are caused by factors outside of a tooth. Intrinsic discolorations are caused by internal factors.

10.2.2 Extrinsic Discolorations

Extrinsic discolorations consist of a discolored superficial layer on the surface of the teeth. They are removed primarily by conventional means such as prophylaxis, ultrascaling, abrasive pastes or root planing. Extrinsic staining occurs due to lifestyle habits and/or poor oral hygiene. Therefore patients require proper instruction as to how to avoid, where possible, those habits that cause extrinsic staining. It is possible to distinguish between several kinds of extrinsic discolorations.

Plaque. Dental plaque can only be observed when it reaches a certain thickness. It appears as white-yellow to green-brown.

Tartar. As dental plaque can accumulate on a tooth surface over a long period of time it can calcify to create tartar. Tartar can appear both supra- and sub-gingivally. The absorption of pigments found in various foods can change the inherent yellow to white color of tartar to brown and black.

Deposit of tar. Smokers and people chewing tobacco often show a brown to black deposit of tar, especially on the lingual surfaces. By dissolving in the saliva, tar decreases the pH, thereby facilitating the penetration of pit and fissures. The dyes of the tar dissolved in the saliva are absorbed by enamel defects and exposed dentin.

Tea and wine. Both contain tannins, causing a brown-black staining.

Chlorhexidine. It is often used as a disinfectant for the mouth causing a brown staining.

Tin fluoride. Tin fluoride, SnFl 8%, is used as a treatment for hypersensitivity and caries prevention. Prolonged use creates a deposit of tin sulfide, detectable by X-rays, and causes light brown to gold-yellow staining.

Food supplements and medications. Medication containing iron in the treatment of anemia causes black staining. Medications such as manganese oxide, potassium chlorate or silver nitrate cause dark stains.

Industrial deposits. Incorporation in the enamel of floating metallic- or nonmetallic dust causes several kinds of staining. A black color is caused by the dust of iron and silver, grey by mercury and lead, blue to green by copper and nickel. Para-aminosalicylic acid causes green, and red to orange staining. Chromic acid produces a deep orange staining.

Betel chewing. Chewing on a combination of betel nut, tobacco and clove is mostly practised by elderly people in South East Asia causing a black staining of the teeth and a red-brown staining of the lips, tongue and cheek mucosa.

Nutritions. The ink from squids and the juice of bilberries cause a grey to black staining.

Chromogenic bacteria

- Black staining following the contour of the gingiva is caused by a higher than normal concentration of Gram+ rods (90% as against 30%) with a domination of the Actinomycetes. Hydrogen sulfide produced by the microorganisms combines with the iron in the saliva to produce iron sulfide which causes the black color.
- Green staining on the labial surfaces of primary teeth caused by poor oral hygiene affects twice as many boys as girls. This condition causes plaque accumulation, and rough and demineralized enamel. The plaque bacteria, such as *Bacillus pyocyaneus*, cause a garlic odor. Fungi, such as *Aspergillus* and *Penicillium glaucum*, are also found in the plaque. Their hydrogen sulfide production combines with blood breakdown products resulting in Cu- and Fe-ions, which causes the green color.
- Orange staining can be seen on the labial and lingual surfaces of children with poor oral hygiene. Several micro-organisms can be identified as well as demineralization of enamel.

10.2.3 Intrinsic Discolorations

Intrinsic discolorations originate from discolorations incorporated inside the teeth during the formation phase. These are called formative discolorations. Discolorations originating after tooth development is complete, are called post-formative discolorations.

10.2.3.1 Discolorations in the Formative Phase

During dentinogenesis, pre- and post-natal, several discoloring substances can be incorporated into the dental structures.

Chemical Agents and Medications.

Fluorosis. Fluorosis is caused by an excessive intake of fluoride during the formation and calcification of enamel, which is approximately from 3 months to 8 years of age. It can cause discolorations, surface alterations and defects. The type and severity of the damage caused by fluorosis depends on the genetic predisposition, concentration of the fluoride, duration of administration and the stage of enamel development during uptake.

- Fluorosis simplex shows a sound enamel surface with a brown pigmentation probably caused by secondary infiltration of pigments from food.
- Opaque fluorosis appears as dull, grey or white spot lesions.
- Pitting fluorosis is characterized by a dark pigmentation and enamel defects. Demineral-

zation ranges from surface roughness to true hypoplasia and pitting.

Tetracycline staining. Tetracyclines are produced by the bacterium, *Actinomyces streptomyces viridifaciens*. The broad-spectrum tetracycline group of antibiotics was first introduced in 1948 for use in the treatment of respiratory illnesses. However, tooth discoloration caused by the incorporation of systemic tetracycline into tooth structure was not reported until 1956. The exact mechanism of tetracycline staining is not completely understood. It is hypothesizsed to occur by the joining of the tetracycline molecule with calcium through a chelation process and a subsequent incorporation into the hydroxylapatite crystal of the tooth during the mineralization stage of development. A second theory maintains that the discoloration involves a binding of the tetracycline to tooth structure by a metal-organic matrix combination of the tetracycline complex. Although some tetracycline accumulates within the enamel it is primarily deposited into the dentin because of the large surface area of the dentin apatite crystals compared to enamel apatite crystals. Enamel hypoplasia can also occur. Tetracycline discoloration may be yellow, yellow-brown, brown, grey or blue. The intensity of the staining varies widely. Distribution of discoloration is usually diffuse and severe cases may exhibit banding. Staining is usually bilateral and affects multiple teeth in both arches. The hue and severity of tooth discoloration depends upon four factors associated with tetracycline administration.

- **Age and time of administration.** Anterior primary teeth are susceptible to discoloration by systemic tetracycline from 4 months in utero through to 9 months postpartum. Anterior permanent teeth are susceptible from 3 months postpartum through to 7 years of age.
- **Duration of administration.** The severity of the staining is directly proportional to the duration of administration of the medication.
- **Dosage.** The severity of the staining is directly proportional to the administered dosage.
- **Type of tetracycline.** Coloration has been correlated to the specific type of tetracycline administered.
  - Chlortetracycline (Aureomycin): grey-brown stain.
  - Dimethylchlortetracycline (Ledermycin): yellow stain.
  - Oxytetracycline (Terramycin): yellow stain.
  - Tetracycline (Achromycin): yellow stain.
  - Doxycycline (Vibramycin): no staining.

Yellow tetracycline staining slowly darkens to brown or grey-brown when exposed to sunlight. Therefore, the anterior teeth of children often darken first, while the posterior teeth, because of reduced exposure to sunlight, darken more slowly. In adults, however, natural photobleaching of the anterior teeth can be observed, particularly in individuals whose teeth are excessively exposed to sunlight because of maxillary lip insufficiency[4]. Hypocalcified white areas of varying opacity, size and distribution may also be present.

Jordon and Boksman[5] classified tetracycline staining into three groups.

- *First degree stains.* First degree stains are light yellow, light brown or light grey and are uniform throughout the clinical crown. No banding is present.
- *Second degree stains.* Second degree stains are more intensive than first degree stains. No banding is present.
- *Third degree stains.* Third degree stains are intense dark-grey, blue to purple discolorations and the clinical crown exhibits horizontal color banding mostly in the cervical third.

Pre-eruption trauma. A local injury or inflammation of a primary tooth may cause deficient enamel formation and white spots in the following permanent tooth. Secondary brown staining is due to the infiltration of food pigments.

Systemic diseases.

- *Erythroblastosis fetalis.* Erythroblastosis fetalis is a syndrome resulting from Rh incompatibility in an infant and is characterized by the hemolysis and breakdown of the infant's blood, producing jaundice. These pigments may produce an intrinsic blue, brown or grey discoloration inside the dentinal tubules.
- *Jaundice.* The incorporation of bilirubine, oxydating into biliverdin inside the dentin, causes staining with different tints. Green, blue, yellow, grey or brown can be apparent.
- *Erythropoietic porphyria.* Erythropoietic porphyria is a congenital disorder of the metabolism with the deposition of porphyrin into developing dentin resulting in a red, purplish brown or brownish discoloration. UV light produces a red fluorescence.
- *Hemolytical anemia.* Thalassemia and sickle-cell anemia produce blood pigments circulating in the blood flow and capable of being incorporated into the dentin. They result in blue-green, brown and grey-black staining.
- *Hyperoxaluria and oxalosis.* Chromic uremia resulting from congenital kidney disorders disturbs the glyoxylate metabolism resulting in a grey staining. Deposits of calcium oxalate cause oxalosis.
- *Ochronosis.* Ochronosis is a congenital metabolic disorder with a malformation of the amino acids tyrosine and phenylalanine. The produced homogentisic acid accumulates in the bone, urine and dentition resulting in a severe arthrosis and a blue-black staining of the teeth.
- *Crigler-Najjar Syndrome.* A congenital deficient excretion of bile resulting in a green to yellow discoloration of the primary dentition.
- Metabolic disorders interfering with a normal enamel matrix formation and calcification, resulting in enamel hypoplasia and hypocalcification with secondary staining. They can be caused by diabetes mellitus and vitamin D deficiency in the pregnant mother, by congenital syphilis, hypoxy and a low weight at birth, a shortage of vitamin A, D, C or E, rubella, measles, high fever, endocrinic disorders of the hypophysis, or the thyroid and parathyroid glands, or a shortage of calcium, phosphorus, magnesium, iron or other minerals needed for normal growth.

Congenital Disorders of Normal Dentinogenesis.

- *Amelogenesis imperfecta.* Amelogenesis imperfecta is the collective noun for several hereditary developmental disorders of the enamel. The enamel may be partially or completely absent or show hypomaturation or hypocalcification. White, yellow and brown staining is dominant.
- *Dysplasia of the dentin.* There are two types of dentin dysplasia. Both are hereditary disorders and may be present in the primary as well as in the permanent dentition.
- *Type I or radicular dysplasia.* Type I shows normal crowns but with too short roots and obliterated pulp chambers. Teeth appear yellow-brown, sometimes blue-brown.
- *Type II or coronal dysplasia.* Primary dentition shows short and spherical crowns with obliterated pulp chambers and a yellow-brown color. The spherical crowns in the permanent dentition mostly present a normal color but some grey or brown staining is possible. Pulp chambers start to obliterate after eruption and multiple pulp stones are formed.
- *Dentinogenesis imperfecta.* Dentinogenesis imperfecta is a hereditary developmental disorder of the dentin. The spherical crowns are amber or opal colored. The roots are thin, too short and transparent, and pulp chambers start to obliterate after eruption.
- *Odontodysplasia or "ghost teeth".* Odontodysplasia is a developmental disorder where both enamel and dentin show hypoplasia. X-ray images show vague, ghostly images. Teeth, if they appear at all, are discolored yellow to brown.

10.2.3.2 Discolorations in the Post-Formative Phase

Staining of pulpal ethiology. Pulpal trauma or caries can lead to pulpal necrosis. Intrinsic staining results from the deposition of hemorrhagic byproducts into the dentinal tubules. At first a hematoma can show a light pink discoloration. Through the hemolysis of the red blood cell, hemoglobin is released and dissolved into hematoidine and hemosiderine. Color changes from blue to dark-blue and finally blue-black.

- Hemoglobin shows a yellow-red hue and colors teeth orange-pink.
- Methemoglobin is red-brown.
- Hematoidin contains no iron and deposits as yellow-brown crystals.
- Hematoidin is identical to bilirubin and is excreted by the bladder of the bile. It colors teeth orange.
- Hemosiderin is an iron-containing derivative of hemoglobin, and the golden to brown particles produce a brown discoloration. The interaction of hemosiderine and ammonium sulfide produces iron sulfide which is responsible for the black staining.
- Hematin is also a hemoglobin derivative. This brown, non-crystallized pigment induces dark brown to black staining.
- Hemin is produced by a further breakdown of hematine, and the dark brown crystals color the teeth black.
- Ammonium sulfide and hydrogen sulfide are byproducts of proteinolysis inside the pulp. They interact with hemoglobin derivatives to produce sulfur methemoglobin and a red-green to green discoloration.

Chemical processes of this kind can also occur when, in an endodontic treatment, the pulp chamber and the pulp horns have not been throughly cleaned.

Hemorrhagic discolorations. A minor pulpal trauma may lead to a localized pulpal bleeding and exposure of erythrocytes into the dentinal tubules. In time, tooth color changes from red-pink to blue-grey and heavy dark grey after several weeks. Teeth remain vital but the pulp chamber starts to obliterate and dentinal tubules become calcified.

Granuloma interna or pink spot. Internal resorption of the dentin enlarges the pulp chamber, producing a pink discoloration of the tooth.

Iatrogenic discoloration. *Endodontic treatment.* Many materials used in an endodontic treatment may cause a tooth discoloration.

- Diaket, a slightly pink staining.
- AH26, a moderate grey staining.
- Rieblerpaste can induce a mildly pink staining at first, resulting in a heavy red discoloration after 6 months.
- Grossman cement, N2, Tubliseal, endomethasone, zinc-oxide eugenol, a moderate orange-red staining.
- Pink gutta percha, a slightly pink staining.
- Silver points and silver-containing sealers induce a grey-black staining.

Corrosion of amalgam, of pins and posts, produces fine metal particles capable of penetrating the dentinal tubules and inducing a grey, grey-black discoloration. Silver alloy and gold fillings may shine through the remaining cavity walls causing poor esthetics.

Caries. Caries is still one of the main causes of tooth discoloration.

Aging. The ongoing sclerotical process in the dentin and the retraction of the pulp chamber causes a darkening of the teeth with age. It is also probable that there is a darkening of the enamel through the penetration of pigments from particular food and drinks into enamel fractures and defects.

10.2.4 Treatment Options

As with any therapeutic treatment, proper diagnosis should be attempted before a course of treatment is promulgated[1]. Although the etiology of a specific tooth discoloration may be difficult to discern, an accurate history as well as an evaluation of the causative factors help in establishing a differential diagnosis. The presence or absence of pulp tissue is also a treatment-planning factor. Four methods of stain removal and improving esthetics are available.

10.2.4.1 Polishing

Hand scalers, ultrasonic scalers, abrasive pastes and airflows allow the removal of superficial, extrinsic staining.

10.2.4.2 Micro-Abrasion

If there is a superficial penetration of staining pigments, acid-abrasion techniques are enticingly efficient because of the short treatment times. However, the non-selective, destructive nature of this procedure limits its application to only the most superficial discolorations and those cases in which treatment time and subsequent cost is a factor. Obviously, whether or not a discoloration is superficial enough to be treated in this way can only be determined through trial and error.

10.2.4.3 Bleaching

Bleaching systems can be used to treat superficial staining and are of a non-destructive nature. They are the only technique available for deeper enamel stains and for staining of the dentin.

10.2.4.4 Restoration

If the structural integrity of teeth is compromised due to defects in enamel or dentin or both, or if bleaching techniques fail, restoration through direct or indirect composite veneers, porcelain veneers or crowns is indicated.

Table 10-1 Extrinsic Discolorations.

Cause	Staining	Treatment			
		Polishing	Micro-abrasion	Bleaching	Restoration
Plaque	white-yellow	X	(X)	(X)	
Tartar – supragingival – subgingival	white-yellow brown-black	X X	(X)	(X)	
Deposits of tar	brown-black	X	(X)	(X)	
Tea and wine	brown-black	X			
Chlorhexidine	brown	X	(X)	(X)	
Tin fluoride	light-brown gold-yellow	X	X	X	
Food supplements and medication	black	X	(X)	(X)	
Industrial deposits	variable				
Betel chewing	black	X			
Nutrition	grey-black	X			
Chromogenic bacteria	brown-black green orange	XXX			X

10.2.4.5 Overview of Treatment Options in Relation to Causes of the Discoloration

Tables 10-1 to 10-3 illustrate the most common discolorations, together with their treatment of choice.

Table 10-2 Intrinsic Discolorations in the formative phase.

Cause	Staining	Treatment			
		Polishing	Micro-abrasion	Bleaching	Restoration
Fluorosis	brown opaque pitting		(X)	X X	 (X) X
Tetracyclines	first degree second degree third degree			X X X	 X
Trauma	brown				X
Erythroblastosis	blue-green				X
Jaundice	green				X
Porphyria	red-brown				X
Anemia	blue-green grey-black				X X
Hyperoxaluria and oxaluria	grey				X
Ochronosis	blue-black				X
Crigler-Najjar syndrome	green-yellow				X
Enamel hypoplasia and hypocalcification	brown-black				X
Amelogenesis imperfecta	white, yellow, brown				X
Dentin displasia	yellow-brown grey-brown				X X
Dentinogenesis imperfecta	amber, opal				X
Odontodysplasia	yellow-brown				X

Table 10-3 Intrinsic Discolorations in the post-formative phase.

Cause	Staining	Treatment			
		Polishing	Micro-abrasion	Bleaching	Restoration
Pulpal necrosis	variable			X	
Hemorrhagic discolorations	dark-grey				X
Internal resorption	pink				X
Iatrogenic - root canal filling - crown filling	 variable variable			 X	 X X
Caries	brown-black				X
Aging	yellow-brown			X	

10.3 Bleaching

Bleaching is a chemical process for whitening materials, which is widely used in industry. In dentistry, bleaching usually refers to products containing some form of hydrogen peroxide.

The best known commercial bleaching processes are peroxide, sodium perborate, chlorine, and chloride, in descending order of use.

Peroxide bleaching requires the least time and is most commonly used. The strength can be designated by volume and by percentage of peroxide. These are interrelated proportionately, where by 27.5% hydrogen peroxide is termed 100 volume, 35% is 130 volume and 50% is 200 volume. Volume indicates the volume of oxygen released by one volume of the designated hydrogen peroxide.

Although bleaching processes are complex, the vast majority work by oxidation, the chemical process by which organic materials are eventually converted into carbon dioxide and water. Wood burning in a fireplace is a common example of oxidation. The differences between the oxidation that occurs with bleaching and that of burning wood are the rate of each reaction and the number of intermediate products produced. Burning rapidly transforms a substance into carbon dioxide, water, and heat. In comparison, bleaching slowly transforms an organic substance into chemical intermediates that are lighter in color than the original. Corrosion of metal is an example of a slow oxidation process. If allowed to progress long enough, however, both burning and bleaching will result in the conversion of organic materials into carbon dioxide and water.

The oxidation-reduction reaction that takes place in the bleaching process is known as a redox reaction. In a redox reaction the oxidizing agent, e.g., hydrogen peroxide, has free radicals with unpaired electrons which it gives up, becoming reduced. The reducing agent, the substance being bleached, accepts the electrons and becomes oxidized.

10.3.1 Chemistry of Hydrogen Peroxide

Hydrogen peroxide is an oxidizing agent and has the ability to produce free radicals, which are very reactive. The perhydroxyl radical, $HO_2^{\cdot}$ is the stronger free radical compared to the oxygen radical, $O^{\cdot}$. In a pure aqueous form, hydrogen peroxide is weakly acidic to reduce breakdown and extend shelf life and ionizes in producing mostly the weaker oxygen free radical, $O^{\cdot}$ (Fig 10-1)[6]. In order to promote the formation of the more potent perhydroxyl free radical, $H_2O^{\cdot}$, the hydrogen peroxide solution needs to be made alkaline (Fig 10-2)[6]. The optimum pH in achieving the productiong of the $H_2O^{\cdot}$ ions is between 9.5 and 10.0. In the ionization of buffered hydrogen peroxide in this range, a greater amount of perhydroxyl $H_2O^{\cdot}$ free radicals are produced, which results in a greater bleaching effect in the same time than at other pH levels[7,8]. Thus hydrogen peroxide is most effective between pH 9.5 and pH 10.8.

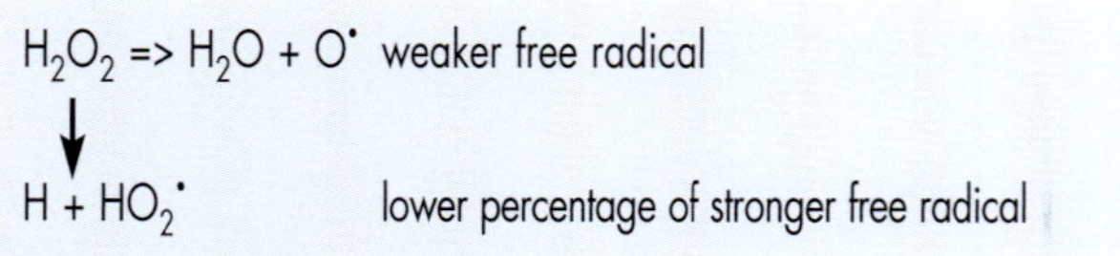

Fig 10-1 Ionization of hydrogen peroxide at acidic pH (According to Frysh[6]).

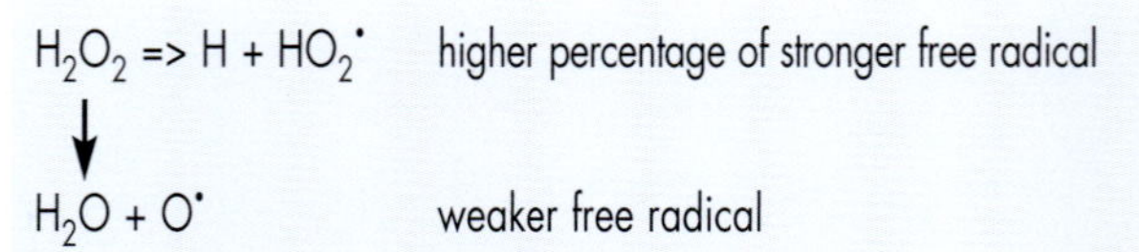

Fig 10-2 Ionization of buffered hydrogen peroxide, pH 9.5 to 10.8 (According to Frysh[6]).

In the presence of decomposition catalysts and enzymes, the hydrogen peroxide ionization occurs as[9]:

$$2\,H_2O_2 \rightarrow 2\,H_2O + O_2$$

This reaction produces no free radicals, rendering the hydrogen peroxide ineffective as a bleaching agent. These enzymes, some of which are present in the mouth, are an important part of the body's defense against oxygen toxicity. It is important to have teeth dry and free of debris when applying a bleaching agent.

10.3.2 Bleaching Mechanism of Teeth

In dental bleaching, hydrogen peroxide diffuses through the organic matrix of the enamel and dentin (Fig 10-3)[6, 10–14]. It increases the permeability of tooth structure, increasing the movement of ions through the tooth. This probably occurs because of the low molecular weight of hydrogen peroxide and its ability to denature proteins[15].

The free radicals have unpaired electrons and are extremely electrophilic and unstable and will attack most other organic molecules to achieve stability, generating other radicals. These radicals can react with most unsaturated bonds resulting in the disruption of electron conjugation and a change in the light absorption energy of the organic molecules in tooth enamel and dentin. Simpler molecules that absorb less and reflect more light are formed, creating a successful whitening action. This process occurs when the oxidizing agent, hydrogen peroxide, reacts with organic material in the spaces between the inorganic crystals in enamel and dentin.

A simple example of this reaction is the oxidation of the deep red, betacarotene molecule. When oxidized, this molecule is split in half to produce two molecules of vitamin A, which are colorless (Fig 10-4)[6].

However, not all oxidizing or bleaching reactions are that simple. A more extensive bleaching process has been described by Albers[16]. "The extent of bleaching is determined by the amount of whitening compared to the amount of material loss. During the initial bleaching process, highly pigmented carbon-ring compounds are opened and converted into chains that are lighter in color. Existing carbon double-bound compounds, usually pigmented yellow, are converted into hydroxy groups, alcohol-like, which are mostly colorless. As these processes continue the bleached material continually lightens". Tetracycline staining, may, more specifically, be bleached through an oxidative degradation of the quinone ring[4,17,18]. The bleaching reaction will differ according to the type of discoloration involved and the chemical and physical environment present at the time of action, i.e., pH, temperature, co-catalysts, lightening and other conditions[19].

As bleaching proceeds, a point is reached at which only hydrophilic colorless structures exist. This is a material's saturation point. Lightening then slows down dramatically and the bleaching process, if allowed to continue, begins to break down the carbon backbones of proteins and other carbon-containing materials. Compounds with

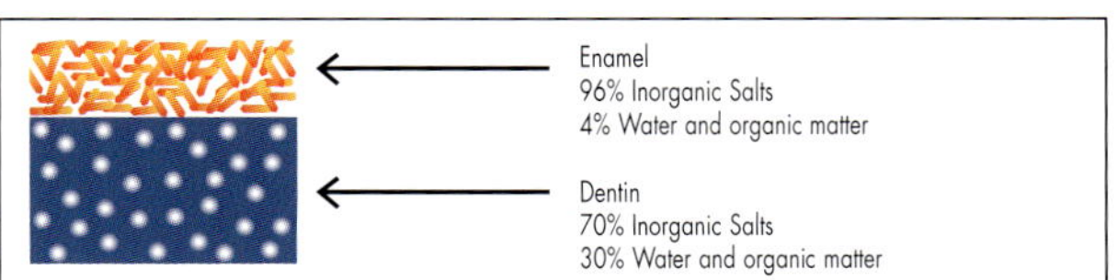

Fig 10-3 Diffusion of hydrogen peroxide through the organic matrix of enamel and dentin in teeth (According to Frysh[6]).

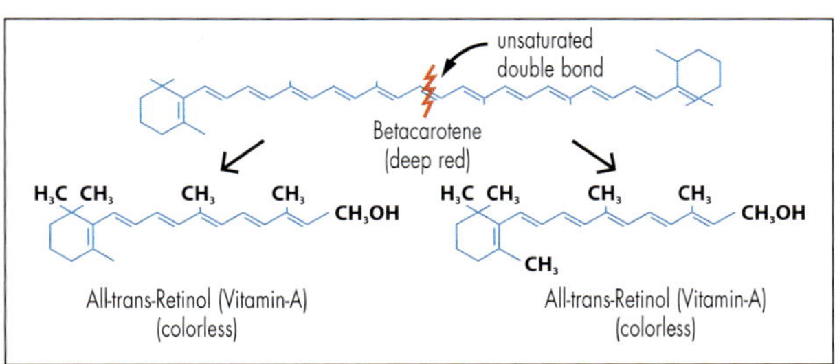

Fig 10-4 Oxidation of beta carotene. A free radical acts at the unsaturated (double) bond (jagged line), producing two molecules of colorless vitamin A (According to Frysh[6]).

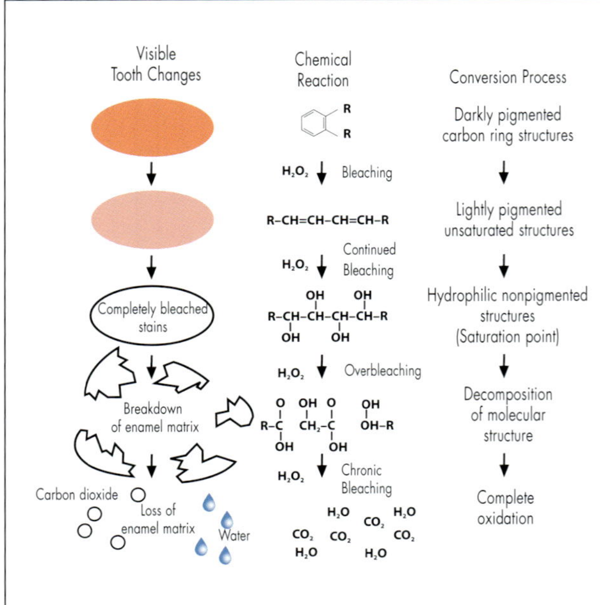

Fig 10-5 Common oxidation processes associated with bleaching teeth. The saturation point, at which the optimal amount of bleaching has occurred, is located in the middle of the diagram. (Reprinted with permission from: Lightening natural teeth. ADEPT Report 1991;2-1:1-24), (According to Frysh[6]).

hydroxy groups, usually colorless, are split, breaking the material into yet smaller constituents. Loss of enamel becomes rapid, with the remaining material being quickly converted into carbon dioxide and water (Fig 10-5)[6,16].

During bleaching, all of these reactions occur at the same time, since most materials contain varying amounts of simple and complex chemical components. However, since some processes occur more easily and quickly than others, the rate of each chemical reaction changes as the bleaching process continues. Figure 10-5[6] illustrates the most common oxidation processes associated with bleaching organic materials. These reactions are common to all proteins, including those of the enamel and dentin matrix[16]. The saturation point is located in the middle of the illustration. The ultimate result of bleaching processes is, like other oxidation processes, breakdown and loss of tooth enamel. It is therefore critical to know that tooth bleaching must be stopped at or before the saturation point.

The price of material loss, of tooth brittleness with increased porosity, is then greater than any marginal gain in tooth whitening. Optimal bleaching achieves maximum whitening, while overbleaching degrades tooth enamel without further whitening.

10.3.3 Safety of Bleaching

The use of any of the current bleaching agents is not totally without risk, and care must be taken in their storage, application and monitoring. Protection of the patient's eyes, skin and soft tissues from potential damaging effects of either light, heat or the bleaching agent itself is an essential part in the in-office treatment process. However, the lack of anesthesia during the bleaching treatment assures patients' feedback to potentially damaging stimuli.

The efficacy of bleaching teeth with hydrogen peroxide and externally applied energy is well documented[5,20–25]. Most of the earlier studies of in-office bleaching during the late 1970s and 1980s focused on possible damage to the pulp in vital teeth. It has been known for more than 40 years that substances can penetrate through enamel and dentin into the pulp. The low molecular weight of hydrogen peroxide and its capacity to denature proteins probably enhances its ability to penetrate teeth[15,26]. Numerous studies of canine, bovine and human teeth have looked at various solutions of hydrogen peroxide, heat and light application and combinations of them in potential damage[13,23,27–82]. The earliest results were positive but cautionary, demonstrating that a technique of low heat application and 30% to 35% hydrogen peroxide solution can cause histologic changes within the dental pulp, but the damage always appears to be reversible[29,36,83,84]. Histologic changes in enamel and dentin have been demonstrated[23]. However, spectroscopic analysis reveals no change in surface chemistry of enamel after exposure to hydrogen peroxide[85]. The scarcity of any negative clinical sequelae over the long term, however, is well- established[86,87]. The findings have encouraged the establishment of current protocols involving shorter bleach time and restricted heat use. Sakagushi and Hampel[34] pointed out that there have been only a few reports of side-effects resulting from bleaching therapy of vital teeth. These include mild inflammatory responses in teeth treated with heat and hydrogen peroxide, while the controlled use of saline and heat, or hydrogen peroxide without heat, did not cause a significant number of inflammatory responses.

Safety issues may be more pressing when bleaching pulpless teeth. Although this treatment offers the most dramatic changes in appearance, it offers the greatest potential hazard, the cervical resorption and the loss of the tooth[84].

Finally, the rapid increase in home bleaching causes an increased concern for safety. Teeth can be more susceptible to caries during the home-bleaching process because of the acidity of many bleaching solutions. The caries process starts when the pH is below 5.5 for enamel[88] and 6.0 for dentin[89].

Another concern for overnight bleaching of healthy teeth is the potential for hydrogen peroxide and the breakdown product of carbamide peroxide to cause soft tissue changes promoting cancer. A review by the World Health Organization of the potential for carcinogenicity of hydrogen peroxide and its derivates concluded that, in the absence of epidemiological data, no evaluation could be made of the carcinogenicity of hydrogen peroxide in humans[90]. But, hydrogen peroxide has been implicated as a potentiator of known carcinogens such as those found in cigarette smoke (DMBA). Smoking or the use of tobacco products has to be refrained from during home bleaching[90]. And home bleaching is carried outproceeded in the absence of professional control.

10.4 Laser versus Conventional Means

There are several factors that affect the bleaching reaction. Surface debridement, time of exposure, the hydrogen peroxide concentration, a sealed environment, the pH, the rate of the chemical reaction and the energy source used to promote it, may all influence the bleaching process and the efficiency and safety of tooth bleaching.

Teeth should be thoroughly cleaned, as the remaining organic material will interact with the bleaching agent resulting in an inadequate chemical reaction, useless in achieving teeth whitening[6]. Overall exposure time of the teeth to the bleaching agent should not exceed 30 minutes, as prolonged exposure times may affect the enamel surface in an adverse way[1]. The active hydrogen peroxide concentration should be between 30% and 35%, resulting in the most effective bleaching reaction but without surface alterations to the enamel, as higher concentrations may cause[1,6]. Most commonly used nowadays are gels rather than aqueous solutions of hydrogen peroxide. By mixing liquid and powder prior to application, the hydrogen peroxide concentration will decrease by 25%[6]. And gels are more effective in achieving a sealed environment promoting the efficiency of the whitening reaction[2]. Critical parameters in achieving not only an efficient and profound but certainly a safe and long lasting tooth whitening are the pH of the gel applied, the rate of the chemical reaction, the radicals produced, and the energy source used. The bleaching gel should have a basic pH in the range of 9.8 to 10.5[6]. In this range, there is not only the production of the far more active perhydroxyl radical $H_2O^{\cdot}$as against the less effective oxygen radical, $O^{\cdot}$. In the chemistry of bleaching, the perhydroxyl radicals interact with the organic molecules, which cause the discoloration, resulting in an opening of the highly pigmented carbon-ring compounds and converting them into chains, which are much lighter in color. The perhydroxyl radicals convert into hydroxy molecules, capable of stabilizing the open bonds produced and thus leading to a whitening that is more likely to last[91,92]. Furthermore, a basic pH of the gel, applied to the enamel or dentin surface, will not cause any surface alterations or demineralization[45,93]. Hydrogen peroxide in an acid mixture, however, will etch the exposed enamel or dentin layer during the time of application, causing loss of material, demineralization and surface alterations[91,92]. Finally, the rate of the chemical reaction within the bleaching gel, and whether this reaction is promoted by externally applied energy, will be responsible for both the effective-

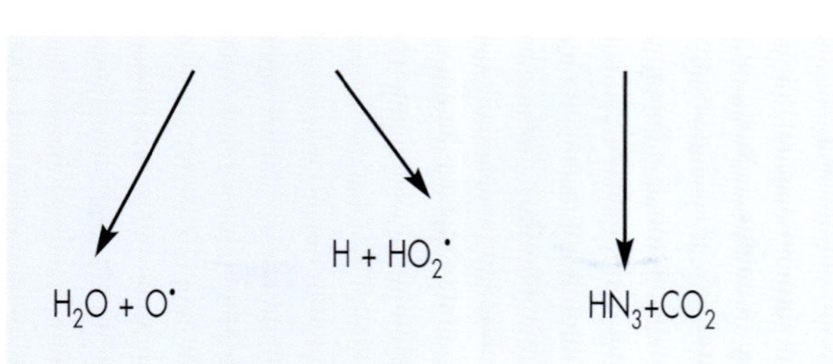

Fig 10-6 Chemical breakdown of carbamide peroxide.

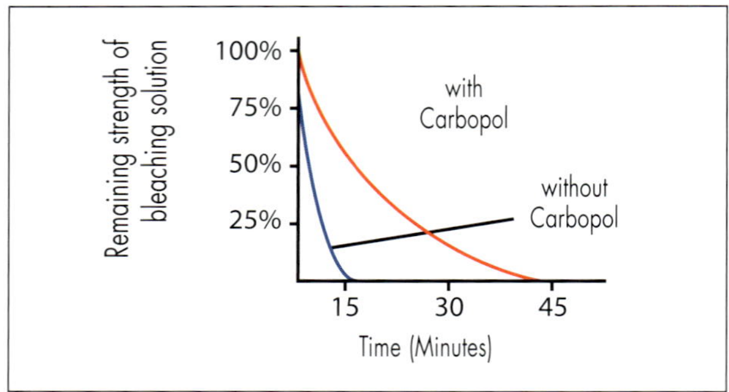

Fig 10-7 Extended performance of bleaching solution for carbamide peroxide bleaching preparations with carbopol. (Reprinted with permission from: Lightening natural Teeth: ADEPT Report 1991;2-1:1-24) (According to Frysh[6]).

ness and safety of the tooth whitening procedure.

Home bleaching procedures never make use of additional applied energy to increase the release of the active bleaching radicals. Instead they use lower concentration of the hydrogen peroxide but with a prolonged exposure time. Fitted trays containing the bleaching gel remain in contact with the teeth to be bleached for a period of time ranging from several hours through to overnight. Treatment is usually performed during the night, which is why home bleaching is also defined as nightguard vital bleaching or NGVB.

Bleaching gel may contain hydrogen peroxide in concentrations of 2–6%, or carbamide peroxide in concentrations of 10–15%. The carbamide peroxide dissolves in hydrogen peroxide and urea during the bleaching action (Fig 10-6)[92].

10–15% carbamide peroxide promotes 3–5% hydrogen peroxide and 7–10% urea.

Carbopol may be added to increase the viscosity of the gel and to increase the releasing of the peroxide (Fig 10-7)[6].

To increase the shelf-life of the home bleaching gels and to increase the stability of the hydrogen peroxide, phosphoric- or citric- acid is added. Prolonged use of home bleaching products will therefore cause enamel and dentin surface alterations, etching, and demineralization. High concentrations of these acids, used in several of the available products, cause carious lesions to occur, due to the high degree of demineralization, especially in the cervical region. Home bleaching should always be performed under professional supervision because of several possible risks, e.g., the carcinogenicity of the hydrogen peroxide in combination with smoking during treatment. Home bleaching can only effectively treat mild discolorations, mostly in the yellow range.

In-office bleaching procedures make use of different kinds of energy sources to increase the rate of the chemical release of bleaching radicals. The use of direct heating has gradually decreased over recent years. It has been replaced by other energy sources, such as plasma-arc devices, halogen lamps, InGaN LEDs or light emitting diodes, and other light sources. Lamps emitting long wavelengths, i.e., visual spectrum or the larger invisible infrared spectrum, have lower energy photons with a high thermal character, and these may induce unfavourable thermal effects. Shorter wavelengths, such as the argon laser (λ = 514.5 nm) or KTP laser (532 nm) have higher energy photons with less direct thermal characteristics.

Energy sources other than lasers are questionable in achieving a positive effect on the bleaching process. Clinical Research Associates (CRA), published several reports regarding in-office vital tooth bleaching and the significance of the heat and light energy produced by halogen lamps, plasma-arc devices, and LEDs[94,95]. They stated that all products tested effectively lightened teeth by one or two shades, and no one product caused better results than others. The use of light did not result in perceptibly brighter teeth. In the tooth whitening procedure, the contact time and concentration of hydrogen peroxide were more critical factors in producing more effective results. It appeared that light and heat do not increase tooth lightening and therefore are not necessary in the procedure[94].

On the other hand, the specific features of the light energy produced by a laser appears to add beneficial effects to the rate of the chemical bleaching reactions[93,96]. As laser light has the unique property of being absorbed by chromophores, emulsions can be added to the bleaching gel, capable of absorbing the laser energy and inducing and promoting a fast, effective and safe redox-reaction, as shown by Wernisch and Moritz (Fig 10-8 to 10-14)[96].

As different lasers produce different wavelengths, not all lasers are suitable for bleaching treatments. Wavelengths absorbed by, scattered in, or transmitted through the tooth structure can not be used for bleaching as they will damage the enamel and dentin or may even cause adverse effects in the vital pulp structures leading to irreversible damage and even necrosis of the tooth.

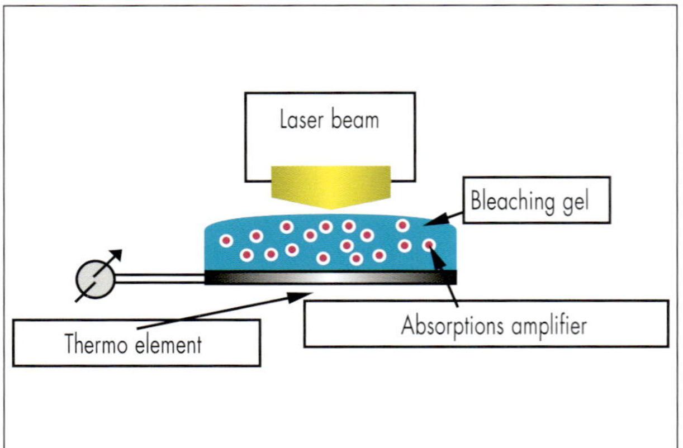

Fig 10-8 Study design.

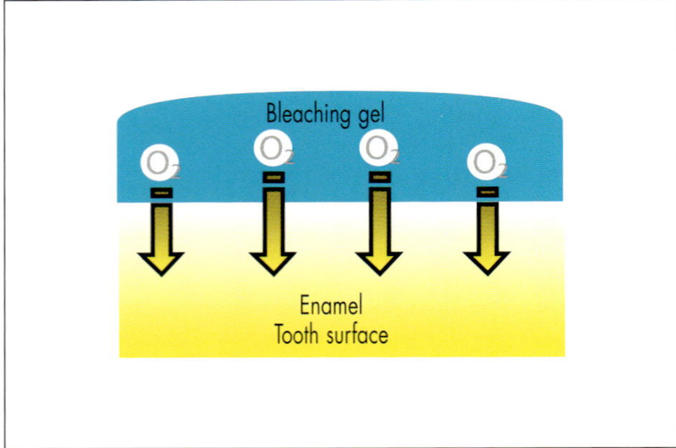

Fig 10-9 Bleaching effect: superficial bleaching activity in the absence of laser energy.

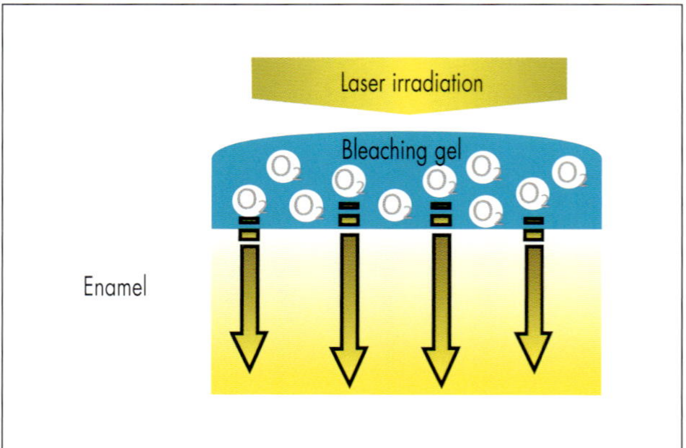

Abb. 10-10 Bleaching effect: "in-depth" bleaching activity by activation of the bleaching gel by laser irradiation.

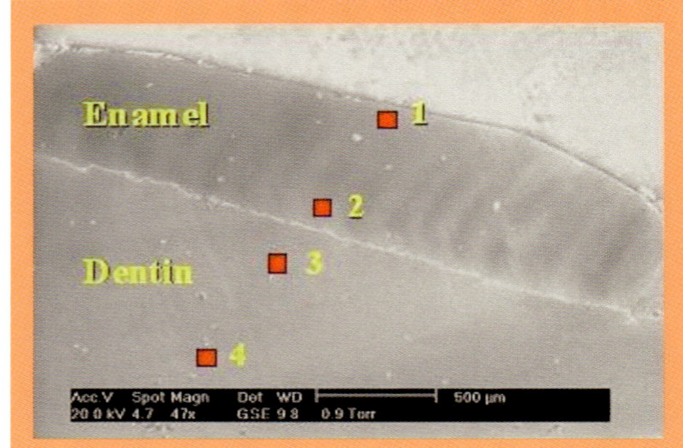

Abb. 10-11 EPMA-analysis of the oxygen distribution at the surface of the enamel (1), in the depth of the of the enamel (2), in the dentin (3) and the deeper dentin layers (4).

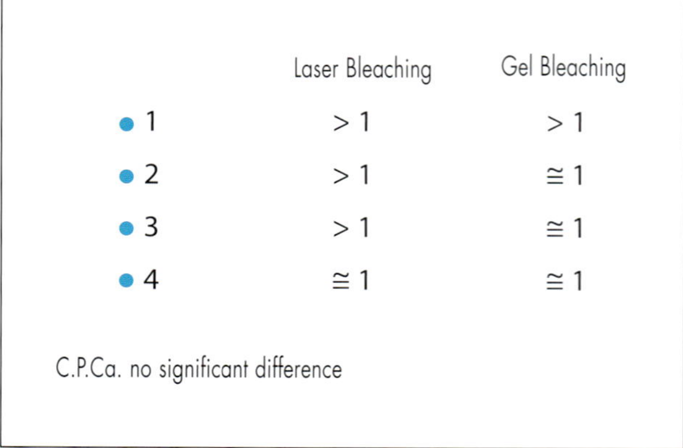

	Laser Bleaching	Gel Bleaching
• 1	> 1	> 1
• 2	> 1	≅ 1
• 3	> 1	≅ 1
• 4	≅ 1	≅ 1

C.P.Ca. no significant difference

Fig 10-12 Results of the EPMA measurements of the oxygen distribution at the different depths.

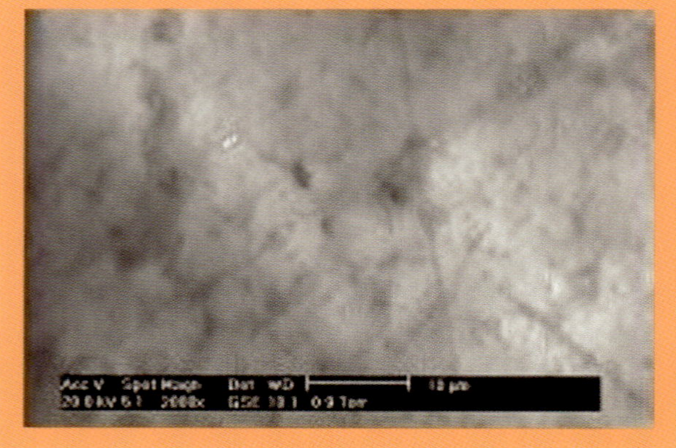

Fig 10-13 Surface of the enamel after interaction with the bleaching gel without laser irradiation. Demineralization with dissolution of the interprismatic substance and free enamel prisms.

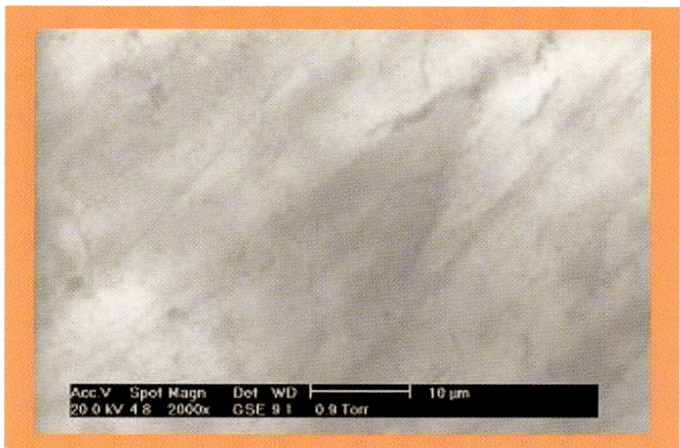

Fig 10-14 Surface of the enamel after interaction with the bleaching gel and laser energy shows an intact surface without any alterations.

KTP, argon, and diode lasers are commonly used for in-office bleaching treatments. Additional benefits of the use of a KTP or argon laser are the complete safety of these wavelengths for both vital and non-vital tooth structures (see chapter 4), and their feasibility for photobleaching[4]. Extracted tetracycline-stained rat, dog and primary human teeth have been shown to darken when exposed to sunlight[97–99]. Interestingly, further exposure produces a subsequent lightening of the tetracycline stain[97,99–101]. It has been postulated therefore, that tetracycline incorporated into hydroxylapatite, when oxidized by light (photo-oxidation), produces the red quinone product 4-α,12-α anhydro-4-oxo-4-dedimethylaminotetracycline (AODTC)[4,17,18]. Continued photo-oxidation of AODTC photolyses, or bleaches, the red quinone[17]. Efficient wavelengths inducing photo-oxidation are λ = 290 nm and λ = 365 nm, both in the UV range, and λ = 532 nm, visible green light[4]. The addition of diluted hydrogen peroxide yields an irreversible bleaching of the red quinone as well[17].

In addition, the energy of a KTP laser induces a photochemical reaction in the bleaching gel, similar to the photochemical reaction induced by argon laser light in the photopolymerization of light-cured materials[91,92].

It has been found that this photochemical activation provides a higher intrinsic overall radical yield than thermal activation, and that the rate at which radicals are generated is higher than with thermal activation. Heating of the teeth is minimized, thus higher energies can be used, so the overall radical yield per time unit can be further increased. Research by Walsh et al. stated that diode lasers give the greatest thermal changes at the level of the dental pulp with a rapid temperature rise during the first 30 seconds. Moreover, with diode lasers there is limited heating of the surface gel, typically 4°C. The KTP laser gives more modest and gradual temperature changes at the level of the dental pulp, and is more efficient at heating the surface gel.

The Smartbleach gel also retained its elevated temperature for an extended period. With all laser systems, intra-pulpal thermal changes were related proportionately to both laser power and irradiance, as well as inversely to tooth thickness. Greater pulpal and surface thermal changes occurred in all systems when the appropriate gel was omitted. The absorbing properties of the gel play an important role in influencing both surface and intra-pulpal thermal effects (Fig 10-15) (Table 10-4)[93,102].

The KTP laser can be used with high energy densities, decreasing the time needed for bleaching teeth, thus leading to a method with improved efficiency. Research by Walsh and Liu[103] has shown that the whitening effect of photochemical KTP laser bleaching is greater than that of diode laser photothermal bleaching. The effect of the 532-nm KTP laser can be explained by synergy effect. Besides the fact that this laser energy appears to be capable of providing a high radical yield of the oxidizing agent, it also appears to be capable of inducing a decomposition reaction of the staining agent. The conjugated electron system of the staining agent, which is responsible for the tooth discoloration, can be at least partly broken down by the irradiation of laser energy, resulting in a first whitening of the tooth. After this first breakdown has occurred, the at least partly decomposed staining agent molecules are capable of reacting with the oxidizing agent radicals, thus inducing a further breakdown of the

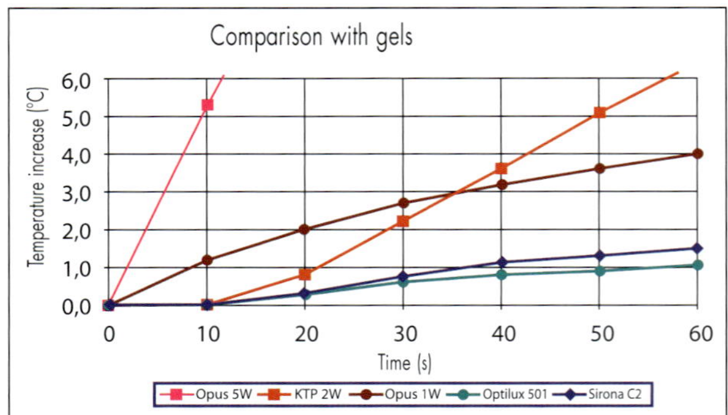

Fig 10-15 Intrapulpal temperature increase with different types of light sources and their corresponding bleaching gels (According to Walsh et al.[102]).

conjugated electron system (Fig 10-16). As the radicals of the oxidizing agent can be built into the molecular structure of the decomposed staining agent, stabilized reaction products can be obtained, which are no longer reactive and are substantially free of conjugated π-electron systems capable of absorbing visible light. As these molecules no longer contain a conjugated π-electron system, capable of absorbing visible light, they will reflect visible light rather than absorbing it. Besides this, the use of a laser source emitting energy outside the UV wavelength range, and outside the near-infrared and infrared wavelength range, minimizes the risk of damaging the tooth structures such as enamel, dentin, and the vital pulp system[91,92]. So the use of specific wavelengths of laser energy together with an appropriate chemical agent will enhance both efficiency and safety of in-office bleaching treatments.

Wernisch and Moritz demonstrated the importance of the use of an absorption agent in controlling the temperature increase inside the pulp, and in maintaining an enamel surface without alterations. When passing through a tissue or a material, the attenuation of a laser beam increases exponentially with the transmission depth. The

Experiment				Average Intrapulpal Temperature Change at 30 seconds of light application (°C)
ID	Light Source	Power	Gel	
1	Opus 10	5.0 W	No gel used	18.3
2	ADT DioLase	1.5 W	No gel used	3.2
3	Optilux 501	1,000* mW/cm²	No gel used	1.5
4	Sirona C2	Not available	No gel used	1.2
5	KTP laser	2.0 W	No gel used	7.6
6	Opus 10	5.0 W	OpusWhite	12.9
7	Optilux 501	1,000* mW/cm²	HiLite	0.6
8	Sirona C2	Not available	HiLite	0.7
9	KTP laser	2.0 W	Smartbleach	2.2
10	Opus 10	1.0 W	No gel used	3.8
11	Opus 10	1.0 W	OpusWhite	2.7

Table 10-4 Results for average temperature change in each experiment at 30 seconds of light application (According to Walsh et al.[102]).

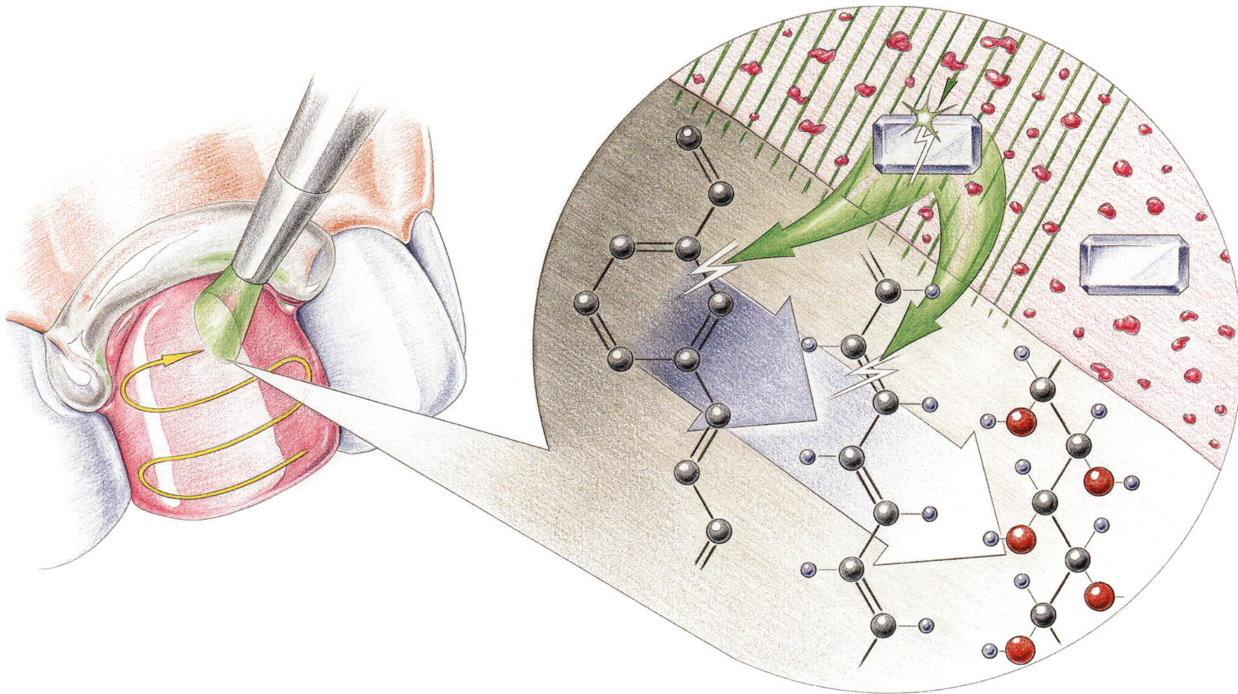

Fig 10-16 Disintegration reaction of the discoloring molecules.

attenuation, when passing through a bleaching gel and the hard tooth structures, can be calculated by the formula:

$$I = I_0 \, e^{-(\mu_1 D_1 + \mu_2 D_2)}$$

where μ_1 is the linear absorption coefficient of the gel, μ_2 the linear absorption coefficient of the enamel and dentin, D_1 the thickness of the gel layer and D_2 the distance between the tooth surface and the pulp. I_0 is the initial intensity of the laser beam when hitting the exposed surface (Fig 10-17).

The degree of attenuation depends on the different absorption coefficients, μ_1 and μ_2, where only μ_1 can be changed or manipulated. And on the overall material thickness D_i, which is D_1+D_2, and where again, only D_1 can be altered.

In their experimental set-up, they used a diode laser with a wavelength of $\lambda = 810$ nm, together with OpusWhite gel. Their experimental design,

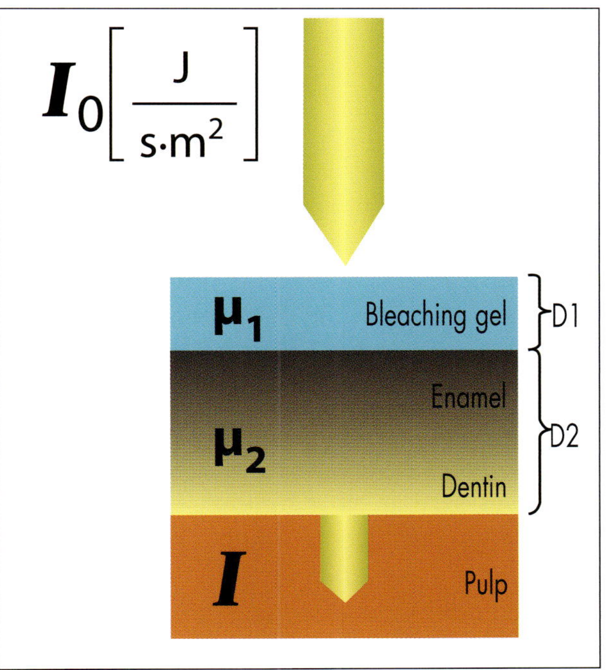

Fig 10-17 Attenuation of the laser beam with increased transmission depth.

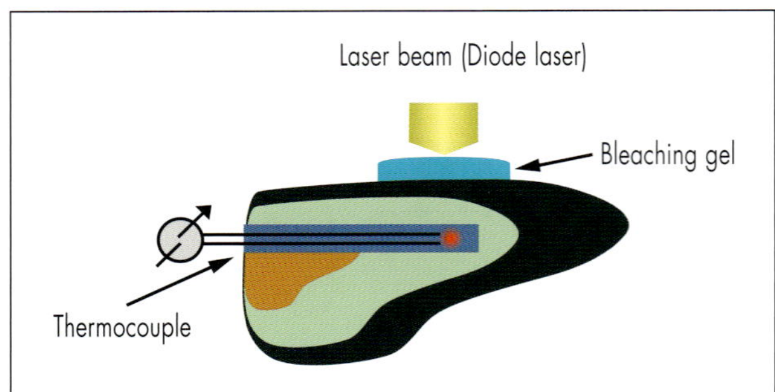

Fig 10-18 Experimental design for measuring temperature changes inside of pulp.

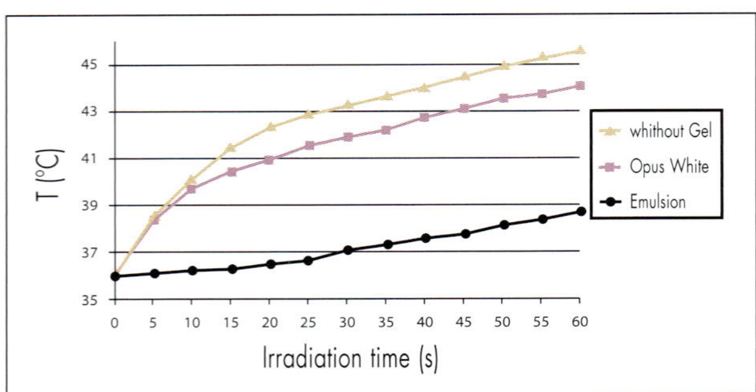

Fig 10-19 Pulpal temperature change. Course of temperature increase in the pulp chamber at an output power of 2 Watt, without gel, with OpusWhite gel, and with OpusWhite and TiO_2 (emulsion).

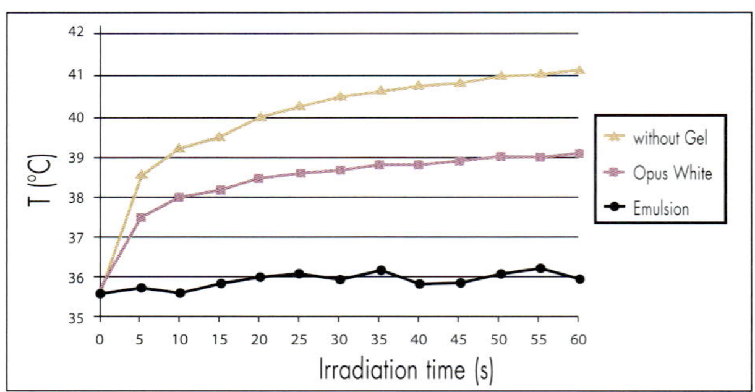

Fig 10-20 Pulpal temperature change. Course of temperature increase in the pulp chamber at an output power of 1 Watt, without gel, with OpusWhite gel, and with OpusWhite and TiO_2 (emulsion).

to accurately measure temperature changes inside the pulp, is shown in Figure 10-18.

Temperature changes inside the pulp, depend upon the degree of attenuation of the laser beam, the initial intensity of the laser beam, and the time of irradiation. They used two different power settings, 1 W and 2 W, and an overall irradiation time of 60 seconds. Temperature measurements were made at intervals of 5 seconds. Titanium dioxide, TiO_2, was used as an absorption agent in a ratio of 1:1 by percentage of weight (Figs 10-19 and 10-20).

When using an average output power of 2 Watt and the OpusWhite gel, the temperature increase in the pulp is about 8°C, which is far too high to be safe[27]. By adding TiO_2, temperature increase can be reduced to about 2.5°C. With an output power of 1 Watt, pulpal temperature increase is shown to be about 3°C with the OpusWhite gel, confirming the previous results of Walsh[93]. The emulsion shows almost no temperature changes in the pulp at this power setting.

Variations in the gel ratio: Changes in the percentage by weight of TiO_2 showed different results in the pulpal temperature increase after 30 seconds of irradiation with a power setting of 1 Watt (Fig 10-21). But the thicker the gel, the more difficult it becomes to handle it and to apply it to the tooth surfaces.

The pulpal temperature increase at different exposure times and with different gel ratios: TiO_2 shows an optimum ratio of 1:1 in percentage by weight (Fig 10-22). Thus, by adding TiO_2 to the OpusWhite gel in a ratio of 1:1, the diode laser may be used as a safe tool in vital tooth bleaching, as the pulpal temperature increase can be reduced in this way to safe levels; this means, less than 5°C.

And scanning electron microscope pictures demonstrate it to be safe for the enamel surface as well. Pictures were made with an environmental scanning electron microscope, ESEM, without gold coating, at magnifications of 25x, 300x and 2000x. In vitro, tooth surfaces were divided in half, whereby one half remained untreated as a control, and the other half was exposed to the 1:1

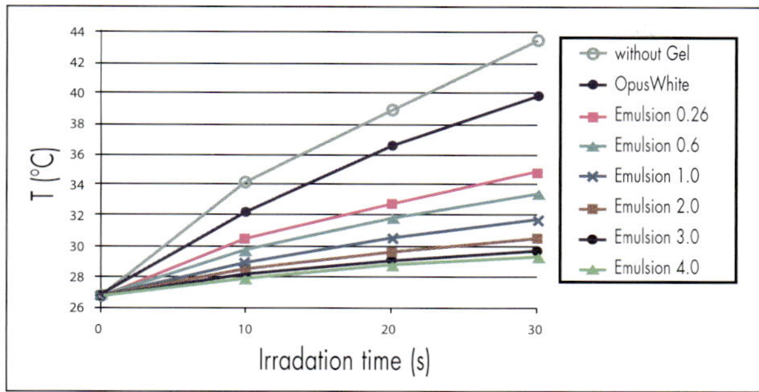

Fig 10-21 Temperature changes at variable ratios of OpusWhite and absorption enhancers.

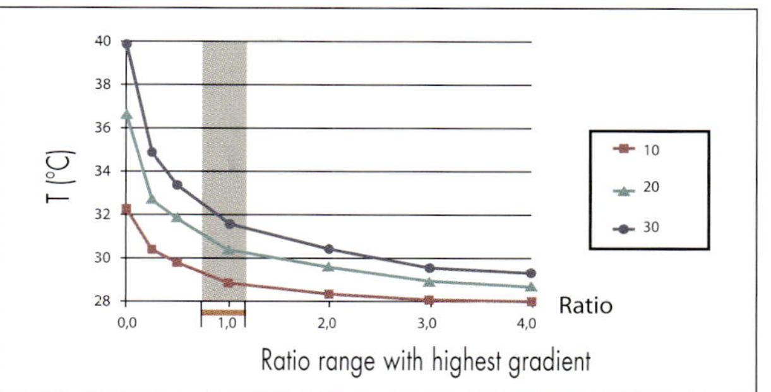

Fig 10-22 Optimization of the ratio between OpusWhite and absorption enhancers.

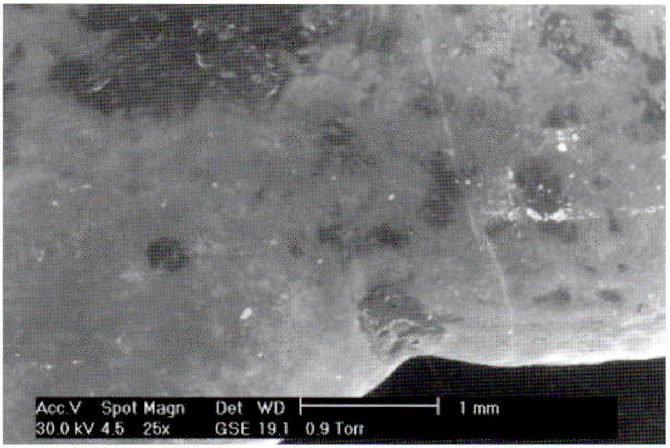

Fig 10-23 Enamel surface at a magnification of 25x without bleaching.

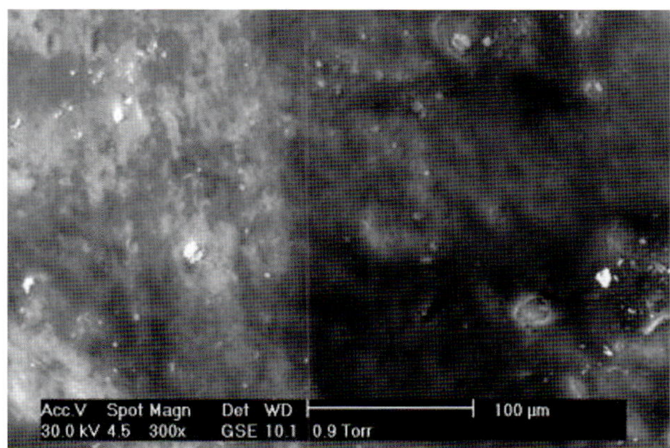

Fig 10-24 Enamel surface at a magnification of 300x without bleaching.

emulsion and irradiated with a diode laser beam (Fig 10-23 to 10-28).

The untreated parts show residues of plaque, the dark areas, at magnifications of 25x and 300x. At a magnification of 2000x, even the clean surfaces show enamel prisms surrounded by dark plaque residues. After bleaching, no plaque can be detected any more at any magnification. The dark area at the treated surface at a magnification of 2000x is the remains of the bleaching gel. More important, after bleaching, even at a magnification of 2000x, no surface alteration of the enamel can be detected and there are no exposed enamel prisms.

Nevertheless, more research is needed to indicate the effectiveness of tooth whitening when this emulsion and a diode laser are used for bleaching.

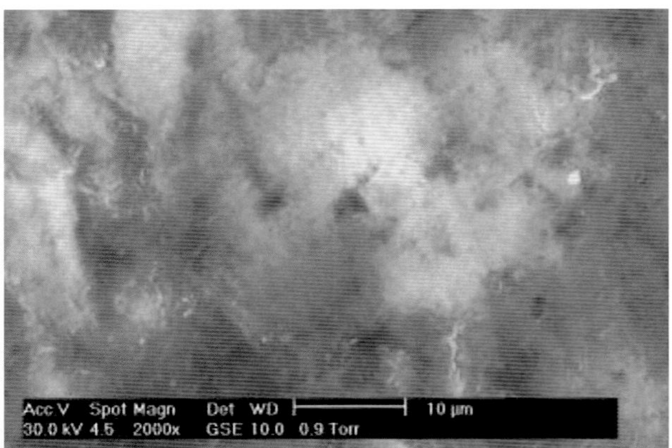

Fig 10-25 Enamel surface at a magnification of 2000x without bleaching.

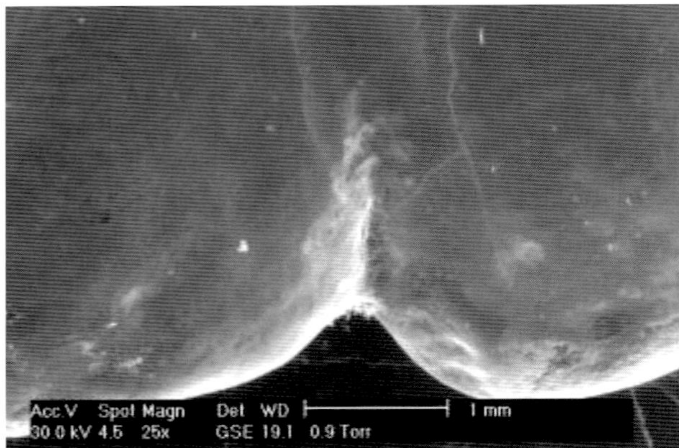

Fig 10-26 Enamel surface at a magnification of 25x after bleaching with the TiO_2 emulsion and diode laser.

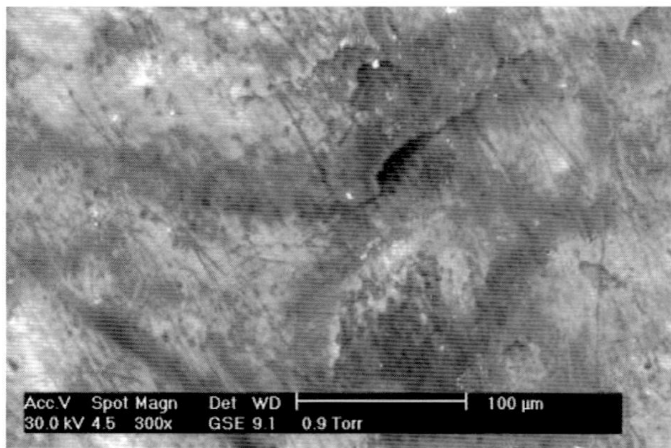

Fig 10-27 Enamel surface at a magnification of 300x after bleaching with the TiO_2 emulsion and diode laser.

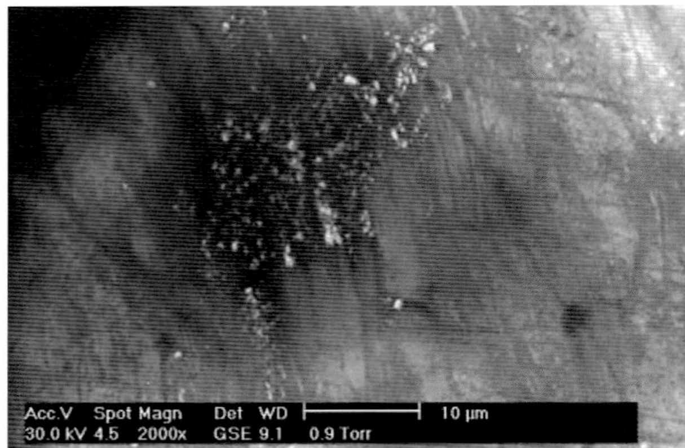

Fig 10-28 Enamel surface at a magnification of 2000x after bleaching with the TiO_2 emulsion and diode laser.

10.5 Clinical Procedure

10.5.1 Diagnosis and Treatment Planning

Since different etiologies causing different kinds of discoloration respond differently to bleaching techniques, diagnosis of the etiology of tooth discoloration is the most important determinant for the success of tooth bleaching. The next most important predictive factor is the condition of the teeth and mouth, especially the presence of compromised teeth that would prohibit the use of either bleaching agents or increased temperatures. But success with bleaching, as measured by immediate and longer-term patient satisfaction, will also depend on many other personal factors.

The individual patient's desires and expectations must be carefully assessed and it must be emphasized that sometimes it is not possible to fulfil these expectations and a compromise must be reached. The patient must also accept responsibility to modify any behaviour that may be causing their tooth discoloration.

After discussing with the patient what they expect from the treatment, and their willingness to cooperate in all aspects of the proposed treatment plan, a visual examination should determine the following:

- The cause of the dental staining
- The extent and depth of discoloration
- Whether a bleaching treatment is indicated

Next, a behavioural and medical history has to be compiled, together with a recording of the baseline data. A general oral examination, including X-rays, and vitality and sensitivity tests, should detect enamel cracks, caries or secondary decay, deficient restorations and soundness of all teeth.

It is important to perform a complete prophylaxis to see the extent of deep stains and to prepare the teeth for the actual bleaching procedure.

Finally, once the dentist has the full picture before him, the patient can now be informed of the expected outcome of the bleaching treatment and the possible side effects, with emphasis placed upon proper oral hygiene habits.

10.5.2 Clinical Procedure

Different laser-assisted bleaching techniques tend to have similar clinical procedures. The guidelines laid down by the manufacturers must be strictly followed, to achieve success. As an example, the clinical procedure of a KTP laser-assisted bleaching system will be discussed (Figs 10-29 to 10-40)[91,92].

Position a cheek-retractor and cotton mouth dry-field system in the patient's mouth. Connect this to the aspiration system. Make sure that the patient has safety glasses on. Perform thorough cleaning of the teeth: all plaque and debris has to be removed in order to obtain optimal results. Use airflow or pumice and water. Polishing pastes may not be used because they contain oils, which inhibit laser energy and the redox reaction (Fig 10-30)[91,92].

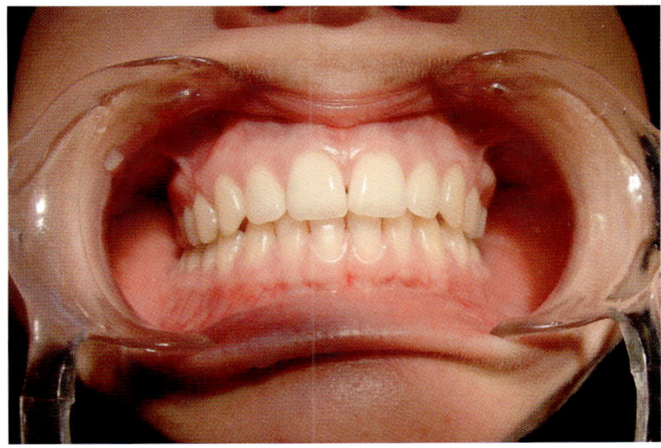

Fig 10-29 Situation before treatment.

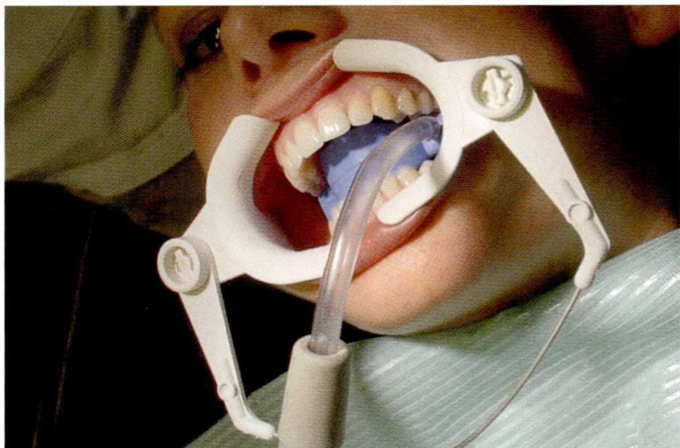

Fig 10-30 Protection appliance in situ.

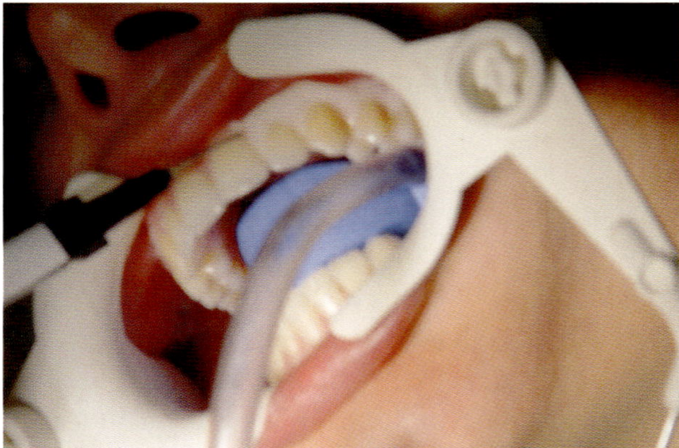

Fig 10-31 Application of the gingival protection.

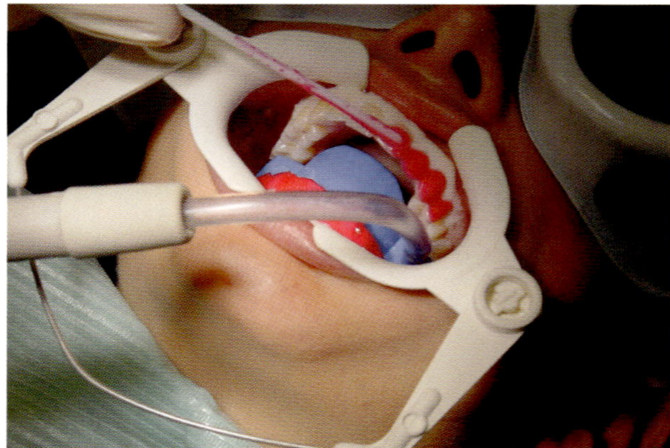

Fig 10-32 Application of the bleaching gel.

Dry teeth and gums thoroughly using compressed air. Apply the gingival protection material and polymerize. Follow the gingival margins and squirt into the sulcus, cover the cervix and about 1 mm of the teeth. Do the same for exposed dentin or spots that do not need to be bleached. Accidental spots have to be removed carefully because inhibition of the whitening reaction will occur wherever the blocking material is present (Fig 10-31)[91,92].

Prepare the gel. Shake the powder well before use. Mix about 5 ml of peroxide with the powder. The viscosity of the gel can be adapted if required by changing the volume of peroxide. Mix powder and liquid well, close the lid and let rest for 5 minutes to allow the pH to rise. After removing gel for each application, close the lid and seal well. The gel has a pH value of ~10 after laser irradiation.

Apply the gel on the teeth with a brush or spatula. Because upper teeth are bigger and have a thicker layer of enamel, particularly the front teeth, always start with the upper front teeth. Apply the gel on the 11, then 21, 12-22, 13-23, 14-24, 15-25, followed by 41-31, 42-32, 43-33, 44-34, 45-35 (Fig 10-32)[91,92].

Irradiate every tooth for 30 seconds in the same sequence as the gel application. Use an average power setting of about 1 Watt. Energy densities on the surface of the gel can be decreased, by increasing the distance of the fiber tip from the surface. If unfavourable or unacceptable sensitivity occurs, decrease energy densities or reduce the average power setting (Figa 10-33a,b)[91,92].

Aspirate the gel, rinse thoroughly and dry gently. If accidental contact of the gel with the soft tissues or the skin occurs, immediately apply a thick layer of vit. E gel. This is a very strong antioxidant which stops the irritating and burning sensation almost immediately (Fig 10-34)[91,92].

Apply new gel in a slightly different mode. Start in the upper arch with tooth 21, then 11, 21-12, ... In the lower arch with 31-41, 32-42, ... Irradiate each tooth again for 30 seconds in the same sequence as applying the gel and with the same power setting of the laser, rinse thoroughly and dry gently. Check the color of the teeth and decide whether to continue or not. If so, restart the procedure in the same sequence as with the first application (Fig 10-35)[91,92].

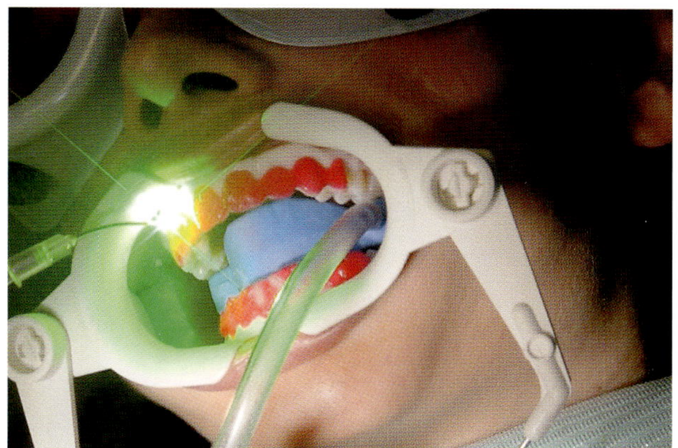

Fig 10-33a Activation of the bleaching gel.

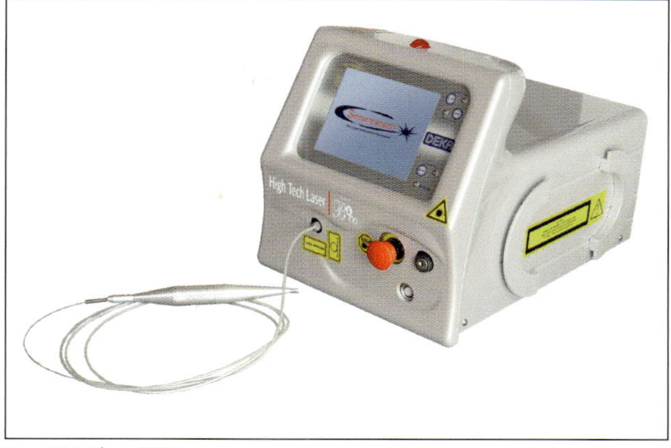

Fig 10-33b KTP-Laser.

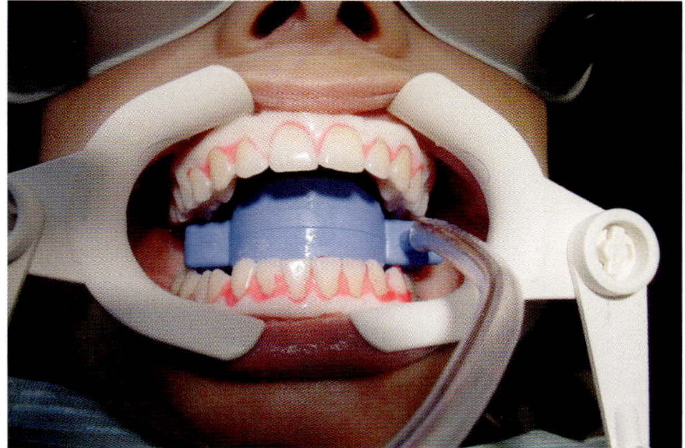

Fig 10-34 Result after the first cycle.

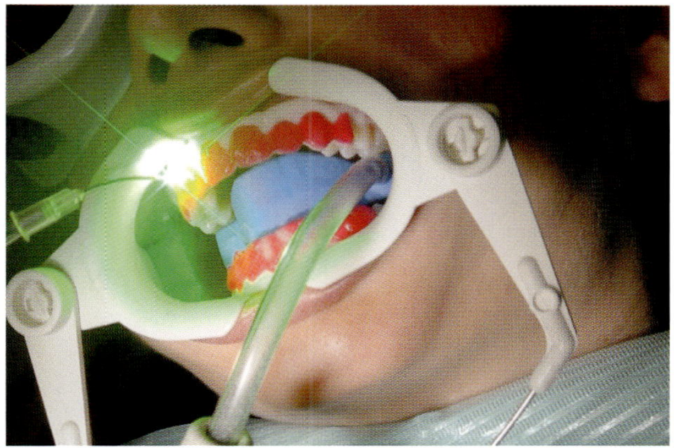

Fig 10-35 Second 10 min. application of gel and laser energy.

Selective application of several teeth is possible, as well as selective application to restricted areas on a single tooth or teeth, if these show more intense discolorations. Always respect the 30 seconds of irradiation time per tooth and the 10 minutes overall interaction time before sucking off the gel and rinsing. A maximum of four 10 minute passes can be performed in one treatment session (Fig 10-36)[91,92].

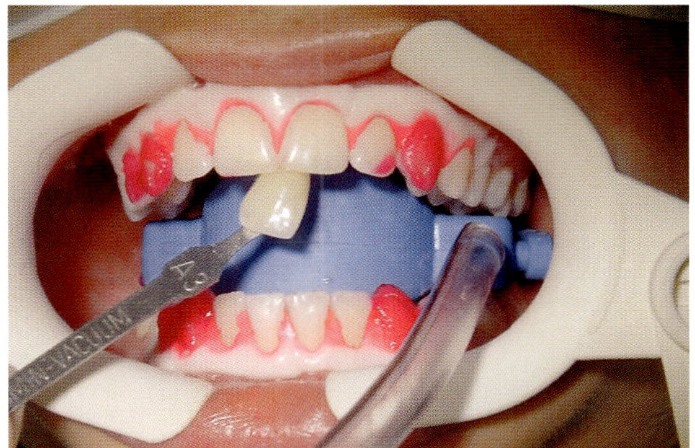

Fig 10-36 Result with color comparison after additional selective application at the darker canines.

Remove the gingival protection, apply fluoride gel liberally with a brush or spatula. Irradiate every tooth for 15 seconds. The fluoride and laser energy provides a profound resistance for the enamel and dentin to future acid attacks (see chapters 4 and 5) (Fig 10-37)[91,92].

Remove cheek-retractor, cotton mouth dry-field system and glasses, and discuss with the patient the result of the treatment. Give instructions for the use of the maintenance gel. Make an appointment for a control session after 2 weeks and one after 6 months (Fig 10-38)[91,92].

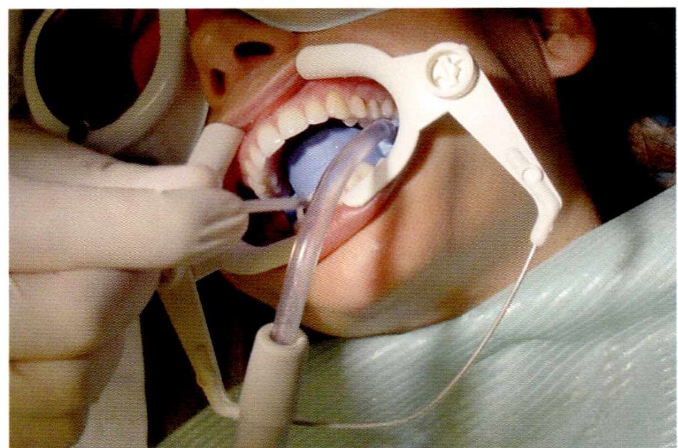

Fig 10-37 Fluoride application followed by the activation with laser light.

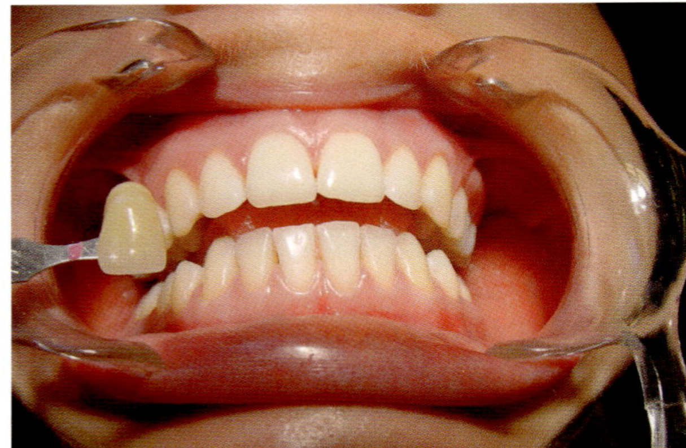

Fig 10-38 Situation after treatment.

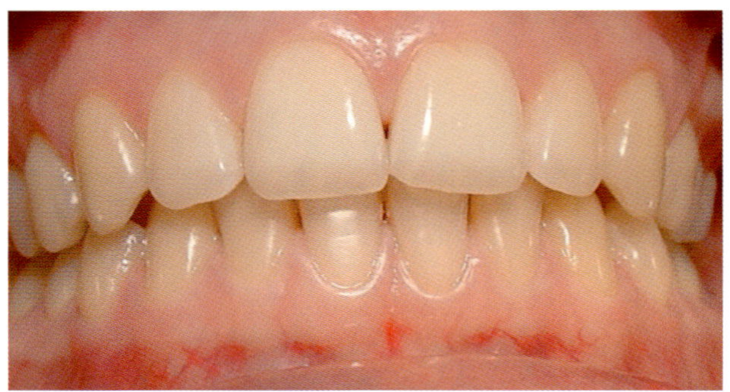

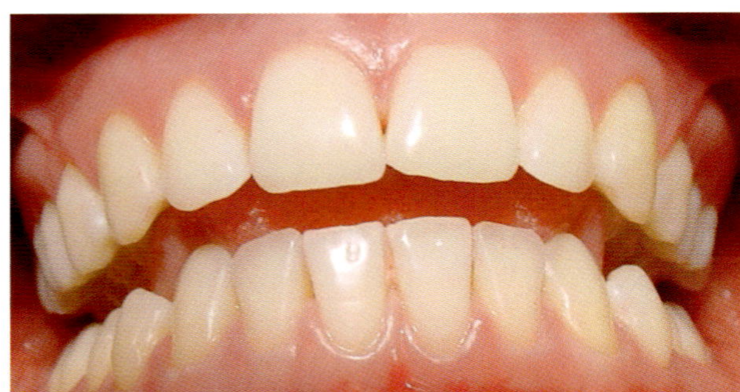

Fig 10-39 and 10-40 Before and after treatment.

10.6 Clinical Cases

10.6.1 Introduction

Walsh et al. compared several bleaching techniques and concluded laser-assisted bleaching to be far more effective than to night guard vital bleaching, NGVB (Table 10-5 to 10-7)[93].

In a publication in the Australian Dental Journal, 2003[104], Walsh showed the superior result of a laser-assisted bleaching, compared to the traditional modes, in a young patient (Fig 10-40a to c).

Table 10-5 The result of tooth whitening treatments for the NGVB patient with PolaNite (According to Walsh et al.[93]).

	Before Tooth Whitening		After Tooth Whitening		
Blue Channel	Intensity Level	Mean Ratio	Intensity Level	Mean Ratio	Changes
5M3	104.69	0.00	152.07	0.00	0.00
12	159.51	62.11	189.84	68.67	6.56
11	167.81	71.52	200.08	87.29	15.77
21	163.24	66.34	196.16	80.16	13.83
22	1532.72	55.55	170.,50	33.51	-22.04
32	136.18	35.68	187.03	3.556	27.88
31	144.03	44.57	193.,66	75.62	31.05
41	139.29	39.20	193.09	74.58	35.38
42	236.16	35.66	189.19	67.49	31.83
XW	192.95	100.00	207.07	100.00	0.00
Denominator XW-5M3	88.26		55.00		

Table 10-6 Results of tooth whitening treatment for the Smartbleach patient (According to Walsh et al.[93]).

	Before Tooth Whitening		After Tooth Whitening		
Blue Channel	Intensity Level	Mean Ratio	Intensity Level	Mean Ratio	Changes
5M3	83.67	0.00	96.28	0.00	0.00
12	114.68	25.59	154.07	59.31	33.71
11	129.08	37.48	169.40	75.04	37.56
21	132.10	39.97	161.26	66.69	26.72
22	127.47	36.15	141.00	45.89	9.74
XW	204.83	100.00	193.72	100.00	0.00
Denominator XW-5M3	121.16		97.44		

Table 10-7 DOTCAM comparison of the effectiveness of bleaching with KTP Smartbleach, OpusWhite and PolaNite NGVB (According to Walsh et al.[93]).

DOTCAM comparison (N=4) Change in ratio of blue channel intensity	
* KTP-Smartbleach 33.71–37.56	Using this objective method, greater whitening effects could be shown for photochemical laser bleaching (KTP laser/Smartbleach) compared with photothermal laser bleaching (diode laser/OpusWhite)
* OpusWhite 8.10–11.58	
* PolaNite NGVB 13.83–15.77	

Figs 10-41a–c KTP laser photochemical bleaching.

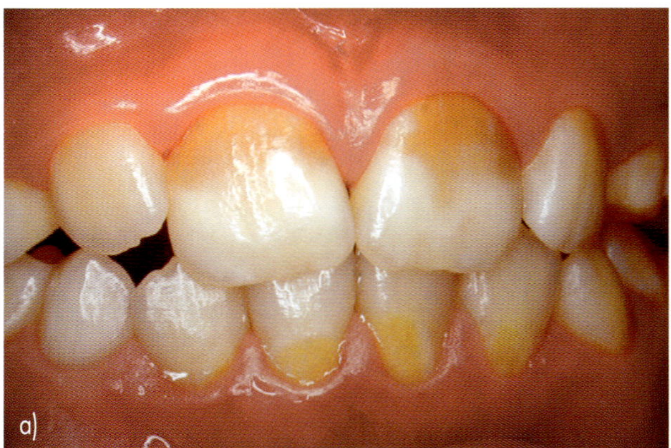

Fig 10-41a Initial clinical appearance of the dentition in a 9-year-old patient with intense discoloration of the incisor teeth caused by prolonged childhood illnesses and associated medications.

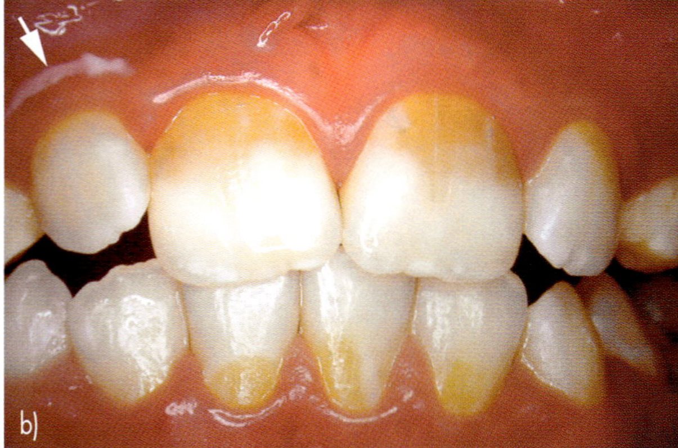

Fig 10-41b The situation immediately after three 60-minute appointments of power bleaching using a conventional quartz tungsten halogen curing lamp and 35% hydrogen peroxide gel. The incisal enamel shade has improved somewhat, but the areas of discoloration at the gingival third are unchanged. The arrow indicates a residue of the protective gingival dam.

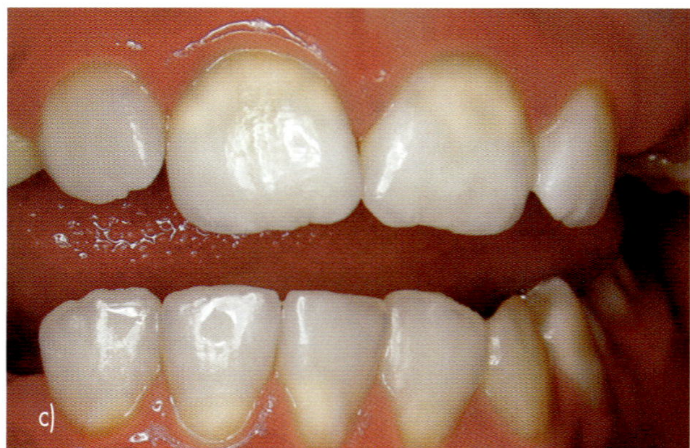

Fig 10-41c Clinical appearance immediately after one session of photochemical bleaching using the KTP laser and proprietary alkaline hydrogen peroxide (Smartbleach®) gel. The laser treatment was targeted to the gingival third. The patient and her parents were pleased with the immediate post-operative result and did not request any additional treatment.

Dotcom analyses as an objective measurement of bleaching result.

"The study confirms the key finding of Bentley's study in 1999 that the blue channel is the best descriptor for tooth colour changes. This is because blue is the complementary colour to yellow, which is the major colour in teeth. It has been thought that tooth colour whitening procedures result in an increase in the brightness of a tooth; however, this is not necessarily so. In this study, the greatest difference in the intensity levels between two different shade tabs, for example XW and DY, were in the blue channel, followed by the green channel, the luminosity channel, and lastly the red channel".

Tooth darkness standard ratio %
= Lightness standard – Darkness standard x 100%

Fig 10-42 DOTCAM analysis as an objective measurement of bleaching results.

To measure the effectiveness of the whitening result, they used the DOTCAM analysis or Digital Objective Tooth Color Analysis Method, providing accurate and reproducible measurements (Fig 10-42)[93]. During treatment, it is very important not to dehydrate the teeth. Tam[105] suggested that the majority of the initial color relapse after treatment is due to an acid-etch pre-treatment and dehydration of the teeth during isolation with a rubber dam[115].

When, after a first application of bleaching gel and laser energy, no substantial effect is obtained, it is best to stop the treatment and restart after a period of ~2 weeks. Effective results will then occur[91,106]. If sensitivity occurs during treatment, power setting and energy density must be decreased[91,106]. While treating pulpless teeth, special precautions for internal isolation have to be made in order to prevent internal resorption of the root[92]. Different kinds of discolorations respond differently to a bleaching treatment. Yellow discolorations are the easiest to whiten. Brown discolorations are more resistant to bleaching, and the grey discolorations are the most difficult to treat. A guideline to predict a possible outcome of a laser-assisted bleaching treatment is shown in Table 10-8[92].

Table 10-8 Effectiveness and number of treatment sessions.

Discoloration		1 Treatment Session	2 Treatment Sessions	3 Treatment Sessions
Yellow	mild	X		
	moderate	X		
	intense	X	(X)	
Brown	mild	X		
	moderate	X	(X)	
	intense	(X)	X	
Grey	mild	X	(X)	
	moderate	(X)	X	
	intense		X	(X)
Tetracycline degree I		X	(X)	
Tetracycline degree II			X	(X)
Tetracycline degree III			(X)	X

10.6.2 Yellow Discolorations

Figs. 10-43 to 10-48 represent clinical cases of typical yellow discolorations. All results were obtained after one in-office treatment session: the mild discolorations after two or three applications of the bleaching gel and laser energy the intense discolorations after four passes[91,106].

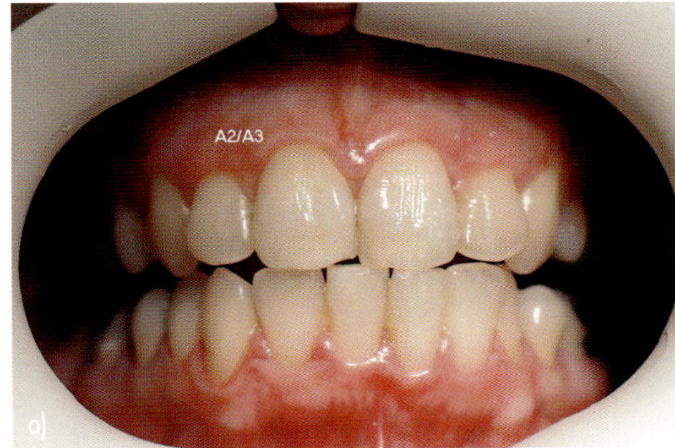

Fig 10-43a Yellow discoloration before treatment.

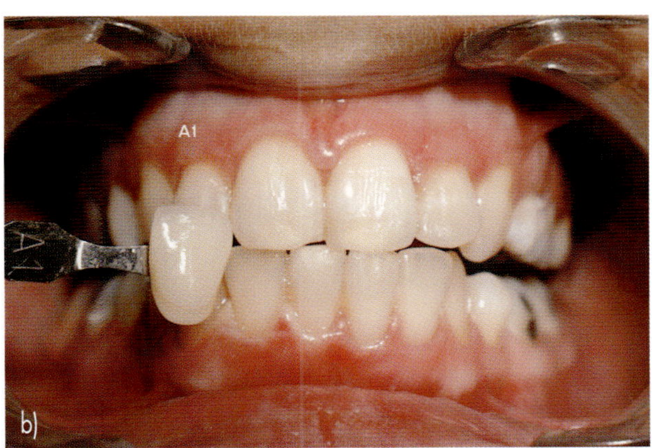

Fig 10-43b After the treatment.

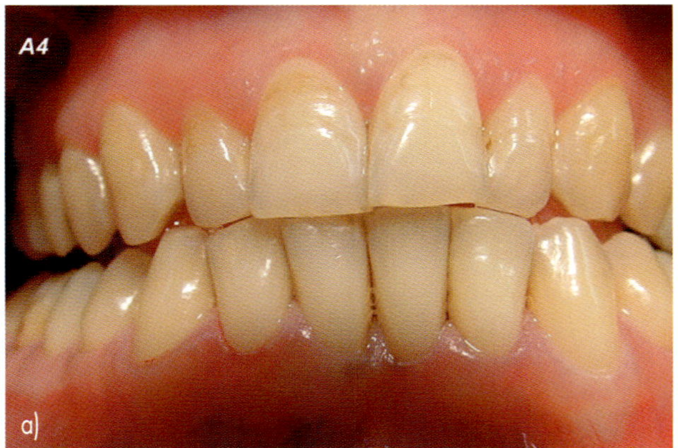

Fig 10-44a Before treatment.

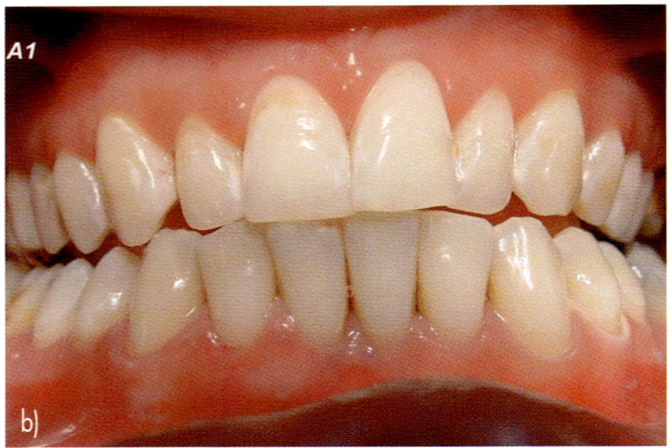

Fig 10-44b After treatment.

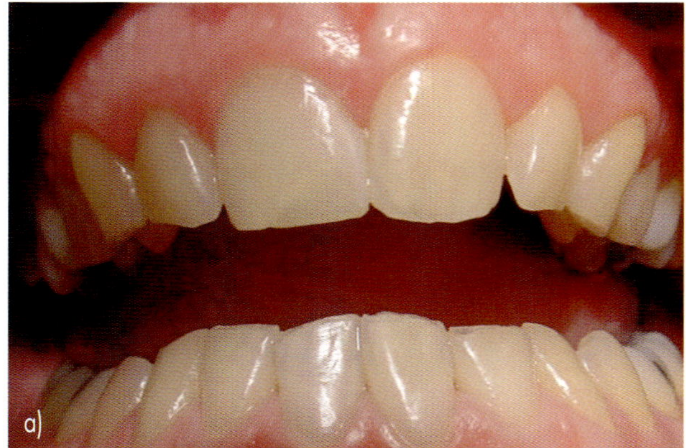

Fig 10-45a Before treatment.

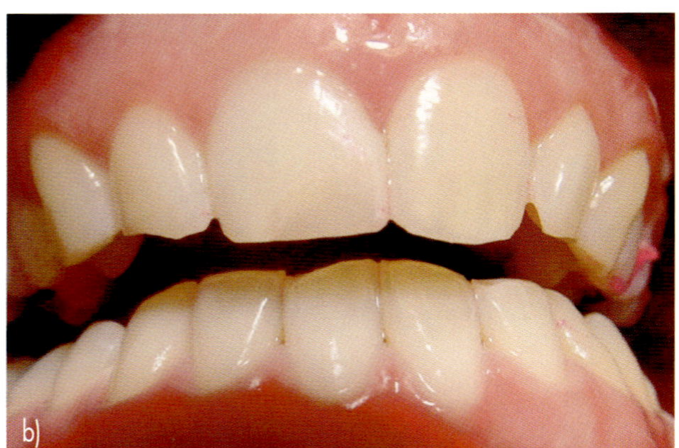

Fig 10-45b After the treatment. The composite filling in tooth 11 has to be renewed, respecting a waiting time of 2 weeks.

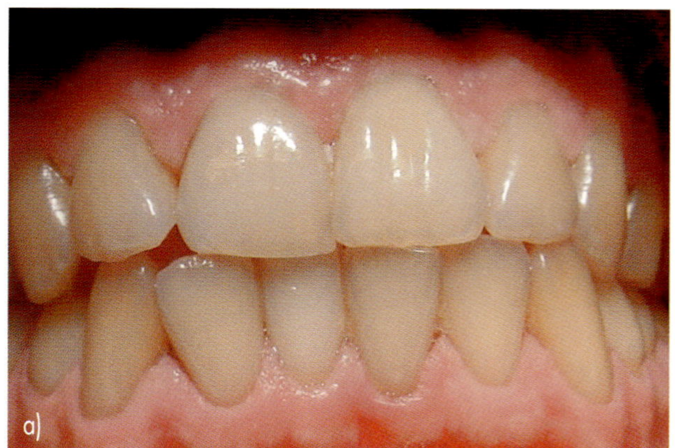

Fig 10-46a Before treatment.

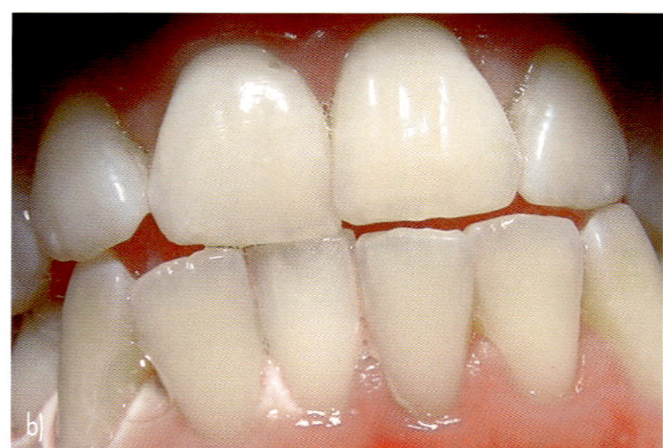

Fig 10-46b After treatment.

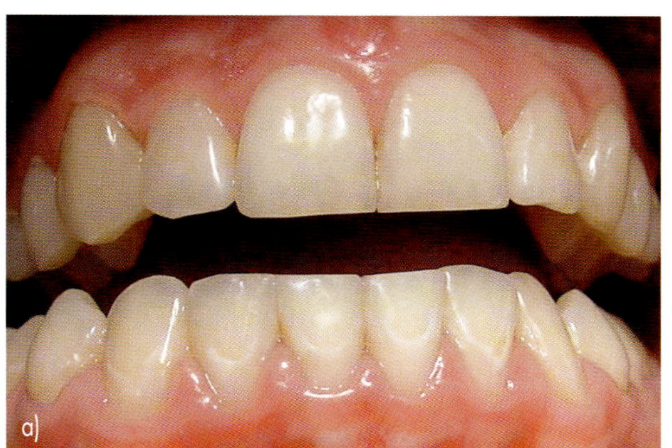

Fig 10-47a Before treatment.

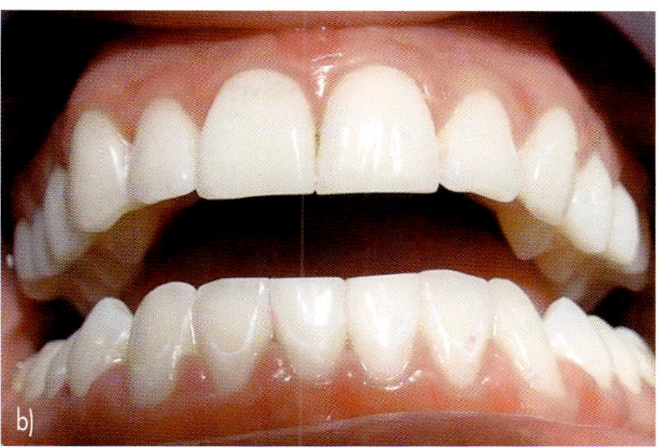

Fig 10-47b After treatment.

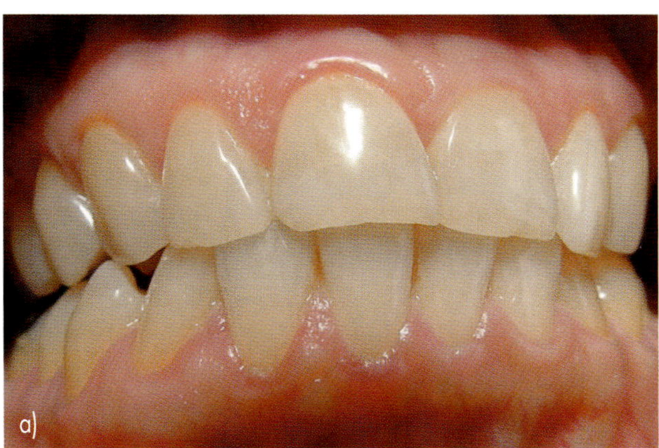

Fig 10-48a Before treatment.

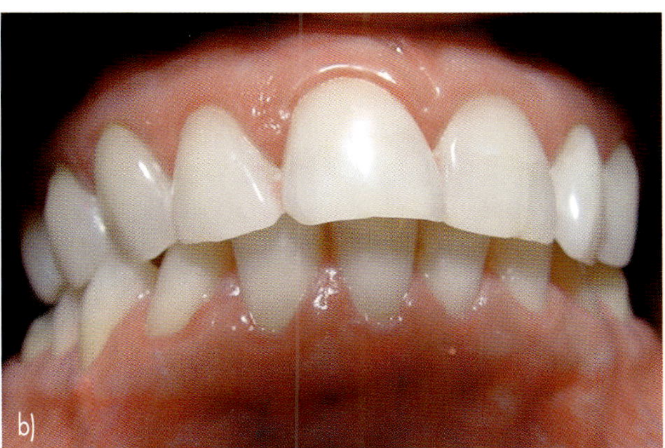

Fig 10-48b After completing the first bleaching session.

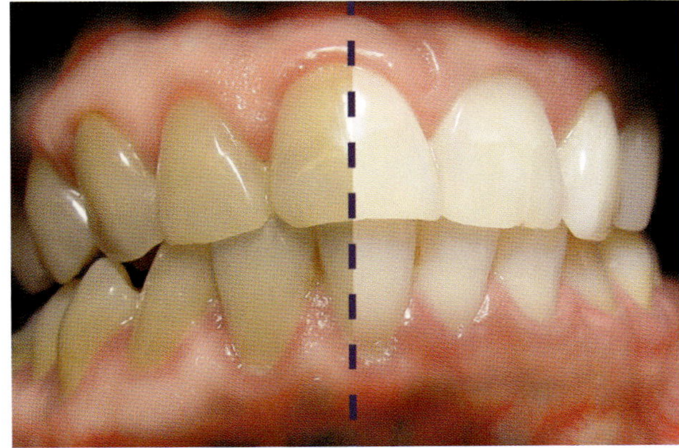
Fig 10-48c Comparison of the situations before – after.

10.6.3 Lightening of a Single Tooth and Internal Bleaching of a Single Dead Tooth

Single tooth treatment (Figs 10-49a,b) is easy to achieve as the bleaching gel can be applied to a tooth without affecting the adjacent teeth. This is the same for applied laser energy.

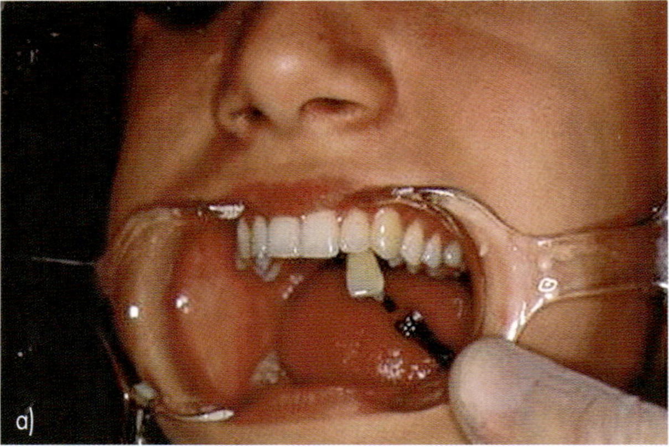

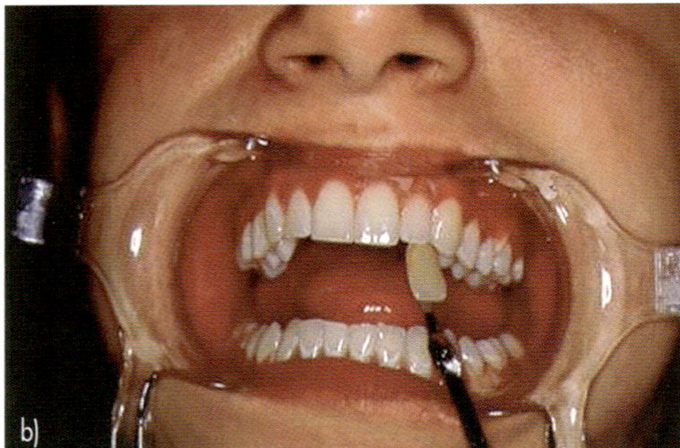

Figs 10-49a and b Selective treatment of the upper canines in a young female patient[91,106].

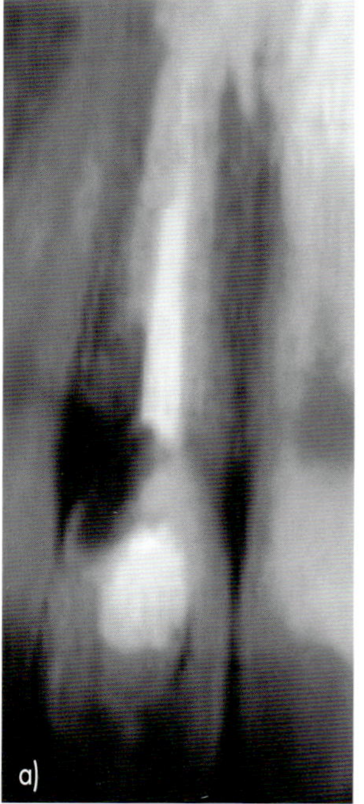

Fig 10-50a Internal bleaching of a single tooth.

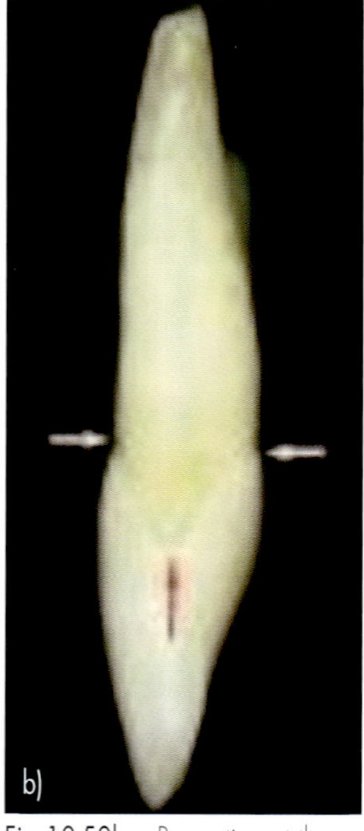

Fig 10-50b Resorption at the distal side.

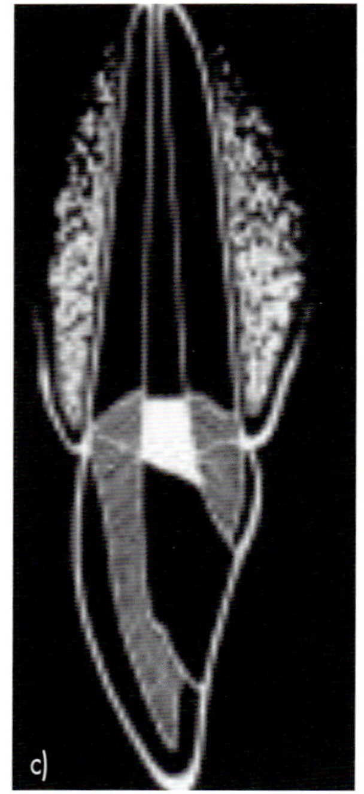

Fig 10-50c and d Isolation of the dentin tubuli, reaching the area of the root surface.

Non-vital, internal bleaching of a single tooth always holds certain risks for internal resorption of the root (Fig 10-50a)[92,107–117].

This resporption most often occurs at the distal side of the tooth, as the cemento-enamel junction extends the most to the incisal region in this area (Fig 10-50b). Special precautions and effective isolation of the dentin tubuli, reaching the area of the root surface, should be performed (Figs 10-50c,d)[92].

Figs 10-50e,h shows a non-vital bleaching of a central incisor, where bleaching gel has to be

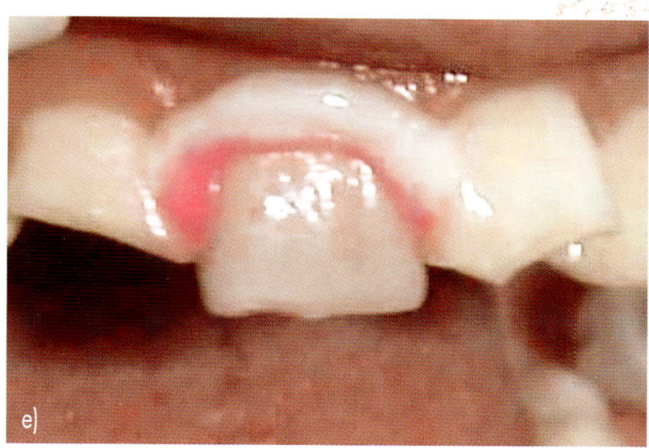

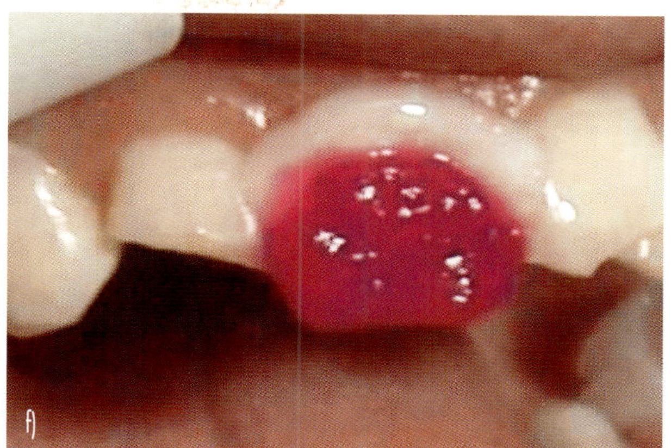

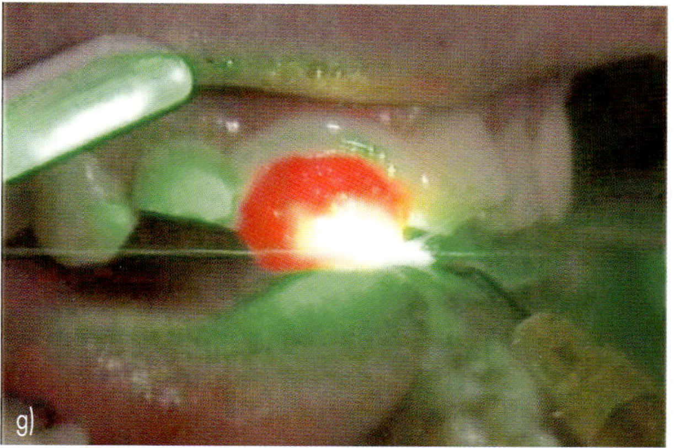

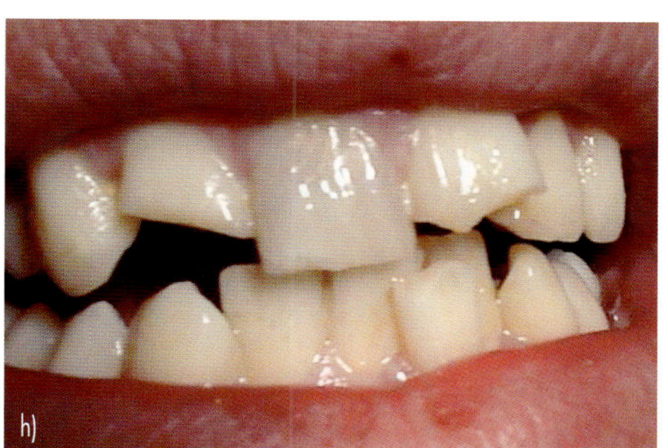

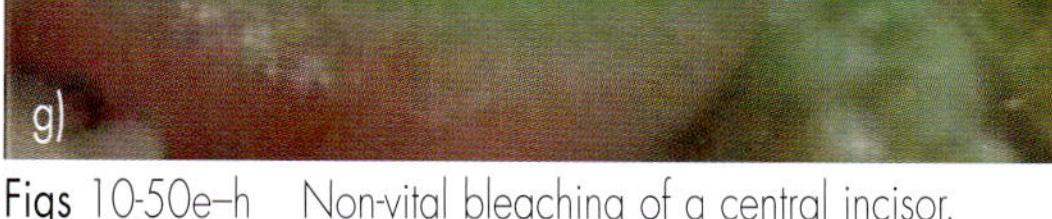

Figs 10-50e–h Non-vital bleaching of a central incisor.

applied to the labial side, as well as to the palatal/lingual side, and inside the prepared cavity. For each application, the gel must remain on the tooth for the full 10 minutes. Laser energy has to be applied to the labial, as well as to the palatal/lingual side. During the 10 minutes of application, two to three 30-second cycles of lasering may be done. Treatment should be stopped while the affected tooth is still a bit darker than adjacent teeth, because inside the more porous dentin, the bleaching effect is continuous for several hours after treatment[91,106].

10.6.4 Brown Discolorations

Brown discolorations are more resistant to whitening and always require the maximum of four full passes of bleaching gel and laser energy. Figs 10-51 to 10-53 are the results obtained in one treatment session[91,16].

Figs 10-54 to 10-55 show the treatment of more intense, brown discolorations in two treatment sessions, with three applications in each of them, of the maximum of four[91,116].

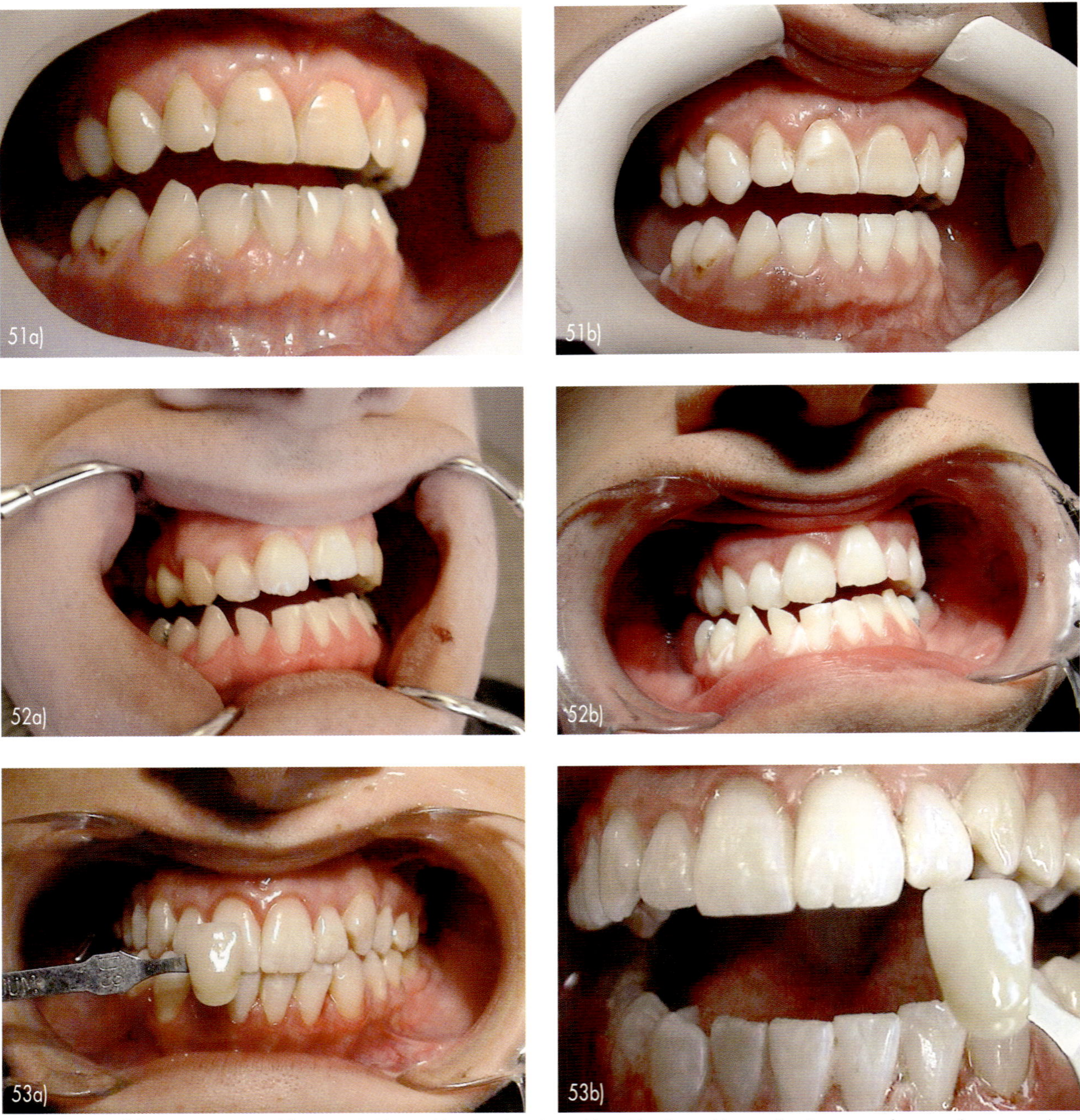

Figs 10-51a and b, Figs 10-52a and b, Figs 10-53a and b Results achieved from bleaching of brown discolorations in four complete passes during one treatment session.

10.6.5 Grey Discolorations and Tetracycline Staining

The treatment of moderate to intense grey discolorations, as well as tetracycline staining degree II and III, is hardly possible without the application of laser energy. Moreover, traditional treatments could result in an adverse affect[91,92,106].

Figures 10-56a and 10-56b show the outcome of a single session treatment, with four applications of bleaching gel and laser energy, of a tetra-

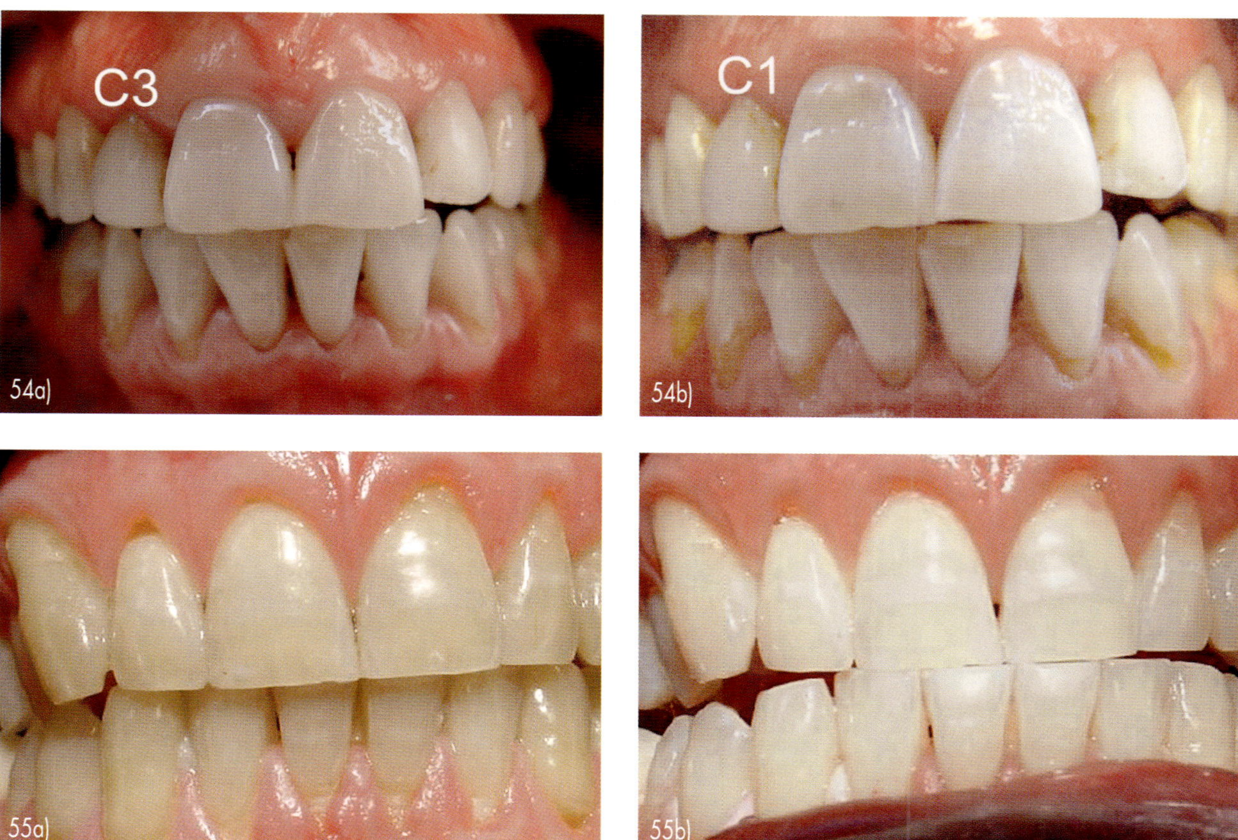

Figs 10-54a and b, Figs 10-55a and b Results achieved from bleaching of brown discolorations in two treatment sessions, each of three passes.

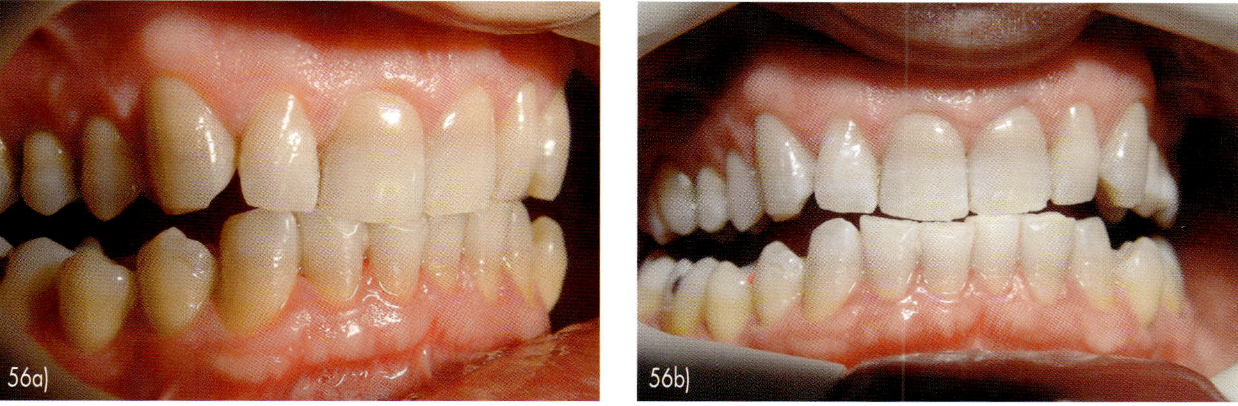

Figs 10-56a and b Results achieved from four passes of bleaching gel and laser light on a tetracycline staining grade II in a single treatment session.

cycline staining degree II. In a possible second treatment session, selective application and treatment of the cervical regions could be done. But the patient was perfectly satisfied with the result achieved in the first one.

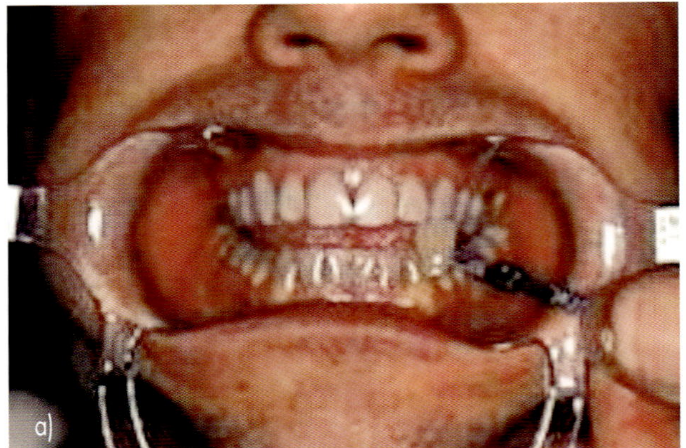

Fig 10-57a Situation before the treatment of a tetracycline discoloration grade III.

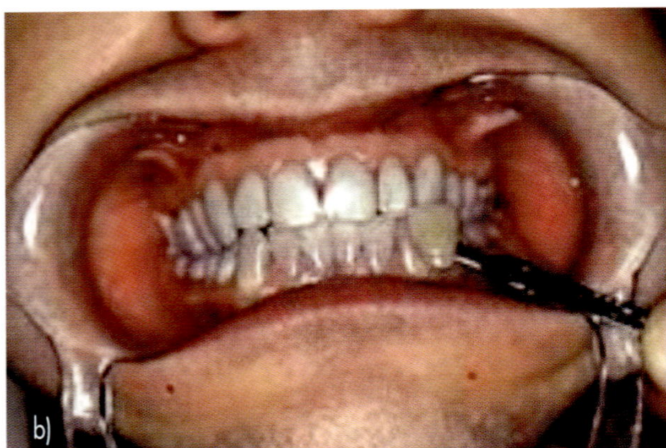

Fig 10-57b Improvement by in-office treatment using Smartbleach in four sessions.

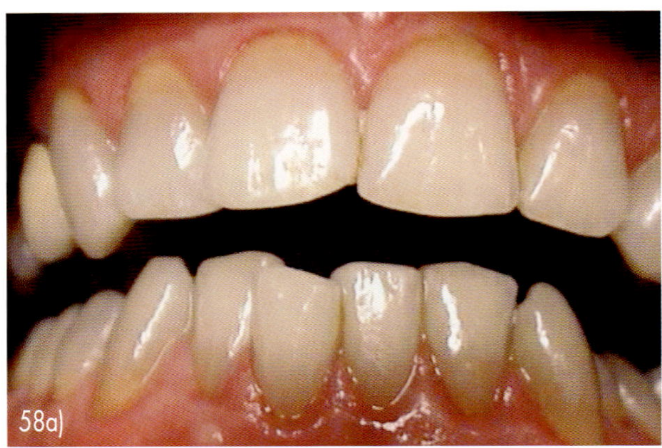

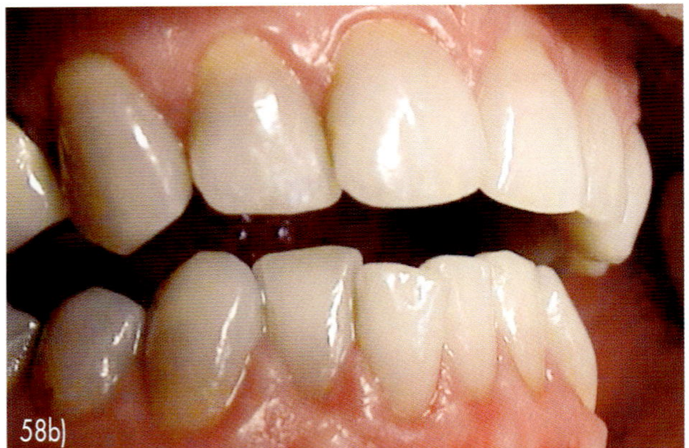

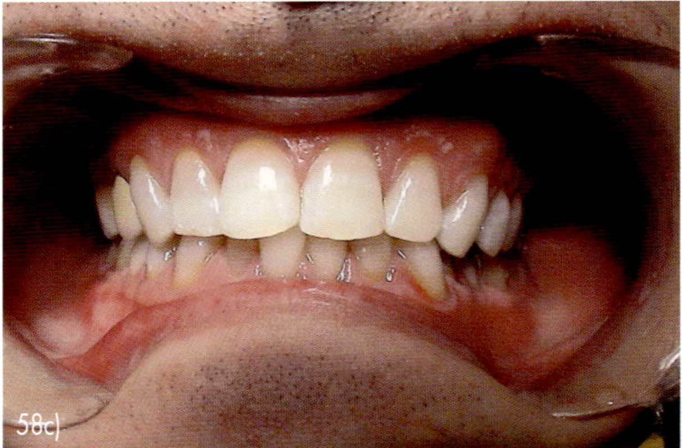

Figs 10-58a–c Result achieved by treating a tetracycline discoloration grade III in two sessions with four cycles each.

Figure 10-57a shows the dramatic situation of a patient (dentist) before treatment. Several home- and in-office bleaching treatments had not improved the generalized tetracycline staining degree III, and this had lead to the application of direct composite veneers in the upper arch. One in-office Smartbleach treatment, with four applications, resulted in a substantial improvement (Fig 10-57b), where the teeth in the lower arch showed the same appearance of those in the upper arch, with the composite veneers.

The treatment of a tetracycline staining degree III , in four passes during two in-office sessions is shown in Figs 10-58a to 10-58c. Dr. L. Cheng, Melbourne, obtained a superior result in a male patient with the same kind of discoloration. Every possible bleaching treatment before had failed. Dr. Cheng applied three treatment sessions within a period of one week each (Figs 10-59a, b).

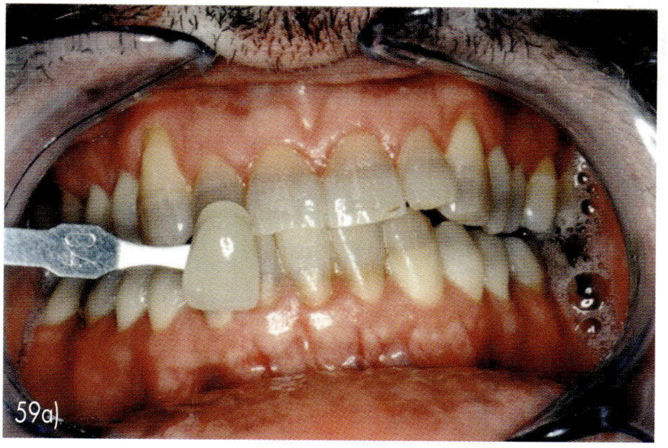

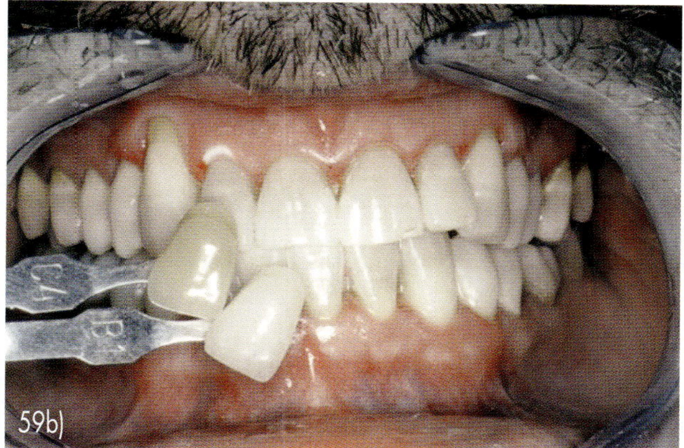

Figs 10-59a,b Result achieved by treating a tetracycline discoloration grade III in three sessions (with kind permission of Dr. L. Cheng, Melbourne).

10.6.6 Trouble-sshooting

Transient hyperemia with sensitivity of one or more teeth is possible during the first 48 hours. Teeth involved often show an occult defect, allowing the bleaching gel to penetrate deeper than needed inside the tooth. Other possible problems and their solutions are discussed in Figs 10-60 to 10-63[106].

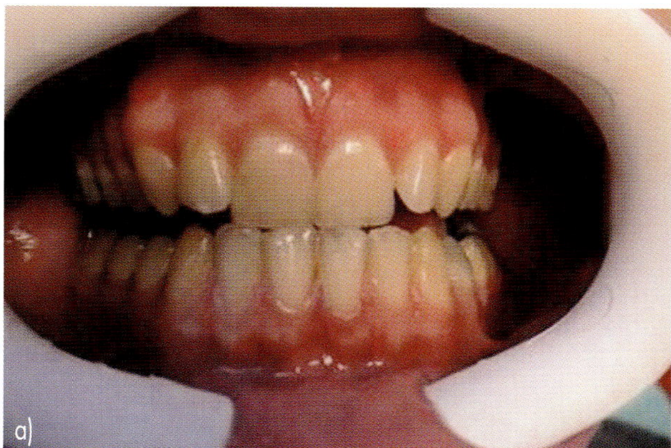

Fig 10-60a Situation before treatment.

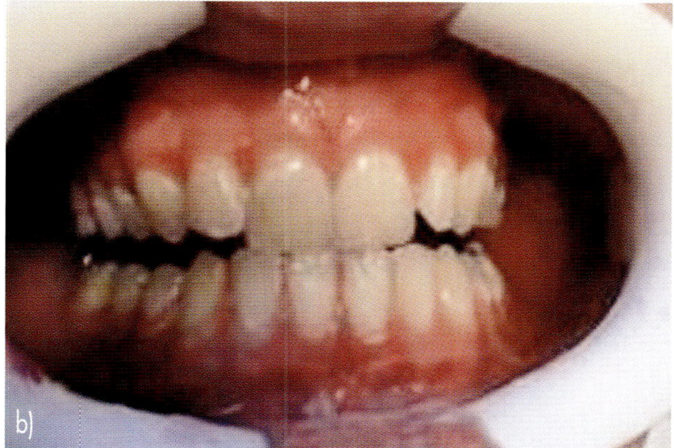

Fig 10-60b After two applications, treatment had to be stopped because of sensitivity. Notice the cervical demineralization which appears clearly with the bleaching process. After preventive treatment with fluoride and laser, another bleaching treatment was conducted 2 weeks later.

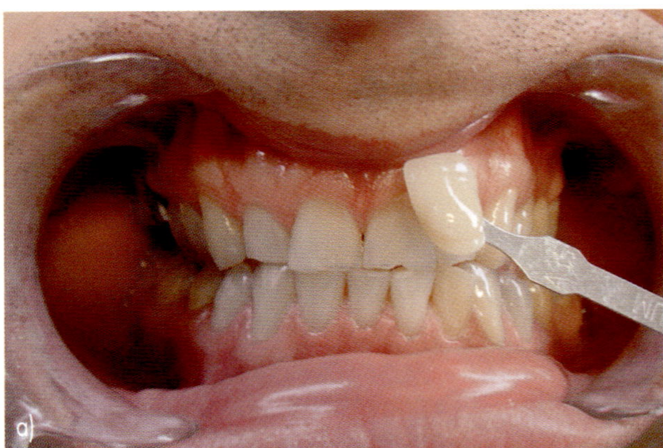

Fig 10-61a Severe loss of hard tooth structure on the incisal part of the upper incisors with the exposure of dentin can cause sensitivity during treatment. Care must be taken not to apply gel on the exposed dentin, or the dentin can be covered up with blocking material. The same applies to exposed root surfaces. It is best to cover them with protective ma-terial just up to the enamel margin.

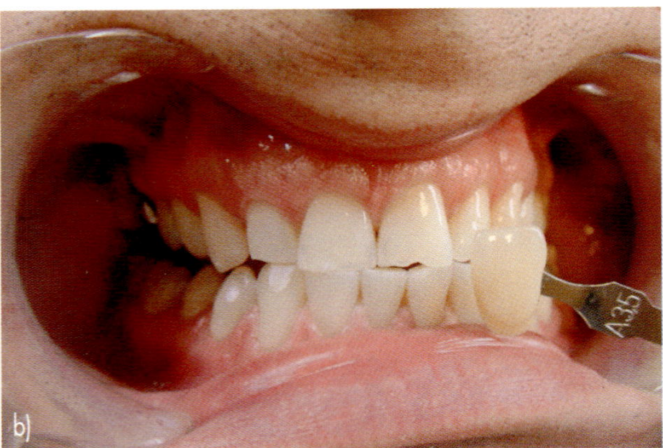

Fig 10-61b Situation after a successful treatment with 3 applications.

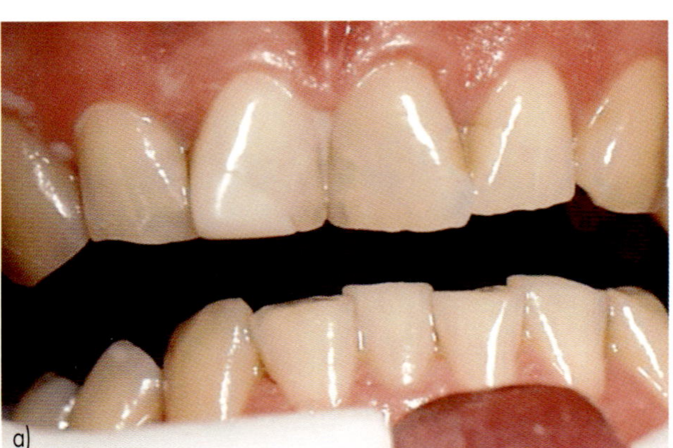

Fig 10-62a Large restorations in the front region are often a contraindication for bleaching. The restorations can not be bleached. Bevels and bonding materials can be spread over large areas, inhibiting the bleaching process.

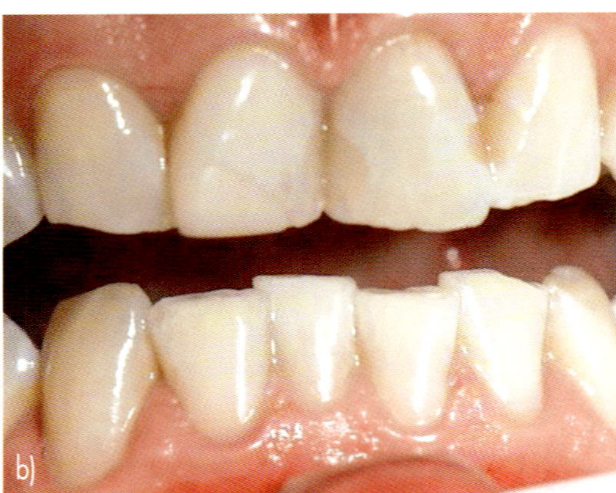

Fig 10-62b A substantial improvement of the color after three3 applications. A period of at least 2 weeks is required before replacement of the composite fillings. The residual oxygen has to dissipate completely out of the dental tissue. Otherwise it will inhibit the polymerization reaction of the composite materials.

Laser-assisted bleaching treatments entail no high risks either to the hard tooth structures or to the vital pulp or soft tissues. No adverse effects or irreversible damage have yet been reported. Hence, bleaching treatments should always be the first treatment of choice, if possible, to treat tooth staining. Unlike other cosmetic treatments, they do not affect the hard or soft oral structures, because they are completely non-invasive in nature.

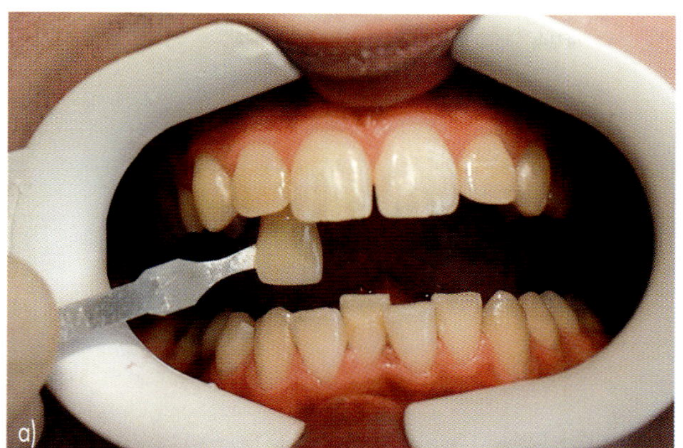

Fig 10-63a Situation before treatment.

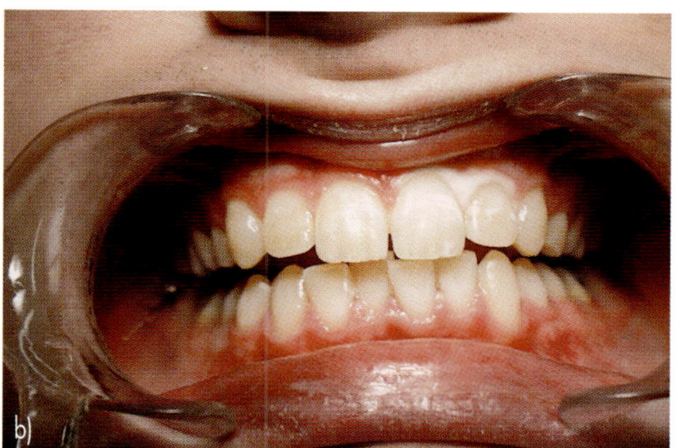

Fig 10-63b Notice the white gingival lesion cervical from the left first and second incisor after treatment. This is caused by poor fitting of the gingival protection material. Leakage of the H_2O_2 burned the gingiva. Symptoms are easily relieved by applying vitamin E gel.

10.7 References

1. Yudhira R F T, Peumans H, Tudts M: Optimaliseren van esthetiek met: Bleaching and microabrasie. Permanente vorming. Katholieke Universiteit Leuven 1999
2. Goldstein R E, Garber D A: Complete Dental Bleaching. Quintessence Publishing Co Inc, Chicago 1995
3. Dale B G: Bleaching and related agents. In: Dale B G, Aschheim K W: Esthetic Dentistry. A clinical approach to techniques and materials. Lea & Febinger, Philadelphia, London 1993, 205–227
4. Lin L C, Pitts D L, Burgess L W: An investigation into the feasibility of photobleaching tetracycline-stained teeth. J Endod 14: 293–299, 1988
5. Jordon R E, Boksman L: Conservative vital bleaching treatment of discolored dentition. Compend Contin Ed Dent 5: 803, 1984
6. Frysh H: Chemistry of Bleaching. In: Goldstein R E, Garber D A: Complete Dental Bleaching. Quintessence Publishing Co Inc, Chicago 1995, 25–33
7. Frysh H, Bowles W, Baker F, Rivera-Hidalgo G, Guillen G: Effect of pH on bleaching efficiency. J Dent Res 72: 384, 1993
8. Zagarosa V M T: Bleaching of vital teeth: Technique. Estomedico 9: 7–30, 1984
9. Carlsson J: Salivary peroxidase: An important defense against oxygen toxicity. J Oral Pathol 16: 412–416, 1987
10. Bowles W H, Ugwuneri Z: Pulp chamber penetration by hydrogen peroxide following vital bleaching procedures. J Endod 13: 375–377, 1987
11. Fuss A, Szajkis S, Tagger M: Tubular permeability to calcium hydroxide and the bleaching agents. J Endod 15: 362–364, 1989
12. Bartelstone H J: Radio-iodine penetration through intact enamel with uptake by bloodstream and thyroid gland. J Dent Res 30: 728–733, 1951
13. Bowles W H, Thompson L R: Vital Bleaching: the effect of heat and hydrogen peroxide on pulpal enzymes. J Endod 12: 108–112, 1986
14. Cooper J S, Bokmeyer T J, Bowles W H: Penetration of the pulp chamber by carbamide peroxide bleaching agents. J Endod 18: 7: 315–317, 1992
15. Arwill T: Penetration of radioactive isotopes through the enamel and dentin. II Transfer of 22 Na in fresh and chemically treated dental tissues. Odontol RW 20: 47, 1969
16. Albers H: Lightening natural teeth. ADEPT Report 2(1): 1–24, 1991
17. Davies A K, McKellar J F, Phillips G D, Reid A G: Photochemical oxidation of tetracycline in aqueous solution. J Chem Soc Perkin Trans II 369–375, 1979
18. Davies A K, Cundall R B, Dandiker Y, Slifkin M A: Photooxidation of tetracylcine absorbed on hydroxyapatite in relation to the light-induced staining of teeth. J Dent Res 65: 936, 1985
19. Feinman R A, Madray G, Yarborough D: Chemical, optical and physiologic mechanisms of bleaching products: a review. Pract Periodont Esthetics 3: 32, 1991
20. Cohen B A, Parkins F M: Bleaching tetracycline-stained teeth. Oral Surg Oral Med Oral Pathol 19: 465, 1970
21. Christensen G J: Bleaching vital tetracycline-stained teeth. Quintessence Int 9: 13, 1978
22. Ingle J I, Taintor J F: Endodontics, 3rd ed. Lea & Febinger, Philadelphia 1965, 607
23. Ledoux W R: Structural effects of bleaching on tetracycline-stained vital rat teeth. J Prosthet Dent 54(55), 1985
24. Reid J S, Newman D: A suggested method of bleaching tetracycline-stained vital teeth. Br Dent J 142: 261, 1977
25. Wilson C F, Seal N S: Color change following vital bleaching of tetracycline-stained teeth. Pediat Dent 7: 205, 1985
26. Pearson H: Bleaching of the discolored pulpless tooth. J Am Dent Assoc 56: 64–68, 1958
27. Zach L, Cohen G: Pulp response to externally applied heat. Oral Surg 19(4): 515–530, 1965
28. Baumgartner J C, Reid D E, Pickett A: Human pulpal reaction to the modified Melnnes bleaching technique. J Endod 9: 527–529, 1983
29. Cohen S C, Chase L: Human pulpal response to bleaching procedures on vital teeth. J Endod 5: 134–138, 1979
30. Griffin R E, Grower M F: Effects of solutions used to treat dental fluorosis on permeability of teeth. J Endod 11: 391, 1977
31. Lisanti V F, Zander H A: Thermal injury to normal dog teeth. J Dent Res 31: 548–558, 1952
32. Nyborg H, Branstrom M: Pulp reaction to heat. J Prosthet Dent 19: 605–612, 1968
33. Postle H H: Pulp response to heat. J Dent Res 38: 740, 1959
34. Sakagushi R L, Hampel A T: Bleaching of vital teeth. Clark's Clin Dent 4: 1–10, 1991
35. Haywood V B: Bleaching of vital and nonvital teeth. Curr Opin Dent: 142–149, 1992
36. Seal N S, McIntosh J E, Taylor A N: Pulpal reaction to bleaching of teeth in dogs. J Dent Res 60: 948–953, 1981
37. Walsh L J: Safety issues relating to the use of hydrogen peroxide in dentistry. Aust Dent J 45(4): 257–269, 2000
38. Matis B A, Cochran M A, Eckert G, Carlson T J: The efficacy and safety of a 10% carbamide peroxide bleaching gel. Quintessence Int 29(9): 555–563, 1998
39. Thitinanthapan W, Satamanont P, Vongsavan N: In vitro penetration of the pulp chamber by three brands of carbamide peroxide. J Esthet Dent 11(5): 259–264, 1999
40. Ernst C P, Marroquin B B, Willershausen-Zönnchen B: Effects of hydrogen peroxide containing bleaching agents on the morphology of human enamel. Quintessence Int 27(1): 53–56, 1996
41. Flaitz C M, Hicks M J: Effects of carbamide peroxide whitening agents on enamel surfaces and caries-like lesion formation: an SEM and polarized light microscopic in vitro study. ASDC J Dent Child 63(4): 249–256, 1996

42. Tong L S M, Pang M K M, Mok NY C, Wei S H Y: The effects of etching, microabrasion, and bleaching on surface enamel. J Dent Res 72(1): 67–71, 1993
43. Hedegüs C, Bistey T, Flóra-Nagy E, Keszthelyi G, Jenei A: An atomic force microscopy study on the effect of bleaching agents on enamel surface. J Dent 27(7): 509–515, 1999
44. Zalkind M, Arwaz J R, Goldman A, Rotstein I: Surface morphology changes in human enamel, dentin and cementum following bleaching: a scanning electron microscopy study. Endod Dent Traumatol 12(2): 82–88, 1996
45. Lewinstein I, Hirschfeld Z, Stabholz A, Rotstein I: Effect of hydrogen peroxide and sodium perborate on the microhardness of human enamel and dentin. J Endod 20(2): 61–63, 1994
46. Potocnik I, Kosec L, Gaspersic D: Effect of 10% carbamide peroxide bleaching gel on enamel microhardness, microstructure, and mineral content. J Endod 26(4): 203–206, 2000
47. Shannon H, Spencer P, Gross K, Tira D: Characterisation of enamel exposed to 10% carbamide peroxide bleaching agents. Quintessence Int 24(1): 39–44, 1993
48. Seghi R R, Denry I: Effects of external bleaching on indentation and abrasion characteristics of human enamel in vitro. J Dent Res 71(6): 1340–1344, 1992
49. Pinheiro Junior E C, Fidel R A, da Cruz Filho A M, Silva R G, Pécora J D: In vitro action of various carbamide peroxide gel bleaching agents on the microhardness of human enamel. Braz Dent J 7(2): 75–79, 1996
50. Van der Vyver P J, Lewis S B, Marais J T: The effect of bleaching agent on composite/enamel bonding. J Dent Assoc S Afr 52(10): 601–603, 1997
51. Titley K C, Torneck C D, Ruse N D, Krmec D: Adhesion of a resin composite to bleached and unbleached human enamel. J Endod 19(3): 112–115, 1993
52. Garcia-Goday F, Dodge W W, Honohuc M, O'Quinn J A: Composite resin bond strength after enamel bleaching. Oper Dent 18(4): 144–147, 1993
53. Dishman M V, Covey D A, Baughan L W: The effects of peroxide bleaching on composite to enamel bond strength. Dent Mater 10(1): 33–36, 1994
54. Torneck C D, Titley K C, Smith D C, Adibfar A: The influence of time on the adhesion of composite resin to bleached bovine enamel. J Endod 16(3): 123–128, 1990
55. Josey A L, Meyers I A, Romaniuk K, Symons A L: The effect of a vital bleaching technique on enamel surface morphology and the bonding of composite resin to enamel. J Oral Rehabil 23(4): 244–250, 1996
56. Sung E C, Chan S M, Mito R, Caputo A A: Effect of carbamide peroxide bleaching on the shear bond strength of composite to dental bonding agent enhanced enamel. J Prosthet Dent 82(5): 595–599, 1999
57. Arends J, Jongebloed W L, Goldberg M, Schuthof J: Interaction of urea and human enamel. Caries Res 18(1): 17–24, 1984
58. Titley K, Tomeck C D, Smith D C: Effect of concentrated hydrogen peroxide solution on the surface morphology of cut human dentin. Endod Dent Traumatol 4(1): 32–36, 1988
59. Rotstein I, Dankner E, Goldman A, Heling I, Stabholz A, Zalkind M: Histochemical analysis of dental hard tissues following bleaching. J Endod 22(1): 23–25, 1996
60. Rotstein I, Lehr Z, Gedalia I: Effect of bleaching agents on inorganic components of human dentin and cementum. J Endod 18(6): 290–293, 1992
61. Pécora J D, Cruz Filho A M, de Sousa Neto M D, Silva R G: In vitro action of various bleaching agents on the microhardness of human dentin. Braz Dent J 5(2): 129–134, 1994
62. Spyrides G M, Perdigáo J, Pagani C, Araújo M A M, Spyrides S M M: Effect of whitening agents on dentin bonding. J Esthet Dent 12(5): 264–270, 2000
63. Titley K C, Torneck C D, Smith D C, Applebaum N B: Adhesion of a glass ionomer cement to bleached and unbleached bovine dentin. Endod Dent Traumatol 5: 132–138, 1989
64. Hanks C T, Fat J C, Wataha JC, Corcoran J F: Cytotoxicity and dentin permeability of carbamide peroxide and hydrogen peroxide vital bleaching materials, in vitro. J Dent Res 72(5): 931–938, 1993
65. Haywood V B, Heymann H O: Nightguard vital bleaching: how safe is it? Quintessence Int 22(7): 515–523, 1991
66. Bowles W H, Burns H Jr: Catalase/peroxidase activity in dental pulp. J Endod 18(11): 527–534, 1992
67. Anderson D G, Chiego D J, Glickman G N, McCauley L K: A clinical assessment of the effects of 10% carbamide peroxide gel on human pulp tissue. J Endod 25(4): 247–250, 1999
68. Zwahlen B J, Fife C G, Ludlow T N: Absorbance of light and heat by tooth bleaching agents. J Dent Res 77 (Spec. iss. A): 134, 1998
69. Sterrett J, Price R B, Bankey T: Effects of home bleaching on the tissues of the oral cavity. J Can Dent Assoc 61(5): 412–420, 1995
70. Rotstein I, Mor C, Arwaz J R: Changes in surface level of mercury, silver, tin, and copper of dental amalgam treated with carbamide peroxide and hydrogen peroxide in vitro. Oral Surg Oral Med Oral Pathol Oral Radiol Endod 83: 506–509, 1997
71. Rotstein I, Dogan H, Avron Y, Shemesh H, Mor C, Steinberg D: Protective effect of Copalite surface coating on mercury release from dental amalgam following treatment with carbamide peroxide. Endod Dent Traumatol 16(3): 107–110, 2000
72. Rotstein I, Dogan H, Avron Y, Shemesh H, Steinberg D: Mercury release from dental amalgam after treatment with 10% carbamide peroxide in vitro. Oral Surg Oral Med Oral Pathol Oral Radiol Endod 89: 216–219, 2000
73. Crim G A: Prerestorative bleaching: effect on microleakage of class v cavities. Quintessence Int 23(12): 823–825, 1992
74. Bowles W H, Lancaster L S, Wagner M J: Reflectance and texture changes in bleached composite resin surfaces. J Esthet Dent 5: 229–233, 1996
75. Gökay O, Tunçbilek M, Ertan R: Penetration of the pulp chamber by carbamide peroxide bleaching agents on teeth restored with a composite resin. J Oral Rehabil 27(5): 428–431, 2000

76. Fay R M, Servos T, Powers J M: Color of restorative materials after staining and bleaching. Oper Dent 24(5): 292–296, 1999
77. Rotstein I, Cohenca N, Mor C, Moshonov J, Stabholz A: Effect of carbamide peroxide and hydrogen peroxide on the surface morphology and zinc oxide levels of IRM® fillings. Endod Dent Traumatol 11: 279–283, 1995
78. Tipton D A, Braxton S D, Dabbous M K H: Effects of a bleaching agent on human gingival fibroblasts. J Periodontol 66: 7–13, 1995
79. Tipton D A, Braxton S D, Dabbous M K H: Role of saliva and salivary components as modulators of bleaching agent toxicity to human gingival fibroblasts in vitro. J Periodontol 66: 766–774, 1995
80. Curtis J W Jr, Dickinson G L, Downey M C, Russell C M, Haywood V B, Myers M L, Johnson M H: Assessing the effects of 10 percent carbamide peroxide on oral soft tissues. J Am Dent Assoc 127(8): 1218–1223, 1996
81. Curtis J W Jr, Dickinson G L, Myers M L, Russell C M: Evaluating the effects of a dentist-supervised, patient-applied carbamide peroxide bleaching agent on oral soft tissues. J Esthet Dent 7(1): 18–25, 1995
82. Giberson T P, Kern J D, Pettigrew D W, Eaves C C, Haynes J F: Near-fatal hydrogen peroxide ingestion. Ann Emerg Med 18(7): 778–779, 1989
83. Robertson W D, Helfi R C: Pulpal response to vital bleaching procedures. J Endodont 6: 645, 1980
84. Seal N S, Wilson C F: Pulpal response to bleaching of teeth in dogs. Pediat Dent 7: 209, 1985
85. Torneck C D, Titley K C, Smith D C, Adibfar A: The influence of time of hydrogen peroxide exposure on the adhesion of composite resin to bleached bovine enamel. J Endod 16: 132, 1990
86. Feinman R A, Goldstein R E, Garber D A: Bleaching teeth. Quintessence Publishing Co Inc, Chicago 1987, 12
87. Goldstein R E: Bleaching teeth, new materials – new role. J Am Dent Assoc 115: 44E, 1987
88. Schmidt-Nielsen B: The solubility of tooth substance in relation to the composition of saliva. Acta Odont Scan 7(2): 1–13, 1946
89. Hoppenbrouwers PMH, Driessens FCM, Borggreven JMPM: The vulnerability of unexposed human dental roots to demineiralization. J Dent Res 65: 955–958, 1986
90. I ARC Monograph. Evaluation of carcinogenesis risk of chemicals in humans. 36: 285–314, 1985
91. Verheyen P: Laser-assisted Bleaching: Smartbleach™. Jola 1(3): 207–213, 2001
92. Verheyen P: Lasers in Dentistry and Maxillo-facial Surgery. Belgium: European Laser Users and Research Association 2000
93. Vital tooth bleaching, in-office. CRA Newsletter 24: 4, 2000
94. Why resin curing lights do not increase tooth lightening. CRA Newsletter 8: 2000
95. Walsh L J, Wong K L, Liv J Y: Safety and Effectiveness of Tooth Whitening by in-office vital tooth bleaching. School of Dentistry, University of Queensland, Brisbane, Australia 2001
96. Goharkay K, Moritz A, Stoop U, Sperr W, Wernisch J: Laser assisted Bleaching. Effiziensssteigerung durch Zusatz eines Absorbers. 12. Internationaler Jahres Kongress der DGL, Berlin 2003
97. Bridges J B, Owens P D A, Stewart D J: Tetracycline and teeth – an investigation into five types in the rat. Br Dent J 1: 306, 1969
98. Walton R E: External bleaching of tetracycline stained teeth in dogs. J Endod 8: 536, 1982
99. Stewart D S: Teeth discoloured by tetracycline bleaching following exposure to daylight. Dent Practitioner 20: 309, 1969
100. Stewart D J: The effects of tetracyclines upon the dentition. Br J Dermatol 76: 374, 1964
101. Wallman I S, Hilton H B: Teeth pigmented by tetracycline. Lancet 1: 827, 1962
102. Walsh L J, Wong K L, Liu J Y: Surface and intra-pulpal changes during laser photochemical and photothermal bleaching. Esola, 2nd Laser Congress, Florence, Italy 2003
103. Walsh L J, Liu J Y: Digital image analysis of changes in tooth shade with laser photochemical and photothermal bleaching. Esola, 2nd Laser Congress, Florence, Italy 2003
104. Walsh L J: The current status of laser applications in dentistry. Aust Dent J 2003 (preprint)
105. Tam L: Vital tooth bleaching: review and current status. J Can Dent Assoc 58(8): 654–663, 1992
106. Overloop K, Blum R, Verheyen P: Esthetic Dentistry with Smartbleach: An Overview of Clinical Laser. J Oral Laser Appl 2: 129–134, 2001
107. Lado E A, Standley H R, Weisman M I: Cervical resorption in bleached teeth. Oral Surg 55: 78, 1983
108. Taylor G N, Madonia J V, Wood N K, Heuer M A: In vivo autoradiographic study of relative penetrating abilities of aqueous 2% parachlorophenol and camphorated 35% parachlorophenol. J Endod 2: 81, 1976
109. Harrington G M, Natkin E: External resorption associated with bleaching of pulpless teeth. J Endod 5: 344, 1979
110. Kehoe J C: PH reversal following in vitro bleaching of pulpless teeth. J Endod 13: 6, 1987
111. Freccia W, Peters D, Lorton L, Bernier W: An in vitro comparison on non vital bleaching techniques in the discolored tooth. J Endod 8: 70, 1982
112. Holmstrup G, Palm A M, Lambjerg-Hansen H: Bleaching of discolored root-filled teeth. Endod Dent Traumatol 4: 197, 1988
113. McCornick J E, Weine F S, Maggio J D: Tissue pH of developing periapical lesions in dogs. J Endod 9: 47, 1983
114. Steiner D R, West J D: A method to determine the location and shape of an intracoronal bleach barrier. J Endod 20: 304–306, 1994
115. Leman R: Bleaching and restoring endodontically treated teeth. Curr Opin Dent 1: 754–759, 1991
116. Caldwell C B: Bleaching vital or nonvital teeth. J Calif Dent Assoc 42: 234–235, 1966
117. Smith J J, Cunningham G J, Montgomery S: Cervical canal leakage after internal bleaching procedures. J Endod 18: 476–481, 1992

11

Laser-Atlas Surgery

F. Beer

with contributions from C. Maiorana, G. E. Romanos

11.1 Introduction

General Remarks. Surgical indications were the first dental applications for which newly developed lasers were used[1,2]. After initial attempts, the laser was also used routinely within the field of surgery[3,4].

At least 10 different wavelengths for surgical indications. A large number of devices operating with different wavelengths, and innumerable publications, are available that treat diverse partial aspects of this subject. The indication spectrum in the oral-surgical sector is just as varied as the suitable wavelengths that can be selected. If the recommended wavelengths can be reduced to two to three for other dental indications, the list of those that can be chosen in surgery, depending upon the tissue and its localization, is about ten different laser types of various wavelengths. In oral surgery, the hard laser is used routinely.

Four surgical methods. Thus, beside "traditional methods" such as the scalpel, cryo-surgery and electrical surgery in the sense of diathermy (= endothermy), laser surgery can be considered as the fourth option at the dentist's disposal. For which indication each of these four methods should be preferred used, has not yet been clarified definitively; the laser represents, however, in each case, a passable alternative. With the increasing importance of forensics in our field, and with the obligation to explain to the patient, the obligatory offering of laser as a treatment alternative has to be taken into consideration.

Surgical methods today:
scalpel
diathermy
cryotherapy
Laser
Laser used routinely since ca. 1965

11.2 Specific Problems in the Context of Surgical Indications

Sterility, Duration of Operation and Re-invasion of Germs. Due to the special milieu in the oral cavity, the establishment of sterile conditions during operational interferences causes a problem almost impossible to solve; the intraoral flora consists of ~ 50 million germs, representing over 300 different species. Of course, not all of them are potentially pathogenic. Even after a "lege artis" accomplished operation preparation, only reduction of bacteria is achievable, and there will never be absolutely sterile conditions. With increasing operation duration, there is the danger of a re-invasion of the OP-area from the remaining microorganisms (Fig 11-1).

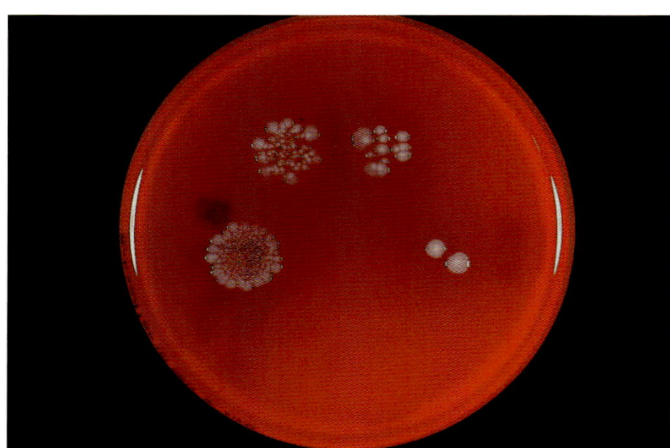

Fig 11-1 Cultivated bacteria in nutrient medium.

Restricted Spatial Conditions. The natural orifice of the mouth constantly limits the unhindered view of the operating surgeon to the area of operations. That means that the necessary simultaneous employment of several instruments is limited. Especially with very young patients (palate clefts in babies), this lack of space places enormous burdens on the surgeon. Control of intraoperative bleedings, as they arise, or other problems that occur, are also more difficult due to the size-restraint of the OP-area (Fig 11-2).

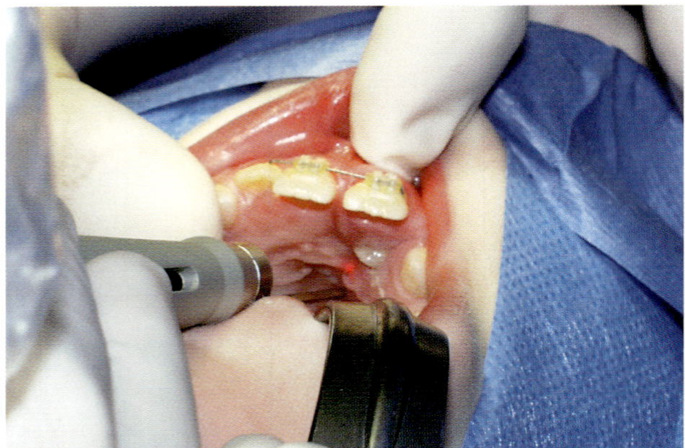

Fig 11-2 Limitation of surgical access.

Direct Neighborhood of Different Tissues. On closer examination we discover, even while performing simple routine operations, tissues of very different hardness, changing water content and differing pigment content in very rapid succession. This necessitates either a very frequent instrument change or a very narrow spectrum of the wavelength used, in order to obtain only the desired effects in the specific tissues.

Using laser types that interact with all dental tissues, in principle, but with different quality and with different efficiency, the correct choice of power settings regulates the effect that can be obtained in the single tissue.

Intraoperative Bleedings. Even with very careful preparation, the anatomic variants of some vessels in the maxillo-facial region offer, as well as rich collateralization, a permanent source for the risk of intraoperative bleeding in almost all tissues of this region. The extent of the bleeding, though usually representing no direct danger to the patient, however, considerably limits the view of the operating surgeon and causes an additional psychological stress, and through the extension of the operation time also often a physical stress on the surgeon and the patient. Postoperatively, the hematoma leads to additional edema and swelling, forming the ideal nutrient medium for bacteria that cause postoperative infections. The postoperative, frequently necessary, antibiotic therapy is for its part subject to considerable risks. The occurrence of resistances, hypersensitivity reactions and colitis, as well as the cost factor, which cannot be ignored, should be mentioned here.

Scars. Scar formation represents one of the most substantial postoperative problems. Conventional surgery can normally not be done without sutures at the end. If the operation area lies on a normally visible part of the body, scars are considered by the patients to be even more disturbing. The development of scars is not totally predictable and occasionally patients develop excessive, keloid-like scars. Scar formation after oral surgery often creates a problem for the following prosthodontic care. In the context of maxillo-facial interventions, often functionally important regions in the mouth are concerned. Restrictions on phonetics, food intake and mimic are to be feared. All these facts together reduce the quality of life of our patients considerably, and may lead to malnutrition or psychological defects due to social isolation (Fig 11-3).

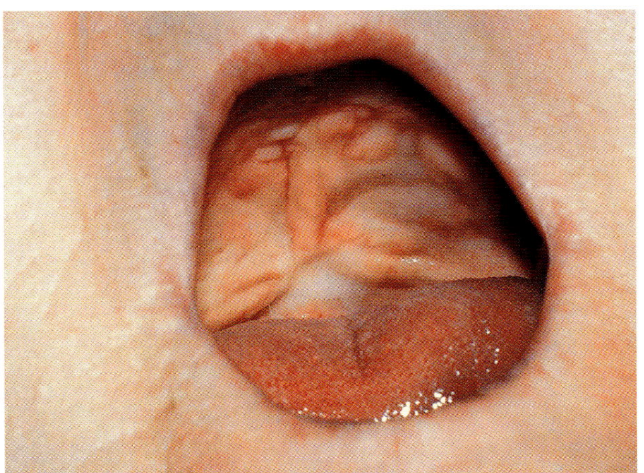

Fig 11-3 Pronounced scars after recurrent operations on a cleft lip and palate.

Reduced Operability Due to Systemic Diseases. Different internal systemic diseases represent a contraindication to surgery. Thus some urgently indicated, elective interventions cannot be accomplished in patients undergoing anticoagulation therapy, or only after a long conversion of the basic therapy. However, going off the established standard medication for anticoagulation represents a higher risk with regards to the patient's basic illness; high-grade blocking of arteries in the heart or cerebral circulation, as well as patients that have experienced thrombotic or embolic disease are examples.

In this context, also patients with hemophilia, status after radiation/chemotherapy – with the resulting reduction of thrombocytes – and patients with hematological malignomas should be considered.

Complications in the Wound-Healing Process. Another group of patients with higher operation risks are those who might develop wound-healing complications due to their internal diseases: diabetes mellitus, uremia, vitamin deficiency syndromes, as well as diseases with chronic hypoxemic conditions (obstructive lung illnesses) or chronic anemia (inflammatory intestine syndromes) often lead to deficits in the healing process. Corticosteroids, which are today commonly applied in almost all medical fields, decrease the synthesis of collagen and cause an inhibition of proliferation; thus they prepare the ground for pronounced disturbances of wound healing.

Surgical problems:
- Sterility and its maintenance during surgery
- Restricted spatial conditions
- Intraoperative bleeding
- Complications in wound healing
- Scars
- Systemic diseases

11.3 Conventional Therapy

Conventional therapy includes the use of scalpel, eletrotomy and cryosurgery, which are described separately below and shown as a survey in table 11-1.

Scalpel. The use of the scalpel offers the advantages of easy handling, as well as minimal trauma of the surrounding tissue. The main problem with traditional intraoral surgery remains the maintenance of sterile conditions. First of all, even under adherence to a standardized preoperative treatment, only germ reduction in the oral cavity is achievable. Secondly, dependent on the surgery duration, the germ population in the area of intervention increases during surgery. Bleeding must be stopped by surgical procedures or by means of electrocoagulation. In the field of oral as well as maxillo-facial surgery, the preparation of different tissues is only possible by using a larger quantity of necessary equipment (scalpel, shears, milling tool, drill, chisel…) (Fig 11-4).

The operation wound must be closed with sutures or through bandage plates created by the technician. The plates are created from a cast, or a pre-existing prosthesis of the patient is used. In the maxilla these bandage plates are fixed with one or two mini-osteosynthesis screws at the vomer and removed after 1 week.

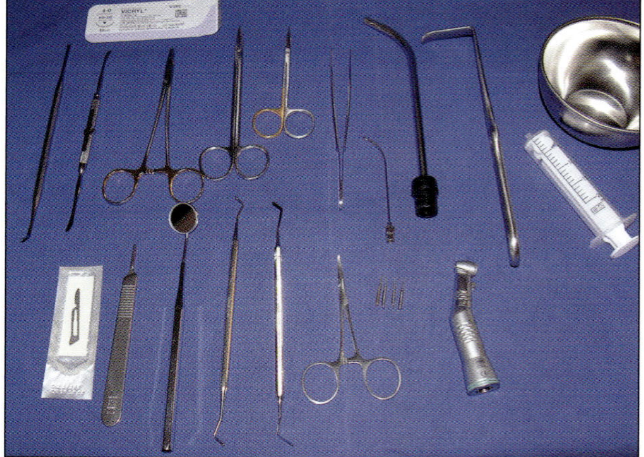

Fig 11-4 Surgical instruments; many different instruments are needed for preparation, hemostasis, and wound closure.

Table 11-1 Conventional Therapy.

	Sterility	Precision	Bandage	Healing
Scalpel	–	+	necessary	+
Diathermy	(+)	–	necessary	–
Cryotherapy	(+)	(+)	necessary	(+)

In the lower jaw, these wound-coverings are fixed by peri-mandibular-led wires for the duration of the wound healing time[5].

This leads, particularly with large defects, to an often time-consuming, complex mobilization of the surrounding tissues creating mucogingival interpolated flaps and/or distant flaps. In the 1950s, free epithelialization was favored after excisional surgery[6] followed by free skin transplants[7] and later on, by free gingival grafts[8]. Furthermore, changes in the mucosa quality can be achieved by conditioning or excision and replacement by new tissues. Both the secondary epithelialization, as well as the sub-mucus preparation, or gingival graft can complete the job. Wound closure in extended defects is achieved by means of suture-fixed iodoform-strips, which support the process of granulation on the one hand, and provide wound-protection during nutrition on the other hand, or by the previously mentioned bandage-plates. The result of this method is a partial re-epithelialization after 3 and more weeks (Fig 11-5).[9]

A favorable side effect of the conventional method is the limitation of expenses, a fact worth considering in times of increasing costs for medical services (initial costs, maintenance costs, etc.).

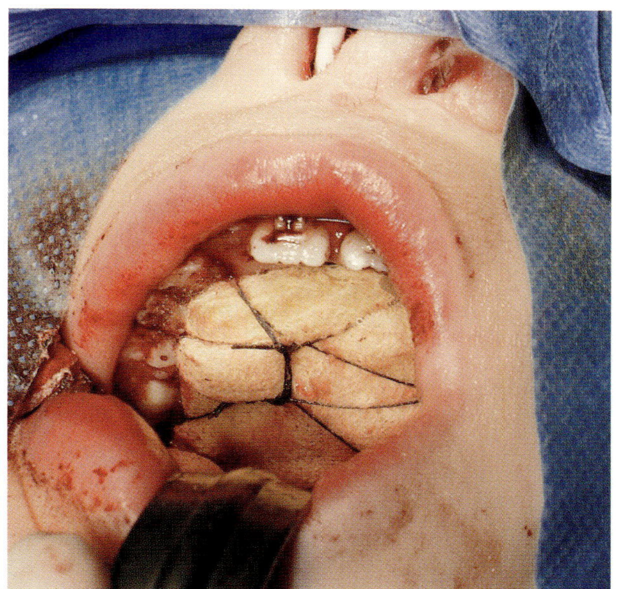

Fig 11-5 Wound closure with an iodoform-strip after excision of a palatal, pleomorphic adenoma.

Electrotomy. The main advantage of electrotomy lies in perfectly unstressed cutting in the soft tissue. The hemostasis due to heat development causes a very clear view of the operation field, suggesting the primary area of application of this technology to be strongly vascularized tissues and/or tumors (e.g., strongly vascularized soft fibromas). The Joule's heat developing at the electrode is responsible for the decreased bleeding, the increased asepsis and less tumor cell spreading. The heat, which is responsible for the desiccation effect, causes, however, necrosis of the surrounding tissue, which is not of predictable depth. This can particularly produce noticeable effects if one of the principles of electrotomy – never repeat a cutting within 20 s – remains unconsidered. Only after this short period will the directly surrounding tissue be sufficiently enriched with intercellular liquid that damage to far distant tissue portions will be avoided. Mainly due to the extended trauma of the surrounding tissue, healing after electro-surgery, in relation to scalpel-accomplished surgery, is clearly retarded. An advantage of electrical surgery is the execution of excision and coagulation with one instrument. Ending electro-surgical interventions also means application of bandage-plates, as described before, or iodoform-strips for wound closure.

Cryosurgery. Hemangiomas represent the main operational area for cryosurgery. A disadvantage of this technique is the multiple sessions, performed every 4 weeks, which permit a prognosis only from session to session. Hemangioma in the maxillary-facial area, which is treated frequently in childhood, requires the compliance of very young patients, which is difficult. Also, hyperkeratosis can be eliminated by cryosurgery[9]. The usually small defects are entrusted to granulation.

11.4 Laser Therapy

Advantages of Laser Therapy. The advantages of laser therapy are similar to electrical surgery concerning coagulation of the wound area combined with the precise cutting force of scalpels.

In contrast to electrical surgery, the necrosis zones are accurately assignable for the respective wavelengths, and/or the power density applied in each case.

Comparable to diathermy (electrotomy), only one instrument is necessary for the excision and coagulation. In the case of the laser, completely different effects can be obtained by simple changes of pulse duration, average power and pulse repetition rate by the same laser, which means one tool acts as several "instruments" for the operator[10]. The chance to execute several necessary surgical steps with only one tool is of major importance in the very narrow space relations of the oral cavity (babies, OP at the soft palate/uvula)[11].

It is, therefore, accepted that the necessary time exposure will be lowered for each patient by omission of the instrument change during the OP, as well as the clearly shortened pre- and post-processing time. This will have to be evaluated in the light of changing financial and personnel resources.

Usually surgery can be done, even in large wound areas, without a surgical bandage or a plastic graft. One advantage of the laser as an "optical scalpel" is the minimization of the expansion of post-operational edema.

Sterility in the Operational Area. It has been documented in numerous studies that the laser creates locally (in the processing region) sterile conditions. The lasting sterility in the OP area results in a reduction of the bacteraemia concomitant to the operation.

A special situation is represented by quasi-intraosseous wounds, as in apicoectomy. The use of a laser, and especially the use of the Er:YAG laser, leads to a very low microbiological contamination in the resection cavity, which is not obtainable with conventional rinsing solutions[12]. Komori et al.[13] assessed the attainable sterility in the lesion as comparably positive, but considered also parameters such as contact-free preparation, absence of vibrations, postoperative reduction of pain, with all of these parameters being very important for patient comfort. In these cases, the use of the Er:YAG laser leads to the possibility of working on all tissues involved (soft tissue, bone, dentin) equally well; possibilities which the CO_2

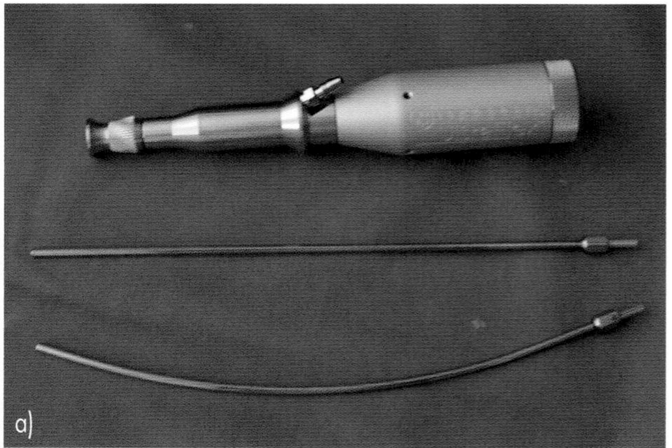

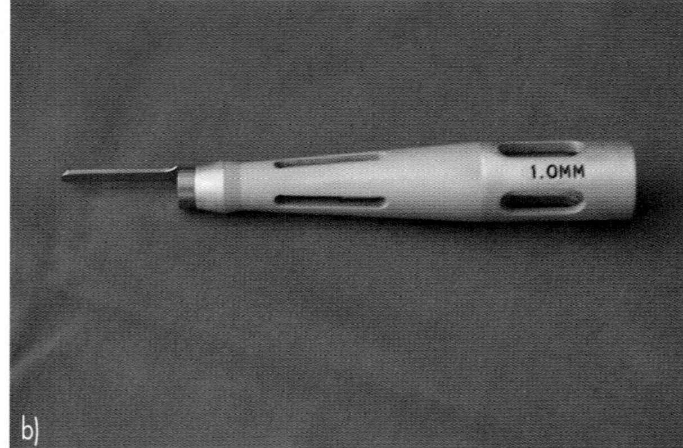

Figs 11-6a and b Different handpieces allow easy access to various operation areas.

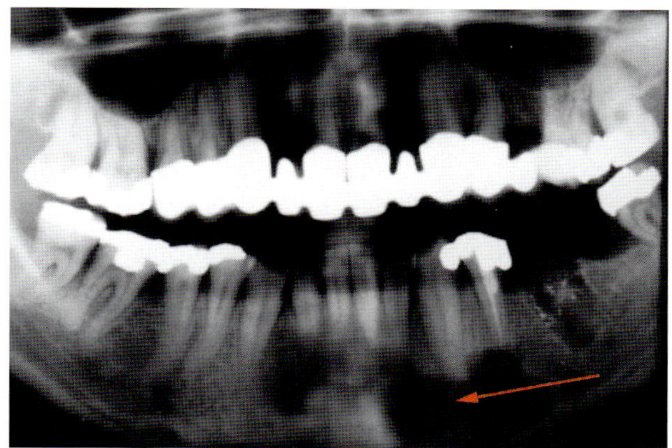

Fig 11-7 Cyst in region 34 (OPG).

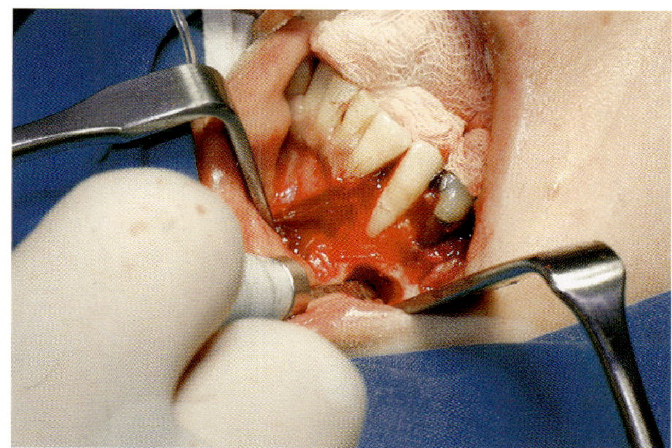

Fig 11-8 Sterilizing the cavity of the cyst after cystectomy and apicoectomy.

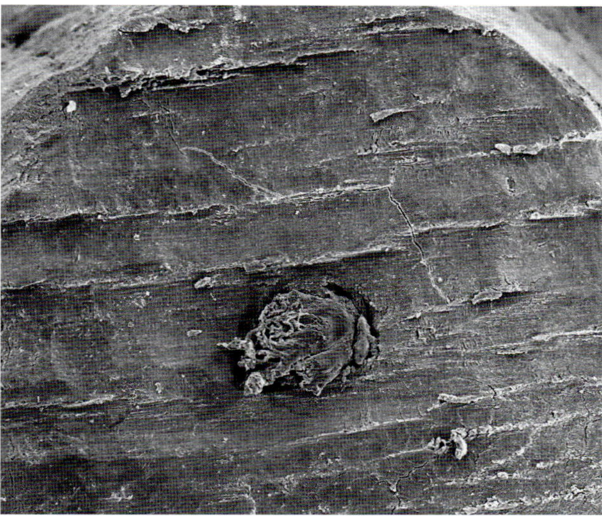

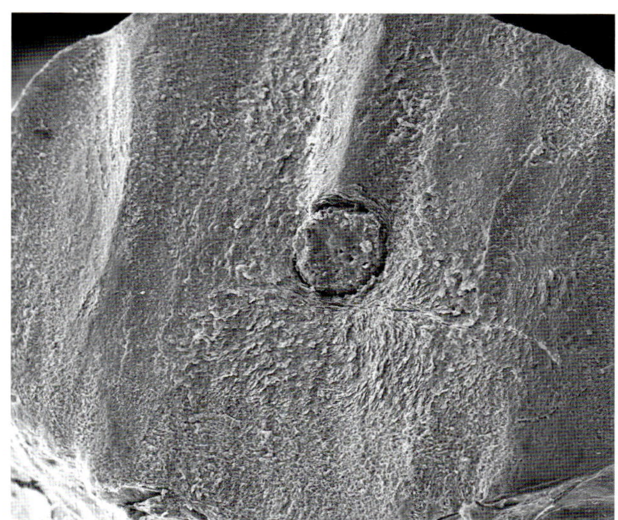

Fig. 11-9a and b REM picture of a resected tooth after Er:YAG laser treatment (a) or after conventional apicoectomy (b).

laser can only offer in a very reduced way and diodes and Nd:YAG laser cannot offer at all.

Blanc et al.[14] found (in vitro), even for *Enterococcus faecalis* – the problematic germ par excellence – 100% eradication after CO_2 laser irradiation, corresponding to the proven operational parameters.

Ando[15] proved the bactericidal effect also for the Er:YAG laser, whereby destruction of bacteria occurred already at power densities far below the clinical operational parameters. Already at an energy density of 0.3–0.4 J/cm^2, he found areas of inhibition of bacterial growth on the tested agar plates.

The bactericidal characteristics of the different lasers were investigated, particularly in endodontology and periodontology. Almost all of the wavelengths used produced excellent results[16].

Surgery of septic wounds also benefits from the advantages of lasers (Figs 11-10 to 11-13).

Pain Reduction Intra- and Post-operative. Many international studies have shown further advantages of laser surgery compared to conventional surgery, such as the lowering of the pain level (intra- and post-operative), an almost bleeding-free operation field, as well as a low incidence of postoperative hemorrhages, all of which reduce

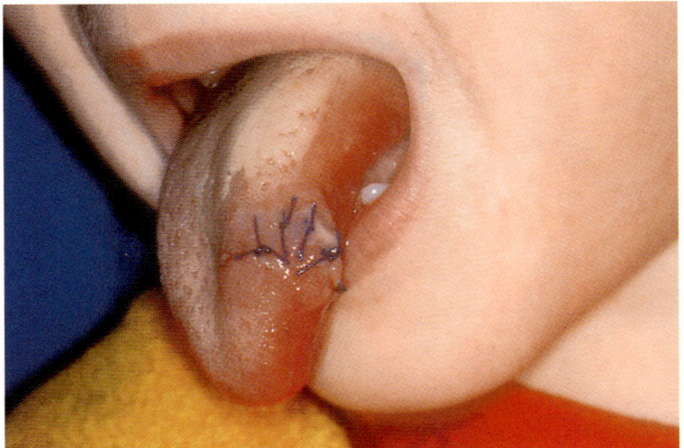

Fig 11-10 A 6-year-old patient suffering from a bite in the tongue after a fall, primarily closed with sutures 1 week before, excessive granulation, dolor, signs of inflammation and infection.

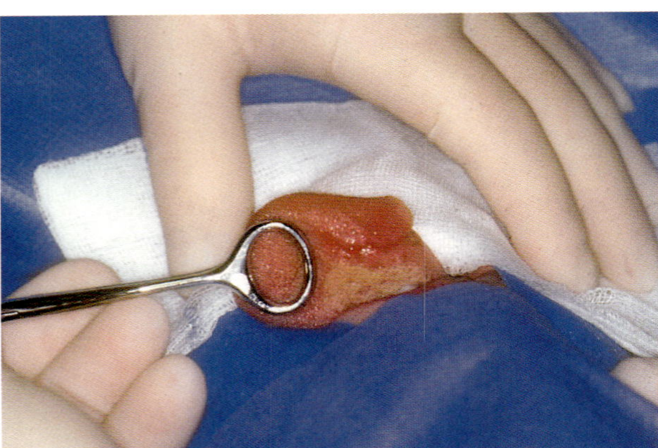

Fig 11-11 After removing the sutures, dehiscence of the wound is clearly to be seen.

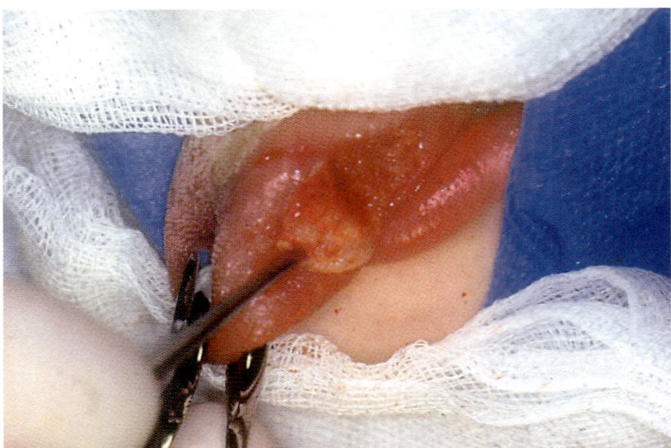

Fig 11-12 Debridement, contouring of the wound surface, CO_2 laser, pulsed mode, 3 W.

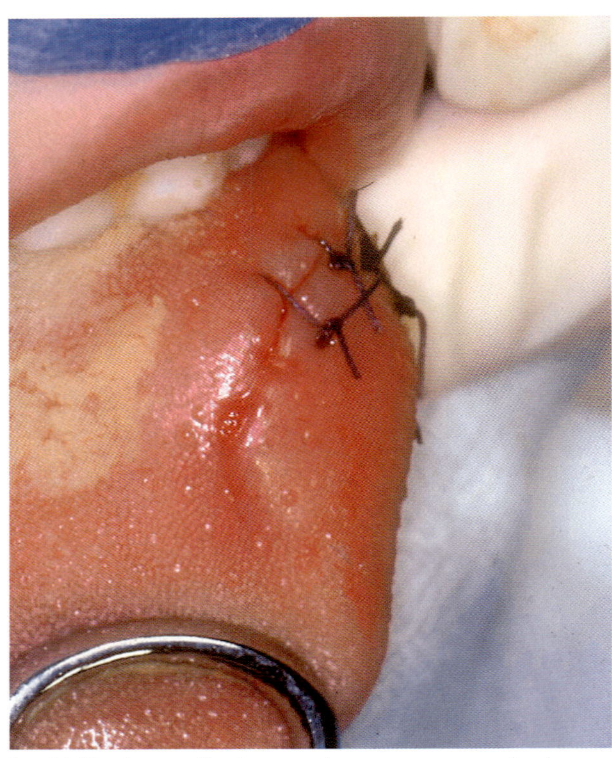

Fig. 11-13 In cases like this, wound management cannot be done without sutures.

the psychological load for both the patient and the surgeon[17,18].

Salina et al.[19] observed, in 50 patients with various types of fibromas, a striking reduction of intra- and postoperative pain. Furthermore, they documented the reduction of local anesthetics, as well as the relief of the strain on the surgeon by the absence of bleeding and time saved through omission of wound closure with sutures.

Pogrel[20] indicated in his patients, treated with CO_2 laser (frenotomies, plastic tuber reduction, hyperplasias, periodontal surgery), a significant reduction of the postoperative pain experienced, registered by the VAS-linear pain scale. In cases of preprosthetic surgery (vestibuloplasty, fibromas due to irritation by prosthesis, etc.) postoperative painlessness permits insertion of the prosthesis immediately after surgery.

A problem of many study settings is the fact that the applications of the lasers are not compared with interventions that were accomplished with traditional surgical technology, thus being "one armed" studies[21].

Even studies with very large patient collectives – as for example Gaspar et al.[22], who describe a total collective of 789 patients operated on with lasers – do not use control groups.

Furthermore, parameters like post-surgical pain, impairment with food intake or comfort of using artificial dentures, are subjective criteria and only meaningful with patients who experienced comparable interferences with the application of both operation techniques.

In a study by Richter[23], such a pool of patients was examined. He reports that all patients preferred laser surgery to conventional surgery. After the laser operation all patients clearly indicated fewer complaints, and/or expressed complete freedom of post-surgical afflictions.

White et al.[24] treated a group of 29 patients with periodontological indications on two OP-sites with the Nd:YAG laser, on one hand, and conventional surgery on the other. Patients could not avoid anesthesia in the scalpel-treated areas, but reported only discrete pain in the lased sites, even without anesthesia. They also graded the postsurgical pain as lower in the laser-treated OP-sites.

Reduction of the Incidence of Bleeding. A major advantage of the use of lasers in surgery is the reduction of the incidence of bleeding complications and/or the substantially reduced blood loss. The reduction is indicated in some studies at up to 36%[25,26].

Especially when operating in babies and small infants, one has to keep in mind that those patients tolerate blood loss considerably less than adults. Even at a blood loss of ca. 50 ml, life-threatening, hypovolemic shock can be provoked. Clinical studies showed that laser application in operations of cleft lip and palate patients, treated with von Langenbeck palatoplasty or interpolated flaps, reduces the intra-operative blood loss (13.4% in conventional surgery, 8.6% in laser surgery) and therefore lowers the frequency of transfusions[27].

It has to be noted that the different lasers show a very unequal coagulative capacity. For treatment of richly perfused tissues (e.g., tongue) or the excision of hemangiomas, many authors prefer the Nd:YAG laser[28]. Thus, for example, in patients with massive gingiva hyperplasia due to cyclosporine medication following organ transplantation, the ablation of tissue by lasers is regarded as the preferred treatment, since only that way can massive bleeding be avoided (Figs 11-14a–c).[29]

Therapy in Patients with Coagulopathies. Laser therapy is used for patients with coagulopathies and in some clinical centers is used preferentially for this indication[30]. Ackermann[31] reports on a collective of 1000 patients, predominantly carriers of hemophilia A and B, thrombastheny, thrombocytopeny, as well as other rare hemophilia inhibitor diseases, who could be treated in most instances under ambulant conditions, often without substitution therapy.

It must be pointed out, however, that in recent times the risk of the transmission of AIDS and hepatitis in the course of a substitution therapy must be calculated. In particular, this holds true for patients with anticoagulative therapy, who could acquire these infections during thrombocyte transfer. Every opportunity to avoid the additional application of human blood components is appreciated.

Patients with high-grade hemophilia must be substituted according to the severity of the illness and supported perioperatively with desmopressin (DDAVP). Above all, the substitution with coagulating factors is very cost-intensive and must be continued until complete wound healing. So, special attention should be paid to a rapid, uncomplicated healing, which is to be expected generally after laser surgery.

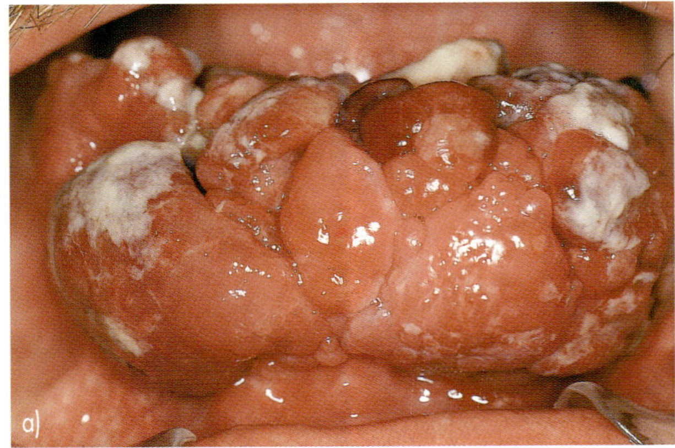

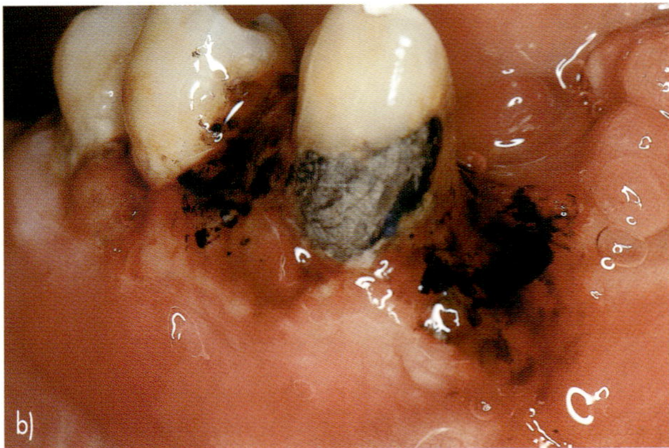

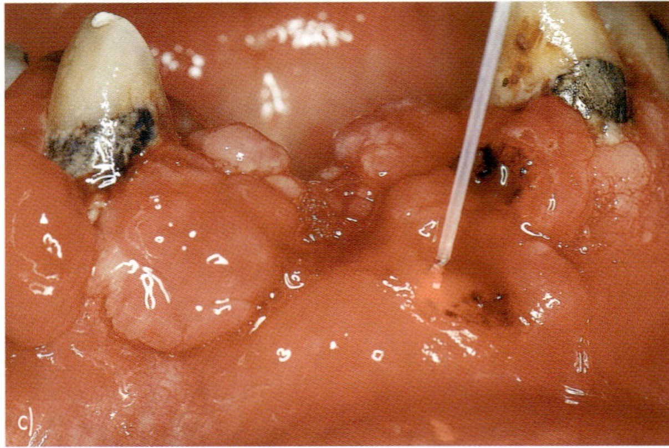

Figs 11-14a to c Excision of the cyclosporine-induced hyperplasia was done with a CO_2-laser. The surgical procedure was carried out without disturbing bleeding, and the postoperative process was uneventful.

Wound Healing. In analyzing the effects of lasers on wound healing, there must be differentiation between two kinds of application. On the one hand, different lasers are used as so-called hard lasers (i.e., "optical scalpel"), on the other hand, the possibility exists to use lasers with low energy in the sense of "low level laser therapy" (LLLT). The latter are said to have a positive influence on healing by the stimulation of metabolic processes in the surgical area (see chapter 13).

Hard laser. The influence of the use of a hard laser on the surrounding (vital) tissue and the associated side effects on the healing represent an important aspect, which affects the decision pro and versus laser application in oral surgery.

Not only wavelength and energy density influence the collateral damage of the surrounding tissue. This kind of damage is reducible through the use of an energy density as high as possible at a pulse duration as short as possible. The configuration of the necrosis zones can not be influenced exclusively by the choice of operative parameters. Laser incisions with the same wavelength, same energy density but different beam deliverance systems or different hand pieces, cause completely different configuration of necrosis in collateral tissue (Figs 11-15, 11-16). The form and width of collateral necrosis influences the appearance of scars, as well as the duration of the wound healing period.

Scholz and Grothues-Spork[32] reported on an explicit reduction of collateral damage when using a CO_2 laser with continuous irrigation of the incision gap with gas, where the kind of gas has no influence on the result. They described an increase of cutting depth by up to 100% and decrease of thermal effects less than to 10%. Inflating the incision gap enables the laser beam to penetrate unimpeded to the bottom of the incision without ablating or injuring parts of the tissue protruding from the margins.

One of the critical topics in the first studies on CO_2-laser application in maxillo-facial surgery[33] was the damage to the bone in the area of operation (within the scope of the incision). Minimal damage to the bone was observed, the healing process of the gingiva seemed however not to be endangered, although the duration of the healing period was retarded compared with conventional

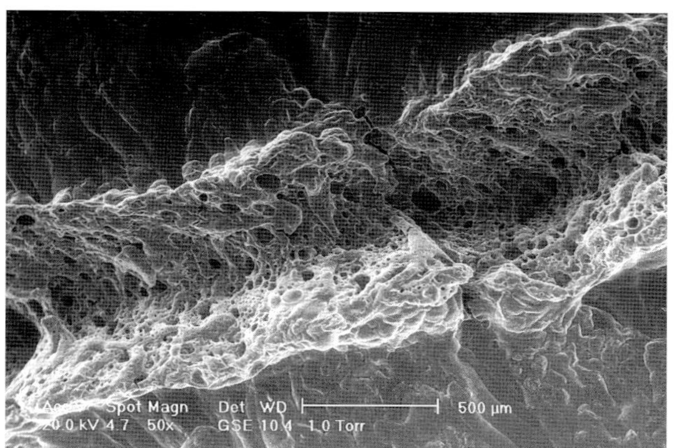

Fig 11-15 Different configuration of incision using identical wavelength (λ = 10,600 nm), energy (3 W) and application mode (cw), but different beam deliverance systems. Beam via hollow conductor.

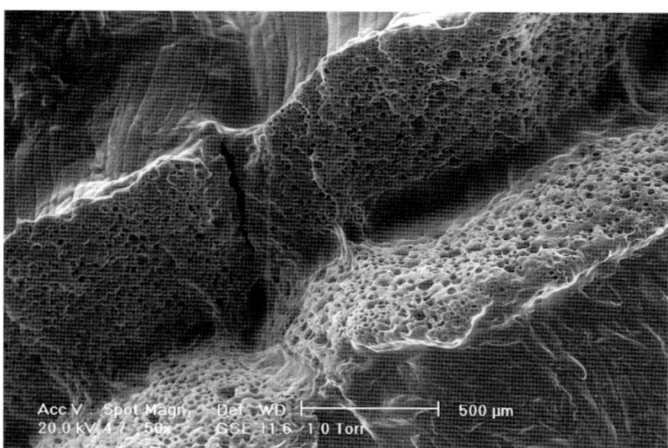

Fig 11-16 Free running beam via articulated mirror arm.

technology (scalpel). Later investigations confirmed this presumption.

Clayman et al.[34] found in comparative investigations on the cutting capacity of cw, superpulsed CO_2 lasers, that the superpulsed mode requires considerably less energy for cutting, but that bone regeneration proceeds equally fast and regularly – via the deposition of trabecular, followed by lamellar, bone.

Recent results of an in vitro study with a Q-switched CO_2 laser lead to the hope that also in bone surgery a breakthrough can be expected[35].

Today's standard in the use of lasers in bone surgery are Er:YAG, Er:YSGG, and to a certain extent also the Ho:YAG laser.

Nearly all early studies on bone surgery with lasers deal with the CO_2 laser, with which in the beginning extremely high energy levels were applied. All authors report healing retardation after laser osteotomies[34,36–38]. Already, however, the sterilizing effect of lasers was recognized[39].

An improvement of coupling of the laser light into the bone tissue is reported by Müller et al.[40], using a wavelength modification of the CO_2 laser to $\lambda = 9.6$ µm.

The Er:YAG laser achieves even higher absorption rates in bone. Numerous studies conclude that the Er:YAG laser is particularly suitable for bone and cartilage treatment. Walsh et al.[41,42] found excellent ablation rates for the Er:YAG laser up to energy densities of 20 J/cm^2. Energy increase beyond this level caused plasma formation and decrease of ablation[43].

Scholz and Grothues-Spork[32] showed very low plasma formation using this special wavelength, which means no "glazing" at the incisional margins. Likewise, they found no carbonization products in the incision cleft. This implies less healing retardation than in conventional osteotomy.

In animal experimental studies, the effects of laser application were examined for the cells and the cellular matrix, which are responsible for the healing process in the epithelium as well as the connective tissue, and compared with conventional scalpel incisions[44–46]. Due to heat development, clear differences showed in the reaction of the tissues. The result is a clearly slower healing after laser interventions compared with incisions with a scalpel. An advantage of laser surgery lies, however, in the fact that it seals capillaries and lymphatic vessels directly while cutting, and thus the expansion of postoperational edema can be diminished[17].

Kirschner and Low[47] used the dye-laser for elimination of capillary tumors in combination with conventional surgical methods (shaving for harvesting histological samples and afterwards photocoagulation of the remaining tumor). With this method, they observed in all cases only punctual, barely visible scars; a fact which is even more important as most of those lesions are located in the face/mucosa with special cosmetic relevance.

The differing temperature development is not only correlated to the wavelength used, but also to the energy density and pulse configuration. Thus, Buccalo and Moy[48] reported a significant increase of inflammatory cells in the wound area after the use of a 900-μs dwell-time laser in comparison to the use of a 90-μs pulsed laser. The clinically observable erythema after the use of the 900-μs dwell-time laser correlates with those findings.

Luomanen[49] states that in the laser wound, including the boundary regions, extracellular proteins of the connective tissue, which play an important role in the avoidance of contractions, were found without the presence of necrotic tissue. In the immunofluorescence analysis, they appear as type IV collagen and β–fibronectin and in the immunoperoxidase stain as laminin. Following Gaspar[50], this is a probable explanation for the smaller scar formation after interventions by means of laser surgery compared with traditional procedures.

The desirable reduction of the hematoma, and thus the danger of infection, results in reduced antibiotic use and all its disadvantages (hypersensitivity and allergic reactions, colitis, cost factor).

Low Level Laser Therapy. Apart from the application of hard lasers for surgical interventions, laser technology is also applied as a soft laser (so called "cold lasers"; low energy laser) in "low level laser therapy". The proliferation of fibroblasts can be increased by irradiation with a soft laser, as was shown in in vitro studies[51–53].

Furthermore, the transformation from fibroblasts to myofibroblasts could be proven. In epithelial cells, irradiation by laser increased the motility of the epithelial keratinocytes. The effects of the laser on wound healing are dose-dependent. While low dosage results in stimulation, higher dosages inhibit the healing process[53].

Van Breugel[54] documented that when he used the same wavelength – in this case $\lambda = 632.8$ nm – simply varying the irradiation time determined whether cell cultures of human fibroblasts were stimulated or inhibited.

In further studies it could be shown that LLLT leads to an increase of the granulation tissue, to an early epithelialization, to an increased proliferation of fibroblasts and enhanced matrix synthesis as well as to an increased neovascularization[55]. Also, the mitotic index in epithelial cells is substantially increased by LLLT. Takeda[56] achieved an increase in the mitotic index of salivary gland epithelial cells up to five times the rate of the control group. For an optimal effect it is necessary to provide a daily treatment[53]. In view of these data, it must be mentioned that these results come primarily from animal experimental studies[56–58]. Only lately have there been clinical investigations of this subject[59]. Meanwhile, multi-center studies have proven that treatment of mucositis in patients with tumors of the oral cavity, arising following chemo and/or irradiation therapy, is particularly successful with "low level laser therapy" (HeNe lasers). Compared with conventional working methods, a substantially more rapid recovery and/or a clearly lower pain level is observed. In this study, patients had manifest problems after LLLT in only 1.9% of cases, while patients of the control group (non-lased) had manifest problems in 23.8% of cases[60].

Penetration Depths. In numerous investigations, it has been documented that the damage of the surrounding tissue due to the heat effect can be minimized by the optimization of the application mode (continuous wave or pulsed wave)[41,61,62]. Special care has to be taken for the teeth and any dental restorations present, as particularly composites can be destroyed by accidental irradiation with lasers[63]. Especially, the direct neighborhood of different tissues in the oral cavity requires a calculable penetration depth. Krause et al.[64] investigated the consequences of laser irradiation (CO_2) on alveolar bone in simulations of muco-

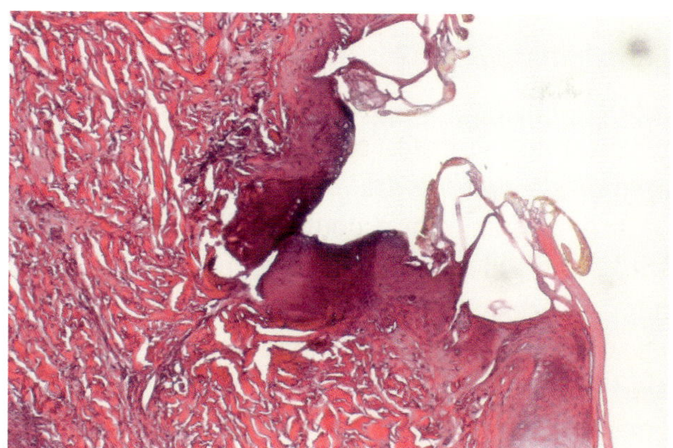

Fig 11-17 Histological specimen after incision with CO_2 laser.

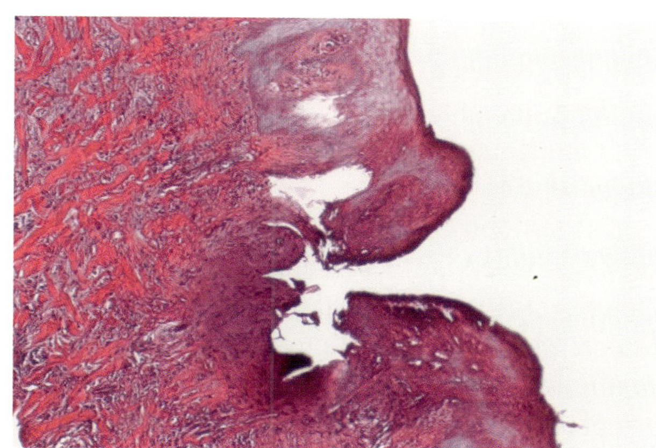

Fig 11-18 Histological specimen after incision with diode laser.

gingival surgery. They found thermal injury to the underlying bone even after only three passages at 1.032 J/cm^2, which was just enough energy to cut the mucosa.

Goharkhay et al.[65,66] found, during histological investigations of oral soft tissue after laser irradiation with different lasers, that the obtained effect depends primarily on the beam characteristics as well as on the laser parameters used, however not on the wavelength applied.

In the pulsed mode the laser achieved a higher cutting depth with minor damage to the collateral tissue than in continuous wave mode using the same performance adjustments (Figs 11-17, 11-18).

Rossmann et al.[67] showed in gingival mucosa, by variation of the irradiation duration between 0.2 s and 0.5 s, while maintaining the other parameters (CO_2, 10 W, 2.0 mm spot, 400 mm focus length, cw, 90° irradiating angle), histological changes of the start of deepithelialization up to complete epithelial destruction.

Stock and Hibst[68] investigated the different penetration depths of diode ($\lambda = 940$ nm) and Nd:YAG laser in soft tissue. They observed a decreasing penetration depth at increasing carbonization and demand carbonization be achieved as quickly as possible to protect the underlying tissue.

Rosenberg et al.[69] compared the Nd:YAG and Ho:YAG laser – both outstanding in the vaporization of soft tissue – with regard to their penetration depth: for the Ho:YAG laser, they measured penetration depths of only 140 μm. That offers the possibility to accomplish rapid and, above all, very precise excisions with relatively low total energies.

Walsh et al.[70] investigated the effect of identical irradiation (CO_2) on various soft tissues. They report a significant dependence on the tensile strength of the tissues. The water content, responsible for optical and thermal features of the tissue, was also measured and considered to be not significantly different for various soft tissues. These findings suggest that the effects of various lasers in soft tissue correlate with their mechanical features to a large extent.

When performing operations with lasers it must also be considered that, through reflections due to metallic instruments, lesions can occur even in mucosal areas far distant from the actual operation field. Neiburger et al.[71] indicates tissue lesions up to 7 cm away from the focus when using a CO_2 laser (7–10 W)[71] To avoid such lesions, the use of matt-finished instruments is recommended[72].

In the field of bone surgery, a compromise is desired between sufficient ablation and cutting speed, and minimal collateral damage. The excimer laser would enable a more or less athermal ablation but, due to its inferior ablation rate, it will never be applicable in practice. Scholz et al.[73] reported on a comparative in-vitro study investigating thermal damage zones in bone created by different lasers. In doing so they tried to select optimal parameters for the different lasers for cutting with minor thermal damage at major cutting velocity. Within the scope of this study, the lowest thermal damage zones resulted for TEA-, CO_2-, excimer and Er:YAG lasers (all presenting damage zones between 30 µm and 40 µm). Stein et al.[74], with osteotomies using a Ho:YAG-laser, found the smallest thermal damage (130–220 µm) when using power densities slightly over the ablation threshold of 11 J/cm^2.

Increase of Temperature in the Tissue. Surgery of the oral cavity frequently concerns several different tissues; tissues exist at least in the direct neighborhood and/or within the range of the direct zone of thermal alteration by the laser. Knowledge about the temperature rise in different, adjacent tissues is of essential importance for minimizing the risk of thermal damage. Usually the tissue shows a linear temperature rise with increasing duration of the irradiation[75].

Economic Considerations. Apart from medical factors, (possibly in the future even more) the cost factor already plays an important role today. The very high cost of laser use represents a relevant problem; this must, however, be put into perspective in the context of saving medical costs and reducing the duration of the patient's hospitalization/period of disability. Gaspar and Szabo[76] found a significant reduction of absences at work following laser surgery.

Beyond that the question, in principle, is how far the employment of the laser can be designated as the "state of the art", or whether it represents only a further option, to be used possibly with specific problems, for example, in patients with hemangioma or hemophilic patients. Further clarification of these aspects has also to be considered in the face of the ever more important obligation to explain the undesirable risks and side-effects[77]. It is assumed that patients have to be informed about the alternative of laser treatment even today, as this special dental therapy has risen above the level of "experimental therapy"[78].

Advantages of laser surgery

- Maintenance of sterile conditions
- Reduction of bleeding
- Good possible estimation of cutting depth
- Precision of cutting
- Reduction in the number of instruments
- Often no need for suturing or bandages
- Pain reduction intra- and post-operatively
- No inhibition of, and perhaps even promotion of wound healing
- Less scars
- Less costs by reduction of material, staff and time

11.5 Lasers Used in Dental Surgery

More or less at the same time, several lasers were developed for medical applications (Javan[79]: HeNe laser, Johnson[80]: Nd:YAG laser, Patel[81]: CO_2 laser). The first reported clinical laser applications in dentistry were for treating surgical indications[82,83].

Several medical disciplines began applying lasers very early (e.g., surgery, ophthalmology, gynecology, otolaryngology, dermatology, esthetic surgery); the maxillo-facial use began only in the late 1970s and early 1980s, and use in dentistry was even later. Since that time, the spectrum of indications has been extended steadily and certain wavelengths have been allocated to defined indications.

11.5.1 Surgical Lasers Used at Present

11.5.1.1 Gas Lasers

The CO_2 laser: 10,600 nm, cw, pulsed, superpulsed. The absorption maximum lies in the range of the same spectral line as that of water, therefore it is used primarily in soft-tissue surgery[26,75].

The CO_2 laser is also used for treatment of hypersensitive dental necks[84–86] and direct pulp capping[87,88], with the CO_2-TEA-laser also used in the "drilling" of enamel and dentin[89–91].

In the special field of maxillo-facial surgery, the flexibility of the articulated arm, which is missing, is a disadvantage, as well as the high weight of the arm in many laser models. The beam is led by an articulated arm, which means that the laser light is deviated by mirrors and so led on to the focused or non-focused hand piece and to the destination. Thus, use in the "non contact mode" is possible. By using curved hand pieces with built-in deflecting mirrors it is also possible to reach areas which are not directly visible to the surgeon. The latest generation of CO_2 lasers is equipped with hollow conductors and facilitates, in this way, precise handling in narrow operation sites, although the flexibility is achieved at the price of precision of beam guidance (Figs 11-19, 11-20).

In superpulsed mode the CO_2 laser is used for skin resurfacing and gives comparable results to the Er:YAG laser, whereby through an alteration of dermal collagenous fibers, an increase of elasticity of up to 18% has been reported[92]. Very optimistic studies even report 100% good/very good results after resurfacing with the CO_2 laser, wherein discrete hypopigmentation occurred in 5.6% of the documented cases[93].

Argon laser: $\lambda = 488$, $\lambda = 514$ nm, cw, chopped. The superior high absorption in hemoglobin, hemosiderine and melanin predestined the argon laser to eliminate pigmented or strongly vascularized pathologies[94–96]. Some authors also use the argon laser in soft-tissue surgery with great benefit[97]. Its domain in the dental field is the use for composite curing and bleaching[98,99].

Helium-neon laser: $\lambda = 633$ nm, cw. This laser is used as a pilot laser for other hard lasers or as a soft laser for wound healing improvement or pain therapy[56,100,101]. HeNe lasers are largely employed in photodynamic therapy, in which the reaction of photo-sensitive, interstitially-applied substances is used to destroy malignant cells by laser light.

Biel[102] reported complete remissions of carcinoma in situ and TI after only one therapy session. In this study also, 10 patients with extensive carcinomas received PDT as adjuvant therapy, following tumor resection. Only three patients showed recurrence. Also, more recent studies show remission rates of up to 100% in early cancer in the head and neck and up to 75% palliative

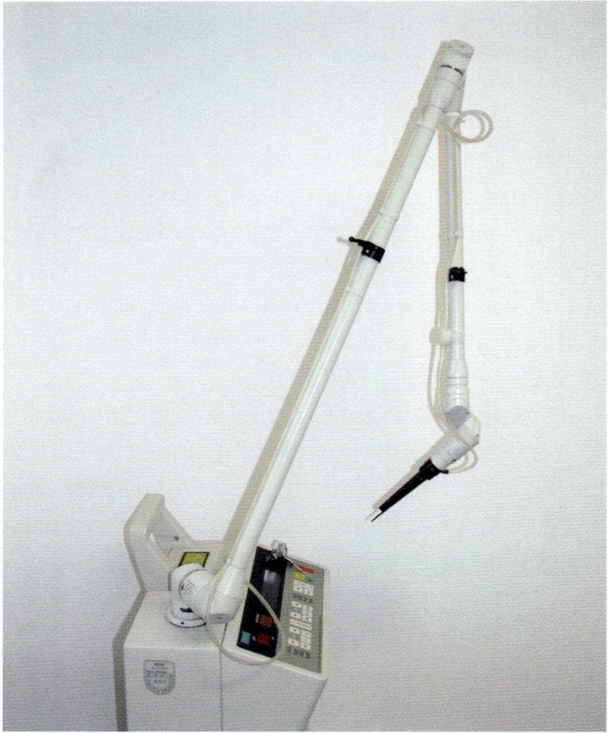

Fig 11-19 Articulated mirror arm.

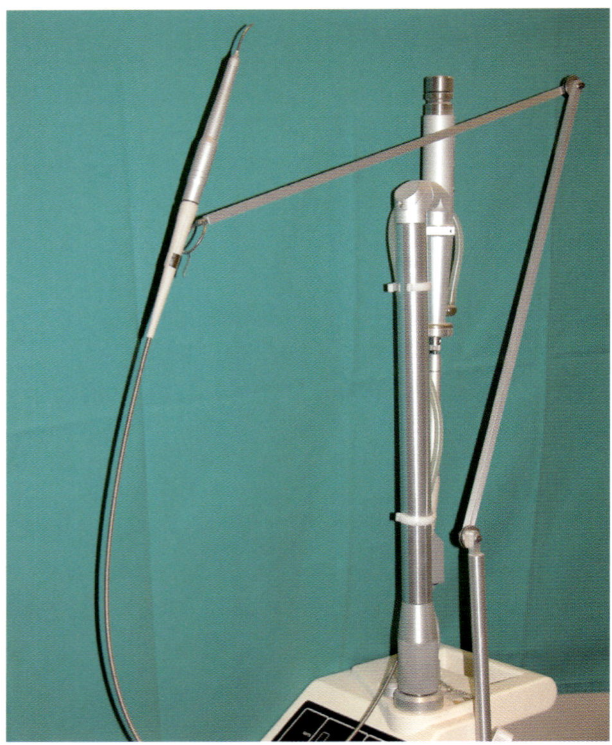

Fig 11-20 Hollow conductor.

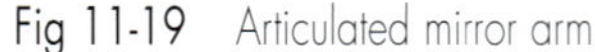

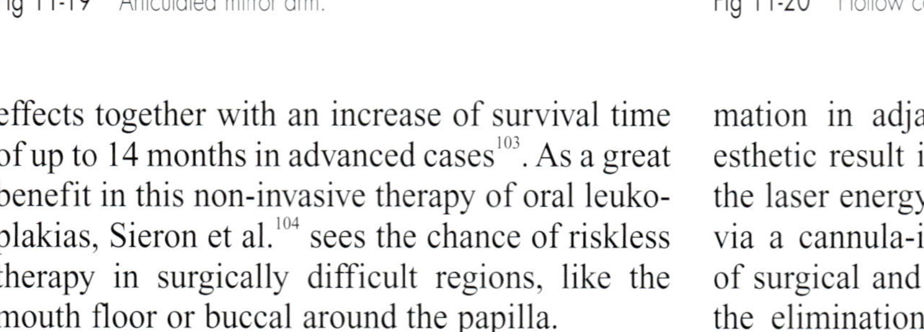

effects together with an increase of survival time of up to 14 months in advanced cases[103]. As a great benefit in this non-invasive therapy of oral leukoplakias, Sieron et al.[104] sees the chance of riskless therapy in surgically difficult regions, like the mouth floor or buccal around the papilla.

The laser machine matches the handpiece. Direct coupling is only applicable with extremely compact systems, like the soft laser.

11.5.1.2 Solid State Lasers

Nd:YAG laser: λ = 1064 nm, cw, pulsed. This laser shows low absorption in water and nevertheless has a large heating effect in the tissue and therefore good coagulation characteristics, which is why its main surgical operational indication is strongly vascularized tissues[105,106]. In percutaneous therapy of hemangiomas, after Berlien et al[107] and Romanos[108], the laser beam is led through an ice cube for sufficient cooling. Using this therapy, hemangiomas are selectively irradiated, scar formation in adjacent tissues is avoided and the esthetic result is excellent. In interstitial therapy, the laser energy is directly applied into the tissue via a cannula-inserted fiber[109]. The combination of surgical and laser therapy has proved itself in the elimination of residual hemangiomas[110] (see chapter 6).

With endodontic interventions for gangrenous teeth, it has been shown clearly that the periapical healing of radiological, clearly visible, pathological changes occurs substantially more rapidly than with conventional endodontic therapy. The deep penetration and the flexible light conductor makes it particularly suitable for this kind of treatment[111–113].

Light transport by flexible quartz glass fibers makes this laser favorable for use in the narrow space of the maxillo-facial area. The high power loss in the fiber, and the reduced focusing ability, has an unfavorable effect. Nevertheless, only fiber systems make laser application possible within unobservable areas (endodontology, periodontology). The flexible fibers are used almost exclusively in the "contact mode"; only a few recent scientific investigations report on the use of Nd:YAG lasers in non-contact mode, concerning sealing of apices in relation to apicoectomy. The fiber tip must be re-cut regularly, since the power density decreases with fiber abrasion[114].

Holmium:YAG laser: λ = 2100 nm, pulsed. The absorption in water lies between the CO_2 and Nd:YAG laser, and therefore the coagulation ability approximates the average value between CO_2 and Nd:YAG. Today's main application field is arthroscopical TMJ surgery[115–117]. The use of arthroscopes with a diameter of only 1.9 mm enables the surgeon to do interventions in areas that are difficult to access. Furthermore, there is almost no scarring, which unavoidably occurs after open surgery between the dissected tissue layers, even if the incision is made in invisible areas[118].

Erbium:YAG laser: λ = 2940 nm, pulsed. This laser exhibits a high absorption in water, with small penetration depth in the tissue (about 1 μm). Thus, besides the use in soft tissue surgery, the preparation of dental hard tissue is possible (enamel, dentin, bone). As mentioned before, selective photo-ablation of different tissues is possible with the Er:YAG laser, with special weighting on a good conditioning effect ("etching") in the enamel (fissure-sealing), and in addition for the ablation of soft tissue in the sense of "skin resurfacing". It is necessary to take care that there is sufficient water cooling because of a high thermal reaction in the surroundings[119–122]. In recent years, the Er:YAG laser has been increasingly used in the field of oral surgery (apicoectomy, etc.). Gouw-Soares et al.[12] found that the results after laser-surgical apicoectomy exceed the results after conventional surgery and trace this back to the fact of almost complete eradication of bacteria in the resection socket.

Osteotomies in orthognathic surgery are, meanwhile, routinely accomplished with lasers. This laser has a special value in implantology; incisions in the muco-periosteum, and pilot drillings for implants, can be done without difficulty[123].

Er,Cr:YSGG laser: λ = 2780 nm, pulsed. Its wavelength predestined it for the treatment of hard tissue in dentistry. This laser is, comparable to the Er:YAG, applicable in soft tissue surgery[124,125] as well as in hard tissue preparation and bone surgery[126]. Eversole and Rizoiu[127] used this type of laser for hard tissue preparation (bone) in a clinical trial in apicoectomies. Although a rather young representative of the laser spectrum for dental use, it has already achieved its place in the clinical routine.

Dye laser: λ = 510 nm (green light), λ = 577 or λ = 585 nm (yellow light), λ = 620 nm (red light), cw, pulsed. Dye lasers are liquid lasers with a variable wavelength. The Q-switched alexandrite laser (wavelength 755 nm) also belongs to this group. These machines are used for removal of tattoos, pigmented lesions and vascular anomalies[128,129]. They are also the first choice in the therapy of pyogenic granuloma[47].

Diode laser: λ = 810–930 nm, cw or pulsed. Diode lasers have the widest range of applications in dentistry. They are used in endodontology and periodontology for their capacity in bacterial reduction, but also in surgery, soft laser therapy and peri-implantitis therapy[130–138]. Beam transmission is conducted by flexible quartz glass fibers, a circumstance which makes the broad use of this laser so easy.

11.5.2 Summary

The properties of lasers used in dental surgery are compiled in Table 11-2.

Table 11-2 Properties of lasers used in dental surgery.

Laser	Wavelength(λ)	Mode	contact/ non contact	Beam deliverance	Surgical indication
CO_2	10,600 nm	cw, pulsed, superpulsed	non contact	Articulated arm, hollow conductor	Soft tissue
Argon	488 nm 514 nm	cw, chopped	non contact	Flexible fibers	Pigmented lesions Vascular anomalies Plastic surgery
He-Ne	633 nm	cw	contact, non contact	Direct coupling, flexible fibers, articulated arm	Pilot beam, soft laser therapy, Photodynamic therapy
Nd:YAG	1,064 nm	cw, pulsed	contact, non contact	Flexible fibers	Soft tissue, Periodontal surgery, Pigmented lesions
Ho:YAG	2,100 nm	Pulsed	non contact	Articulated arm, hollow conductor, flexible fibers	Arthroscopic surgery (soft tissue surgery)
Er:YAG	2,940 nm	Pulsed	non contact	Flexible fibers	Bone-surgery, Periodontology, Skin resurfacing, Lithotripsy
Er,Cr:YSGG	2,780 nm	Pulsed	non contact	Flexible fibers	Bone-surgery, Periodontal surgery
Dye	510 nm (green) 577 nm, 585 nm (yellow) 620 nm (red)	cw, pulsed	non contact	Flexible fibers	Pigmented lesions, Tattoo-removal, Vascular anomalies, Photodynamic therapy
Diode	670–900 nm	cw, pulsed	contact, non contact	Flexible fibers	Soft tissue, Periodontal surgery, Bleaching, Photodynamic therapy, Soft laser therapy

11.6 Indications

From a historical point of view it is understandable that the focus in laser use internationally varies to a great extent (e.g., CO_2 laser used in pigmented lesions in Asian countries, in contrast to argon and Nd:YAG in Europe) [39,140].

Table 11-3 Indications for lasers used in dental surgery

Indication	Laser
Gingival surgery	CO_2, Nd:YAG, Diode, Argon
Preprosthetic surgery	CO_2, Nd:YAG, Diode, Er:YAG, Er,Cr:YSGG
Decontamination in Peri-implantitis	CO_2, Diode, Er:YAG, Er,Cr:YSGG
Hyperkeratosis	CO_2, Nd:YAG, Diode, Dye
Precancerous lesions	CO_2, Nd:YAG, Diode, PDT (He-Ne)
Benign tumors	CO_2, Nd:YAG, Diode, Argon, Er:YAG
Cysts in bone, Cysts in soft tissue	Er:YAG, Er,Cr:YSGG, CO_2-TEA, CO_2, Nd:YAG, Diode, Argon
Malformations	CO_2
Scar corrections	Er:YAG, CO_2
Skin resurfacing	Er:YAG, (CO_2)

11.7 Frequently Asked Questions When Using a Laser

Usability of Histological Specimens. As the excision of benign tumors in the oral cavity, such as leukoplakias and lesions of uncertain dignity (such as PE), is one of the main indications for laser use, the indisputable evaluation of the resection borders is of great importance. In experimental studies in animals, but also in clinical trials, it was documented that the thermal damage zone is precisely calculable and therefore a certain histological evaluation is possible if the additional security zone of 1 mm is respected. Analyzing excidates, Fleiner and Plath found a mean damage zone of 0.5 mm at the resection border, whereas epithelium and basal membrane stayed unaffected. In animal experiments, the ATPase-activity of cells was measured after excision with a CO_2 laser, pulsed mode, with differing energy from 1 to 5 W. On average, the width of the ATPase-negative zone was 200 µm, and using cw-mode they measured 500 µm, reaching up to 800 µm maximum[141]. It has to be mentioned that the ATPase-negative zone is much wider than the histologically evaluable zone of carbonization effects. The latter is limited to less than 100 µm, this result also correlating with the findings of Goharkhay et al.[66].

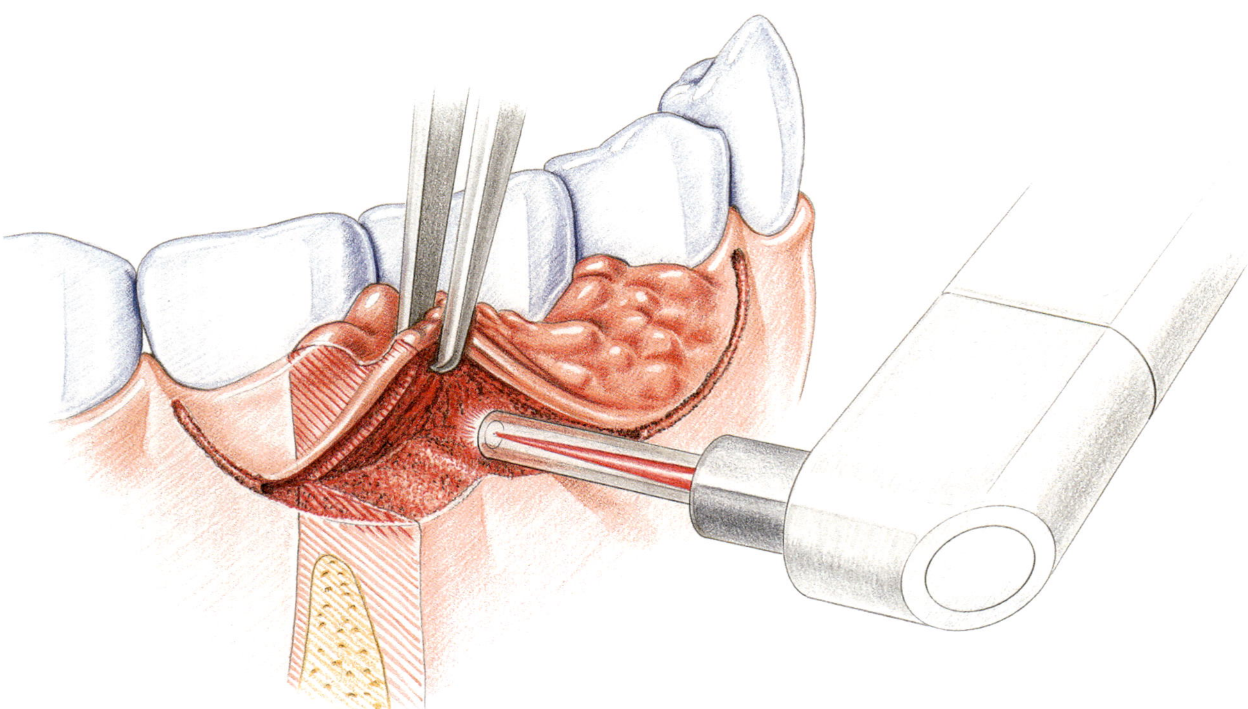

Fig 11-21 Graphic: excision; straining the tissue, incision is made with movements similar to the use of a scalpel. Choosing the exact parameters, each single muscle fiber or connective tissue fiber can be dissected.

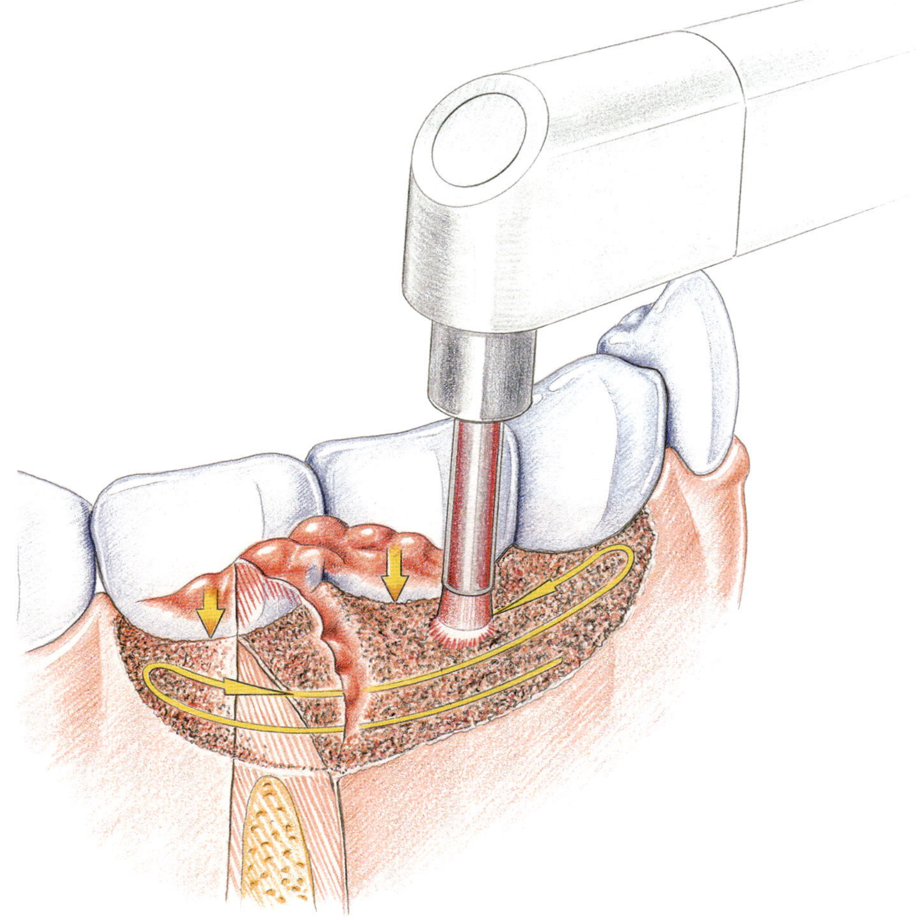

Fig 11-22 Graphic: vaporization; the laser is used in a sweeping motion, passing over the tissue in meanders. The most superficial tissue layers are vaporized at a time. This way contouring the tissue is possible. Highest esthetic demands can be satisfied using this procedure.

Vaporization or Excision. Only with a non-ambiguous histological result or clinically unsuspicious appearance, have we the choice between the two alternatives, e.g. the elimination of ranulae. Studies showed a slightly higher incidence of scars after vaporization compared to excision, where the higher thermal incrimination of the tissue using the cw-mode for vaporization might be responsible[142].

11.8 Practical Proceedings

11.8.1 Preparation of the Patient

General medical aspects: Interventions in **local anesthesia** do not need internistic preparation, as long as the medical history did not reveal a hint of a systemic disease which could restrict the patient's operability in general.

Only patients with anticoagulative therapy would have their medication preoperatively changed from Marcoumar to low-molecular heparin, after consideration of their individual risk concerning their basic disease. The operation is carried out beyond a TT-level of 20%. Patients with ASS-therapy have to pause their therapy for 7 days. The medication of high-risk patients stays unchanged, and patients are treated under stationary observation. Patients suffering from diabetes mellitus are controlled concerning dietary compliance, such as insulin medication, thus minimizing wound healing complications.

Patients treated under **general anesthesia** are prepared following the anesthesiological "state of the art" (X-ray, ECG, laboratory tests, internistic survey, sometimes other necessary examinations).

Information on the operation is given at the time of the first appointment and the operation date is fixed so as to give the patient time enough for deliberation and not put psychological pressure on him due to an immediately following operation.

Content and result of the briefing are documented in the patient's history.

Directly Preoperative, Standardized Procedures:

Operations in local anesthesia

1. Patient is given Chlorhexidine mouth wash.
2. If necessary, depending on the patient's compliance and the operation planned, surface analgesia with, e.g., Xylocain Pumpspray, 1 pump-shot = 0.1 ml = 10 mg Lidocain (Astra GmbH, Linz) or Xylogel enfant (Septodont, Vertrieb Austrodent, A-4021 Linz), local or conduction anesthesia with, e.g., Xylanaest dental 3% or Scandicain 3%.
3. Patient and medical staff are given protective goggles appropriate to the wavelength.
4. Chair/OP is provided with laser safety equipment (danger sign, door-contact-circuit-breaker), their function is controlled. The whole laser treatment is executed following the safety guidelines of the international norm IEC 60825-1, called EN 60825-1 in Europe[143].
5. Again rinsing with Chlorhexidine, perioral disinfection with, e.g., Octinisept farblos (Schülke & Mayr, D-22840 Norderstedt).
6. Sterile covering (e.g., Raucodrape, Rauscher, 1140 Vienna).

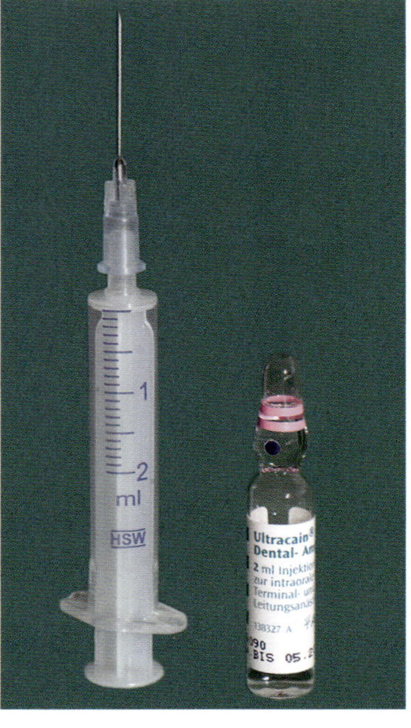

Fig 11-23 Local anesthesia with 3% Scandicain (if necessary).

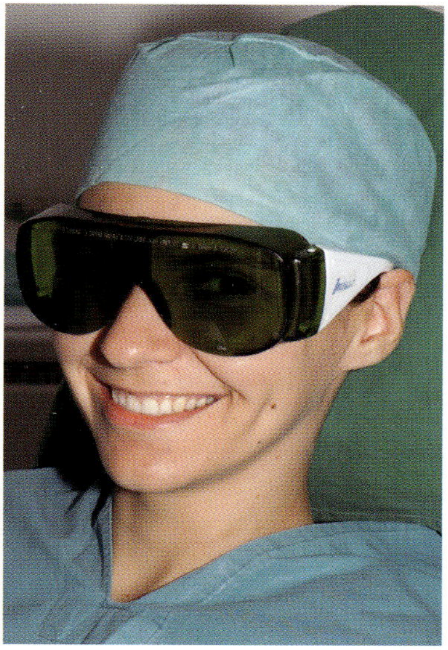
Fig 11-24 Patient wearing protective goggles, sterile covering, cap.

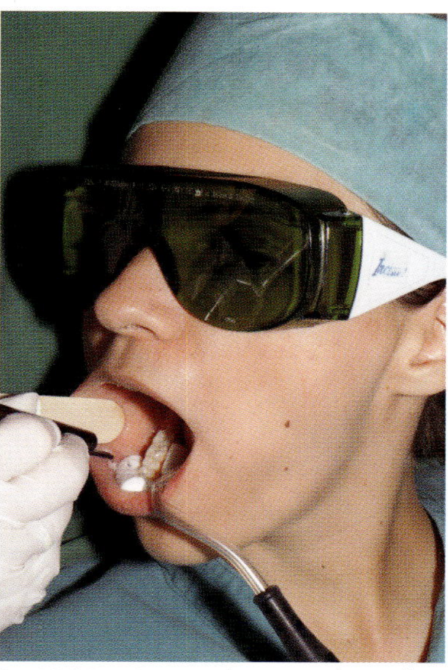
Fig 11-25 Covering the surroundings of the operation area with moist cotton wool rolls or gauze to avoid reflections.

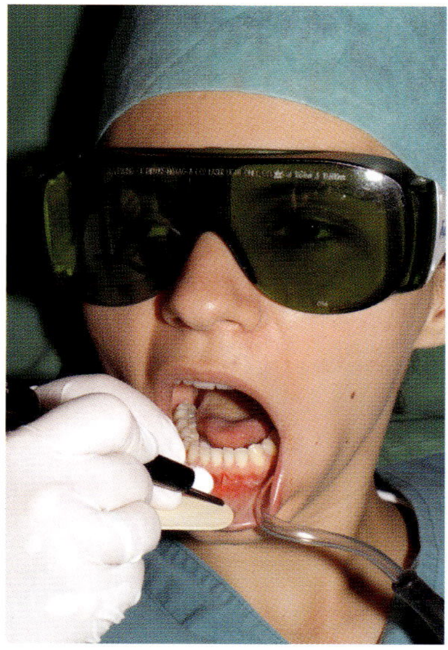
Fig 11-26 Using non-metallic or matt-finished instruments also minimizes possible lesions due to reflections.

Interventions under general anesthesia

1. Bedding of the patient following safety standards (use of supporting rests, electric insulation, cooling-protection).
2. Sterilization of the operation area following the standards of the surgical unit.
3. All medical staff are given protective goggles.
4. OP is provided with laser safety equipment (danger sign, door-contact-circuit-breaker), their function is controlled. The whole laser treatment is executed following the safety guidelines of the international norm IEC 60825-1, called EN 60825-1 in Europe[143].

11.8.2 Laser Surgical Interventions

The exact procedure of the interventions is described in the cases following. The choice of the power settings depends on the clinical appearance of the lesion on one hand, and on international standards on the other hand[65]. Treating superficial, soft lesions needs low energy levels, while indurated, hard tissues require higher energy levels. To avoid reflections, matt-finished instruments should be used and the surrounding tissue is covered up with moist gauze or absorbent cotton rolls. This also avoids reflection on metallic fillings.

Coagulation of the intraoperative bleeding that occurs is accomplished by variation of the working distance, thus producing a different energy density, or carbonization of the wound surface at the end of the operation, using cw-mode. Ending the operation, the wound is rinsed with physiological NaCl solution, wound are closed with sutures (only necessary in wide gaping wounds), and finally application of Solcoseryl Dental adhesive paste (Solco Basel, CH-4127 Birsfelden) is applied.

Wound control should be done 2 and 8 days postoperatively, with further appointments depending on histology and status of the patient.

11.9 Indications and Cases

11.9.1 Benign Tumors

Epulides. In removing epulides, all of the benefits that lasers provide can be utilized (hemostasis, no wound closure, sterility)[144]. Especially when this lesion occurs during pregnancy, the possible reduction of local anesthetics would be desirable. In addition, fewer recurrences are reported after laser surgery of these lesions[145].

Case 1

A 73-year-old male patient, partially edentulous, inappropriate oral hygiene, 15 cigarettes/day.

Medical history: hypertonia, on medication (Figs 11-27 to 11-30).

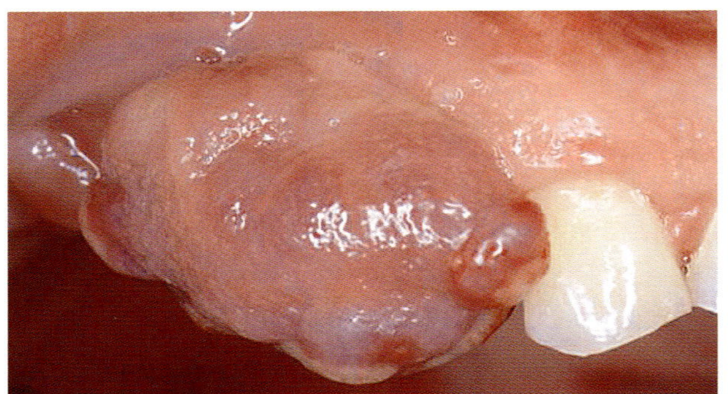

Fig 11-27 Epulis on the gingival tissue of the upper jaw.

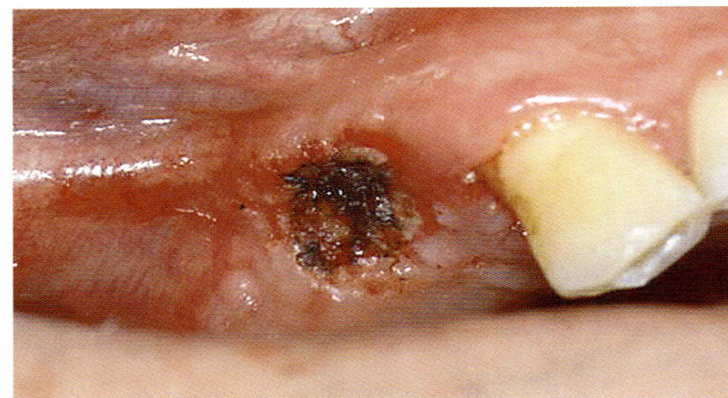

Fig 11-28 After the surgical laser, exeresis with an $\lambda = 810$ nm diode laser, 4 W, cw.

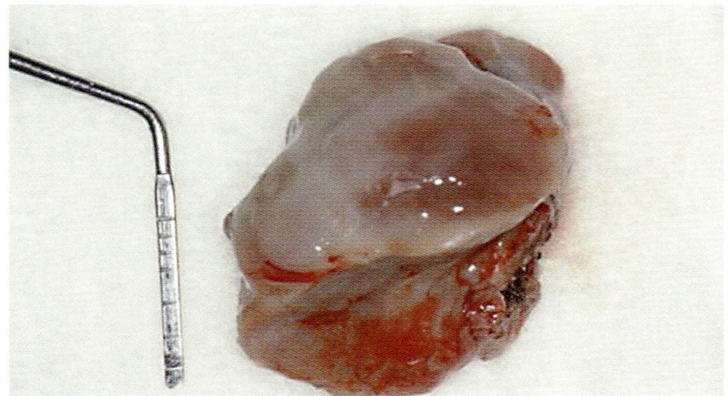

Fig 11-29 The histologic specimen.

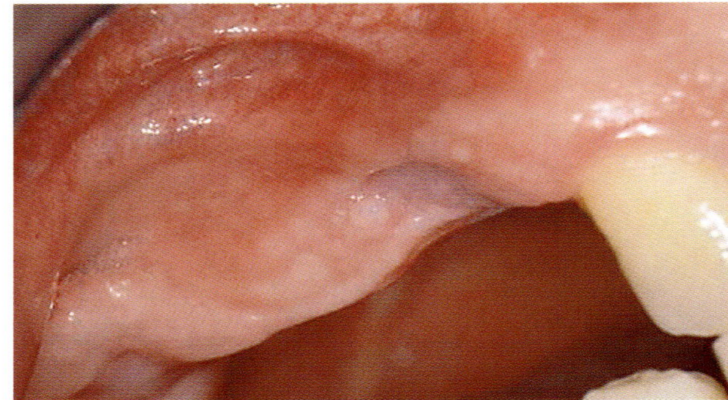

Fig 11-30 Postoperative condition after 18 days .

Case 2

A 65-year-old male patient, totally edentulous with an upper ill-fitting complete old denture; terrible oral hygiene. In the right upper vestibulum an *epulis fissurata* is located due to the non-fitting prosthesis. The patient suffers from diabetes mellitus and is a non-smoker (Figs 11-31 to 11-38).

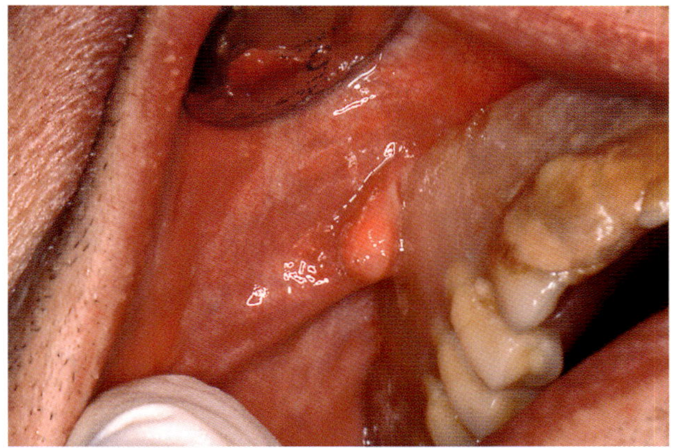

Fig 11-31 The epulis fissurata caused by the ill-fitting upper denture.

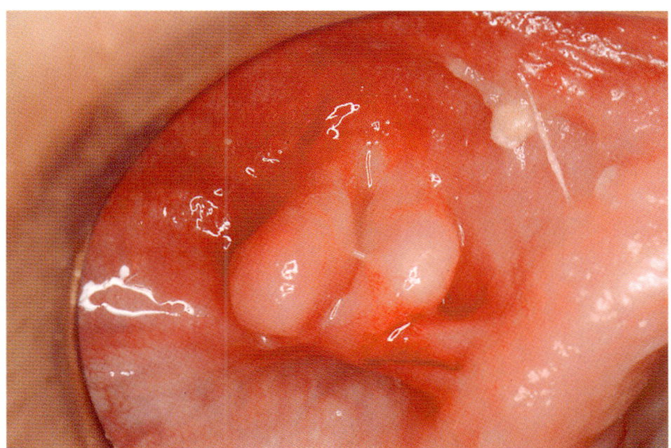

Fig 11-32 The particulars of the lesion.

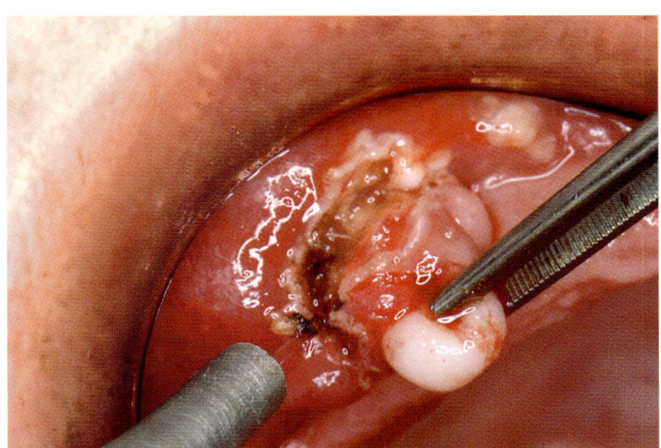

Fig 11-33 During the surgical laser procedure, Nd:YAG laser, 6 W, 150 mJ, 40 Hz, local anesthesia.

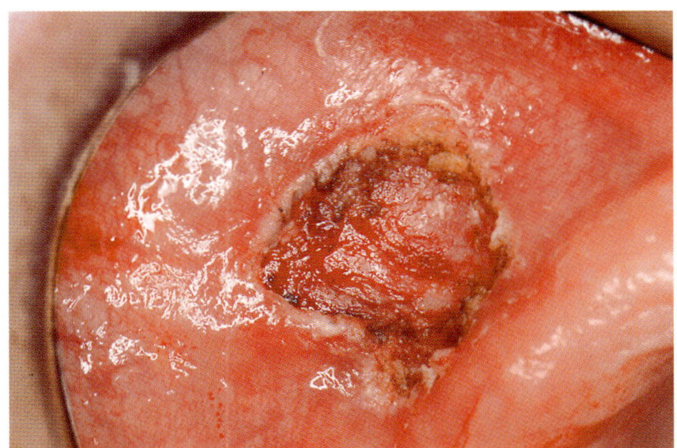

Fig 11-34 Immediately after treatment with an Nd:YAG laser.

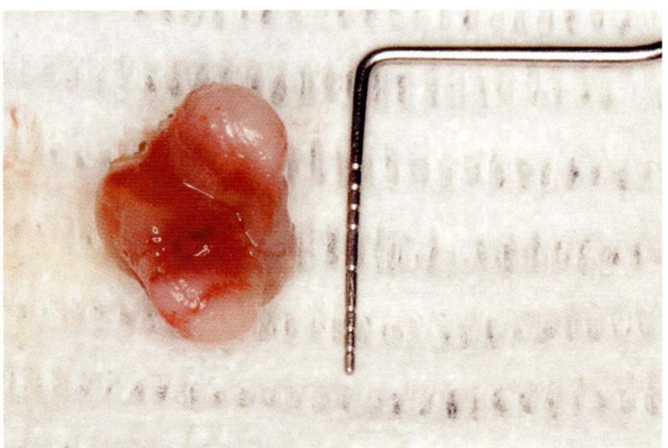

Fig 11-35 Histologic specimen.

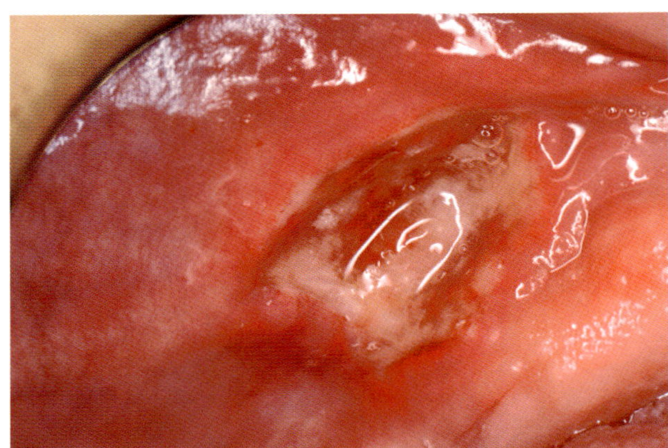

Fig 11-36 One week post-operation.

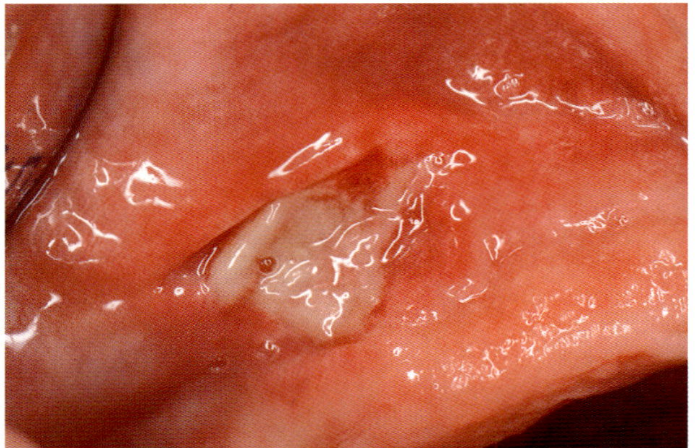

Fig 11-37 Two weeks post-operation.

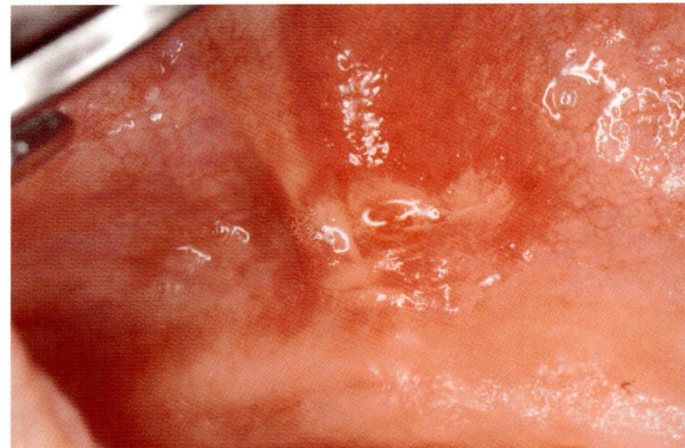

Fig 11-38 Final control after one month, patient was also provided with a new prosthesis.

Hemangiomas are the domain of the Nd:YAG laser. Small lesions are vaporized or excized; bigger, cavernous hemangiomas, which often destroy adjacent, important structures (orbital floor, nose, tongue) due to their massive growth, can be treated with interstitial therapy. The fiber of the Nd:YAG laser is directly inserted via a cannula into the hemangioma and pushed forward under continuous coagulation. Reduction of the hemangiomas reaches up to 100% in some cases[146]. Maiorana et al.[147] reports exceedingly good results in a big clinical study. First and foremost, he states the low rate of complications and the high patient comfort as an advantage of laser surgery in comparison to conventional scalpel surgery. To reach an optimal result, the technique with the ice cube is appropriate[108].

Case 3

A 52-year-old female patient, presenting a 2-mm micro-hemangioma on the lower lip, which is considered mechanically and esthetically disturbing (Figs 11-39 to 11-41).

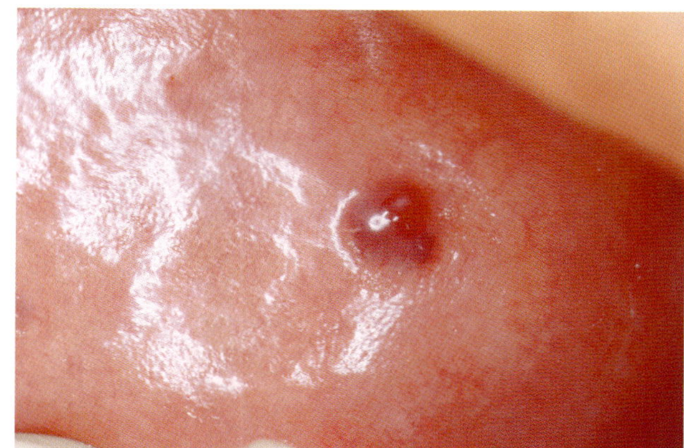

Fig 11-39 Hemangioma of the lower lip, 2 mm.

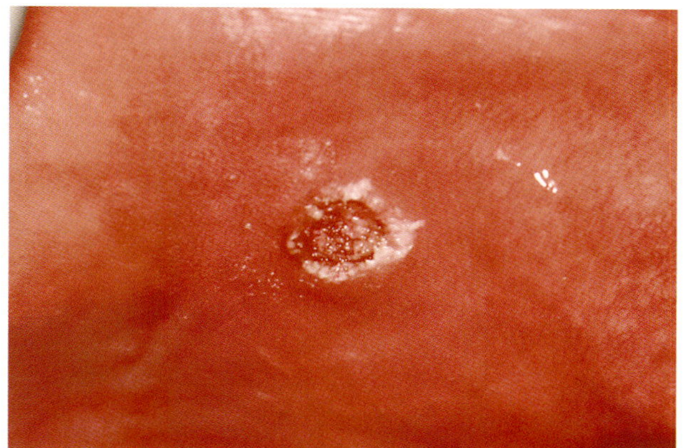

Fig 11-40 Immediately after vaporization with the Nd:YAG laser.

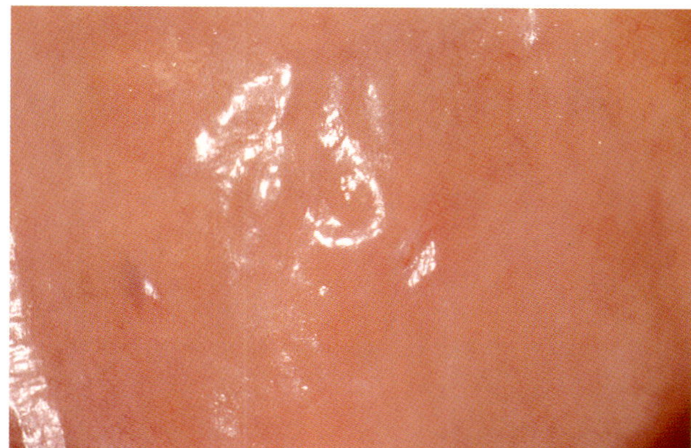

Fig 11-41 14 days postoperatively.

Case 4

A 54-year-old male, moderate diabetic, partial dentition, oral hygiene very bad, smoker: 15–20 cigarettes/day (Figs 11-42 to 11-45).

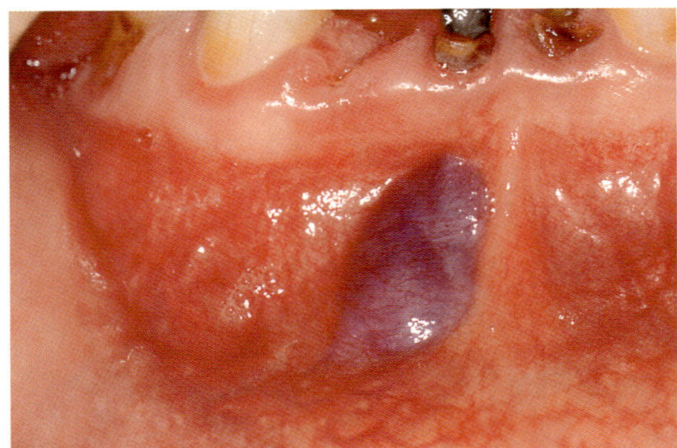

Fig 11-42 Hemangioma of the vestibulum of the lower jaw.

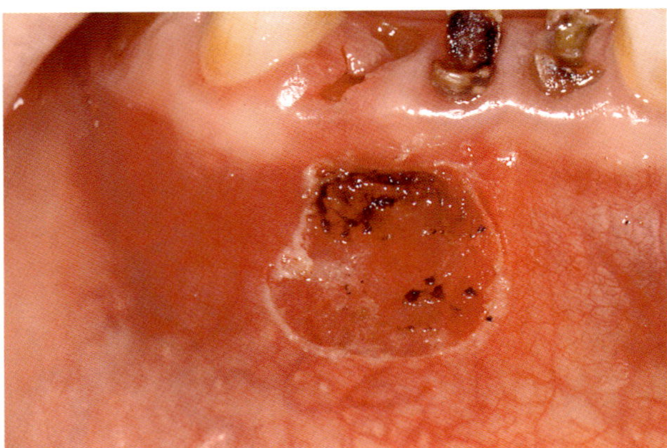

Fig 11-43 The op site after the Nd:YAG laser excision: 4 W (100 mJ and 40 Hz); anesthesia: local infiltration.

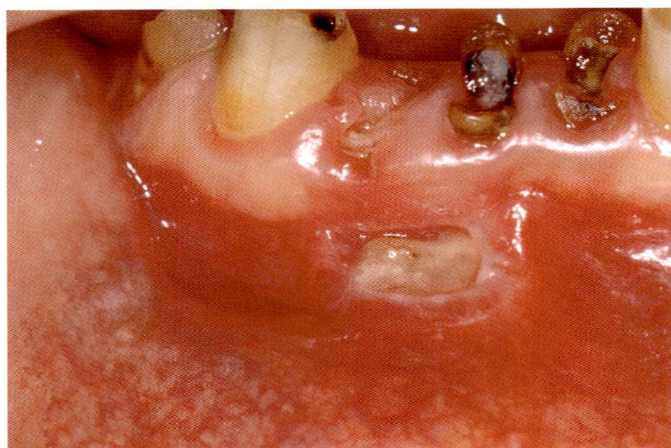

Fig 11-44 After 10 days the epithelial deficiency due to the operation looks already covered by newly formed tissue.

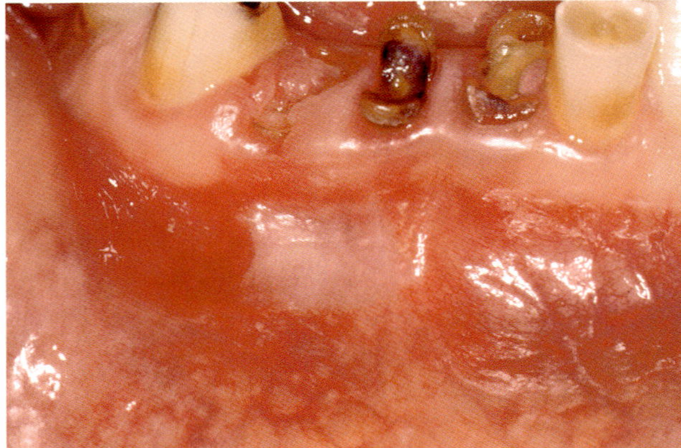

Fig 11-45 After 30 days the treated area appears healed.

Case 5

Hemangioma of the lower lip, destined to be eliminated by Nd:YAG laser (Figs 11-46a–c).

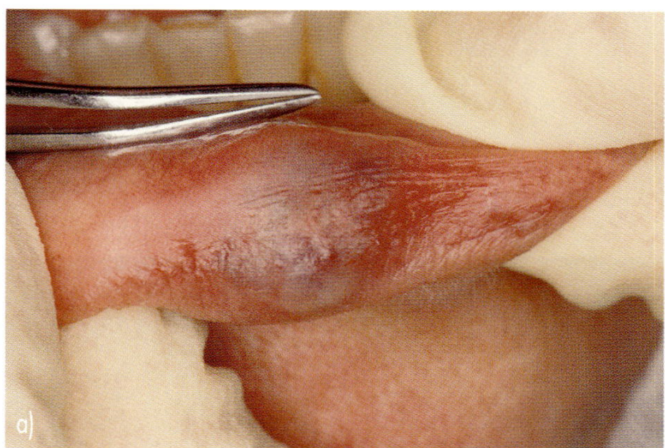
a)

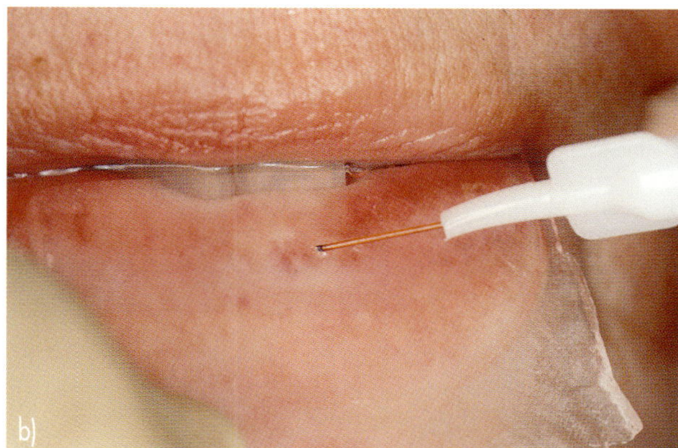
b)

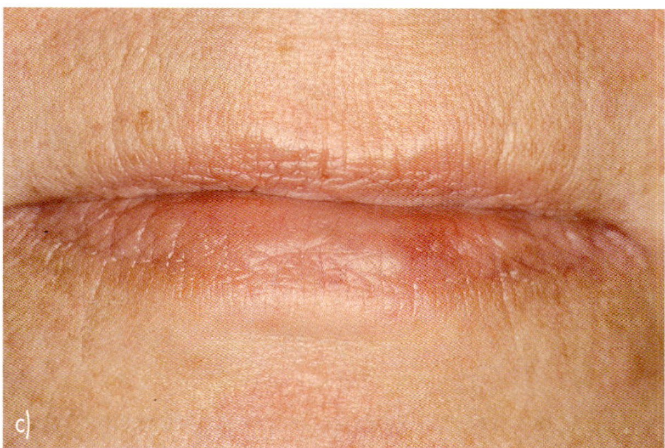
c)

Figs 11-46a–c Preoperative situation of a hemangioma of the lip (a); ice cube-technique and laser treatment (b); postoperative result after Nd:YAG laser application (c).

Case 6

A 68-year-old female patient, good general condition, non-smoker. Sent to the hospital because of a tumor in the right upper vestibulum. Sonographic examination suggests it to be a lipoma (Figs 11-47 to 11-55).

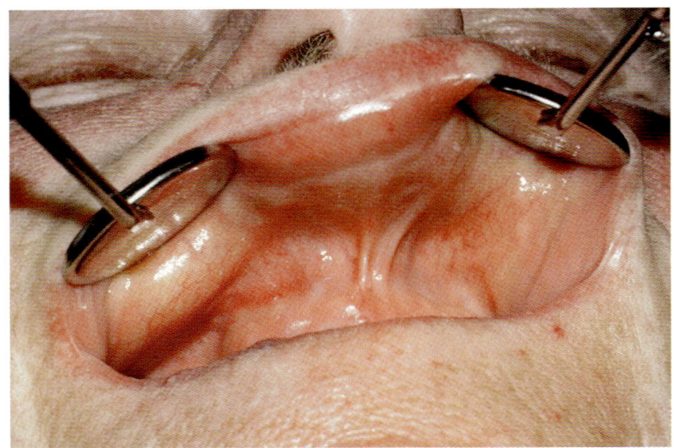

Fig 11-47 Clearly visible tumor in the right upper vestibulum.

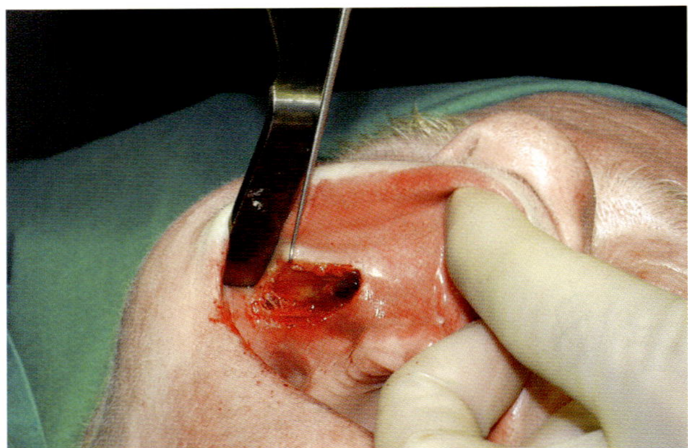

Fig 11-48 Incision with the CO_2 laser, superpulsed mode, 5 W, focused.

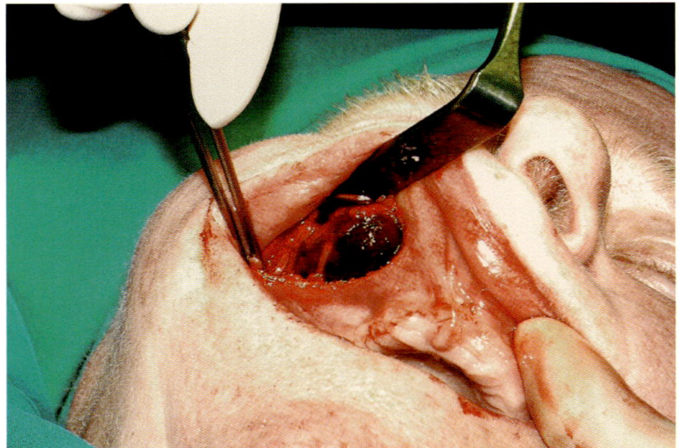

Fig 11-49 The sonographically-assessed lipoma intraoperatively turns out to be a cavernous hemangioma.

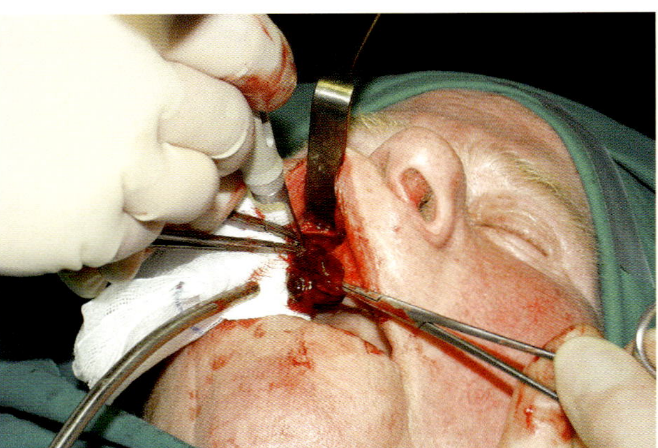

Fig 11-50 Further preparation with the laser and exposition of the hemangioma.

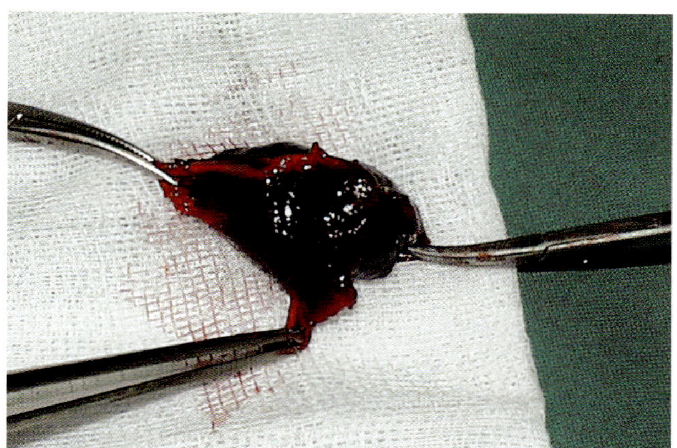

Fig 11-51 Histologic specimen.

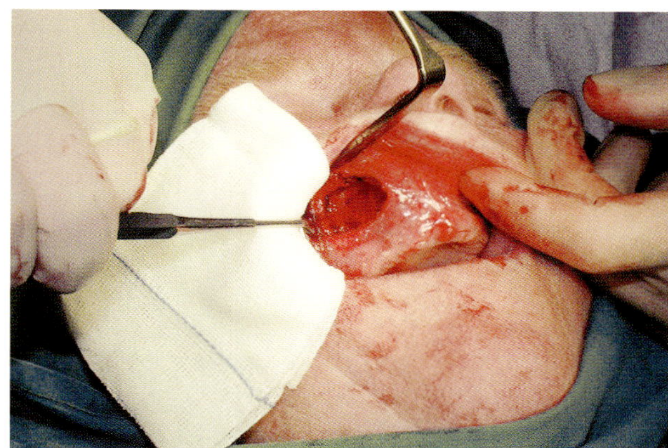

Fig 11-52 Resection socket.

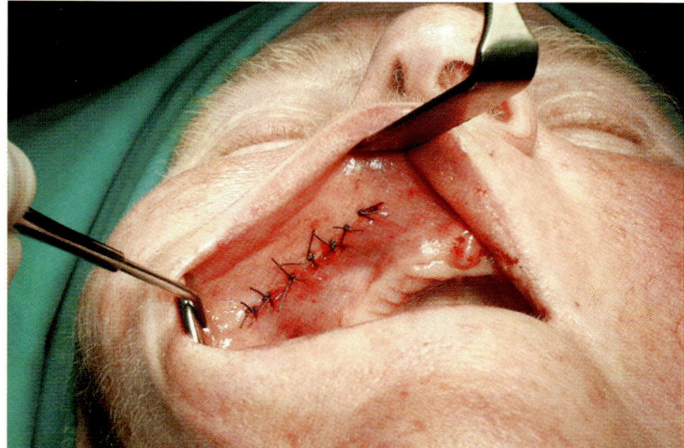

Fig 11-53 In such cases wound closure with sutures is inevitable.

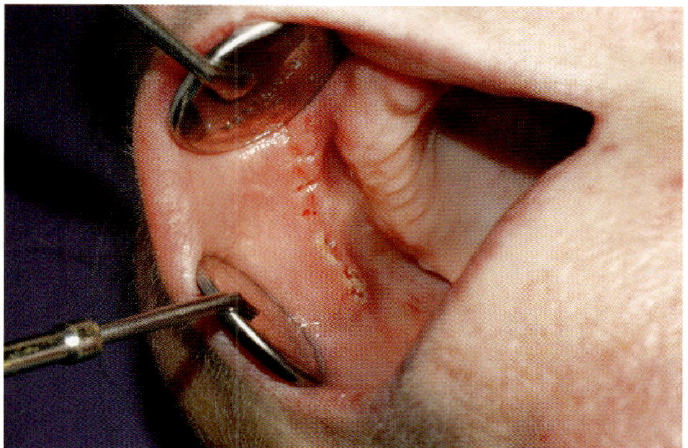

Fig 11-54 5 days post OP, removal of sutures is already possible – in comparison to conventional surgery where the retention period for sutures is ~10 days. Prosthesis is worn from the first day on without pain.

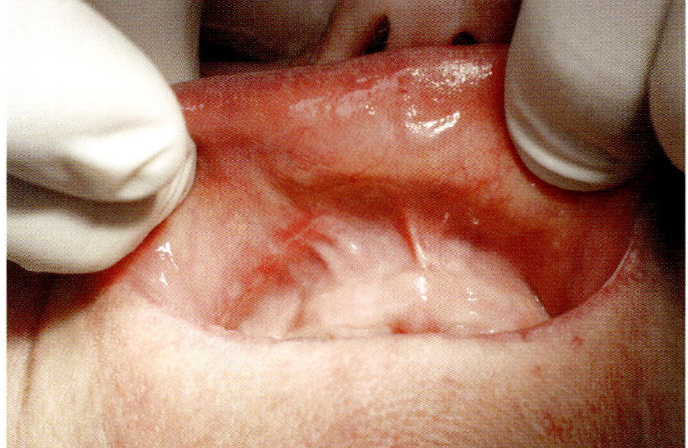

Fig 11-55 14 days post OP.

Fibromas are the most frequent benign neoplasms in the oral mucosa. They are formed by fibroblasts. Particularly often they appear on the mucosa of lips, lingual margins and gingiva, thus related to strongly irritated areas. The therapy of these lesions is simple excision[148].

Case 7

A 71-year-old female patient, partially edentulous, non-smoker, adequate oral hygiene.

Unremarkable medical history. For two years has a fibroma on the mucosa of the right cheek (Figs 11-56 to 11-59).

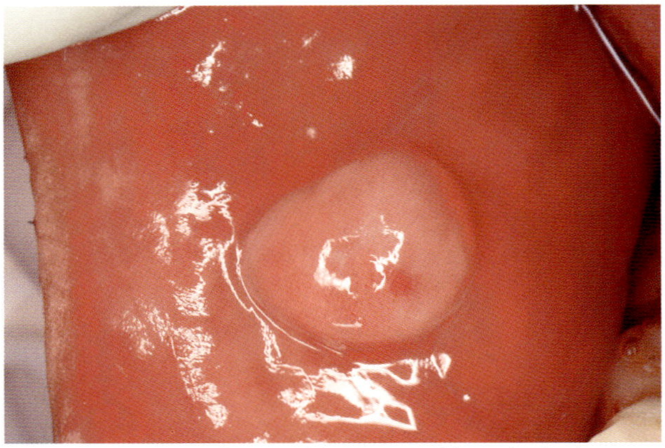

Fig 11-56 Traumatic fibroma of the mucosa of the right cheek.

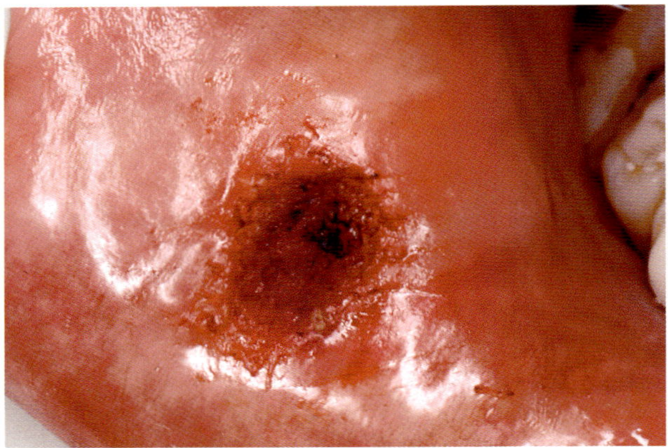

Fig 11-57 OP site with a light scar after the diode laser excision (λ = 980 nm, 4 W, cw mode). Anesthesia: local infiltration of 1/2 tube-ampoule of ecocain 2%.

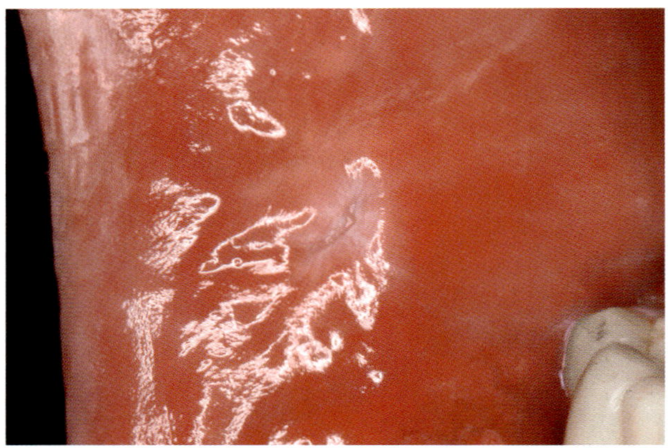

Fig 11-58 After 2 weeks the epithelial deficiency due to the operation appeared already covered by newly formed tissue.

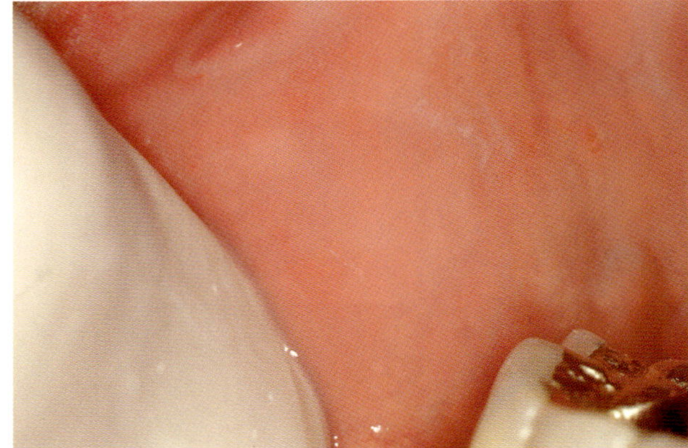

Fig 11-59 After 30 days, nearly scarless healing has resulted.

Case 8

A 39-year-old female patient shows up with an ovoid fibroma at the tip of the tongue, 4 mm in diameter, complete dentition, oral hygiene satisfactory, smoker (15 cigarettes/day), no known diseases in the patient's history (Figs 11-60 to 11-63).

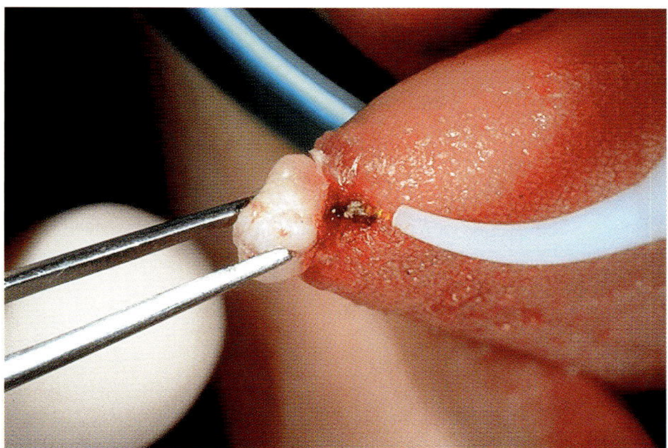

Fig 11-60 Traumatic fibroma located on the tip of the tongue for almost 1 year. At the moment of the surgical operation with an Nd:YAG laser (4 W, 100 mJ, 40 Hz), local anesthesia.

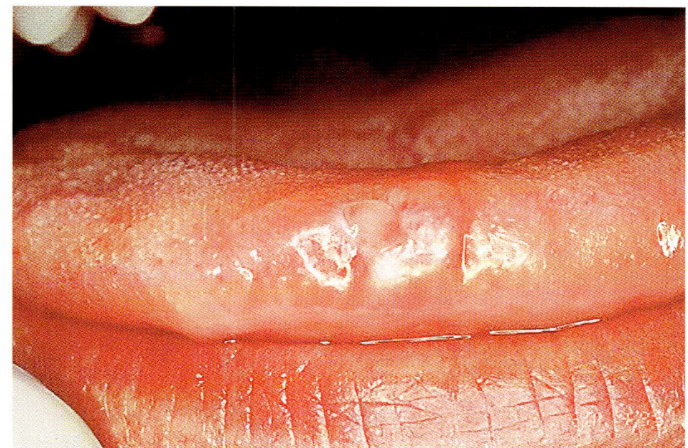

Fig 11-61 After one week the epithelial deficiency due to the operation seemed already covered by newly formed tissue.

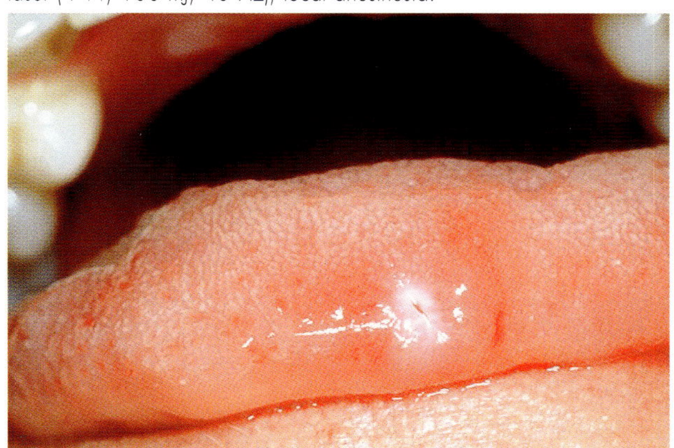

Fig 11-62 After one month the restitution ad integrum of the area treated is complete.

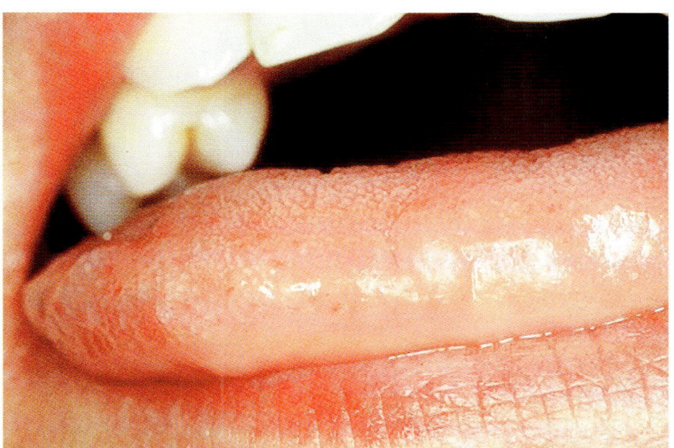

Fig 11-63 The follow-up control after one year, no recurrence.

Case 9

A 57-year-old male patient, completely edentulous, non-smoker, fibroma at the upper alveolar ridge due to non-fitting prosthesis, sufficient oral hygiene. No systemic diseases (Figs 11-64 to 11-68).

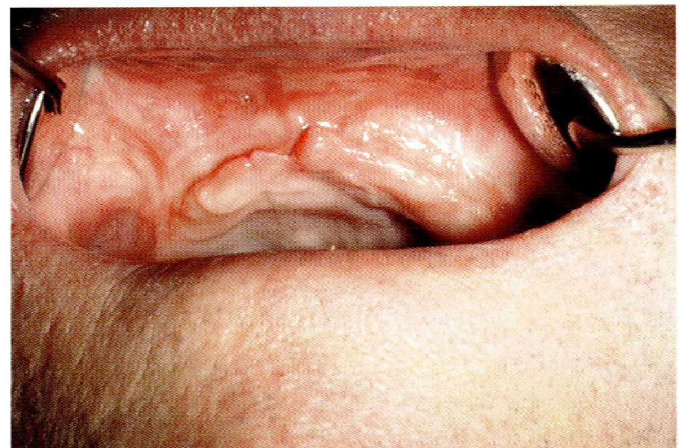

Fig 11-64 Fibroma at the alveolar ridge due to irritation by non-fitting prosthesis.

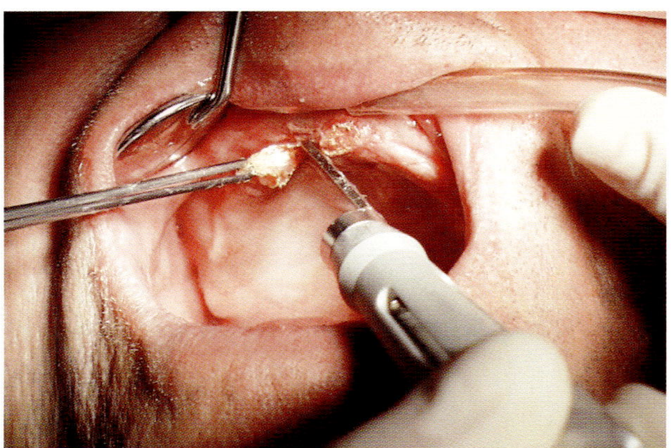

Fig 11-65 Excision of the fibroma with CO_2 laser, superpulsed mode, 5 W focused.

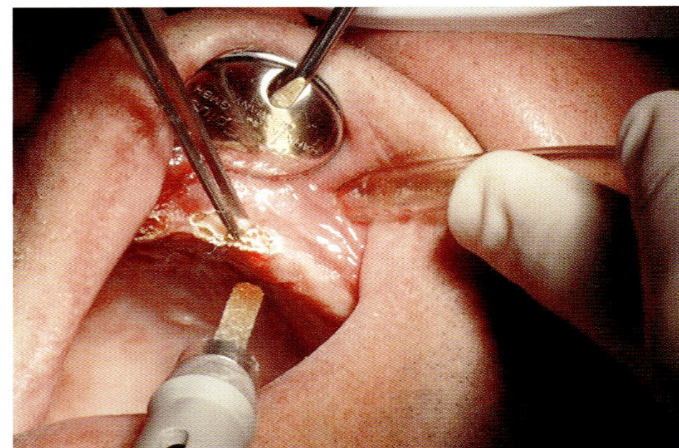

Fig 11-66 Absolutely bloodless operation field, contouring of the alveolar crest.

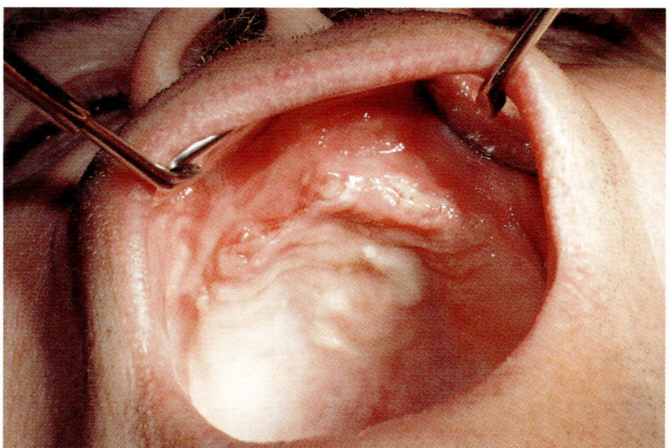

Fig 11-67 Two days post OP, fibrinous coverage of the wound, beginning granulation.

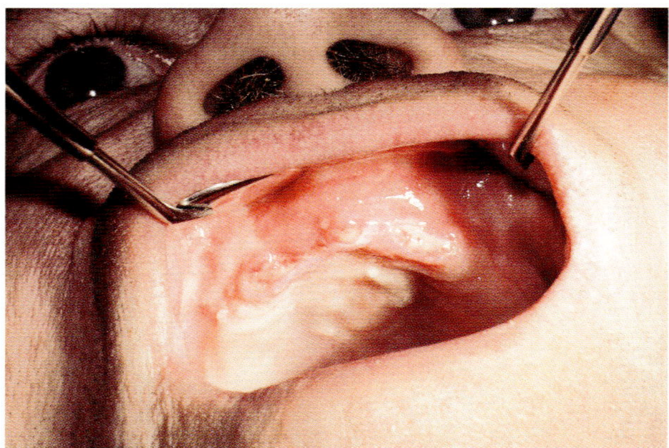

Fig 11-68 Eight days post OP, nearly complete wound healing, subsequently setting up of a new prosthesis.

Papillomas are epithelial tumors with a whitish, rough surface, which can have leukoplasia-like appearance and are able to degenerate to carcinomas. They consist of multilayered squamous cell epithelium with exophytic growth[149].

Case 10

A 72-year-old male patient, partial dentition, oral hygiene not satisfactory, non-smoker; large Papilloma Verrucosus steadily located on the palate for almost 3 years, mechanical interference, no growing tendency(Figs 11-69 to 11-72).

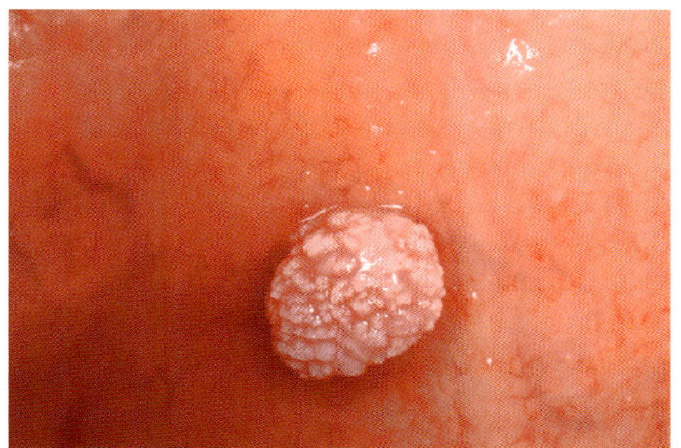

Fig 11-69 Large Papilloma Verrucosus steadily located on the palate.

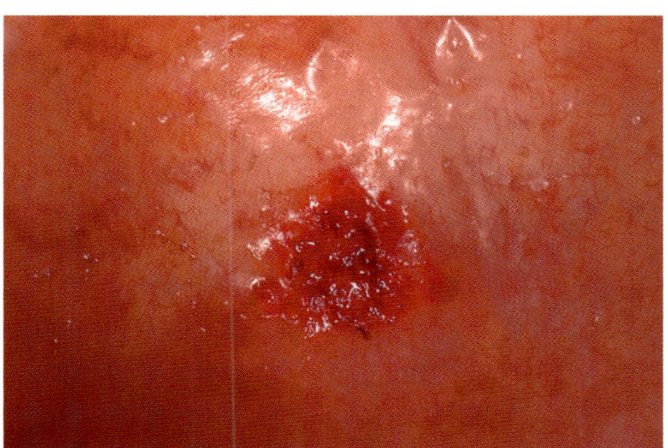

Fig 11-70 After the surgical excision with an Nd:YAG laser, 4 W, 100 mJ and 40 Hz, the post OP site was ensanguine and steadily covered by a thin and light scar.

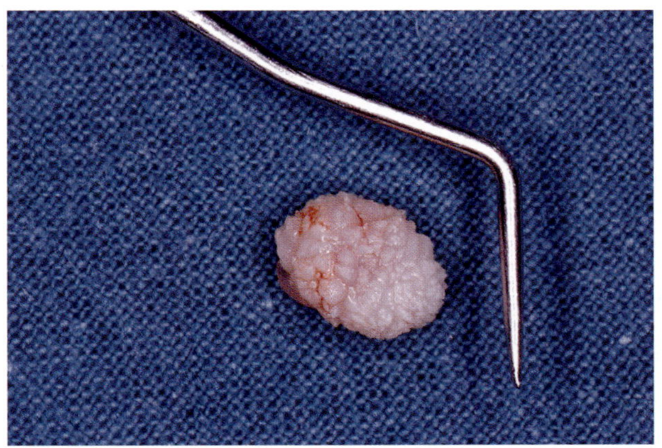

Fig 11-71 The histological specimen.

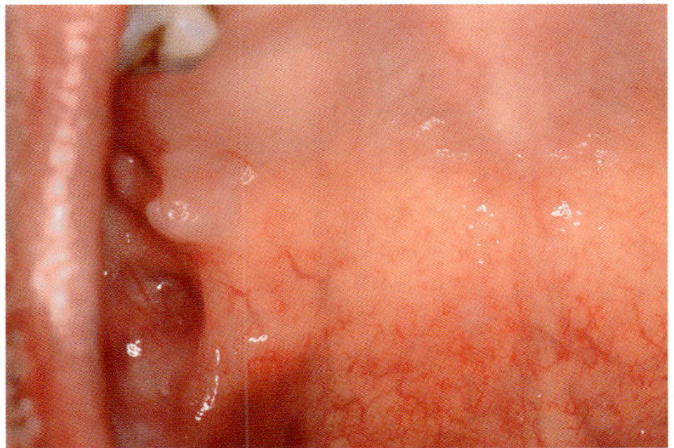

Fig 11-72 The follow-up control after 6 months.

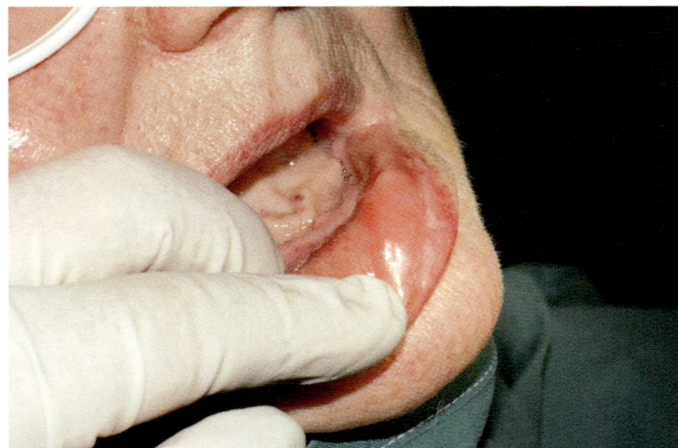

Fig 11-73 Papilloma on the lower lip, without inflammation at this time.

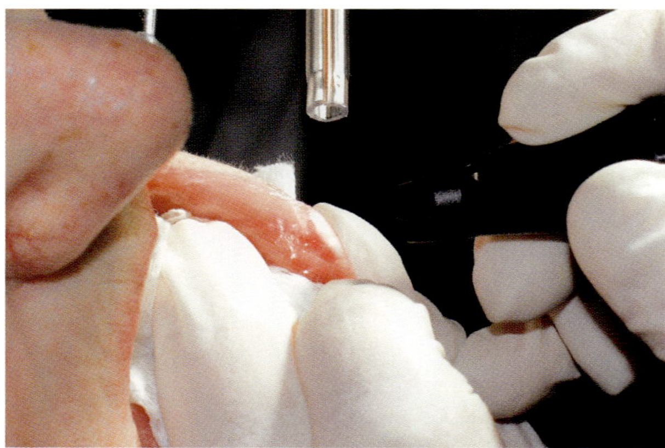

Fig 11-74 Vaporization with the CO_2 laser, cw, 4 W.

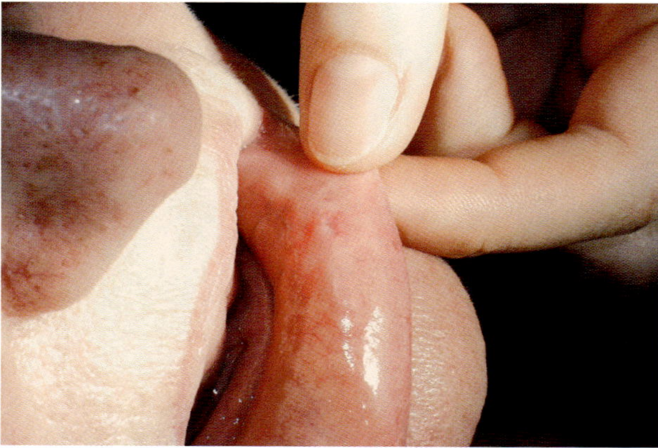

Fig 11-75 Residuum 7 days post OP, due to her poor general condition she did not show up for further controls.

Case 11

A 75-year-old female patient, edentulous, oral hygiene satisfactory, non-smoker, diabetes mellitus, medication-controlled hypertonia, Statex post apoplexia. Papilloma on the lower lip, which tends to inflammation due to mechanical irritation. Exeresis with superficial anesthesia (Xylocain-gel) (Figs 11-73 to 11-75).

11.9.2 Leukoplakias and Precancerous Lesions

Leukoplakias represent a very common indication for oral/maxillo-facial surgical interventions. Regarding the morphology, they are divided as follows. *Leukoplakia simplex/plana* (49%): homogenous, whitish, sharp margins, smooth to slightly wavy surface. *Leukoplakia verrucosa* (27%): slightly spotted, gray-red, irregular, nodular surface. *Leukoplakia errosiva* (24%): highly spotted, irregular surface with erosions.

The incidence of malignant degeneration is indicated as 0.1% to 28% in the literature[150–153], some authors even find 38% of malignant degeneration[154]. Leukoplakia errosiva has therefore to be regarded as very suspicious, whereas in recent studies only inhomogeneous leukoplakias are regarded as suspect[155,156]. Keeping to the same recall intervals and follow-up schemes as in conventional surgery, laser surgery of leukoplakias seems to be an equivalent[157] or even superior treatment alternative[158]. Even during long follow-up periods (more than 38 months) the incidence of recurrences after laser surgical elimination of leukoplakias (22%), and other precancerous lesions (13%), in comparison to vitamin A therapy (40–55%) and conventional surgical methods (33%) is significantly reduced[159]. Other authors found reduced recurrence rates between 5.9% and 18% for leukoplakias after laser surgery[160–162].

The vaporizing ablation of leukoplakias should proceed only after histological verification, and then it is available particularly for multicentric, large leukoplakias. Definitely favorable is the total excision of the leukoplakia, most of all with the CO_2 laser, which also allows a histopathologic clarification. For smaller leukoplakias, other wavelengths may also be clinically appropriate.

Gooris et al.[163], investigating leukoplakias of the lip, found the same results. Besides the general absence of relapses, they mentioned the nearly invisible scar formation, which is of great importance in the highly sensitive area of the lips to maintain esthetics and function.

Other studies, like the one of Burkey and Garett[164], find the results after laser surgical excisions of precancerous lesions and carcinomas of the mouth to be not superior, but equivalent to conventional surgical procedures, where the majority of cases were treated with the CO_2 laser, and only strongly vascularized tissues with the Nd:YAG laser. The 5-year survival rate and the functionality after resections was assessed.

Extremely dangerous is the **erythroplakia**, which corresponds to a carcinoma in situ or an early invasive carcinoma. The floor of the mouth, ventrolateral area of the tongue, as well as the soft palate are high-risk regions for erythroplakias. These form as deep-red and fine-grained, and might be riddled with leukoplakiac stipples, circumscribed or extensive lesions, with the low induration often suggesting benignity. Particularly, the extensive version tends to early, invasive cancerization as well as to regional metastasis[165].

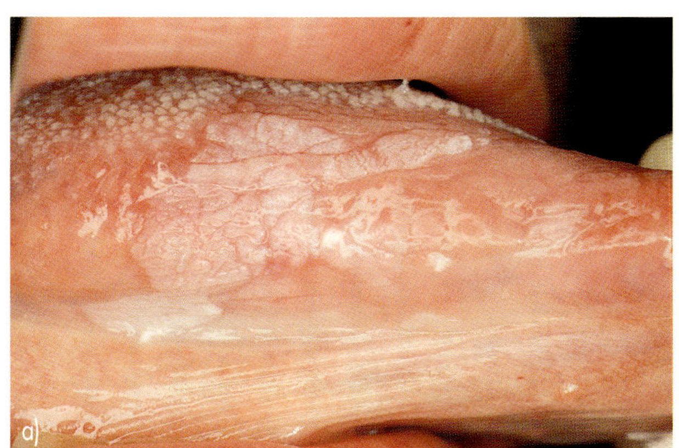

Fig 11-76a Leukoplakial lesion of the tongue margin.

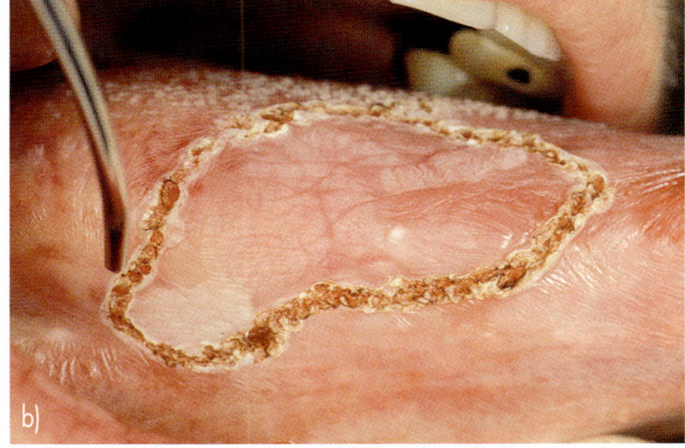

Fig 11-76b Excision with a CO_2 laser and focused mode.

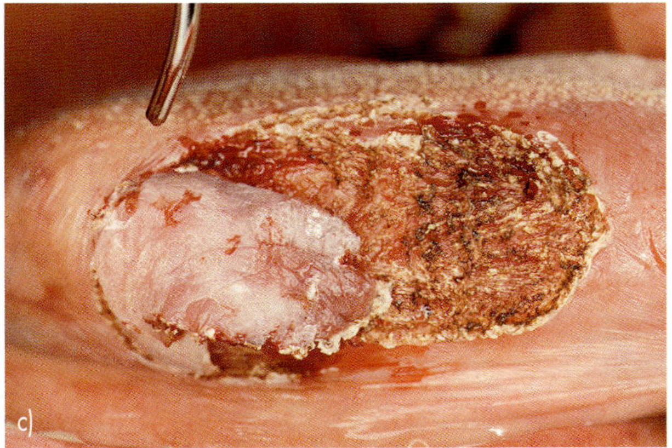

Fig 11-76c Excision of the leukoplakia with satisfying coagulation.

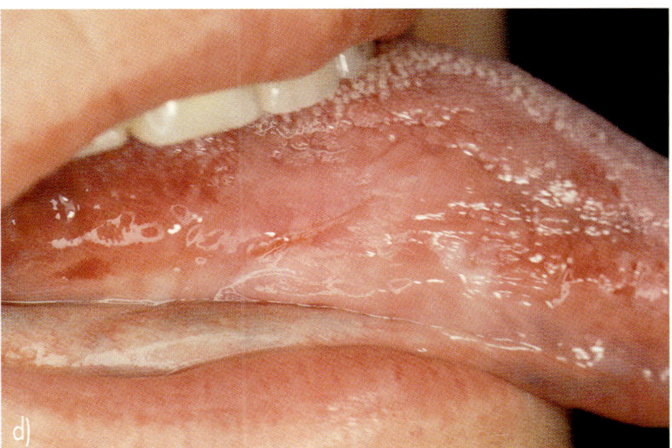

Fig 11-76d Postoperative result, without recurrence after one year.

Case 12

A 52-year-old female patient with erythro/leukoplakia, good general condition, non-smoker, sufficient oral hygiene and periodontal status (Figs 11-77 to 11-81).

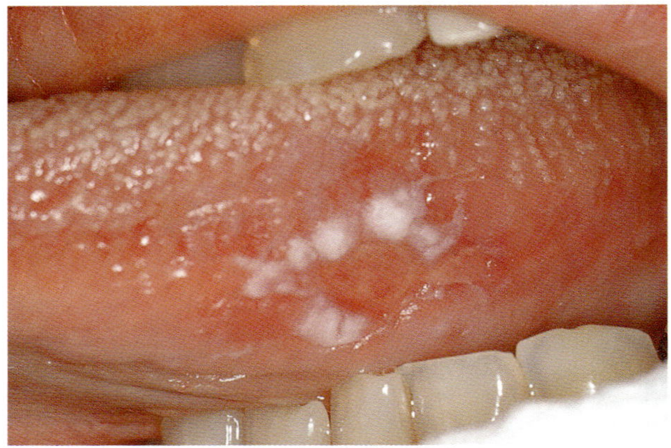

Fig 11-77 Leuko/erythroplakia on left margin of the tongue.

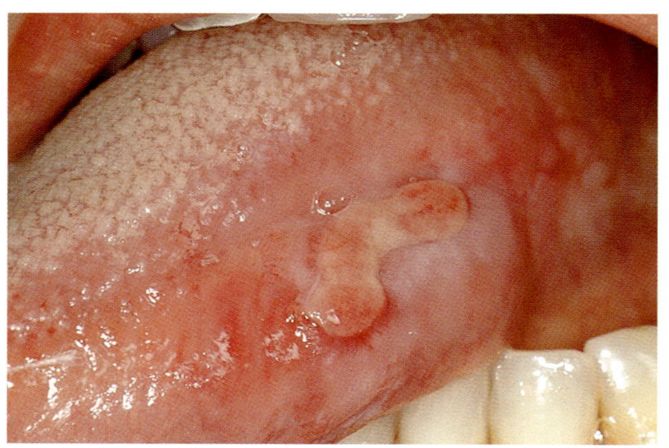

Fig 11-78 Hyperplastic scar after primary scalpel excision.

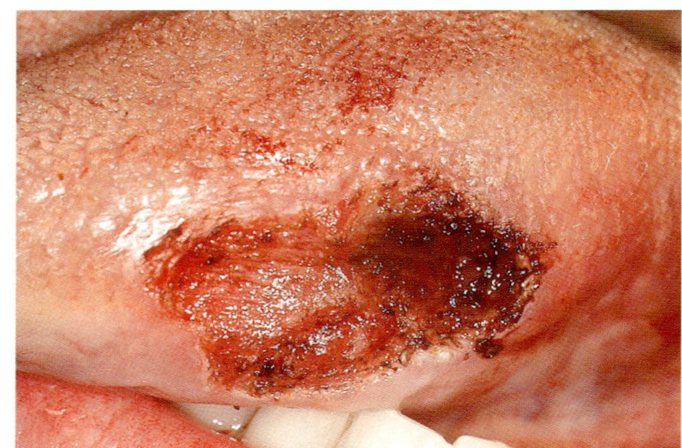

Fig 11-79 Immediately after the exeresis of the lesion with an Nd:YAG laser, 4 W, 100 mJ with 40 Hz.

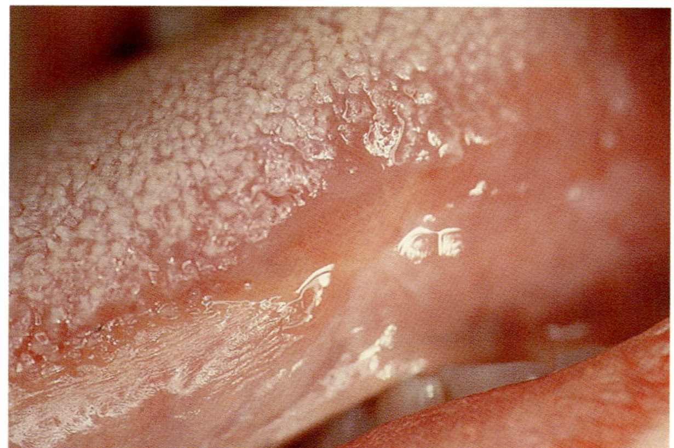

Fig 11-80 Restitution ad integrum after 3 weeks.

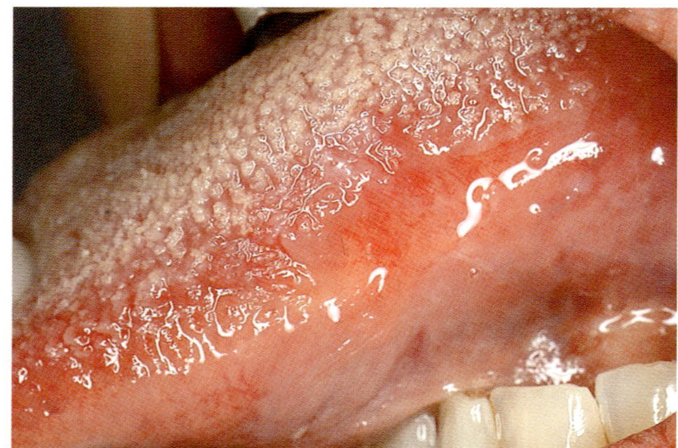

Fig 11-81 The control after 8 months, no recurrence.

Case 13

A 49-year-old male patient, partial dentition, smoker, coronary heart disease known for years, on medication, ASS paused for 1 week, after consultation with the internist no change of medication to heparin indicated. Patient has been operated twice for leukoplakias in the right cheek (conventional surgery). Histology resulted in the statement of high dysplastic cells both times, no sign of malignancy. Now patient showed again with leukoplakia of the right cheek (Figs 11-82 to 11-86).

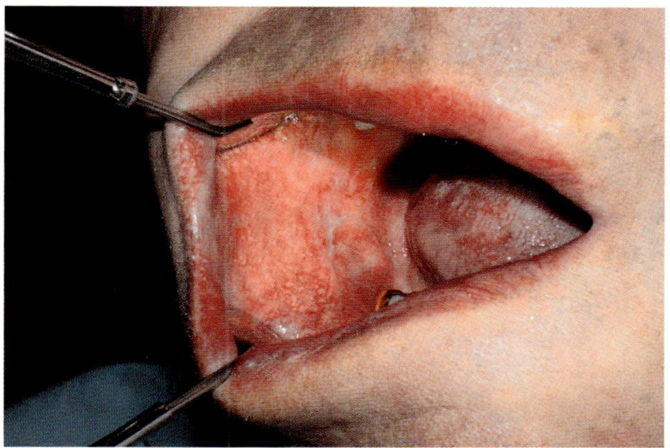

Fig 11-82 Recurrence of leukoplakia on the right cheek mucosa, clearly visible scars after former conventional surgery.

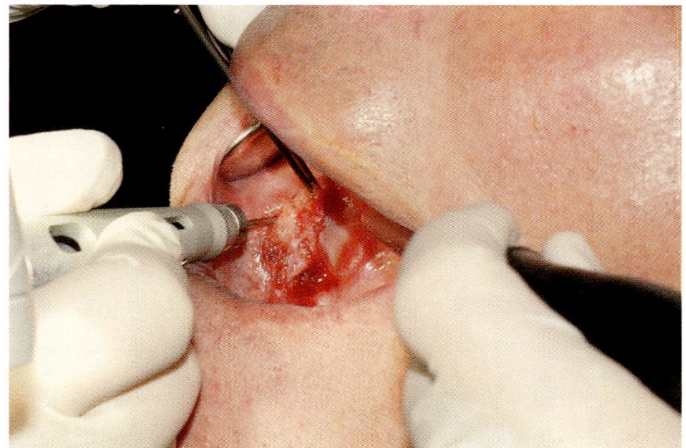

Fig 11-83 Excision of the leukoplakic lesion with CO_2 laser, 4 W focused, to guarantee histological findings, additional safety zone of 0.3 cm is kept.

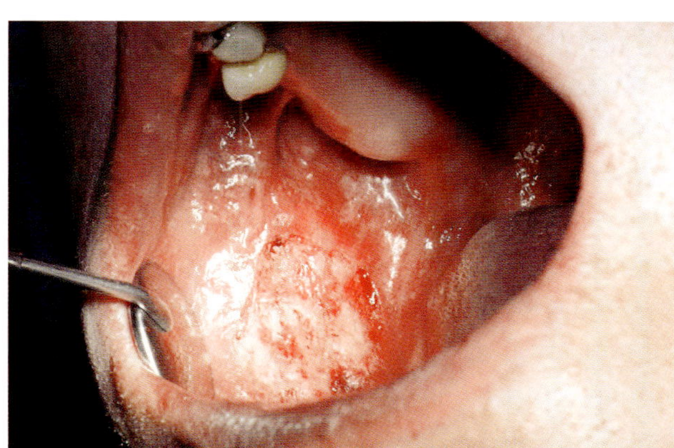

Fig 11-84 Bloodless operation area after excision.

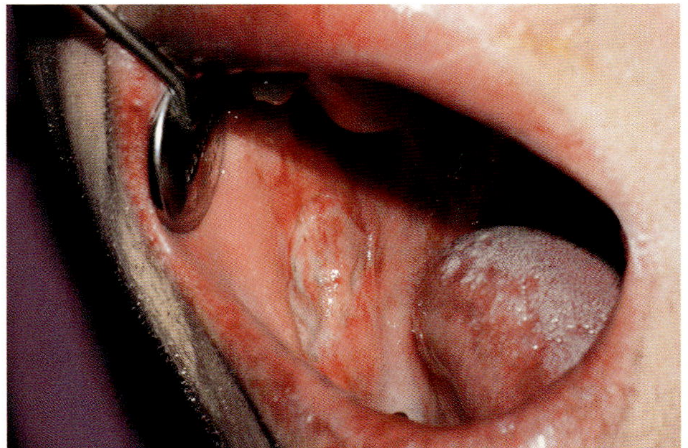

Fig 11-85 7 days post OP, fibrinous coverage, beginning granulation, no signs of inflammation.

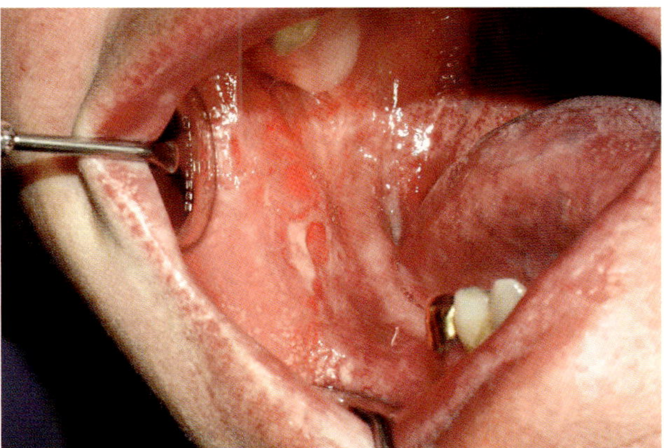

Fig 11-86 14 days post OP, only slight central dent, histology found high grade of dysplasia again.

11.9.3 Oral Lichen Planus

Lichen ruber planus (LRP) is a disease that can occur in skin, as well as in mucosal tissue. LRP shows chronic progression with sometimes spontaneous remissions. Of the adult population, 0.5–2% are affected[166]. Andreasen[167] divides LRP into six different kinds: reticulous, papulous, plaque-like, erosive, atrophic, and bullous. The most frequent form is the reticulous LRP, characterized by the Wickham-signs, a gray-white, fine-meshed, striped pattern[168].

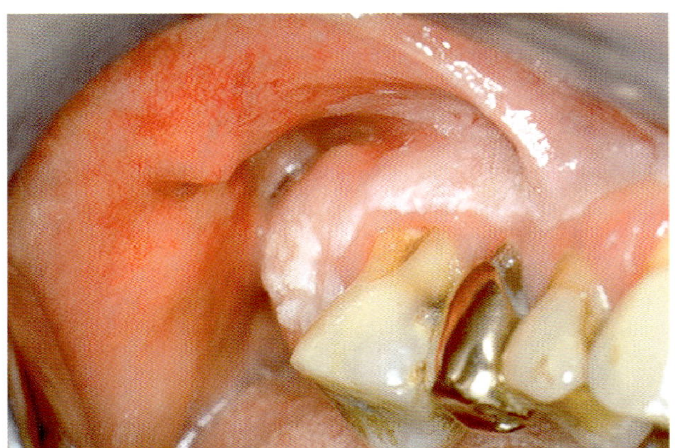

Fig 11-87 Hyperplastic lichen lesion drug-resistant on the right upper fornix and retro-molar area.

11.9.4 Mucocele/Ranula

Every cyst in the secretory ducts of small or major salivary glands, containing mucus, is called a mucocele. Most of the mucoceles are located on the lower lip (45–70%), the cheek, sublingual and in the floor of the mouth. Essentially they are retention cysts based on inflammatory-irritative genesis[169].

Various wavelengths are available for ablation of those cysts. Total elimination is aimed for, not only cystostomy, which could lead to recurrence.

Case 14

A 63-year-old female patient, Hepatitis B positive (HbsAg +), old fillings and crowns; sufficient oral hygiene. Smoker (15 cigarettes/day). She presented OLP lesions absolutely drug-resistant only in the mouth (Figs 11-87 to 11-89).

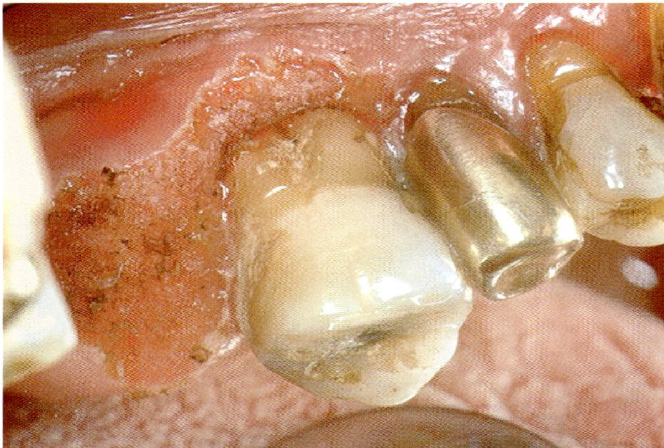

Fig 11-88 Immediately after the laser ablation with an Nd:YAG laser beam powered at 2 W, 20 Hz.

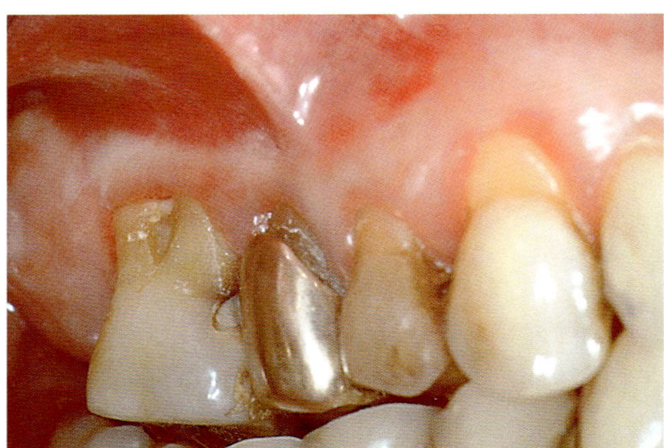

Fig 11-89 The control after 2 months, discrete signs of a recurrence.

Case 15

A 33-year-old male patient, complete dentition, very good oral hygiene, non-smoker, no systemic diseases (Figs 11-90 to 11-94).

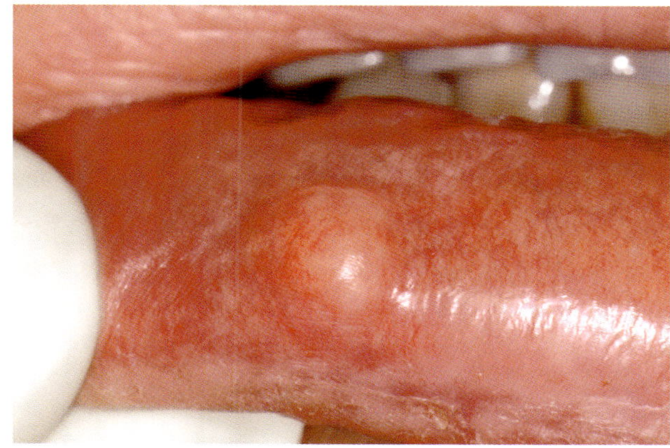

Fig 11-90 Mucocele (5 mm Ø) on the lower lip.

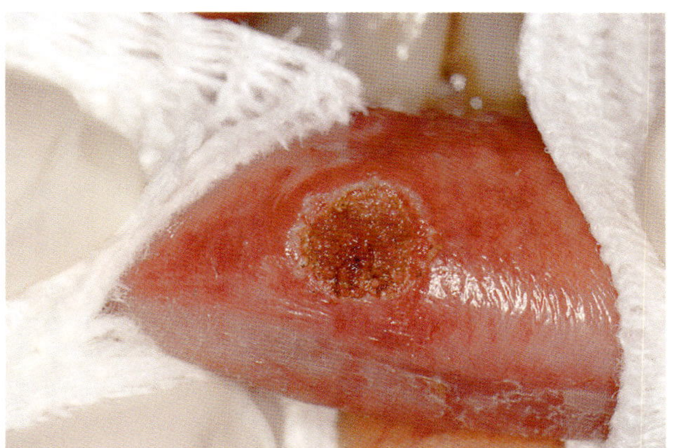

Fig 11-91 Absolute blood-free vaporization with the Nd:YAG laser, 3 W, 150 mJ, 20 Hz.

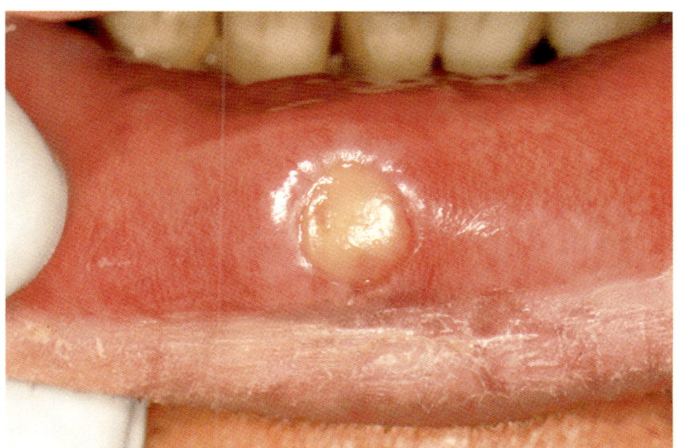

Fig 11-92 1 week post OP.

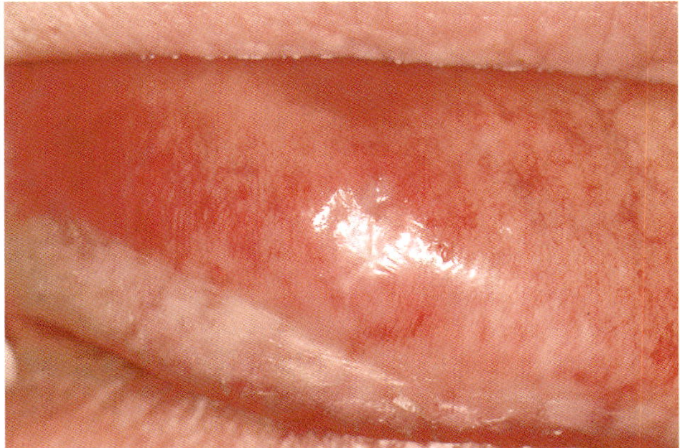

Fig 11-93 4 weeks post OP.

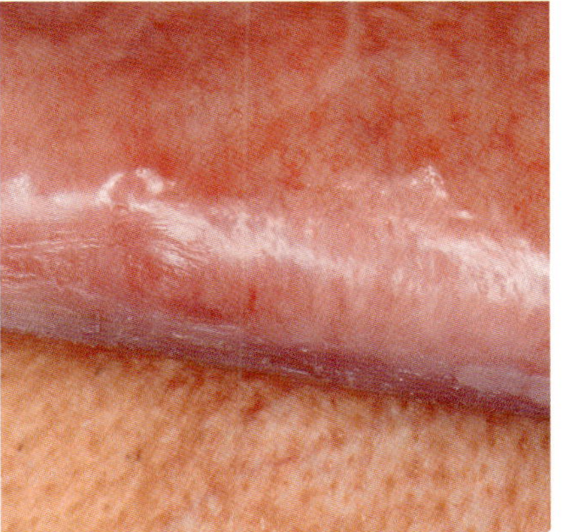

Fig 11-94 Follow-up after 1 year.

Case 16

A 42-year-old male patient, healthy, partial dentition, moderate oral hygiene, smoker (20 cigarettes/day) (Figs 11-95 to 11-99).

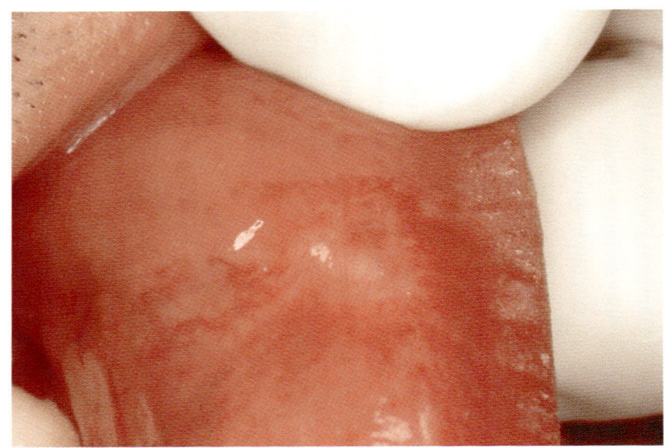

Fig 11-95 Mucocele on the lower lip (6 mm Ø).

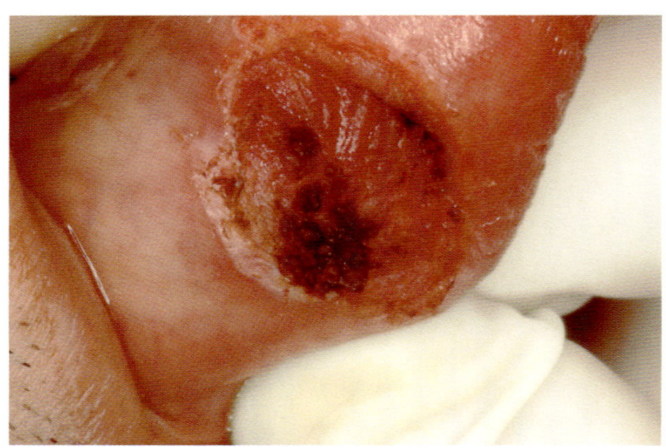

Fig 11-96 Immediately after vaporization with the Nd:YAG laser, 3 W, 150 mJ, 20 Hz. Central carbonized zone after coagulation of a small vessel.

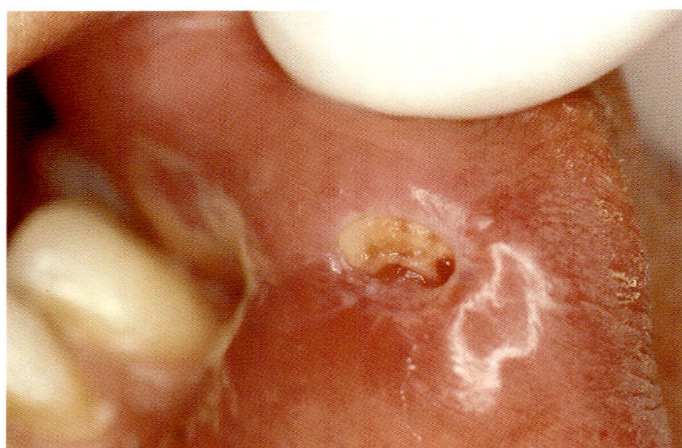

Fig 11-97 1 week post OP.

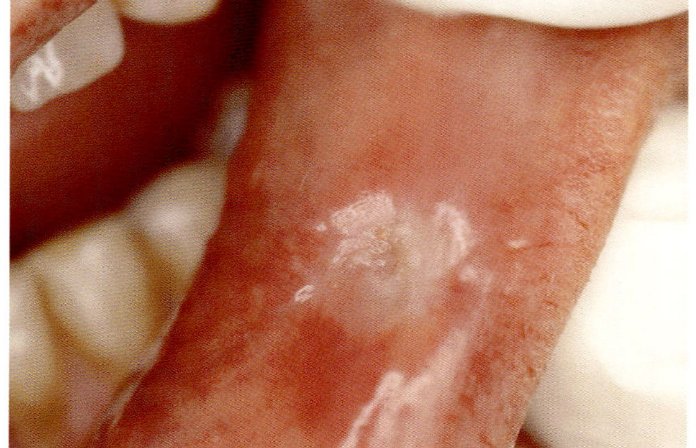

Fig 11-98 1 month post OP.

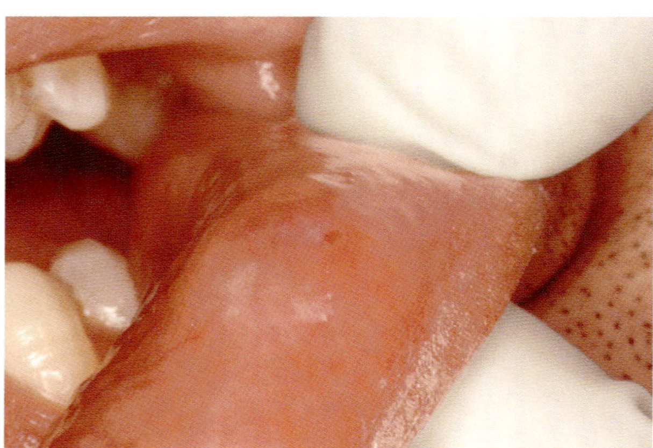

Fig 11-99 Follow-up after 1 year.

11.9.5 Preprosthetic Surgery

Case 17

An 83-year-old male patient, hypertonia, non-smoker, artificial denture in upper and lower jaw, irritation fibroma in upper jaw (Figs 11-100 to 11-103).

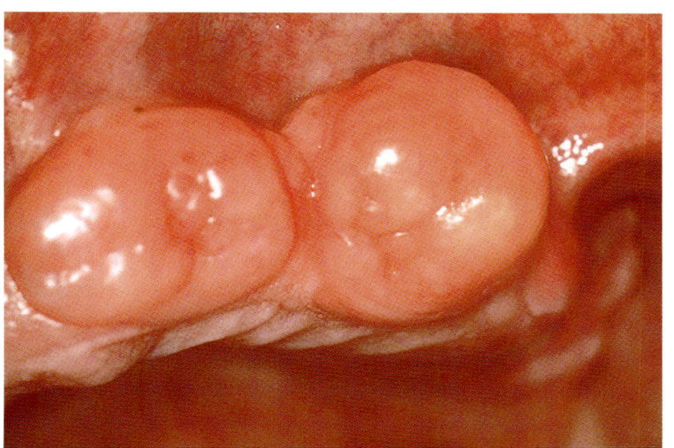

Fig 11-100 Clinical appearance before removal of the fibroma with Nd:YAG laser, local anesthesia with 2% ecocain.

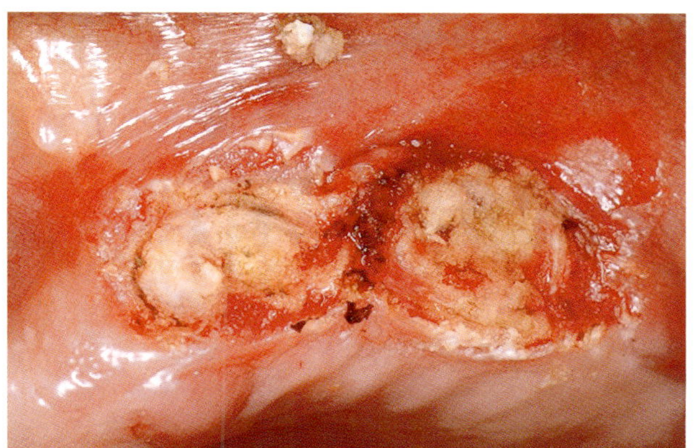

Fig 11-101 Immediately after excision with Nd:YAG, 6 W , 40 Hz, 150 mJ, bloodless operation field.

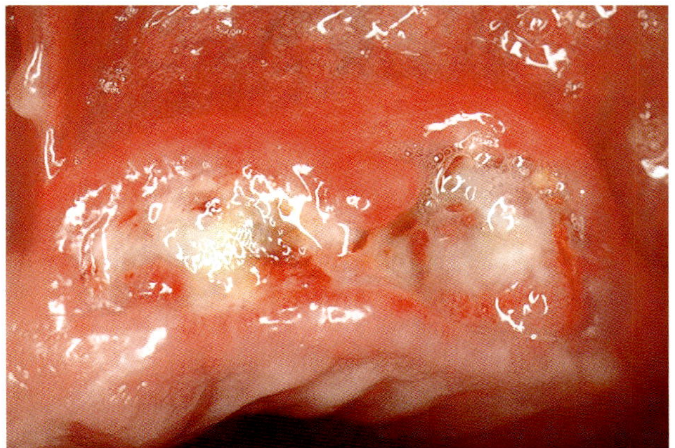

Fig 11-102 2 weeks post OP.

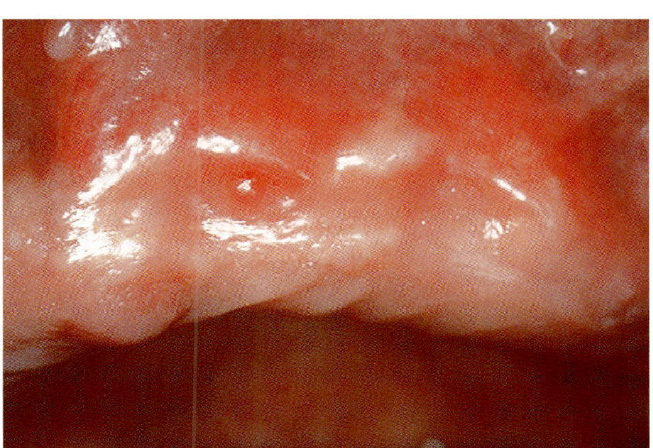

Fig 11-103 Control after 1 month.

11.9.6 Frenotomy

This clinical indication is almost always seen in very young patients. Patients show insufficient oral hygiene due to the strong, abnormal frenulum, inflammation of the gingiva of adjacent teeth, and sometimes a diasthema. Excision is performed after consultation with an orthodontist; patients having speech disorders also see the logopedist. Using a laser enables the surgeon to excise the frenulum painlessly, without bleeding, without sutures and no need of special postoperative care. A fibrinous layer covers the operation area after 3–5 days and the result is favorable (Figs 11-104a–c).

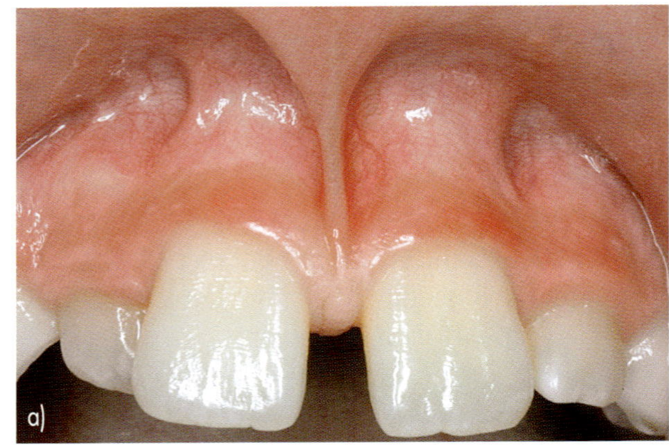

Fig 11-104a Strong frenulum of the upper lip.

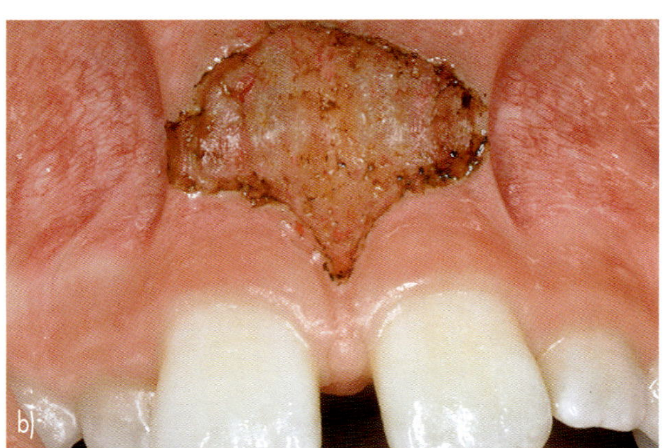

Fig 11-104b Excision with a CO_2 laser.

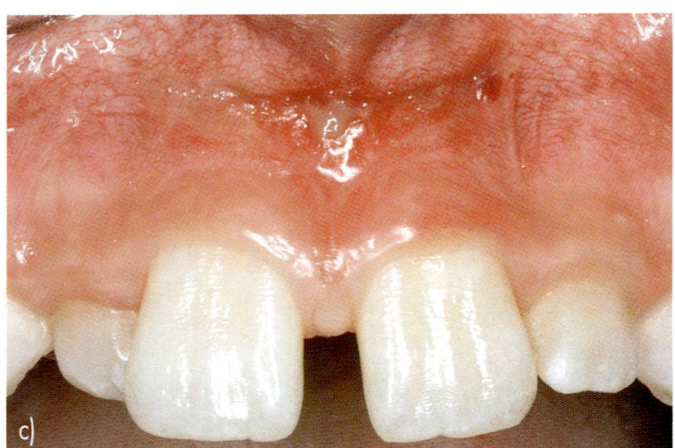

Fig 11-104c Wound healing with slight fibrinous coverage, 3 days post OP.

11.9.7 Implantology/Peri-Implantitis

A borderline between implantology and periodontology is the therapy of peri-implantitis.

The lasers used are mainly the Nd:YAG, diode, Er:YAG and Er,Cr:YSGG or the CO_2[170,171]. Of special interest is not only the bactericidal capacity, which is well-documented for most of those lasers[170], but the way the lasers change implant surfaces as well, which might be important for bone regeneration[170–172].

Salina et al.[176] assessed the effect of the diode laser in peri-implantitis therapy. The bactericidal effect provides a satisfying reduction of bactericidal population and therefore remission of the inflammatory symptoms. This provides an advantageous situation before GBR therapy.

It is relevant for the prognosis to keep the thermal alteration of the adjacent bone as small as possible. Barak et al.[177] found no critical temperature rise at the implant/bone interface using a CO_2 laser, up to energy levels of 4 W in cw mode and 8 W in pulsed mode, both ranges being far higher than the therapeutical energy range.

Kreisler et al.[178] compared the temperature rise at the implant/bone interface in Ti-plasma-sprayed implants using a diode (GaAlAs), and a CO_2 laser. The critical threshold was reached with the diode laser after 8 s at 2.5 W, after 13 s at 2.0 W, and after 18 s at 1.5 W. The CO_2 laser reaches the critical temperature a little later (15 s – 2.5 W; 23 s – 2.0 W; 35 s – 1.5 W). Although the time range seems to be relatively wide using standard power settings, care has to be taken not to damage the surrounding bone.

Wooten et al.[179] compared the temperature rise at the implant/bone interface using the three possible application modes of the CO_2 laser, 2–15 s and 3–15 W. He found the smallest temperature rise in the superpulsed mode, but he stated that in all three working modes, the temperature returns to the baseline within 1 min.

Mouhyi et al.[180] observed that the temperature rise under CO_2 laser irradiation of the implant/bone interface (different power settings, max. 8 W/ 10 ms/ 20 Hz, pulsed mode) stayed below 3°C, if the implant surface was moist, whereas the risky temperature threshold for overheating was reached when dry implant surfaces were irradiated.

The temperature changes at the implant/bone interface were investigated by Kreisler et al. too, using Ti-plasma-sprayed, sandblasted and etched implant surfaces (Er:YAG laser energy 60–120 mJ, 10 pps). Even when irradiated continuously for 120 s, the temperature never exceeded 47°C, stated to be the critical temperature by the authors[181].

Clinical cases (but not evidence based) often favor the Er:YAG laser in implantology. Without thermal damage to the adjacent bone, all tissues (mucosa, periosteum, bone) can be treated with the same laser. Walsh et al.[182] documented an only 5–10 µm deep damage zone when preparing with a

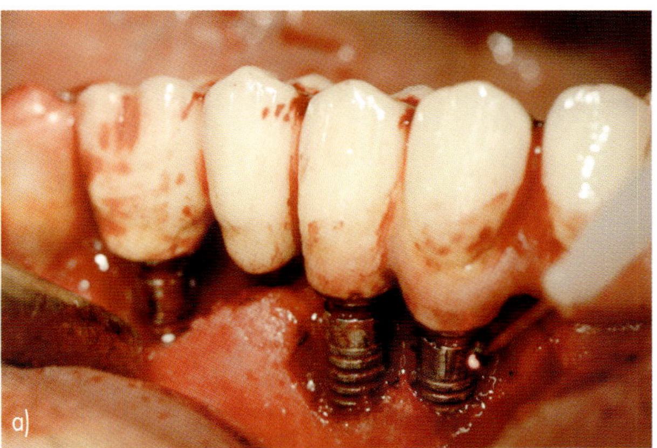

Fig 11-105a Decontamination with diode laser (980 nm, Biolitec, Germany).

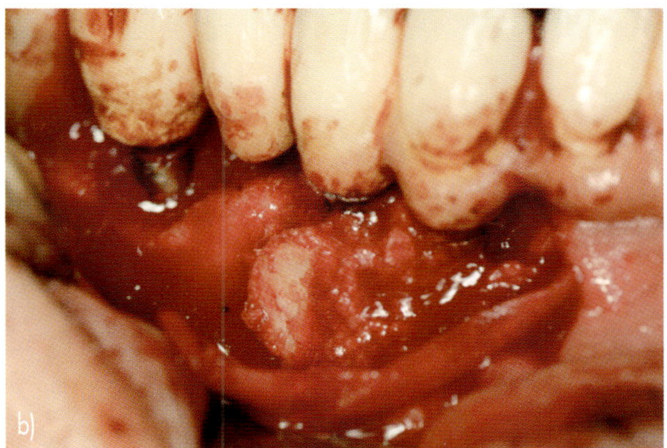

Fig 11-105b Subsequent augmentation of the peri-implantal bony defects with autologous bone and membrane coverage.

Q-switched Er:YAG laser. Using regular Er:YAG laser (max. pulse duration 200 µs) the damage zone reaches not more than 100 µm. The CO_2 laser is preferred if a thick mucoperiostal layer has to be cut and its coagulative capacity is necessary[183]. A therapeutical chance to enhance and speed up the integration of cortico-cancellous transplants is seen in the perforation of the transplants with the Er:YAG laser. Via punctual de-mineralization of the bone, the integration of the transplant is said to be enhanced[184,185]. In comparison, the CO_2 laser causes a significant retardation in the bone healing process[186]. Arnabat et al.[124] used the Er,Cr:YSGG laser for second-stage operations in implantology. Uncovering the implants is possible without anesthesia, and they observed complete wound healing after only 5 days and thereby ideal conditions for a rapid prosthetic solution.

Wang et al.[126] did osteotomies with the Er,Cr:YSGG laser and found only minimal thermal damage in parallel with satisfactory precision of preparation using power settings of 140–200 ms and 160 J/cm^2.

Kimura et al.[187] investigated temperature changes and morphological changes in osteotomies done with the Er,Cr:YSGG laser. They found sharp osteotomy margins and smooth walls in the cutting gap when using 5 W and 8 Hz. Investigations with stereoscopy and spectroscopy revealed no burnings, melting nor changes in Ca/P ratio.

11.9.8 Periodontal Surgery

One of the most important components for a good prognosis of healing of periodontal diseases is the removal of the sulcus epithelium to enable re-attachment. Some studies indicate enhanced re-attachment after de-epithelialization with lasers in the course of a conventional flap-operation[188].

Centty et al.[189] compared the removal of sulcus epithelium by scalpel with the ablation by CO_2 laser. They found (1) ablation of the sulcus epithelium is feasible to a greater extent with the CO_2 laser and (2) the flap was not compromised in its vitality – a certain benefit concerning the healing prognosis.

Rossmann and Israel[190] especially worked on severe periodontal pathologies, which push today's

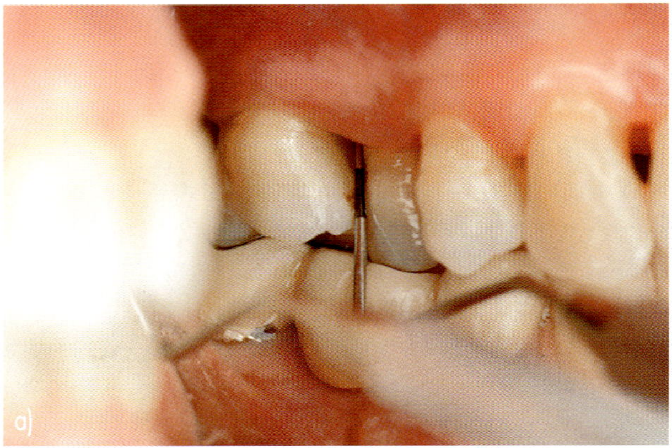

Fig 11-106a Moderate pocket with 8 mm (initial situation).

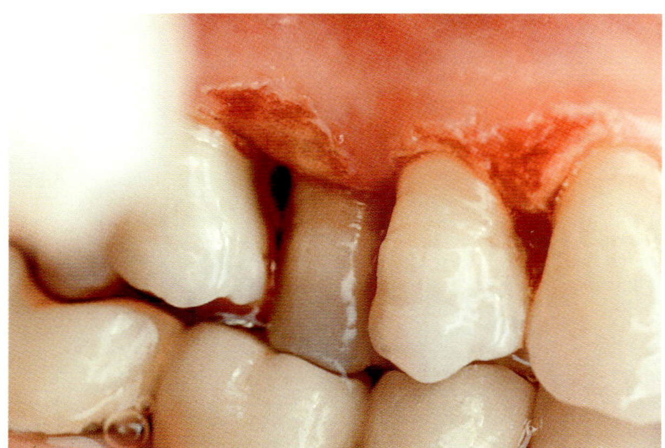

Fig 11-106b Intraoperative situs after root planing and de-epithelialization with Nd:YAG laser.

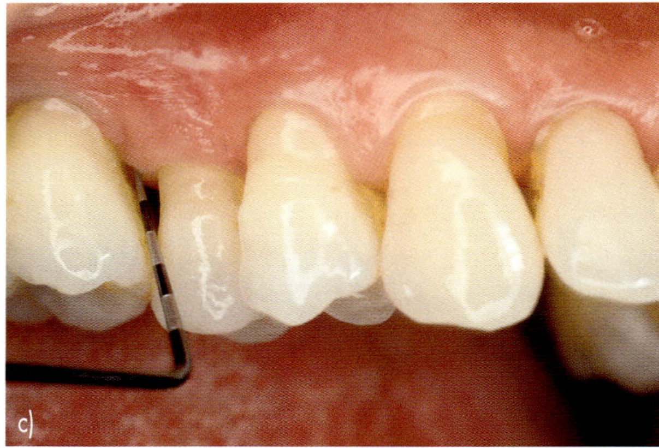

Fig 11-106c Postoperative result after 5 years. See the significant reduction of probing depth (gain of attachment 6 mm), without gingival retraction.

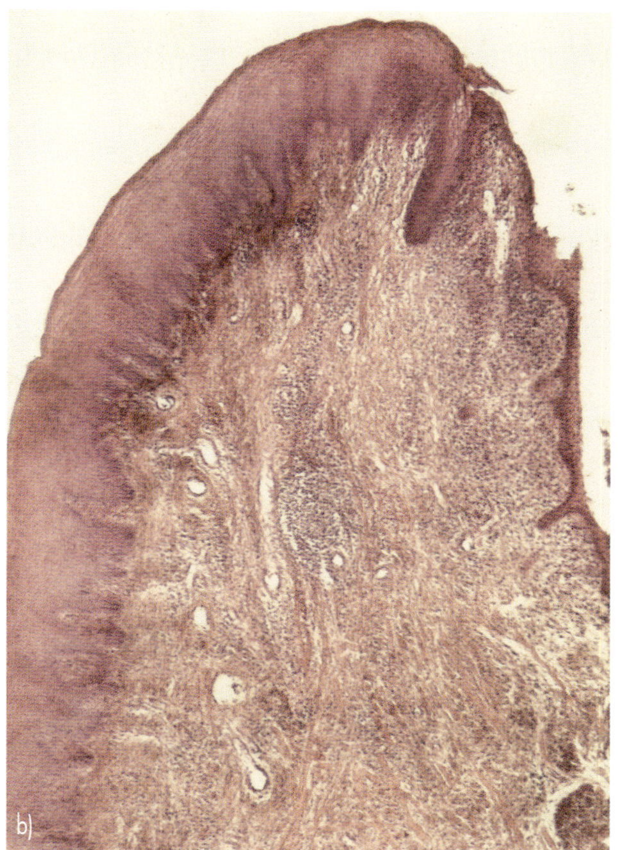

Fig 11-107a Histological preparation of the pocket after root planning (in pig).

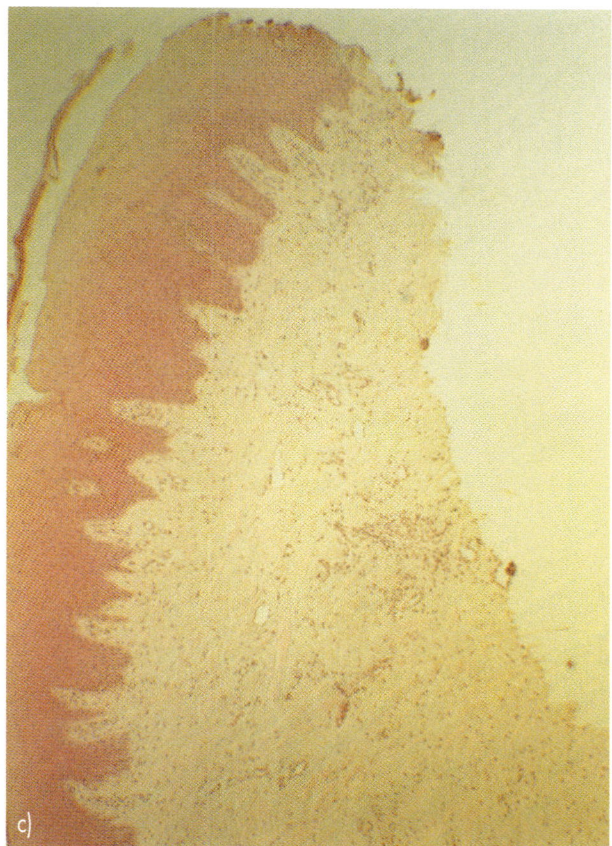

Fig 11-107b Histological specimen after just curettage with a 980 nm diode laser. The removal of epithelium is clearly visible in comparison to the control group.

state-of-the-art therapy – GTR therapy – to its limits. Especially when several locations in one quadrant are incriminated, laser de-epithelialization offers the patient a promising therapy from an economic point of view. On the contrary, some authors find a reduction of fibroblast attachment after debridement with lasers[191].

Friesen et al.[192] carried out a comparative study on the use of CO_2 and Nd:YAG lasers. They used parameters that are qualified for periodontal applications. They found the above-mentioned retardation in bone healing, whether or not rinsing solutions were used, or a carbonized layer was left. After application of Nd:YAG laser plus rinsing, they observed newly formed bone on the lased spots.

Gouw-Soares et al.[193] utilized the special benefits of various lasers (Er:YAG, Nd:YAG, diode) in cases of apicoectomies. The osteotomy was performed with the Er:YAG, apex sealing with Nd:YAG and final decontamination and possibly stimulation of bone regeneration with the diode laser. This represents a therapy combination that offers the greatest safety, even if it involves a rather large technical expenditure.

The often-discussed time factor was investigated by Williams et al.[194]; they found a mean delay of only 55 s per treated pocket if using the CO_2 laser for debridement, in comparison to conventional scaling methods.

The latest investigations on Er:YAG laser in periodontology indicate good results after flap operations and root planning with the laser compared to conventional root planning, which is more difficult and also relatively time consuming. These clinical findings are correlated to the bactericidal effects of the Er:YAG laser[195].

11.10 References

1. Patel C K N: Interpretation of CO_2-optical maser experiments. Phys Rev Lett 12: 588, 1964
2. Geusic J E, Marcos H W, Van Uitert L G: Laser oscillations in Nd-doped yttriumaluminium, yttrium gallium, and gadolinum garnets. Appl Phys Lett 4: 182, 1964
3. Jako F G: Laser surgery of the vocal cords: an experimental study with carbon dioxide laser on dogs. Laryngoscope 82: 2204–2216, 1972
4. Polany T G, Bredmesiser H C, Davis T W: A CO_2 laser for surgical research. Med Bio Eng 8: 541–548, 1970
5. Schettler D, Mohr C: In: Hausamen J-E, Machtens E, Reuther, J: Präprothetische Chirurgie in Mund-Kiefer-Gesichts-Chirurgie. Kirschnersche Operationslehre, Springer Verlag, Heidelberg 1995
6. Rehrmann A: Excision lappiger Fibrome und gleichzeitiger Mundvorhofplastik. Dtsch Zahnärztl Z 7: 133, 1952
7. Schuchardt K: Die Epidermistransplantation bei der Mundvorhofplastik. Dtsch Zahnärztl Z 7: 364, 1952
8. King K O, Pennel B M: Evaluation of attempts to increase the width of attached gingiva. Presented at the Philadelphia Society of Periodontology 1964
9. Sailer H F, Pajarola G F: In: Rateitschak K H, Wolf H F: Orale Chirurgie. Farbatlanten der Zahnmedizin 11, Georg Thieme Verlag, Stuttgart 268–269, 1996
10. Wilder-Smith P, Dang J, Kurosaki T, Neev J: The influence of laser parameter configurations at 9.3 microns on incisional and collateral effects in soft tissue. Oral Surg Oral Med Oral Pathol Oral Radiol Endod 84(1): 22–27, 1997
11. Herford A S, Finn R: Single-stage CO_2 laser assisted uvuloplastic for treatment of snoring and mild obstructive sleep apnoea. Craniomaxillofac Surg 28(4): 213–216, 2000
12. Gouw-Soares S, Tanji E, Haypek P, Cardoso W, Eduardo C P: The use of Er:YAG, Nd:YAG, and Ga-Al-As-Lasers in Periapical Surgery. J Clin Lasers Med Surg 19(4): 193–198, 2001
13. Komori T, Yokoyama K, Takato T, Matsumoto K: Clinical Application of the Er:YAG Laser for apicoectomy. J Endod 23(12): 748–750, 1997
14. Blanc P, Bourgeois P, Doyer J P: Study and Evaluation of Root Canal Sterilization with CO_2 Laser. 4th Int. Congress on Lasers in Dentistry, Singapore 1994
15. Ando Y, Aoki A, Watanabe H, Ishikawa I: Bactericidal effect of Erbium:YAG laser on perodontopathic bacteria. Lasers Surg Med 19: 190–200, 1996
16. Schoop U, Kluger W, Moritz A, Sperr W: The bactericidal Effect of Different Laser Systems in Deep Dentin Layers. Laser Congress, Florence 2003
17. Slutzki S, Shafir R, Bornstein L A: Use of a carbon dioxide laser for large excisions with minimal blood loss. Plast Reconstr Surg 60: 250–255, 1977
18. Wigdor H A, Walsh J T, Featherstone J D B, Visuri S R, Fried D, Waldvogel J L: Lasers in Dentistry. Lasers Surg Med 16: 103–133, 1995
19. Salina S, Maiorana C, Censi R, Betretta M: Treatment of oral fibromata using the Nd:YAG laser. J Oral Laser Applic 1(1): 59–63, 2001
20. Pogrel M A: The carbon dioxide laser in soft tissue preprosthetic surgery. J Prosthet Dent 61(2): 203–208, 1989
21. White J M, Chaundhry S I, Kudler J J, Sekandr, N, Schoelch M L, Silverman S Jr: Nd:YAG and CO_2 laser therapy of oral mucosal lesions. J Clin Laser Med Surg 16(6): 299–304, 1998
22. Gaspar L, Kasler M, Szabo G, Banhidy F: Separate and combined use of Nd:YAG and CO_2 lasers in oral surgery. J Clin Laser Med Surg 9(5): 381–383, 1991
23. Richter W: Die Anwendung eines Kohlendioxid-Lasers bei der Behandlung oraler Weichgewebe. ZWR 99: 969–976, 1990
24. White J M, Goodis H E, Rose C L: Use of the pulsed Nd:YAG laser for intraoral soft tissue surgery. Lasers Surg Med 11(5): 455–461, 1991
25. Horch H H: The use and evaluation of CO_2 laser in cleft palate surgery. Lasers Surg Med 2(1): 15–20, 1982
26. Beer F, Porteder H, Moritz A: Introduction of the CO_2 Laser in Cleft Lip and Palate Surgery. J Oral Laser Appl 1(2); 135–141, 2001
27. Horch H-H, Piel H-E: Der Blutverlust bei Gaumenspaltenplastiken im Kleinkindesalter unter Anwendung des Lasers. In: Scheunemann H, Schmiederer R (Hrsg.): Plastische und Wiederherstellungschirurgie bei bösartigen Tumoren. Springer Verlag, Berlin, Heidelberg, New York 1982, 332–335
28. Bradley P F: A review of the use of the neodymium YAG laser in oral and maxillofacial surgery. Br J Oral Maxillofac Surg 35 (1): 26–35, 1997
29. Pick R M, Colvard M D: Current status of Lasers in soft tissue dental surgery. J Periodontol 64(7): 589–602, 1993
30. Santos-Dias A: CO_2 laser surgery in hemophilia treatment. J Clin Laser Med Surg 10(4): 297–301, 1992
31. Ackermann K: Neodym-YAG Laser in der Zahnheilkunde. Münch Med Wschr 126: 1119–1121, 1984
32. Scholz C, Grothues-Spork M: Knochenbearbeitung. In: Müller-Ertl: Angewandte Laserzahnheilkunde. Knochenbearbeitung. III–2.2: 1–24, 1995
33. Goldman L, Shumrick D A, Rockwell R J, Meyer R: The laser in maxillofacial surgery. Arch Surg 96: 397–400, 1968
34. Clayman L, Fuller T, Beckman H: Healing of continuous-wave and rapid superpulsed, carbon dioxide laser induced bone defects. J Oral Surg 36: 932–937, 1978
35. Horch, H-H: Laser in der oralen Chirurgie. Vortrag bei dem 11. Internationalen Jahreskongress der DGL. Berlin 2002
36. Moore J H: Laser Energy in Orthopedic Surgery. 1. Aufl. Excerpta Medica, Amsterdam 1973
37. Königsmann G, Karbe E, Beck R: Application of the CO_2 Laser and the CO Laser as a Surgical Instrument Compared with other IR Lasers and Conventional Instruments. Proc Symp Laser Med Biol, GSF-Bericht, BPT 5: 38, 1977

38. Gretzbein S D, De Demeter D, Cruikshank B, Kapasouri A: The Effect of Laser-Osteotomy on Bone Healing. Lasers Surg Med 1: 361, 1981
39. Horch H-H: Zum aktuellen Stand der Laser-Osteotomie. Der Orthopäde 13: 125–132, 1984
40. Müller G, Bader H, Greve P: 9,6 µm CO_2 Laser für medizinische Anwendungen. Laser 1, 86, 1985
41. Walsh J T, Deutsch T F: Er:YAG Laser Ablation of Tissue: Measurement of Ablation Rates. Lasers Surg Med 9: 327–337, 1989
42. Walsh J T, Flotte T F, Deutsch T F: Er:YAG Laser Ablation of tissue: Effect of Pulse duration and tissue type on thermal damage. Lasers Surg 9: 314–326, 1989
43. Nelson J S, Orenstein A, Liaw L-H L, Berns M W: Mid-Infrared Er:YAG Laser Ablation of Bone: the Effect of Laser Osteotomy on Bone Healing. Lasers Surg Med 9: 362–374, 1989
44. Luomanen M, Meurman J H, Letho V-P: Extracellular matrix in healing CO_2 laser incision wound. J Oral Pathol 16: 322–331, 1987
45. Luomanen M, Virtanen I: Healing of laser and scalpel incision wounds of rat tongue mucosa as studied with cytoceratin antibodies. J Oral Pathol 16: 139–144, 1987
46. Luomanen M: Oral focal epithelial hyperplasia removed with CO_2 laser. Int J Maxillofac Surg 19: 205–207, 1990
47. Kirschner R E, Low D W: Treatment of pyogenic granuloma by shave excision and laser photocoagulation. Plastic Reconstr Surg 104(5): 1346–1350, 1999
48. Bucalo B D, Moy R L: Quantitative comparison of inflammatory infiltrate and linear contraction in human skin treated with 90-µsec pulsed and 900-µsec dwell time carbon dioxide lasers. Dermatol Surg 24(12): 1314–1316, 1998
49. Luomanen M: Die Anwendung des CO_2 Lasers zur Entfernung von multiplen oralen epithelialen Hyperplasien. Proc Finn Dent Soc 83 (Suppl XII), 1989
50. Gaspar L: Comparative Experimental Study on Wound Healing of Incisions made with Scalpel, Electrocautery and CO_2 Laser in the Oral Cavity. J Clin Las Med Surg 8: 35–38, 1990
51. Loevschall H, Arenholt-Bindslev D: Effect of low level diode laser irradiation of human oral mucosa fibroblasts in vitro. Laser Surg Med 14: 347–354, 1994
52. Yu W, Naim J O, Lanzafame R J: The effect of laser irradiation on the release of bFGF from 3T3 fibroblasts. Photochem Photobiol 59: 167–170, 1994
53. Walsh L J: The current status of low level laser therapy in dentistry. Part 1. Soft tissue applications. Aust Dent J 42: 247–254, 1997
54. Van Breugel H, Bär D: Power dentistry and exposure time of He-Ne Laser irradiation are more important than total energy dose in photo-biomodulation of human fibroblasts in vitro. Lasers Surg Med 12: 528–537, 1992
55. Bisht D, Gupta S C, Misra V, Mital V P, Sharma P: Effect of low intensity laser irradiation on healing of open skin wounds in rats. Indian J Med Res 100: 43–46, 1994
56. Takeda Y: Irradiation effect of low-energy laser on rat submandibular salvary gland. J Oral Pathol 17: 91–94, 1988
57. Porteder H, Strassl H, Stanek G, Vinzenz K: Einsatz des Helium Neon Lasers zur Förderung der Wundheilung. Österr Z Stomatol 80: 333–339, 1983
58. Schenk P, Porteder H. et. al: Helium-Neon-Laser-Effekt auf Haut und orale Schleimhautgewebe. Laryng Rhinol Otol 65: 146–150, 1986
59. Migliorati C, Massumoto C, de Paula Eduardo F, Muller K P, Carrieri T, Haypek P: Low-energy Laser Therapy in Oral Mucositis. J Oral Laser Appl 1(2): 97–103, 2001
60. Bensadoun R J et al.: Low-energy He/Ne laser in the prevention of radiation-induced mucositis. A multicenter phase III randomized study in patients with head and neck cancer. Support Care Cancer 7(4): 244–252, 1999
61. Walsh J T, Flotte T J, Anderson R R, Deutsch T F: Pulsed CO_2 laser tissue ablation: Effect of tissue type and pulse duration on thermal damage. Lasers Surg Med 8: 108–118, 1988
62. Walsh J T, Deutsch T F: Pulsed CO_2 laser tissue ablation: Measurement of and modeling of ablation rate. Lasers Surg Med 8: 264–275, 1988
63. Mazouri Z, Walsh L: Damage to dental composite restorations following exposure to CO_2 laser radiation. J Clin Lasers Med Surg 13(2): 73–76, 1995
64. Krause L , Cobb C M, Rapley J W, Killoy W J, Spencer P: Laser irradiation of bone. I. An in vitro study concerning the effects of the CO_2 laser on oral mucosa and subjacent bone. J Periodontol 68(9): 872–880, 1997
65. Goharkhay K et al.: Effects on oral soft tissue produced by a Diode laser in vitro. Lasers Surg Med 25: 401–406, 1999
66. Goharkhay K, Moritz A, Schoop U, Pattera C, Rumetzhofer A, Wernisch J, Sperr W: Auswirkung unterschiedlicher Laserwellenlängen auf die orale Schleimhaut – eine in vitro Studie. Stomatol 97: 173–179, 2000
67. Rossmann J, Gottlieb S, Koudelka B, McQuade M: Effects of CO_2 Laser Irradiation on Gingiva. J Periodontol 58(6);423–425, 1987
68. Stock K, Hibst R: Comparative in vitro study of Diode Laser (940 nm) and Nd:YAG laser for oral surgery. Lecture Laser Congress, Florence 2003
69. Rosenberg C, Tadir Y et al.: Endometrial laser ablation in rabbits: a comparative study on three laser types. Lasers Surg Med 10: 66–73, 1990
70. Walsh J T, Deutsch T F: Pulsed CO_2 laser tissue ablation: Effect of mechanical properties. IEEE Trans Biomed Engl 36: 1195–1201, 1989
71. Neiburger E J, Miserendino L: Laser reflectance: hazard in the dental operatory. Oral Surg Oral Med Oral Pathol 66: 659–661, 1988
72. Romanos G et al.: Laseranwendung in der Parodontologie-aktueller Stand. Parodontologie 4: 299–312, 1998
73. Scholz C, Grothues-Spork M, Dinkelaker F, Büchle A, Cierpinski T, Meyer D-R, Matthes M, Müller G: Comparison of Experimental Laser Systems for in vitro Osteotomy of Human Bone: Proc IX Int. Congress „Laser 1989", Springer Verlag, Berlin, Heidelberg 1990
74. Stein E, Sedlacek T, Fabian R, Nishioka N: Acute and chronic effects of bone ablation with a pulsed Holmium Laser. Laser Surg Med 10: 384–388, 1990

75. Wilder-Smith P, Arrastis A M, Liaw L H, Berns M: Incision properties and thermal effects of three CO_2 lasers in soft tissue. Oral Surg Oral Med Oral Pathol Oral Radiol Endod 79(6): 685–691, 1995
76. Gaspar L, Szabo G: Manifestation of the advantages and disadvantages of using the CO_2 laser in oral surgery. J Clin Laser Med Surg 8 (1): 39–43, 1990
77. Porteder H: Forensik in der Zahnheilkunde. Ärztewoche Verlag Ed. Zahn und Arzt, Wien 2001, 12–14
78. Beer F, Sperr M: Methodenvergleich der chirurgischen Therapie benigner Mundhöhlentumore: konventionelle versus Laserchirurgie. Dissertation an der Univ. Zahnklinik Wien 2002
79. Javan A, Bennett W R Jr., Herriot D R: Population inversion and continuous optical maser oscillation in a gas discharge containing a Helium-Neon mixture. Phys Rev Lett 6: 106, 1961
80. Johnson L F: Optical maser characteristics of rare earth ions in crystal. J Appl Physiol 34: 897–909, 1961
81. Patel C K N, McFarlane R A, Faust W L: Selective excitation through vibrational energy transfer and optical maser action N_2-CO_2. Physiol Rev 13: 617–619, 1964
82. Stern R H, Sognnaes R F: Laser beam effect on dental hard tissues. J Dent Res 43: 873–876, 1964
83. Goldman L, Gray, J A, Goldmann, J, Goldmann, B, Meyer, R: Effects of laser impacts on teeth. J Am Dent Assoc 70: 601–606, 1965
84. Moritz A, Gutknecht N, Schoop U, Wernisch J, Sperr W: Irradiation Treatment of Hypersensitive Dental Necks – Results of an In-vitro-Study. J Clin Laser Med Surg 13(6): 397–400, 1995
85. Moritz A, Gutknecht N, Schoop U, Goharkhay K, Ebrahim D, Wernisch J, Sperr W: The Advantage of CO_2 Treated Dental Necks in Comparison with a Standard Method: Results of an in-vivo-study. J Clin Laser Med Surg 14(1): 27–32, 1996
86. Moritz A, Schoop U, Wernisch J, Nell A, Sperr W: Ergebnisse einer REM-Untersuchung von freiliegenden Zahnhälsen nach CO_2-Laserbestrahlung in vitro. Z Stomatol 93(5): 243–247, 1996
87. Moritz A, Schoop U, Goharkhay K, Sperr W: Advantages of a Pulsed CO_2 Laser in direct Pulp Capping – a long term in vivo-Study. J Lasers Surg Med 22: 288–293, 1998
88. Moritz A, Schoop U, Goharkhay K, Sperr W: The CO_2-Laser as an Aid in Direct Pulp Capping. J Endod 24(1): 27–32, 1997
89. Gaspar L: The use of high power lasers in oral surgery. J Clin Laser Med Surg 12 (5): 281–285, 1994
90. Fried D, Zuerlein M J, Le C Q, Featherstone J D B: Thermal and chemical modification of dentin by 9–11 µm CO_2 Laser pulses of 5–100 µsec duration. Lasers Surg Med 31(4): 275–282, 2002
91. Fried D, Ragadio J, Akrivou M, Featherstone J D B, Murray M W, Dickenson K M: Dental hard tissue modification and removal using sealed transverse excited atmospheric-pressure lasers operating at lambda = 9.6 and 10.6 µm. J Biomed Opt. 6(2): 231–238, 2001
92. Koch R J, Cheng E T: Quantification of skin elasticity changes associated with pulsed carbon dioxide laser skin resurfacing. Arch Facial Plast Surg 1(4): 272–275, 1999
93. Weinstein C: Ultrapulse Carbon dioxide laser removal of periocular wrinkles in association with laser blepharoplasty. J Clin Lasers Med Surg 12 (4): 205–209, 1994
94. Hobby L W: Further evaluation of the potential of the Argon laser in the treatment of Strawberry hemangiomas. Plast Reconstr Surg 71(4): 481–485, 1983
95. White R A, Abergel R P, Lyons R: Biological effects of laser welding on vascular healing. Lasers Surg Med 6: 134–141, 1986
96. Apfelberg D B, Maser M R, Lash H, Flores J: Expanded role of Argon Laser in plastic surgery. J Dermatol Surg Oncol 9(2): 145–151, 1983
97. Powell G L, Blankenau R J: The use of Argon Laser for soft tissue procedures. J Oral Laser Appl 2(4): 235–239, 2002
98. Verheyen P: Photopolymerisation with the argon Laser. J Oral Laser Appl 1(1): 49–55, 2001
99. Baik J W, Rueggeberg F A, Liewehr F R: Effect of light-enhanced bleaching on in vitro surface and intrapulpal temperature rise. J Esthet Restor Dent 13(6): 370–378, 2001
100. Braverman B, McCarthy R J, Ivankovich A D, Forde D D, Overfield M, Bapna M S: Effect of helium-neon and infrared laser irradiation on wound healing in rabbits. Lasers Surg Med 9: 50–58, 1988
101. Lyons R F, Abergale R B, White R A, Dwyer R M, Castel J C, Uitto J: Biostimulation of wound healing in vivo by helium-neon laser. Am J Pathol 18: 47–50, 1987
102. Biel M A: Photodynamic Therapy and the treatment of head and neck cancers. J Clin Lasers Med Surg 14 (5): 239–244, 1996
103. Lou P J, Jones L, Hopper C: Clinical outcomes of photodynamic Therapy for head-and-neck cancer. Technol Cancer Res Treat 2(4): 311–317, 2003
104. Sieron A, Adamek M, Kawczyk-Krupka A, Mazur S, Ilewicz L: Photodynamic therapy (PDT) using topically applied delta-aminolevulinic acid (ALA) for treatment in oral leukoplakia. J Oral Pathol Med 32(6): 330–336, 2003
105. Goldstein A, White J M, Pick R M: Clinical applications of the Nd:YAG laser. In: Miserendino L J, Pick R M (eds.): Lasers in dentistry. Quintessence, Chicago 1995, 199–216
106. Romanos G E: Clinical applications of the Nd:YAG laser in the oral soft tissue surgery and periodontology. J Clin Laser Med Surg 12: 103–108, 1994
107. Berlien H P, Phillip C, Waldschmidt J: Technique and clinical results of Nd:YAG-laser in plastic surgery. J Lasers Surg Med 6: 68, 1996
108. Romanos G E: Laser - was leisten sie in der Implantologie? Eine Bestandsaufnahme aus Forschung und Praxis. Laser J 2: 17–20, 1999
109. Werner J A, Lippert B M, Gottschlich S, Folz B J, Fleiner B, Hoeft S, Rudert H: Ultrasound-guided interstitial Nd:YAG laser treatment of voluminous hemangiomas and vascular malformations in 92 patients. Laryngoscope 108: 463–470, 1998
110. Gratzow R: Kombination von Nd:YAG-Lasertherapie und chirurgischer Therapie in der Behandlung von Hämangiomen. In: Cremer H: Hämangiome. Springer Verlag, Berlin, Heidelberg, New York

111. Gutknecht N, Moritz A, Conrads G, Sievert T, Sperr W, Lampert F: Bactericidal Effect of the Nd:YAG-Laser in in vitro Root Canals. J Clin Laser Med Surg 14(2): 77–80, 1996
112. Moritz A, Schoop U, Goharkhay K, Jakolitsch S, Kluger W, Wernisch J, Sperr W: The Bactericidal Effect of Nd:YAG-, Ho:YAG- and Er:YAG-Laser Irradiation in the Root Canal: An in-vitro comparison. J Clin Laser Med Surg 17(4): 161–164, 1999
113. Moritz A, Jakolitsch S, Goharkhay K, Schoop U, Kluger W, Mallinger R, Sperr W, Georgopoulus A: Morphologic changes correlating to different sensitivities of *Escherichia coli* and *Enterococcus faecalis* to Nd:YAG-Laser irradiation through dentin. Lasers Surg Med 26(3): 250–261, 2000
114. Baraldi C E, Puricelli E, de Paula Eduardo C: Superficial Smoothness of Resection Surface after Apicoectomy and Nd:YAG Noncontact Laser Irradiation: an in vitro Study. J Oral Laser Appl 2(1): 17–24, 2002
115. Hendler B H H, Cateno J, Mooar P, Sherk H H: Holmium:YAG laser arthroscopy of the temporomandibular joint. J Oral Maxillo Fac Surg 50: 931–934, 1992
116. Gerard N, Hendler B H: Laser arthroscopy of the temporomandibular joint. Compend Contin Educ Dent 16 (4): 350, 352–354, 1995
117. Koslim M G, Martin J C: The use of Holmium laser for temporomandibular joint arthroscopic surgery. J Oral Maxillo Fac Surg 51: 122–124, 1993
118. Undt G: Arthroskopische Chirurgie bei Dysfunktionen des Kiefergelenks. Zahn und Arzt 8(10): 8–9, 2003
119. Kaufmann R, Hibst R: Pulsed Erbium:YAG laser ablation in cutaneous surgery. Lasers Surg Med 19: 324–330, 1996
120. Keller U, Hibst R: Ultrastructural changes of enamel and dentin following Erbium:YAG laser irradiation on teeth. Laser Surgery: Advanced characterization, therapeutics and systems. Proc SPIE 120: 408–415, 1990
121. Keller U, Hibst R, Mohr W: Tierexperimentelle Untersuchungen zur Laserosteotomie mit dem Erbium:YAG Laser. Dtsch Z Mund Kiefer Gesichtschir 15: 197–199, 1991
122. Schoop U, Moritz A, Malleschitz P, Goharkhay K, Kluger W, Wernisch J, Sperr W: The impact of Erbium:YAG irradiation on root surfaces: an in vitro evaluation. J Oral Laser Appl 1: 35–43, 2001
123. Salina S, Maiorana C, Piattelli A, Lezzi G, Colombo A, Fontana F: Analysis of the Implant Site Prepared with the Er:YAG Laser Compared to ones Prepared with Traditional Bur and Following Analysis of the Osteointegration of Mini Implants in Rabbits Fibula. Laser Congress, Florence 2003
124. Arnabat J, Espana A, Satorres M, Berini L, Gay-Escada C: Er,Cr:YSGG laser application in the second phase of implant surgery: a pilot study in 30 patients. Lecture Laser Congress, Florence 2003
125. Rizoiu I M, Eversole L R, Kimmel A I: Effects of an Er;Cr:YSGG Laser on mucocutaneous soft tissues. Oral Surg Oral Med Oral Pathol Oral Radiol Endod 82(4): 386–395, 1996
126. Wang X, Ishizaki N T, Suzuki N, Kimura Y, Matsumoto K: Morphological changes of bovine mandibular bone irradiated with Er,Cr:YSGG laser: an in vitro study. J Clin Laser Med Surg 20(5): 245–250, 2002
127. Eversole L R, Rizoiu I M: Preliminary Investigations on the utility of an Er,Cr:YSGG Laser. J Calif Dent Assoc 23(12): 41–47, 1995
128. Mang W L, Sawatzki K: Laserchirurgische Verfahren in der ästhetischen Chirurgie. Dtsch Z Mund Kiefer Gesichtschir 3 (Suppl 1): 162–167, 1999
129. Barlow R J, Walker N P J, Marey A C: Treatment of proliferative hemangiomas with a 585 nm pulsed dye laser. Br J Dermatol 134: 700–704, 1996
130. Moritz A, Gutknecht N, Dörtbudak O, Schoop U, Schauer P, Sperr W: Bacterial reduction in periodontal pockets through irradiation with a Diode laser: a pilot study. J Clin Laser Med Surg 15(1): 33–37, 1997
131. Moritz A, Gutknecht N, Schoop U, Goharkhay K, Dörtbudak O, Sperr W: Irradiation of infected root canals with a Diode Laser in vivo: Results of microbiological examinations. Lasers Surg Med 21: 221–226, 1997
132. Moritz A, Gutknecht N, Goharkhay K, Schoop U, Sperr W: In-vitro Irradiation of Infected Root Canals with a Diode Laser: Results of Microbiologic, Infrared Spectrometric and Stain Penetration Examination. Quintessence Int 28(3): 205–209, 1997
133. Moritz A, Schoop U, Goharkhay K, Schauer P, Doertbudak O, Wernisch J, Sperr W: Treatment of periodontal pockets with a Diode Laser. Lasers Surg Med 22: 302–311, 1998
134. Gutknecht N, Moritz A, Conrads G, Lampert F: The Diode Laser and its bactericidal effect in root canals: an in vitro study. Endodontie 3: 217–222, 1997
135. Mitamba E D, Haanes H R: Low reactive-level 830 nm GaAlAs Diode laser therapy (LLLT) successfully accelerates regeneration of peripheral nerves in human. Laser Ther 5(3): 125, 1993
136. Bernal G: Helium Neon and diode laser therapy is an effective adjunctive therapy for facial paralysis. Laser Ther 5(2): 79–87, 1993
137. Hartmann HJ, Bach G: Diodenlaser-Oberflächen-Dekontamination in der Periimplantitistherapie. Eine Drei-Jahres-Studie. ZWR 106: 524–526, 1997
138. Romanos G, Nentwig G H: Diode Laser (980nm) in oral and maxillofacial surgical procedures: observations based on clinical applications. J Clin Laser Med Surg 17 (5): 193–197, 1999
139. Nakamura Y, Funato A, Wakabayashi H, Matsumoto K: A Study on the Removal of the Melanin Pigmentation of Dog Gingiva by CO_2 Laser Irradiation. J Clin Laser Med Surg 10(1): 41–46, 1992
140. Nakamura Y, Hossain M, Hirayama K, Matsumoto K: A Clinical Study on the Removal of Gingival Melanin Pigmentation with the CO_2 Laser. Laser Surg Med 25(2): 140–147, 1999
141. Fleiner B, Plath T: Histological Evaluation of Leukoplakia following CO_2 Laser Excision. In: Lasers in Otorhinolaryngology, and in Head and Neck Surgery. Adv Otorhinolaryngol 49: 125–129, 1995
142. Mintz S, Barak S, Horowitz I: Carbon Dioxide Laser Excision and Vaporisation of nonplunging ranulas: A Comparison. J Oral Maxillofac Surg 52: 370–372, 1994

143. Schulmeister K: Lasersicherheit; Arbeitsunterlage zur Ausbildung von geprüften Laserschutzbeauftragten. Austrian Research Centers, 2001
144. Keng S B, Loh H S: The treatment of epulis fissuratum of the oral cavity by CO_2 laser surgery. J Clin Lasers Med Surg 10 (4): 303–306, 1992
145. Gaspar L, Szabo G: Removal of epulis by CO_2 Laser. J Clin Lasers Med Surg 9(4): 289–294, 1991
146. Clymer M A, Fortune D S, Reinisch L: Interstitial Nd:YAG Photocoagulation for vascular malformations and hemangiomas in childhood. Arch Otolaryngol Head Neck Surg 124: 431–436, 1998
147. Maiorana C, Salina S, Censi R, Fontana F, Borgonovo A: Nd:YAG Laser in Soft tissue surgery: A two-year retrosprective study on 130 patients. J Oral Laser Appl 1: 21–27, 2001
148. Bier J: Tumoren im Mund-Kiefer-Gesichtsbereich: Bindegewebstumore. In: Praxis der Zahnheilkunde 10/II, Mund-Kiefer-Gesichtchirurgie. Verlag Urban & Schwarzenberg 1991
149. Märker R, Burkhardt A: Erkrankungen der Mundschleimhaut. In: Praxis der Zahnheilkunde 10/II, Mund-Kiefer-Gesichtschirurgie, Verlag Urban & Schwarzenberg, 1991: 216
150. Maerker R, Burkhardt A: Klinik oraler Leukoplakien und Präkanzerosen. Retrospektive Studie an 200 Patienten. Dtsch Z Mund Kiefer Gesichtschir 2: 206–220, 1978
151. Pindborg J J: Oral Cancer and Precancer. Wright, Bristol, 1980
152. Silverman S, Gorsky M, Lozada F: Oral Leukoplakia and Malignant Transformation. Cancer 53: 563–568, 1984
153. Van der Waal I, Snow G B: Oral Oncology. Nijhoff, The Hague 1984
154. Burkhardt A, Maerker R: Vor- und Frühstadien des Mundhöhlenkarzinoms. Hanser Verlag, München 1981
155. Hogewind W F C, Van der Kwast W A M, Van der Waal I: Oral Leukoplakia, with Emphasis on Malignant Transformation. J Cranio Max Fac Surg 17: 128–133, 1989
156. Tischendorf L, Giehler U: Studien zur Dignität von Leukoplakien der Mundschleimhaut und Lippen. Dtsch Z Mund Kiefer Gesichtschir 14: 301–305, 1990
157. Thomson P J, Wylie J: Interventional laser surgery: an effective surgical and diagnostic tool in oral precancer management. Int J Oral Maxillofac Surgery 31(2): 145–153, 2002
158. Schoelch M L, Sekandari N, Regezi J A, Silverman S Jr: Laser management of oral leukoplakias: a follow-up study of 70 patients. Laryngoskopie 109(6): 949–53, 1999
159. Horch HH, Gerlach K, Schaefer HE: CO_2 laser surgery of oral premalignant lesion. Int J Oral Maxillofac Surg 15: 19–24, 1986
160. Chiesa F, Tradati N, Sala L, Costa L, Podrecca S, Boracchi P: Follow-up of Oral Leukoplakia after Carbon Dioxide Laser Surgery. Arch Otolaryngol Head Neck Surg 44: 425–430, 1990
161. Gerlach K L, Roodenburg J L, Herzog M, Horch HH, Panders A K, Pape HD, Feaux de la Croix W, Vermey A: Die Therapie oraler Leukoplakien mit dem CO_2-Laser. Langzeitergebnisse aus drei Kliniken. Dtsch Zahnärztl Z 48: 48–50, 1993
162. Frame J W: CO_2 Laser Excision of soft Tissue Pathology in the Mouth. Zahnärztl Mitt 80: 238–242, 1990
163. Gooris P J, Roodenburg J L, Vermey A, Nauta J M: Carbon Dioxide Laser evaporation of leukoplasia of the lower lip: a retrospective evaluation. Oral Oncol 35 (5): 490–495, 1999
164. Burkey M D B B, Garrett G: Use of laser in the oral cavity. Otolaryngol Clin North Am 29(6): 949–961, 1996
165. Shafer W G, Waldron C A: Erythroplakia of the oral cavity. Cancer 36: 1021–1028, 1975
166. Jungell P: Oral lichen planus. A review. Int J Oral Maxillofac Surg 20: 129–135, 1991
167. Andreasen J O: Oral lichen planus. A clinical evaluation of 115 cases. Oral Surg Oral Med Oral Pathol 25(1): 31–42, 1968
168. Maiorana C, Spadai F, Salina S, Beretta M: Laser therapies and oral lichen planus. J Oral Laser Appl 2(1): 57–61, 2002
169. Cohen L: Mucoceles of the oral cavity. Oral Surg Oral Med Oral Pathol 19: 365–372, 1965
170. Romanos G E, Everts H, Nentwig GH: Alterations of implant surface after CO_2- or Nd:YAG laser irradiation: A SEM evaluation. J Oral Laser Appl 1, 29–33, 2001
171. Romanos G E: Treatment of periimplant lesions using different laser systems. J Oral Laser Appl 2: 75–81, 2002
172. Romanos G E, Purucker P, Bernimoulin J P, Nentwig G H: Bactericidal Efficacy of CO_2-Laser Against Bacteria-Contaminated Sandblasted Titanium Implants. J Oral Laser Appl 2: 171–174, 2002
173. Block C, Mayo J, Evans G: Effects of the Nd:YAG Dental laser on Plasma-sprayed and hydroxyapatite-coated Titanium Dental implants: Surface alteration and attempted Sterilization. Int Oral Maxillofac Implants 7: 441–449, 1992
174. Romanos G E, Everts H, Nentwig G H: Effects of the diode (980 nm) and Nd:YAG (1064 nm) laser irradiation on titanium discs. A SEM examination. J Periodontol 71: 810–815, 2000
175. Romanos G E: Laser surgical tools in Implant Dentistry for the long-term prognosis of oral implants. In: Ishikawa I, Frame J, Aoki A (eds.): Lasers in Dentistry. International Congress Series 1248: 109–114. Elsevier Science BV, Amsterdam 2003
176. Salina S, Beretta M, Speroni S, Maiorana C: Treatment of peri-implantitis with Diode Laser and GBR: preliminary results. Posters, Laser Congress, Florence 2003
177. Barak S, Horowitz I, Katz J, Oelgiesser D: Thermal Changes in Endosseous Root-Form Implants as a Result of CO_2 Laser Application: an in vitro and in vivo study. Int J Oral Maxillofac Implants 13(5), 666–671, 1998
178. Kreisler M, Al Haj H, Gotz H, Duschner H, d'Hoedt B: Effect of simulated CO_2 and GaAlAs Laser surface decontamination on temperature changes in Ti-plasma sprayed dental implants. Lasers Surg Med 30(3), 233–239, 2002
179. Wooten C A, Sullivan S M, Surpure S: Heat generation by superpulsed CO_2 Lasers on plasma-sprayed titanium implants: an in vitro study. Oral Surg Oral Med Oral Pathol Oral Radiol Endod 88(5), 544–548, 1999
180. Mouhyi J, Sennerby L, Nammour S, Guillaume P, Van Reck J: Temperature increases during surface decontamination of titanium implants using CO_2 Laser. Clin Oral Implants Res 10(1), 54–61, 1999

181. Kreisler M, Al Haj H, d'Hoedt B: Temperature changes at the implant-bone interface during simulated surface decontamination with an Er:YAG laser. Int J Prosthodont 15(6), 582–587, 2002
182. Walsh J T Jr, Flotte T J, Deutsch T F: Er:YAG Laser Ablation of Tissue: Effect of Pulse Duration and Tissue Type on Thermal Damage. Lasers Surg Med 9, 314–326, 1989
183. Chryssikopoulos S: Er:YAG and CO_2 Lasers in oral implantology: a study on 83 implants. J Oral Laser Appl 3, 97–103, 2003
184. Lewandrowski K U, Tomford W W, Schomaker K T, Deutsch T F, Mankin H J: Improved osteoinduction of cortical bone allografts: a study of the effects of laser perforation and partial demineralisation. J Orthop Res 15, 748–756, 1997
185. O'Donell R J, Deutsch T F, Flotte R J, Lorente C A, Mankin H J, Schomaker K T: Effect of Er:YAG Laser holes on osteoinduction in demineralized rat calvarial allografts. J Orthop Res 14, 108–113, 1996
186. McDavid V G, Cobb C M, Rapley J W, Glaros A G, Spencer P: Change in temerature of subjacent bone during soft tissue laser ablation. J Periodontol 69, 1278–1282, 1998
187. Kimura Y, Yu D G, Fujita A, Yamashita A, Murakami Y, Matsumoto K: Effects of Er,Cr:YSGG laser irradiation on canine mandibular bone. J Periodontol 72, 1178–1182, 2001
188. Isreal M, Rossmann J, Froum S: Use of the carbon dioxide laser in retarding epithelial migration: a pilot histological human study. J Periodontol 1995; 66: 197–204
189. Centty I G, Blank L W, Levy B A, Romberg E, Barnes D M: Carbon Dioxide laser for de-epithelialization of periodontal flaps. J Periodontol 68(8), 763–769, 1997
190. Rossmann J A, Israel M: Laser de-epithelialization for enhanced guided tissue regeneration. A paradigm shift? Dent Clin North Am 44(4), 793–809, 2000
191. Trylovich D J, Cobb C M, Pippin D J, Spencer P: The effects of Nd:YAG Laser on in vitro fibroblast attachment to endotoxin-treated root surfaces. J Periodontol. 63, 626–632, 1992
192. Friesen L R, Cobb C M, Rapley J W, Forgas-Brockman L, Spencer P: Laser Irradiation of bone: II. Healing Response following Treatment by CO_2 and Nd:YAG Lasers. J Periodontol. 70(1), 75–83, 1999
193. Gouw-Soares S, Tanji E, Haypek P, Cardoso W, Eduardo CP: The use of Er:YAG, Nd:YAG, and Ga-Al-As-Lasers in Periapical Surgery. J Clin Lasers Med Surg 19(4): 193–198, 2001
194. Williams T M, Cobb C M, Rapley J W, Killoy W J: Histologic Evaluation of alveolar bone following CO_2 Laser removal of connective tissue from periodontal pockets. Int J Periodont Restorat Dent 15(5), 497–506, 1995
195. Sculean A, Schwarz F, Berakdar M, Windisch P, Arweiler N, Romanos G E: Healing of intrabony defects following surgical treatment with or without an Er:YAG Laser. A controlled clinical study. J Clin Periodontol 2004 (in press)

12

Photoactivated Disinfection (PAD)

P. Verheyen, R. Blum, K. Goharkhay, L. J. Walsh,

12.1 Introduction

Certain molecules known as photosensitizers generate cytotoxic species, particularly singlet oxygen, when irradiated with light of an appropriate wavelength[1,2]. On absorbing a photon, the photosensitizer molecule is promoted to a high-energy state (known as the triplet state) which then transfers its energy to an oxygen molecule, resulting in the generation of singlet oxygen. This phenomenon can be used to kill bacteria in a process termed "lethal photosensitization"[2–5], in which the singlet oxygen damages bacterial membranes and DNA[6]. Singlet oxygen has an extremely short lifetime[7], and must be generated in close proximity to cells to produce cytotoxic effects.

Photoactivated disinfection (PAD) can be defined as "a method of disinfecting or sterilizing a hard tissue or soft tissue site by topically applying a photosensitizing compound to the site, and then irradiating this with laser light at a wavelength absorbed by the photosensitizing compound, so as to destroy microbes at the site"[4].

The concept of killing human or microbial cells via photosensitive agents is well established in medicine, and the application of this to the treatment of malignancies (photodynamic therapy, PDT) has proven successful for certain types of tumors. The key principle is that the laser-activated agent must bind selectively to the target cells, rather than to adjacent normal human cells[8].

The applications of PAD in dentistry and medicine are wide, and include the destruction of bacterial, fungal and viral pathogens in a range of clinical settings[2–4,9,10]. The fact that lethal photosensitization is not species-specific is advantageous in that it is possible to kill all the bacteria present in a mixed infection. Where absolute specificity is required, conjugation of the photosensitizer dye to a monoclonal antibody to the target organism offers a suitable strategy to achieve selective PAD[11].

PAD may represent a viable alternative to antibiotics and antiseptics for the treatment of localized infections, particularly for those caused by organisms which are innately resistant or have developed resistance to conventional antimicrobial agents. The oral cavity is a particularly suitable site for this treatment since it is easily accessible, and many key pathogens in oral diseases have been shown to be susceptible to killing by PAD using tolonium chloride dye[12–15]. Because the development of resistance to photochemically-induced killing is very unlikely, PAD treatment can be used on multiple occasions in the same patient or site.

12.2 Photodynamic Therapy – the Origins of PAD

In photodynamic therapy (PDT), laser activation of a sensitizing dye (usually a porphyrin derivative) generates reactive oxygen species (ROS), which directly damage cells and the associated blood vascular network, triggering both necrosis and apoptosis[16,17]. PDT also alters the host anti-tumor immune response. In addition to direct toxicity from ROS, tumor cells can die as a result of damage to the microvasculature, the associated inflammatory reaction and the enhanced host anti-tumor immune response. Arguably, the vascular events are more important than direct toxicity[18–20].

When used for oral mucosal malignancies such as carcinoma in situ and squamous cell carcinoma, PDT has a response rate of ~ 90%[21,22]. The treated sites show erythema and edema, followed by necrosis and frank ulceration. The ulcerated lesions take up to 8 weeks to heal fully, and supportive analgesia is required in the first few weeks. Other than short-term photo-sensitivity, the treatment appears to be tolerated well. PDT is less destructive to normal tissues than the conventional treatments of surgery or radiotherapy, and unlike the latter can be repeated[22].

PDT for tumors is typically undertaken with porphyrin derivatives such as hematoporphyrin 10. One of the newer generation of tumor photosensitizers, aluminum disulfonated phthalocyanine, was found to be an effective photosensitizer of Gram-positive and Gram-negative bacteria[4]. In general, photosensitizers developed for use in PDT of tumors are less effective at sensitizing bacteria to killing by visible red laser light than dyes such as toluidine blue. The latter bind poorly to human cells, a feature of considerable importance since this reduces the possibility of "bystander" injury to human cells.

12.3 Principles of PAD

The principles of photoactivation using lasers to achieve disinfection in selected sites in the oral cavity have been established by the extensive work of Michael Wilson and his colleagues at the Eastman Dental Institute in London. In the past 10 years, numerous laboratory studies conducted by this group, and more recently by others, have explored the effectiveness of photoactivated disinfection (PAD) and demonstrated its use in a variety of dental applications [2–4,6,10–15,23–50].

The mechanism of action of PAD is based on the interaction of a photosensitive antimicrobial agent and a source of light. When the photosensitizing agent is exposed to the light source of a particular wavelength, it absorbs photons of energy with subsequent electronic transition to the next state – the singlet excited state. From here, the electrons may fall back to the ground state and release the gained energy via electronic or physical processes (fluorescence), or they may jump to the next excited state (intersystem crossover) – the triplet excited state. Whether the molecule follows the first or the second path is determined by its molecular structure and also by the surrounding environment[8].

Once in the triplet excited state (which is a more stable species), the molecule may fall back to the ground state or undergo reactions with molecular oxygen, transferring its energy to the molecule. Reactions that take place with oxygen are of two types: (1) those that give rise to hydroxyl radicals, superoxide ions, peroxides and radicals which then instigate redox reactions with the surrounding environment, and (2) those that result in the formation of a labile singlet oxygen or reactive oxygen species[8,51].

Whether bacterial killing is achieved is determined by how many triplet state molecules are generated from the photosensitizer, and this in turn is determined by how long it can stay in the triplet excited state. The formation of labile singlet oxygen and the evoked cascade of redox reactions are the primary mechanisms that destroy bacterial cells and their cellular components[4].

12.4 Photosensitizers

A limited number of bacteria naturally produce endogenous photosensitive agents (such as porphyrins) and can therefore be killed by exposure to laser light alone of the proper wavelength. In contrast, the outer membranes of all bacteria (as well as some fungi and viruses) can be stained with synthetic dyes to allow for their killing by PAD.

There are many types of photosensitizers, both naturally occurring and synthetically produced. Some of the more commonly used sensitizers for PAD are listed in Table 12-1.

Table 12-1 Photosensitizers used in PAD.

Tolonium chloride (toluidine blue O, TBO)
Methylene blue
Azure dyes
Crystal violet
Hematoporphyrins
Aluminum disulfonated phthalocyanine (ADP)
Chlorins (e.g. Photochlorines I, II, III)

As noted above, several oral pathogenic bacteria naturally produce their own photosensitizers. Black pigmented species belonging to the genera *Porphyromonas* and *Prevotella*, contain protohemin and protoporphyrin IX, respectively[52–54]. The work of Konig et al.[54] has shown that for these species, exposure to visible red light from a helium–neon laser (7.3 mW, λ = 632.8 nm) in the absence of an external photosensitizing dye can cause a reduction in viability of up to 50%. However, many key oral pathogens such as *Streptococcus mutans* and *Enterococcus faecalis* do not endogenously produce such porphyrins, and are therefore resistant to killing with red light alone[45,53]. Such bacteria can, however, be successfully killed using external photosensitizers such as tolonium chloride and methylene blue.

Because of their binding properties, some photosensitizers are active against a limited range of microbial species. As well, photosensitizer dyes may interact differently with various species of bacteria because of differences in their electrostatic interactions with the bacterial cell membrane. Thus, a photosensitizer may induce cell damage by binding to the cell wall of one target cell, while in a different target cell it may bind to both the cell wall and the nucleic acids within the cell. Conversely, with a completely different species, it may not have any effect. Of interest, there is some evidence that the photosensitizer does not necessarily have to be present intracellularly in order to exert a bactericidal effect[11].

Many common photosensitizers such as tolonium chloride have a positive charge under physiological conditions since this will enhance their binding to negatively-charged bacterial cell walls.

To achieve optimal results with PAD therapy, the following characteristics of the photosensitizer should be taken into account:
- the cell types to which the photosensitizer binds
- the concentrations at which its actions are most effective
- the wavelength of light required to activate it and the intensity of the light
- the concentration at which it would exhibit any toxic effects and what these would be
- its solubility in water and lipid environments
- its degree of ionization
- the excitation efficiency (how effective it is at reaching the triplet state) and
- how long it can stay in the triplet state[48].

Numerous studies have been conducted to determine not only the most efficient photosensitizer for killing particular oral pathogens, but also the most efficient combination of photosensitizer and wavelength of light. Toluidine blue, methylene blue and azure B chloride have been shown to be effective against a wide range of Gram-positive and Gram-negative bacteria[4]. Studies of 24 other compounds at different concentrations indicated that some 16 other photosensitizers could reduce the viability of some bacteria, but these have little or no effect on some key pathogens[4]. Consequently, these would be of limited clinical use.

Photosensitizing compounds used in PAD typically cause limited killing of the target microbes at concentrations used clinically. One notable exception to this is methylene blue, which shows considerable toxicity to *Candida albicans* and to some species of streptococci, even when there has been limited exposure to light[48,49].

A key property of photosensitizers is that they should absorb laser light in the red portion of the visible spectrum or at longer wavelengths in the near infrared region. Red visible wavelengths will give the greatest penetration of tissues surrounding a wound or lesion, and will also penetrate any blood which may be present.

Common photosensitizer/laser combinations are:

- tolonium chloride with a 635-nm diode laser or a 632.8-nm helium–neon gas laser
- methylene blue with a 670-nm diode laser
- aluminum disulfonated phthalocyanine with a 660-nm diode laser.

Typically, these photosensitizers are used in low concentrations, for example 0.001% to 0.01% w/v in aqueous solution when at their final concentration, i.e., after any dilution in the root canal, periodontal pocket or wound site. The relatively low concentration of dye ensures that soft tissue irritation and staining of hard tissues do not occur. Staining can occur when tolonium chloride or methylene blue are used at high concentrations. Tolonium chloride has been used as a biological stain for the in situ delineation of epithelial malignancies in the oro-pharynx[55,56], and methylene blue has been employed as a caries detector dye; however, there have not been any reported adverse reactions or side effects following topical application of these dyes in these clinical applications.

An additional point to consider is the effect of dye concentration on the effectiveness of PAD. A low dye concentration will mean limited generation of reactive oxygen species and a requirement for a longer irradiation time, while too high a dye concentration may provide an optical barrier because of absorption. The importance of optimizing the dye concentration has been demonstrated in several studies. Bhatti et al.[45] reported that increasing the concentration of tolonium chloride dye resulted in less efficient killing. The explanation for this effect was that saturation of bacterial cells had been achieved, and unbound dye reduced the penetration of laser light, resulting in reduced effectiveness of the whole system.

As well as the photosensitizing dye, other components of the photosensitizing liquid used in PAD may include buffers, salts for adjusting the tonicity of the solution, anti-oxidants, preservatives, and surfactants to ensure surface wetting. Buffers are essential to give a reliable PAD effect in clinical situations. The pH of the medium has been shown to influence the properties and behavior of both photosensitizers and bacteria[14,57,58], by changing penetration and binding of the dye. Alkaline pH environments (pH 8.0) tend to promote photosensitization as opposed to acidic environments (pH 4.0 and 5.0) for several reasons:

- improved penetration of dye into the cells[59]
- increased cytotoxicity of singlet oxygen molecules[57] and
- increased lifetime of the excited triplet state compared with the ground state[60]

12.5 Clinical Aspects of the PAD Technique

When using PAD clinically, the photosensitizer solution must be placed in direct contact with the site for a short period of time (such as 30 s) to enable the microbes to take up some of the photosensitizer and thus become sensitive to the laser light.

The photosensitizer will only be able to efficiently destroy the targeted organism if activated by the appropriate wavelength of light. Using a light source with a wavelength outside the absorption range will result in only a small portion of the laser energy being absorbed by the dye, and thus little if any production of singlet oxygen, leading to minimal killing of the targeted pathogen.

Furthermore, it must be borne in mind that the hard or soft tissue penetration capabilities of light vary enormously according to the wavelength employed[61]. A window of transmissibility in the visible red region, for instance, is exploited by most PAD therapies of interest to dental practice (Table 12-2).

Using a range of laboratory models, including dentin slices and collagen gels, PAD treatment of representative microbes commonly found in the oral cavity and implicated in inflammatory periodontal disease, caries and other dental diseases has been shown to give effective destruction (Table 12-3)[2-4,6,10-15,23-50]. These studies have been complemented by trials in animal models as well as clinical trials in humans[15].

The presence of organic materials (such as blood and saliva) may offer some protection to bacteria against lethal photosensitization[27,28,38,58]. Decreased effectiveness of photosensitization in the presence of saliva and serum is due to several factors:

- partial absorption of laser light, which reduces the yield of cytotoxic molecules produced from the dye
- electrostatic interaction with the dye, thus decreasing the number of photosensitizer molecules available for binding to the target bacteria
- the presence of scavenger molecules such as catalase and lactoperoxidase[40] and
- direct protection from singlet oxygen

Nevertheless, substantial levels of kill (> 5 $\log_{10}$ reductions) can still be achieved using PAD in the presence of saliva or blood, by using an adequate energy dose[14]. Typical microbes killed by PAD are collected in Table 12-3.

Table 12-2 Dental applications of PAD (based on Wilson and Wilson[4]).

Treating periodontal pockets
Treating plaque-infected cervical regions of teeth and dental implants
Disinfecting carious dentine prior to restoration
Destroying cariogenic microbes on a tooth surface in order to treat or prevent dental caries
Disinfecting oral tissues prior to or during surgical procedures
Treating oral candidiasis in immune compromised patients
Treating denture stomatitis

Table 12-3 Typical microbes killed by PAD.

Streptococcus sanguis
Streptococcus mutans
Streptococcus sobrinus
Lactobacillus casei
Lactobacillus fermentum
Actinomyces viscosus
Porphyromonas gingivalis
Fusobacterium nucleatum
Actinobacillus actinomycetemcomitans
Salmonella enteritidis
Staphylococcus aureus
Candida albicans
Pseudomonas aeruginosa
Escherichia coli
Klebsiella pneumonia

12.6 Laser Used in PAD

The laser types most commonly used for PAD operate in the red visible portion of the electromagnetic spectrum, and include gallium aluminum arsenide diode lasers (λ = 633–635 nm, or λ = 660–670 nm wavelengths), and the helium–neon gas laser (λ = 632.8 nm). Because the output parameters (power and wavelength) of diode lasers can be altered by heating, PAD laser systems which use diode lasers typically employ a solid-state Peltier cooling device, which is attached directly to the rear surface of the diode laser.

Typical PAD parameters for effective killing of microbes[4] are of the order of 15 J/cm^2 (ranging from10–20 J/cm^2), delivered using a laser with an output power (measured at the distal end of the optical fiber delivery system) of up to 100 mW. Higher power densities allow the required time of irradiation of the dye to be kept within a clinically usable range, e.g., from 5 s to 60 s.

There are a range of delivery systems for the laser, including simple optical fibers with cloven ends, through to more complex photodynamic therapy diffusers with spherical or cylindrical emission patterns, for use in carious lesions and root canals, respectively (Figs. 12-1 to 12-4).

The use of diffuser tips ensures an even irradiation of the target site. Moreover, the diffusion effect reduces the effective power density and this reduces the risk for optical injury from the laser.

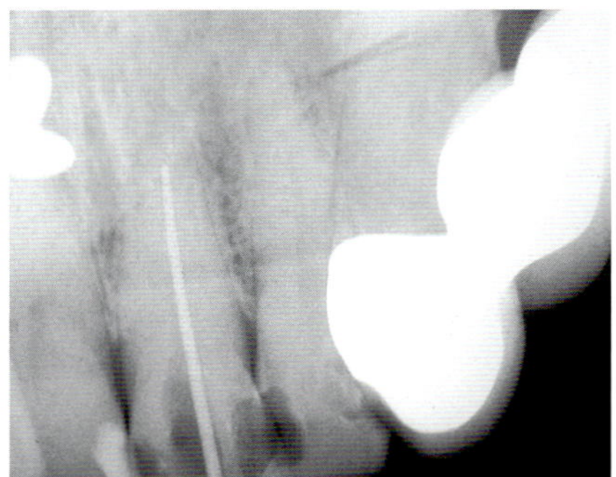

Fig 12-1 An endodontic case with refractory infection and clinical pain.

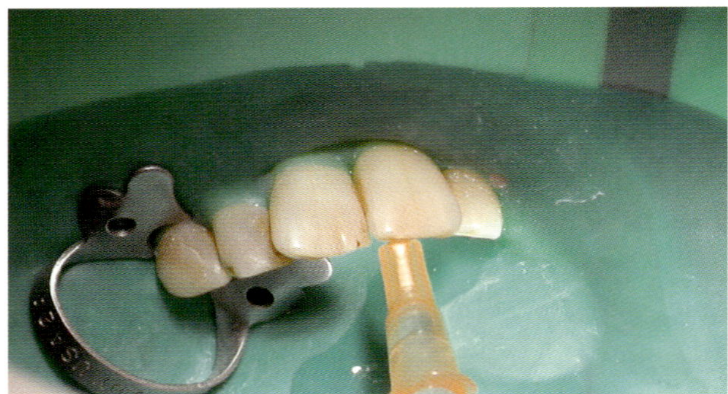

Fig 12-2 After conventional canal preparation has been completed, the root canal system is dried, and tolonium chloride dye placed in the canal.

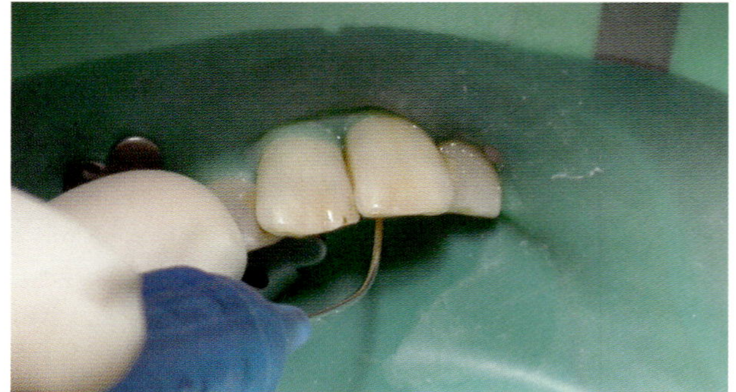

Fig 12-3 The endodontic PAD hand piece in place. The SaveDent system (Denfotex) is being used, which employs a cylindrical diffuser to illuminate the root canal system with 635-nm laser light.

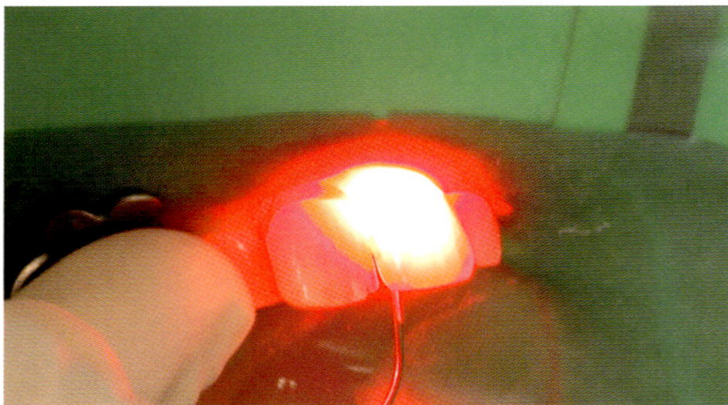

Fig 12-4 Irradiation of the tolonium chloride dye.

12.7 Laboratory and Clinical Studies of PAD

Numerous laboratory studies have shown that the photosensitizing effect in PAD is the result of a specific interaction between the dye and the laser energy, and that use of either component on its own does not result in efficient killing of the target bacteria[2–4,24]. Burns et al.[25] noted that with an extended period of exposure (up to 1 h), tolonium chloride dye at high concentrations (50–100 μg/ml) could cause a significant reduction in the viability of *S. mutans*, *S. sobrinus*, and *L. casei*; however, it must be pointed out that this extended time period would not be of value clinically. Similarly, some degree of killing can occur with methylene blue and with ADP when used without laser irradiation, but this alone cannot provide a useful clinical result[29].

The parameters required for killing bacteria by PAD have been established in independent studies in several university centers. For example, the Wilson research group in London[23–25] showed that for *S. mutans* using tolonium chloride dye and a helium–neon laser, the mean lethal energy dose was 1.22×10^{-4} to 2.42×10^{-4} mJ per bacterial cell. In an independent study, the group in Brisbane[62] calculated that when using methylene blue dye and a diode laser ($\lambda = 670$ nm), the mean lethal dose for the same species (and laboratory strain) was 1.2×10^{-4} to 2.8×10^{-4} mJ per bacterial cell, which corresponds exactly.

With regard to bacteria involved in dental caries, Burns et al.[24] showed that tolonium chloride (25 μg/ml) used with $\lambda = 632.8$ nm laser energy could reduce the viability of *S. mutans, S. sobrinus, L. casei,* and *Actinomyces viscosus*. This was confirmed in independent studies in other countries by Stringer[62,63] and Okamoto[64]. The Eastman group[41] also demonstrated successful killing using the photosensitizer ADP (50 μg/ml) when used with a gallium aluminum arsenide diode laser (11 mW, $\lambda = 660$ nm).

Subsequent studies confirmed that successful killing could be obtained under in vivo simulated conditions using mixed supragingival plaque flora, while several studies using dentin slices or collagen gels[36,63,65] showed that *S. mutans* could be successfully killed up to depths of 1 mm when within dentin. Current clinical protocols for PAD treatment of carious dentin include the use of a 0.8-mm-diameter spherical isotropic diffuser to give even irradiation of the cavity floor[50].

Several studies have addressed the important issue of killing cariogenic bacteria when present within a biofilm, a situation which could potentially confer a greater resistance to a chemically-based killing process. Particular issues with biofilms include penetration of the dye and the laser light, and the growth state of bacteria deep within the biofilm. With some species of bacteria, cells in stationary phase have thicker cell membranes and thus may be somewhat less susceptible to killing by PAD than when in lag or log phase[45], although this effect can be overcome by using PAD under more alkaline pH conditions[14,38]. Several studies have reported that *S. sanguis* when present within a biofilm which mimicked the in vivo situation can be killed by PAD using tolonium chloride, ADP, or methylene blue[41,46]. O'Neill et al.[48] have also reported a 9 × 109 bacterial reduction with PAD in a multi-species biofilm that was intended to simulate in vivo plaque matrix conditions.

In terms of bacteria associated with periodontitis, several photosensitizers have been shown to be effective when tested in laboratory models, including tolonium chloride, dihematoporphyrin ester, ADP, and methylene blue[4,6,11,13–15,26,28,29,31,33]. Typical target bacterial species for these studies have been *Porphyromonas gingivalis, Actinobacillus actinomycetemcomitans*, and *Fusobacterium nucleatum*. Effective killing by PAD (with reductions in viability of 97.2%, 99.9% and 99.4%, respectively) have been obtained using tolonium chloride (25 μg/ml), although methylene blue and ADP give somewhat less uniform results across these species[4].

For example, PAD with methylene blue achieved reductions of 99.9% and 92.6% for *F. nucleatum* and *P. gingivalis*, respectively, but only 64.3% for *Actinobacillus actinomycetemcomitans*, which is much lower than was achieved using tolonium chloride. Moreover, hematoporphyrin ester, which was shown to be effective against *P. gingivalis* in planktonic suspension, had little effect when used in PAD against the same organism in a biofilm[23]. This emphasizes the importance of dye selection for clinical use in PAD. A final and important variation on the PAD concept for periodontal therapy is the use of an antibody to *P. gingivalis* attached to tolonium chloride dye, in order to target the therapy to this one key pathogen[11].

The above studies examined the effectiveness of killing periodontopathic bacteria using PAD applied to pure bacterial cultures. As is the case with dental caries, in a clinical setting the microflora of the plaque is mixed, rather than pure. Subsequent studies have shown that bacteria from subgingival plaque from sites of periodontal destruction or peri-implantitis when grown in mixed cultures and biofilms can be effectively killed using PAD with tolonium chloride dye[26,66].

Further studies have also shown effective killing of the oral opportunistic pathogen *Candida albicans* by PAD using tolonium chloride dye[10,30,67,68], while methylene blue dye has been used for the inactivation of viruses in blood products using a PAD approach[69,70].

More recent work conducted in our laboratory has applied the PAD technique to the root canal system, using first *S. mutans* and then *E. faecalis* as the challenge organisms, both of which lack endogenous porphyrin photosensitizers and are thus resistant to killing by visible red light alone. *E. faecalis* is a common cause of treatment failures in root-filled teeth that have suffered from coronal leakage[71–75], and is a challenge to conventional endodontic medicaments and disinfection approaches[76–80]. Successful killing of *E. faecalis* by PAD using either methylene blue or tolonium chloride has been obtained[81–83]; however, the effect obtained is even more profound with the latter dye when used in combination with a purpose-designed flexible endodontic diffuser which gives even irradiation of the root canal system (Table 12-4). For clinical endodontics, it should also be remembered that acute exacerbations during endodontic therapy typically involve *Porphyromonas* species[78,88], particularly *P. endodontalis*, which as a strict anaerobe is extremely susceptible to killing by singlet oxygen. PAD can be used effectively for canal disinfection, as an adjunct to existing measures such as irrigation with sodium hypochlorite[82]. However, sufficient bacterial elimination in deep dentin layers, especially tubules and side canals, is more efficient with high power dental lasers (see chapter 9).

In an in-vivo study, at the University of Vienna, the effect of photodynamic treatment on bacteria associated with peri-implant disease, especially *Actinobacillus actinomycetemcomitans*, *Porphyromonas gingivalis* and *Prevotella*

Table 12-4 In vitro endodontic disinfection of *E. faecalis* using PAD (according to Lee[83]).

Plain optical fiber delivery system (Omnilase)	Methylene blue dye alone 50 µg/ml: 17% kill Diode laser alone λ = 670 nm, 10 mW, 120 s: 5% kill PAD using methylene blue dye + laser: λ = 670 nm: 99.74% kill
Endodontic diffuser fiber (SaveDent)	Tolonium chloride dye alone 50 µg/mL: 8.4 % kill Diode laser alone λ = 633 nm, 50 mW, 120 s: 10.7% kill PAD using tolonium chloride dye + laser: λ = 633 nm: 99.99% kill

intermedia, indicated that this treatment resulted in a significant bacterial reduction by a maximum of 3 log-steps. It is possible to reduce the periodontal pathogens by more than 92%[84]. However, a complete elimination of all three microorganisms is achieved in none of the cases in contrast to an in-vitro study from Haas et al[85]. The reason for this effect might be that the application of toluidine-blue-O and the irradiation with the laser into the bone pockets is possibly restricted.

A new method in the treatment of peri-implantitis is the combination of toluidine blue and laser irradiation (λ = 906 nm) and the filling of bone defects with autogenous bone using e-PTFE membranes. A mean reduction in the bone defect of 2 mm is achieved[86].

TBO and an irradiation with a diode-laser in-vivo (λ = 690 nm, 7.3 mW) for 1 min provides a significant reduction of bacteria (*A.a.*; *P.g.*; *P.i.*) by a maximum of 4 log steps in patients with progredient periodontal disease. The cell count of reduction by all three microorganisms is more than 99.9%[87]. The photodynamic therapy is merely locally effective and not systemic as antibiotics are. Therefore there are no side effects, allergies or intolerances. It can be suggested that it is a beneficial treatment for pregnant patients and at-risk patients suffering from paradontitis.

Treatment recommendations for PAD applications in dentistry are shown in Table 12-5.

Table 12-5 Treatment recommendations for PAD applications in dentistry.

Periimplantitis	Diode laser, 7.3m W, λ = 690–905 nm, 60s, in combination with toluidin blue, buccal and oral.
Implantation	75m W, λ = 680nm, 2J, 40 s, without photosensitizing dye. Irradiation before starting the implantation, after drilling and after suture. Reduction of pain, edema and hematoma development, and the possibility of infection. Perhaps repetition on the next day and the day after next.
Periodontitis	Diode soft laser λ = 690 nm, 7.3–3.0 mW, 1.6 J/cm^2, 1 min. in combination with toluidine blue, 2–3x / week. Insertion of toluidine blue with a syringe using a soft plastic peak into the pocket or spread the tooth near gingiva with a thin layer of methylene blue (1 min.) and with a special top from girland to girland, buccal and oral, irradiation for 1 min.
Periodontal Operation	75 mW, λ = 680 nm, 2–3 J, 40–60 s, irradiation before, during and after the OP. If the periodontal pocket is deeper than 4 mm, flapping.
Dolor post therapy	Methylen blue soaked stripe into the alveole for 1 min. and after the removal 1 min. irradiation.
Root resection	Toluidin blue in bone cavity and 1 min. irradiation.
Aphtous, herpes, *Candida*	Are also dyed and irradiated.

12.8 Safety Issues with PAD

The most commonly employed dye for PAD is tolonium chloride. As mentioned previously, this dye is widely used as an adjunct to biopsy and other clinical tools, in diagnosing early stages of oral epithelial dysplasia and in situ and invasive squamous cell carcinomas[55,89,90]. Both the concentration and volume of dye utilized for this purpose are several orders of magnitude higher than those used in PAD, yet no adverse effects have been reported over several decades of use. There is direct evidence from animal studies that tolonium chloride is not a carcinogen, co-carcinogen or promoter of cancer, even when used at extreme exposures, e.g., 2% concentration applied three times daily.

In terms of the potential for bystander injury, an important concern is whether PAD dyes can bind to human cells and cause injury or cell death by photosensitization. There is direct laboratory evidence from cell culture studies that human fibroblasts and keratinocytes are not killed by the combination of tolonium chloride and visible red laser light used clinically for PAD[42]. Animal studies of PAD applied in the periodontal pocket environment or onto mucosal soft tissues have confirmed that no adverse effects of photosensitization occur on normal tissues[15,47].

Direct thermal measurements of heating of the dental pulp (during PAD treatment for caries) or of the root surface (during endodontic disinfection with PAD) have revealed that thermal changes are less than 0.5° C[63,81,83]. This is not significant clinically as the critical threshold levels at which irreversible pulpitis occurs is 11 times higher (i.e., an increase of 5.5° C)[91]. The minimal thermal effects of PAD with visible red laser light in the root canal system can be compared very favorably with the thermal changes associated with disinfection using powerful near-infrared lasers such as the Nd:YAG and carbon dioxide lasers[92–96].

12.9 Summary and Conclusions

PAD is a novel form of low power laser therapy in which the laser energy in itself is not particularly lethal to bacteria, but is used to achieve photochemical activation of oxygen-releasing dyes. Singlet oxygen released from the dyes causes membrane and DNA, damage to microorganisms, leading to their rapid death. The most common dyes used for PAD are tolonium chloride (with 633-nm lasers), methylene blue (with 670-nm lasers), and aluminum disulfonated phthalocyanine (with 675-nm lasers). Tolonium chloride is the preferred dye as it gives the most consistent killing effect across a range of bacterial species of importance to dentistry.

The effectiveness of PAD is influenced by the type and concentration of dye, the laser parameters employed, and the local growth environment (biofilm and growth state). Major applications of PAD include the disinfection of deep carious lesions, periodontal pockets and peri-implant sites, mucosal wounds, and root canals. PAD treatment does not give rise to deleterious thermal effects, and does not injure adjacent tissues by thermal or chemical effects. Thus, PAD is a valuable component of the modern practice of laser dentistry[97]. It is expected that further research work will extend the range and usefulness of PAD in preventing or treating infections of the oral cavity and the associated structures.

Acknowledgements

The authors thank Drs P Bird, GJ Stringer, T Silbert, and MT Lee for their important contributions to the PAD research program at the University of Queensland School of Dentistry. This research work has been supported by grants from the Australian Dental Research Foundation, and the Australian Research Council.

12.10 References

1. Ochsner M: Photophysical and photobiological processes in the photodynamic therapy in tumours. J Photochem Photobiol B 39: 1–18, 1997
2. Wilson M, Dobson J, Harvey W: Sensitization of oral bacteria to killing by low-power laser radiation. Curr Microbiol 25: 77–81, 1992
3. Wilson M: Photolysis of oral bacteria and its potential use in the treatment of caries and periodontal disease. J Appl Bacteriol 75: 299–306, 1993
4. Wilson M, Wilson H: Laser treatment. US Patent 5, 611,793. 1997
5. Walsh L J: The current status of low level laser therapy in dentistry. Part 2. Hard tissue applications. Aust Dent J 42: 302–306, 1997
6. Bhatti M, MacRobert A, Meghji S, Henderson B, Wilson M: A study of the uptake of toluidine blue O by *Porphyromonas gingivalis* and the mechanism of lethal photosensitization. Photochem Photobiol 68: 370–376, 1998
7. Moan J, Berg K: The photodegradation of porphyrins in cells can be used to estimate the lifetime of singlet oxygen. Photochem Photobiol 53: 549–553, 1991
8. Wainwright M: Photodynamic antimicrobial chemotherapy (PACT). J Antimicrob Chemother 42: 13–28, 1998
9. Smetana Z, Malik Z, Orenstein A, Mendelson E, Ben-Hur E: Treatment of viral infections with 5-aminolevulinic acid and light. Lasers Surg Med 21: 351–358, 1997
10. Jackson Z, Meghji S, MacRobert A, Henderson B, Wilson M: Killing of the yeast and hyphal forms of *Candida albicans* using a light-activated antimicrobial agent. Lasers Med Sci 14: 150–157, 1999
11. Bhatti M, MacRobert A, Henderson B, Shepherd P, Cridland J, Wilson M: Antibody-targeted lethal photosensitization of *Porphyromonas gingivalis*. Antimicrob Agents Chemother 44: 2615–2618, 2000
12. Komerik N, Hopper C, Wilson M: Lethal photosensitisation of mucositis-associated bacteria. J Dent Res 76: 1024–1026, 1997
13. Komerik N, Wilson M, Poole S: The effect of photodynamic action on two virulence factors of gram-negative bacteria. Photochem Photobiol 72: 676–680, 2000
14. Komerik N, Wilson M: Factors influencing the susceptibility of Gram-negative bacteria to toluidine blue O-mediated lethal photosensitization. J Appl Microbiol 92: 618–623, 2002
15. Komerik N, Nakanishi H, MacRobert A J, Henderson B, Speight P, Wilson M: In vivo killing of *Porphyromonas gingivalis* by toluidine blue-mediated photosensitization in an animal model. Antimicrob Agents Chemother 47: 932–940, 2003
16. Spikes J D, Jori G: Photodynamic therapy of tumours and other diseases using prophyrins. Lasers Med Sci 2: 3–15, 1987
17. Foote C: Future directions and application in photodynamic theory. SPIE 1 (Suppl. 6): 115–126, 1990
18. Michael B P: Effects of photodynamic therapy in the normal mouse tongue. J Oral Maxillofac Surg 51: 1129–1134, 1993

19. Bonnett R: Photosensitizers of the porphyrin and phthalocyanine series for photodynamic therapy. Chem Soc Rev 24: 19–33, 1995
20. Dougherty T J, Gomer C J, Henderson B W: Photodynamic therapy. J Natl Cancer Inst 90: 889–905, 1998
21. Fan K F, Hopper C, Speight P M, Buonaccorsi G, MacRobert A J, Bown S G: Photodynamic therapy using 5-aminolaevulinic acid for premalignant lesions of the oral cavity. Cancer 78: 1374–1383, 1996
22. Fan K F, Hopper C, Speight P, Buonaccorsi G, Bown S C: Photodynamic therapy using mTHPC for malignant disease in the oral cavity. Int J Cancer 73: 25–32, 1997
23. Dobson J, Wilson M: Sensitization of oral bacteria in biofilms to killing by light from a low-power laser. Arch Oral Biol 37: 883–887, 1992
24. Burns T, Wilson M, Pearson G J: Laser induced killing of photosensitised cariogenic bacteria. J Dent Res 71: 675, 1992
25. Burns T, Wilson M, Pearson G J: Sensitisation of cariogenic bacteria to killing by light from a helium-neon laser. J Med Microbiol 38: 401–405, 1993
26. Sarkar S, Wilson M: Lethal photosensitization of bacteria in subgingival plaque from patients with chronic periodontitis. J Periodont Res 28: 204–210, 1993
27. Wilson M, Dobson J, Harvey W: Sensitisation of *Streptococcus sanguis* to killing by low power laser light. Lasers Med Sci 8: 69–73, 1993
28. Wilson M, Dobson J, Sarkar S: Sensitization of periodontopathogenic bacteria to killing by light from a low-power laser. Oral Microbiol Immunol 8: 182–187, 1993
29. Wilson M, Dobson J: Lethal photosensitization of oral anaerobic bacteria. Clin Infect Dis 16 (Suppl. 4): 414–415, 1993
30. Wilson M, Mia N: Sensitisation of *Candida albicans* to killing by low-power laser light. J Oral Pathol Med 22: 354–357, 1993
31. Wilson M, Sarkar S, Bulman J S: Effect of blood on lethal photosensitization of bacteria in subgingival plaque from patients with chronic periodontitis. Lasers Med Sci 8: 297–303, 1993
32. Wilson M, Pratten J: Lethal photosensitisation of *Staphylococcus aureus*. Microbios 78:163–168, 1994
33. Wilson M: Bactericidal effect of laser light and its potential use in the treatment of plaque-related diseases. Int Dent J 44: 181–189, 1994
34. Wilson M, Pratten J: Sensitization of *Staphylococcus aureus* to killing by low-power laser light. J Antimicrob Chemother 33: 619–624, 1994
35. Burns T, Wilson M, Pearson G J: Killing of cariogenic bacteria by light from a gallium aluminium arsenide diode laser. J Dent 22: 273–278, 1994
36. Burns T, Wilson M, Pearson G J: Effect of dentine and collagen on the lethal photosensitization of *Streptococcus mutans*. Caries Res 29: 192–197, 1995
37. Wilson M, Yianni C: Killing of methicillin-resistant *Staphylococcus aureus* by low-power laser light. J Med Microbiol 42: 62–66, 1995
38. Wilson M, Pratten J: Lethal photosensitisation of *Staphylococcus aureus* in vitro: effect of growth phase, serum, and pre-irradiation time. Lasers Surg Med 16: 272–276, 1995
39. Wilson M, Burns T, Pratten J, Pearson G J: Bacteria in supragingival plaque samples can be killed by low-power laser light in the presence of a photosensitizer. J Appl Bacteriol 78: 569–574, 1995
40. Griffiths M A, Wren B W, Wilson M: Killing of methicillin-resistant *Staphylococcus aureus* in vitro using aluminium disulphonated phthalocyanine, a light-activated antimicrobial agent. Antimicrob Chemother 40: 873–876, 1997
41. Wilson M, Burns T, Pratten J: Killing of *Streptococcus sanguis* in biofilms using a light-activated antimicrobial agent. Antimicrob Chemother 37: 377–381, 1996
42. Soukos N S, Wilson M, Burns T, Speight P M: Photodynamic effects of toluidine blue on human oral keratinocytes and fibroblasts and *Streptococcus sanguis* evaluated in vitro. Lasers Surg Med 18: 253–259, 1996
43. Millson C E, Wilson M, MacRobert A, Bedwell J, Bown S G: The killing of *Helicobacter pylori* by low-power laser light in the presence of a photosensitiser. J Med Microbiol 44: 245–252, 1996
44. Millson C E, Wilson M, MacRobert A, Bown S G: Ex-vivo treatment of gastric *Helicobacter* infection by photodynamic therapy. J Photochem Photobiol B 32: 59–65, 1996
45. Bhatti M, MacRobert A, Meghji S, Henderson B, Wilson M: Effect of dosimetric and physiological factors on the lethal photosensitization of *Porphyromonas gingivalis* in vitro. Photochem Photobiol 65: 1026–1031, 1997
46. Wilson M: Lethal photosensitisation of biofilm grown bacteria. Proceedings of photochemistry: photodynamic therapy and other modalities III. SPIE 3191: 68–78, 1997
47. Komerik N, Curnow A, MacRobert A J, Hopper C, Speight P M, Wilson M: Fluorescence biodistribution and photosensitising activity of toluidine blue O on rat buccal mucosa. Lasers Med Sci 17: 86–92, 2002
48. O'Neill J F, Hope C K, Wilson M: Oral bacteria in multi-species biofilms can be killed by red light in the presence of toluidine blue. Lasers Surg Med 31: 86–90, 2002
49. O'Neill J, Wilson M, Wainwright M: Comparative antistreptococcal activity of photobactericidal agents. J Chemother 15: 329–334, 2003
50. Williams J A, Pearson G J, Colles M J, Wilson M: The effect of variable energy input from a novel light source on the photoactivated bactericidal action of toluidine blue O on *Streptococcus mutans*. Caries Res 37: 190–193, 2003
51. Malik Z, Hanania J, Nitzan Y: Bactericidal effects of photoactivated porphyrins - an alternative approach to antimicrobial drugs. J Photochem Photobiol B 5: 281–293, 1990
52. Shah H, Bonnett R, Mateen B: The porphyrin pigmentation of subspecies of *Bacteroides melaninogenicus*. Biochem J 180: 45–50, 1979
53. Henry C A, Dyer B, Wagner M, Judy M, Matthews J L: Phototoxicity of argon laser irradiation on biofilms of *Porphyromonas* and *Prevotella* species. J Photochem Photobiol B 34: 123–128, 1996
54. Konig K, Teschke M, Sigusch B, Glockmann E, Eick S, Pfister W: Red light kills bacteria via photodynamic action. Cell Mol Biol (Noisy-le-grand) 46: 1297–1303, 2000

55. Mashberg A: Final evaluation of tolonium chloride rinse for screening of high-risk patients with asymptomatic squamous carcinoma. J Am Dent Assoc 106: 319–323, 1983
56. Warnakulasuriya K, Johnson NW: Sensitivity and specificity of Orascan toluidine blue mouthrinse in the detection of oral cancer and precancer. J Oral Pathol Med 25: 97–103, 1996
57. Pottier R, Bonneau R, Joussot-Dubien J: pH dependence of singlet oxygen production in aqueous solutions using toluidine blue. Photochem Photobiol 22: 59–61, 1975
58. Nitzan Y, Shainberg B, Malik Z: The mechanism of photodynamic inactivation of *Staphylococcus aureus* by deuteroporphyrin. Curr Microbiol 19: 265–269, 1989
59. Wakayama Y, Takagi M, Yano K: Photosensitized inactivation of *E. coli* cells in toluidine blue-light system. Photochem Photobiol 32: 601–605, 1980
60. Tuite E M, Kelly J M: Photochemical interactions of methylene blue and analogues with DNA and other biological substrates. Photochem Photobiol 21: 103–124, 1993
61. Odor T M, Watson T F, Pitt Ford T R, McDonald F: Pattern of transmission of laser light in teeth. Int Endod J 29: 228–234, 1996
62. Stringer G J, Bird P S, Walsh L J: Lethal laser photosensitization of *Streptococcus mutans* with a visible red diode laser. Aust Dent J 45 (Suppl.): 22, 2000
63. Stringer G J: Lethal laser photosensitisation in the treatment of dental caries. MDSc thesis, Univ. of Queensland, St. Lucia 1999
64. Okamoto H, Iwase T, Morioka T: Dye-mediated bactericidal effect of He-Ne laser irradiation on oral microorganisms. Lasers Surg Med 12: 450–458, 1992
65. Stringer G J, Bird P S, Walsh L J: Laser/dye killing of *Streptococcus mutans* on transverse and longitudinal dentine slices. J Dent Res 78: 951, 1999
66. Haas R, Baron M, Dortbudak O, Watzek G: Lethal photosensitisation, autologous bone and e-PTFE membrane for the treatment of peri-implantitis: preliminary results. Int J Oral Maxillofac Implants 15: 374–382, 2000
67. Ito T, Kobayashi K: In vivo evidence for the photodynamic membrane damage as a determining step of the inactivation of yeast cells sensitized by toluidine blue. Photochem Photobiol 25: 399–401, 1977
68. Paardekooper M, De Bruijne A W, Steveninck J V, Van den Brock P J: Intracellular damage in yeast cells caused by photodynamic treatment with toluidine blue. Photochem Photobiol 61: 84–89, 1995
69. Mohr H, Bachmann B, Klein-Struckmeier A, Lambrecht B: Virus inactivation of blood products by phenothiazine dyes and light. Photochem Photobiol 65: 441–445, 1997
70. Wainwright M: The emerging chemistry of blood product disinfection. Chem Soc Rev 31: 128–136, 2002
71. Kerekes K, Tronstad L: Long-term results of endodontic treatment performed with a standardized technique. J Endod 5: 83–90, 1979
72. Haapasalo M, Orstavik D: In vitro infection and disinfection of dentinal tubules. J Dent Res 66: 1375–1379, 1987
73. Haapasalo M: *Bacteroides* spp. in dental root canal infections. Endod Dent Traumatol 5: 1–10, 1989
74. Lin L M, Pascon E A, Skribner J, Gangler P, Langeland K: Clinical, radiographic, and histologic study of endodontic treatment failures. Oral Surg Oral Med Oral Pathol 71: 603–611, 1991
75. Love R M: *Enterococcus faecalis* – a mechanism for its role in endodontic failure. Int Endod J 34: 399–405, 2001
76. Abbott P V, Hume W R, Pearman J W: Antibiotics and endodontics. Aust Dent J 35: 50–60, 1990
77. Abbott P V: Medicaments: aids to success in endodontics. Part 1. A review of the literature. Aust Dent J 35: 438–48, 1990
78. Dahlen G, Samuelsson W, Molander A, Reit C: Identification and antimicrobial susceptibility of enterococci isolated from the root canal. Oral Microbiol Immunol 15: 309–312, 2000
79. Hancock H H, Sigurdsson A, Trope M, Moiseiwitsch J: Bacteria isolated after unsuccessful endodontic treatment in a North American population. Oral Surg Oral Med Oral Pathol Oral Radiol Endod 91: 579–86, 2001
80. Peters L B, Wesselink P R, van Winkelhoff A J: Combinations of bacterial species in endodontic infections. Int Endod J 35: 698–702, 2002
81. Silbert T, Bird P S, Milburn G J, Walsh L J: Disinfection of root canals by laser dye photosensitization. J Dent Res 79 (Spec. iss.): 569, 2000
82. Seal G J: An in vitro comparison of the bactericidal efficacy of lethal photosensitization or sodium hyphochlorite irrigation on *Streptococcus intermedius* biofilm in root canals. Int Endod J 35: 268–274, 2002
83. Lee M T: Photoactivated disinfection of *E. faecalis* in root canals using lasers. MDSc thesis, Univ. of Queensland, St. Lucia 2003
84. Dörtbudak O, Haas R, Mailath-Pokorny G: Effect of low-power laser irridation on bony implant sites. Clin Oral Impl Res 13: 288–292, 2002
85. Haas R, Dörtbudak O, Mensdorff-Pouilly N: Elimination of bacteria on different implant surfaces through photosensitization and soft laser. Clin Oral Impl Res 8: 249–254, 1997
86. Haas R, Baron M, Dörtbudak O: Lethal photosensitization, autogenous bone and e-PTFE membrane for the treatment of peri-implantitis: preliminary results. Int J Oral Maxillofac Impl 15(3): 374–382, 2000
87. Dörtbudak-Kneissl E, Dörtbudak O, Bernhart R: Die photodynamische Therapie zur Keimreduction bei paradontalen Erkrankungen. Z Stomatol 1: 1–4, 2000
88. van Winkelhoff A J, Carlee A W, de Graaff J: *Bacteroides endodontalis* and other black-pigmented *Bacteroides* species in odontogenic abscesses. Infect Immun 49: 494–497, 1985
89. Onofre M A, Sposto M R, Navarro C M: Reliability of toluidine blue application in the detection of oral epithelial dysplasia and in situ and invasive squamous cell carcinomas. Oral Surg Oral Med Oral Pathol Oral Radiol Endod 91: 535–540, 2001
90. Epstein J B, Zhang L, Poh C, Nakamura H, Berean K, Rosin M: Increased allelic loss in toluidine blue-positive oral premalignant lesions. Oral Surg Oral Med Oral Pathol Oral Radiol Endod 95: 45–50, 2003
91. Zach L, Cohen G: Pulp response to externally applied heat. Oral Surg Oral Med Oral Pathol 19: 515–530, 1965

92. Walsh L J: Pulpal safety parameters for irradiation of dental hard tissues with carbon dioxide lasers. Aust Endod J 19: 21–25, 1993
93. Moshonov J, Orstavik D, Yamauchi S, Pettiette M, Trope M: Nd:YAG laser irradiation in root canal disinfection. Endod Dent Traumatol 11: 220–224, 1995
94. Klinke T, Klimm W, Gutknecht N: Antibacterial effects of Nd:YAG laser irradiation within root canal dentin. J Clin Laser Med Surg 15: 29–31, 1997
95. Le Goff A, Dautel-Morazin A, Guigand M, Vulcain J M, Bonnaure-Mallet M: An evaluation of the CO_2 laser for endodontic disinfection. J Endod 25: 105–108, 1999
96. Amyra T, Walsh L J: An assessment of techniques for dehydrating root canals using infrared laser radiation. Aust Endod J 26: 78–80, 2000
97. Walsh L J: The current status of laser applications in dentistry. Aust Dent J 48: 146–155, 2003

13

Low Level Laser Therapy (LLLT)

L. J. Walsh, K. Goharkhay, P. Verheyen, A. Moritz

13.1 Introduction

Low level laser therapy (LLLT) is also known as "soft laser therapy" and bio-stimulation. The use of LLLT in health care has been documented in the literature for more than three decades. Numerous research studies have demonstrated that LLLT is effective for some specific applications in dentistry[1].

The LLLT literature is large, with more than 1,000 papers published on this topic. A problem in dissecting this literature is the variation in methodology and dosimetry between different studies. Not only have a range of different wavelengths been examined, but exposure times and the frequency of treatments also vary. The inclusion of sham-irradiated controls in clinical studies is an important element since placebo effects can be important, particularly in terms of the level of pain experienced and reported following treatment[1].

While broad band light can exert effects on cells[2,3], interest has been concentrated on using lasers as a light source because of their greater therapeutic effect. While much of the initial work with LLLT used the helium–neon gas laser (λ = 632.8 nm), nowadays most LLLT clinical procedures are undertaken using semiconductor diode lasers, for example, gallium arsenide-based diode lasers operating at λ = 830 nm or λ = 635 nm wavelengths[4]. Since wavelength is the most important factor in any type of phototherapy, the clinician must consider which wavelengths are capable of producing the desired effects within living tissues.

The typical power output for a low level laser device used for this therapy is of the order of 10–50 mW, and total irradiances at any point are of the order of several Joules. Thermal effects of LLLT on dental tissues are not significant[5], and do not contribute to the therapeutic effects seen. The wavelengths used for LLLT have poor absorption in water, and thus penetrate soft and hard tissues from 3 mm to up to 15 mm. The extensive penetration of red and near-infrared light into tissues has been documented by several investigators[6]. As the energy penetrates tissues, there is multiple scattering by both erythrocytes and microvessels. Because of this, both blood rheology and the distribution of microvessels in the tissue influence the final distribution pattern of laser energy[1].

13.2 Mechanism of Action

The mechanisms of low level laser therapy are complex, but essentially rely upon the absorption of particular visible red and near-infrared wavelengths in photoreceptors within sub-cellular components, particularly the electron transport (respiratory) chain within the membranes of mitochondria[2,7]. The absorption of light by the respiratory chain components causes a short-term activation of the respiratory chain, and oxidation of the NADH pool. This stimulation of oxidative phosphorylation leads to changes in the redox status of both the mitochondria and the cytoplasm of the cell. The electron transport chain is able to provide increased levels of promotive force to the cell, through increased supply of ATP, as well as an increase in the electrical potential of the mitochondria membrane, alkalization of the cytoplasm, and activation of nucleic acid synthesis[8]. Because ATP is the "energy currency" for a cell, LLLT has a potent action that results in stimulation of the normal functions of the cell. The specific actions of LLLT are summarized in Table 13-1.

Karu, who has studied the bio-stimulative effects of light on cell cultures in great detail, has demonstrated that cell cultures that are initially irradiated with laser light show a range of biological effects[7,9,10]. Of importance, if these cultures are then irradiated with non-monochromatic and incoherent light, the previous laser-produced biological effects are almost nullified. This suggests that there are more complex mechanisms at work than the simple excitation of polarization-sensitive chromophores in the cell.

Table 13-1 Effect of different wavelengths on biostimulation (modified from the work of Laakso et al.[3]).

Wavelength λ [nm]	Energy Density [J/cm^2]	Effect
540 nm, and 600–900 nm	0–56	dose and light intensity-dependent fibroblast proliferation
632.8 nm	2.4	vasodilation, mast cell exocytosis, interstitial edema and opening of cell membrane pores
632.8 nm	2.4	enhanced neutrophil phagocytosis
632.8 nm	2	improved fibroblast metabolic rate
632.8 nm, and 904 nm	0.25–4	increased keratinocyte proliferation
660 nm, 820 nm, 870 nm and 880 nm	2.4	stimulation of fibroblast proliferation by affecting macrophage responsiveness
660 nm	2.4–9.6	enhanced macrophage responsiveness and proliferation
820 nm	2.4–7.2	increased macrophage responsiveness and fibroblast proliferation
830 nm	10	increased perfusion and angiogenesis in rat skin flaps
830 nm	10	increased phagocytic activity of neutrophils
904 nm	76.4	reduced edema and improved rate of skin wound closure in rats

It is crucial to recognize the optical distinction between irradiating human tissues, in which light will scatter very widely, and a thin transparent monolayer of cells in a laboratory. In this context, a key issue is polarization of the light, since polarized and non-polarized light can bring about different biological responses. In a thin layer of cells in culture, the polarization of laser light is maintained through the entire thickness of the cell layer. The work of Mester et al.[11], which used leukocytes in the laboratory setting, indicates that both polarized laser light and polarized incoherent light can evoke bio-stimulation, whilst no such stimulation occurs with non-polarized incoherent light.

Considerable insight into the effect of wavelength on LLLT has been gained from the work of Karu, who over a period of years[7,9,10] has conducted extensive research using cell cultures of various types. Her work has provided an action spectrum for bio-stimulation of the rate of DNA synthesis in HeLa cells, and for the proliferation of bacteria and yeast colonies. These spectra show peaks in the blue ($\lambda = 404$ nm and $\lambda = 454$ nm), red ($\lambda = 620$ nm), and near-infrared ($\lambda = 760$ nm and $\lambda = 830$ nm) wavelengths. Her findings also reveal that individual spectral bands may give antagonistic effects on the all-important electron transport chain, for example, blue versus red, and ultraviolet versus red, when these respective wavelengths are delivered in sequence[7]. In her own words: "... it is possible to conclude that irradiation with monochromatic visible light in the blue, red and far red regions can enhance metabolic processes in the cell. The photobiological effects of stimulation depend on the wavelengths, dose and intensity of the light".

By increasing the respiratory metabolism of the cell, LLLT can also affect the electro-physiological properties of the cell. This has relevance in terms of cells such as mast cells, which are triggered to respond by ionic gradients.

13.3 Cellular Effects of LLLT During Wound Healing

LLLT has also been shown to cause vaso-dilation, with increased local blood flow. This vaso-active effect is of relevance to the treatment of joint inflammation, such as may occur in the TMJ. LLLT causes the relaxation of smooth muscle associated with endothelium. This vaso-dilation brings in oxygen and also allows for greater traffic of immune cells into tissue. These two effects contribute to accelerated healing.

Furthermore, LLLT can exert vaso-active effects by its actions on mast cells. The effects of different types of light on mast cells are well-recognized[12]. There is direct evidence[13] that 660-, 820-, and 940-nm light can trigger mast cell degranulation. Mast cells are distributed preferentially about the microvascular endothelium in skin, oral mucosa and dental pulp[14,15]. Mast cells in these locations contain the pro-inflammatory cytokine tumor necrosis factor-α in their granules[16]. Release of this cytokine promotes leukocyte infiltration of tissues[17] by enhancing expression of endothelial-leukocyte adhesion molecules.

In addition, mast cell proteases, such as chymase[18], alter basement membranes and facilitate entry of leukocytes into tissues.

Because mast cells play a pivotal role in controlling leukocyte traffic, modulation of mast cell functions by LLLT can be of considerable importance in the treatment of sites of inflammation in the oral cavity.

Laboratory studies of low level laser effects have demonstrated a range of bio-stimulation effects (Table 13-2). For fibroblasts, increased proliferation, maturation and locomotion have been noted, as well as transformation to myofibroblasts, reduced production of pro-inflammatory prostaglandin E_2, and increased production of basic fibroblast growth factor. These effects have been reported for fibroblasts from the skin, buccal mucosa and gingiva, all of which show increased proliferation at low doses (e.g., 2 J/cm^2). Of note, high dose LLLT suppresses both fibroblast proliferation and autocrine production of basic fibroblast growth factor[19].

LLLT effects on macrophages include increased ability to act as phagocytes, and greater secretion of basic fibroblast growth factor. Macrophages resorb fibrin as part of the demolition phase of wound healing more quickly with LLLT, because of their enhanced phagocytic activity during the initial phases of the repair response (for example, 6 h after trauma). More rapid demolition of the wound establishes conditions necessary for the proliferative phase of the healing response to begin.

Table 13-2 Possible mechanisms involved in the acceleration of wound healing by LLLT (according to Walsh[1]).

Cell type	Mechanisms
Fibroblasts	proliferation maturation locomotion transformation into myofibroblasts reduced secretion of PG E_2 and IL-1 enhanced secretion of bFGF
Macrophages	phagocytosis secretion of fibroblast growth factors fibrin resorption
Lymphocytes	activation enhanced proliferation
Epithelial cells	motility
Endothelium	increased granulation tissue relaxation of vascular smooth muscle
Neural tissue	reduced synthesis of inflammatory mediators maturation and regeneration axonal growth

With LLLT, lymphocytes become activated and proliferate more quickly, while epithelial cells become more motile and are able to migrate across wound sites with accelerated closure of defects. Endothelium forms granulation tissue more quickly.

Early epithelialization, increased fibroblastic reactions, leucocytic infiltration, and neo-vascularization are seen in wounds irradiated using LLLT. Because of the overall impact of these influences, the time required for complete wound closure is reduced. Moreover, the mean breaking strength, as measured by the ability of the wound to resist rupture force, is increased[20].

Wound healing consists of several distinct phases[21], all of which can be affected at the cellular level by LLLT. The initial, pro-inflammatory and vaso-active phases of inflammation include clotting of any cut blood vessels and deposition of a platelet plug, after which the site is infiltrated by neutrophils and macrophages. These infiltrating cells, together with resident tissue cells such as fibroblasts, release a variety of biologically active substances such as growth factors. Enhanced production of fibroblast growth factor, for example, can occur with LLLT from fibroblasts and macrophages.

The second phase of wound healing involves proliferation, with the formation of granulation tissue as a result of new blood vessel growth. This angiogenesis combined with the deposition of new connective tissue requires successful degradation of the wound matrix by macrophages. The final phase of wound healing, which is remodeling, can continue for months or years, and in this context accelerated formation of bone is of great clinical interest. Studies by Walsh, Doan and Bartold which have measured DNA synthesis in cell culture have shown that bone-derived cells and fibroblasts are stimulated to grow by low level laser therapy at 630 nm, 670 nm, or 830 nm. Of interest, the 830-nm wavelength exerts greater effects on bone cells than on fibroblasts. Similar findings for fibroblasts were obtained by Karu in her studies on the effect of red light on DNA synthesis[7].

Direct evidence for enhanced collagen gene expression both in skin fibroblast cultures in vitro, as well as in animal models of wound healing in vivo, has been presented[22]. Biochemical assays of wounds have revealed that the amount of total collagen is significantly increased in laser-treated sites, indicating accelerated collagen production. As well, there less pepsin soluble collagen in laser-treated wounds than in wounds, indicating higher resistance to proteolytic digestion. Together, these bio-mechanical and biochemical results suggest that laser photo-stimulation promotes the tissue repair process by accelerating collagen production and promoting overall connective tissue stability[23].

A final aspect of the effect of LLLT on cells relates to the effects of laser light on the cytoskeleton. Several studies have suggested that LLLT can modulate cell behavior by causing rearrangements of the cytoskeleton[24,25]. As shown by Medrado et al.[26], stimulation of connective-tissue cells toward a myoid phenotype can result in the differentiation of myofibroblasts.

It is this cell type which mainly is responsible for the contraction force during wound healing[27–29]. Myofibroblasts share morphologic features in common with fibroblasts and smooth muscle cells[30]. These cells are observed in normal tissue, granulation tissue, and some pathological conditions[31,32]. Because LLLT is an effective stimulator of differentiation to myofibroblasts, the process of wound healing should be accelerated. In the study by Medrado et al.[26], sequential semi-quantitative histological examination revealed that laser treatment shortened the exudation phase of wound healing in skin, and stimulated the reparative process. LLLT showed the greatest wound area reduction between 1 and 3 days after treatment, a finding that correlated with higher numbers of myofibroblasts. Their results confirm numerous earlier studies, such as the seminal investigation of Mester et al.[11], who used photographs to document the faster wound contraction with LLLT.

Faster wound closure is of great importance in compromised patients, such as diabetics, and patients undergoing treatment for malignancies. Because LLLT can enhance the release of growth factors from fibroblasts, and can stimulate cell proliferation, it is able to improve wound healing in such compromised patients. Histological studies have demonstrated that laser irradiation improves wound epithelialization, cellular content, granulation tissue formation, and collagen deposition in laser-treated wounds, compared to untreated sites[8,33]. These findings have been confirmed in oral mucosal wound healing in clinical studies in humans[34].

13.4 LLLT and Neural Tissues

Following LLLT, neural tissues show reduced synthesis of inflammatory mediators, as well as more rapid maturation and regeneration, particularly axonal growth. LLLT has also been proven to reduce pain in patients suffering from post-herpetic neuralgia, from cervical dentinal hypersensitivity[5], or from periodontal pain during orthodontic tooth movement[35].

LLLT may also be of benefit in treating TMJ disorders. Clinical studies of LLLT used on patients with injuries to joints in other locations (ankle, knee, shoulder, and wrist), using either the AlGaAs (λ = 830 nm) diode laser in continuous wave mode or the He–Ne laser (λ = 632.8 nm) combined with a diode laser (λ = 904 nm) in pulsed mode, have shown clinical benefits in terms of a reduction in pain and swelling.

Patients treated with LLLT obtain pain relief and recover function more rapidly compared to untreated patients[36,37]. Identical results have been obtained for LLLT of the TMJ. Active and passive maximum mouth opening, and lateral motion are significantly improved by LLLT, with similar results in myogenic and arthrogenic cases[38]. The number of tender trigger points was also reduced. Clearly, such effects may be mediated by a combination of both local and systemic effects.

Further evidence of the utility of LLLT was shown in a meta-analysis of 13 placebo-controlled clinical trials of LLLT, involving patients with rheumatoid arthritis affecting their hands. The duration of treatment ranged from 4 to 10 weeks. LLLT reduced pain (by 70%) relative to placebo. It also reduced morning stiffness, and increased flexibility, when applied over the joint or over the relevant nerves[39]. Consistent with this, positive reports of the benefit of LLLT used in the dental office to treat disorders including TMJ pain, trigeminal neuralgia, and muscular pain have been presented[40]. Once again, this suggests both a local and a systemic action of LLLT.

LLLT has proven to be very effective when applied to "trigger points", i.e., myofascial zones of particular sensibility and of highest projection of focal pain points, due to ischemic conditions. Results obtained after clinical treatment of patients with pain of varying origin (headaches and facial pain, skeletomuscular ailments, myogenic neck pain, shoulder and arm pain, epicondylitis humery, tenosynovitis, low back and radicular pain, Achilles tendinitis) using LLLT have been particularly promising. In fact, in one study, the author commented that the results "were better than we had ever expected"[36].

An additional area of interest in this field is the use of LLLT to achieve an analgesic effect in the dental pulp prior to restorative procedures. First noted with the Nd:YAG laser in the early 1990s, the clinical use of "pre-emptive laser analgesia" is becoming more widespread now as a clinical technique with the Er:YAG and Er,Cr:YSGG laser.

When operated at pulse rates between 15 and 20 Hz, at pulse energies below the ablation threshold of tooth structure, the erbium laser energy penetrates into the tooth, and is directed along hydroxyapatite crystals (which function like waveguides) towards the dental pulp. Here, the pulses of energy coincide with the natural bio-resonance frequency of Type C and other nerve fibers in the dental pulp. The action of this type of LLLT is to cause a disruption in the action of the Na-K pump in the cell membrane, resulting in a loss of impulse conduction, and thus an analgesic effect.

The duration of this effect is ~ 15 min. Direct examination of teeth lased to achieve this analgesic effect have not shown any evidence of adverse pulpal change at the histological level over the short or long term. There are parallels of the dental laser analgesic effect with several situations in medicine in which simultaneous non-destructive thermal and non-thermal bioactivation occur at the periphery of the target tissue. This phenomenon of "simultaneous LLLT" that may occur along with high level laser treatment has been explained in detail by Ohshiro and Calderhead[6,41].

In vivo studies of the analgesic effect of LLLT on nerves supplying the oral cavity have demonstrated that LLLT decreases the firing frequency of nociceptors, with a threshold effect seen in terms of the irradiance required to exert maximal suppression[42,43]. In vivo, LLLT selectively inhibits a range of nociceptive signals arising from peripheral nerves, including neuronal discharges elicited by pinch, cold, heat stimulation, and chemical irritation[44,45]. In contrast, neuronal discharges induced by brush stimulation are not affected by LLLT. There is some evidence that laser irradiation may selectively target fibers conducting at slow velocities, particularly afferent axons from nociceptors[46,47]. This explains why the LLLT effect of laser "analgesia" is not a complete "anesthesia" of the lased tooth.

13.5 Clinical Applications of LLLT

While there is extensive laboratory evidence on the effect of low level laser therapy on stimulating cells, the major interest in this technique clinically has been for accelerated wound healing or pain reduction. It is thought that the wound healing effects are due to local release of cytokines, chemokines and other biological response modifiers, while analgesic effects may result from both local and systemic effects. The latter may include release of endorphins.

Detailed and critical analysis of the LLLT literature reveals that the treatment exerts a range of effects, which in themselves are responsive to a range of experimental variables. In their classical work, Tuner and Hode[48] critically reviewed the parameter pitfalls found in many of the classic "negative" studies of LLLT. They assessed some 1,200 papers on LLLT, and examined carefully aspects of experimental design in 85 positive and 35 negative double-blind studies. The negative studies contained a variety of factors which in themselves could provide an explanation for a nil effect of the treatment.

Low level laser therapy has a range of dental, medical, physiotherapy, and veterinary applications. The latter group is of some interest, since when used in animals the possibility of any placebo effects of treatment (for example, on the perceptions of pain or discomfort) can be eliminated completely. LLLT benefits have been reported in both small and large animals[49,50].

Low level laser applications in dentistry include the promotion of wound healing in a range of sites[1], including:

- surgical wounds to oral soft tissues
- gingival incisions[51]
- extraction sites (bone fill and soft tissue healing)
- lesions of recurrent aphthous stomatitis (canker sores)[52]
- the dental pulp, with secondary dentin formation after pulpotomy
- oral ulcerations (mucositis) induced by cancer chemotherapy[42]
- TMJ injury or arthritic disease
- neuronal tissue which has been injured or transected, to accelerate regeneration

Table 13-3 Factors affecting the efficacy of LLLT.

Patient selection factors	– standardized clinical presentation – randomization – blinding of the subjects and examiners – sample size (number of patients and sites) – statistical power of the study – confounding factors, such as medications or other treatments – use of anaesthesia – inclusion of controls – "sham" irradiation to identify the size of the placebo effect – optimal "window" for the timing of treatment – length of follow-up
Optical factors	– laser or LED light source – wavelength – spot size – power density – energy density – mode of operation (continuous wave or pulsed) – timing of treatments (single or multiple)

Table 13-4 Current LLLT applications in dentistry.

Soft tissue modulation	– stimuation of wound healing – aphthous stomatitis – pulpotomy – mucositis
Neural modulation	– laser analgesia – neuronal regeneration – post-herpetic neuralgia – TMJ pain – post-surgical pain – bone regeneration

Table 13-5 Treatment recommendations for LLLT applications in dentistry:

Temporomandibular disorders	Ga-Al-As laser, λ = 680 nm, 75 mW, 1.5–2 J, 40 s, 2–3x/week surface irradiation transdermal, perhaps acupuncture points, resulting in a prompt pain reduction.
Trismus	1–2 J, 3–4x/week, perhaps acupuncture points, speedy relaxation of the musculature.
Bone regeneration	Bone matrix production increase with a diode laser λ = 690 nm, 60 s, 1.6 J/cm^2. Osteocyte viability increase with a 100 mW laser, λ = 690 nm, 1 min., 6 J.
Implantation	75 mW, λ = 680nm, 2 J, 40 s, without photosensitizing dye. Irradiation before starting the implantation, after drilling and after suture. Pain reduction, edema and hematoma development as well as the possibility of infection is reduced. Perhaps repetition on the next day and the day after next.
Peri-implantitis	Diode laser, 7.3 mW, λ = 690–905 nm, 60 s, in combination with toluidin blue, buccal and oral.
Periodontal operation	75 mW, λ = 680 nm, 2–3 J, 40–60 s, irradiation before, during and after operation, periodontal pockets deeper than 4 mm should be flapped
Neurosensory recovery	Begin the treatment as soon as possible after the nerve injury. Ga-Al-As laser: 75mW, 680nm, 3J 60s, 5x/week. Direct irradiation of the injured site already during the operation. Afterwards above the region and in the area of sensitivity disorder.
Trigeminus neuralgia and neuralgiform disorders	Irradiation on the site of the nerve exit at the foramina and the points which are painful. 75mW, 680nm, 2-3J, 40s, 2x/week.
Hematoma	75 mW, λ = 680 nm, 1–2 J, 30 s, 2-3x/week. The irradiation accelerates the resorption.
Abscess	2–3 J, 30–60 s on the incision site around the abscess and on the peripheral edema. Maturity is accelerated.
Orthodontic treatment	Increase of the bone formation and the tooth movement with Ga-Al-As laser: λ = 830 nm, 100 mW, 3 min./ 12 days, gingival contact mesial, buccal, lingual.
Pain reduction	Shortly before and after activating orthodontic forces irradiation should be done. He-Ne laser: λ = 832.8nm, 6 mW, labial and lingual at the apex 30 s, Ga-Al-As laser: 75 mW, λ = 680nm, 1–2 J, 30 s in the apex region buccal and palatinal. Repeat the irradiation when pain returns.
Increase of fibroblast activity and higher proliferation	GaAlAs-laser: λ = 809–904 nm, 10–50 mW, 2–8 J/cm^2, He-Ne-laser: 25 mW, 12 J/cm^2
Wisdom tooth removal	75 mW, 1–2 J, 40 s, irradiation before the operation (regio 8), during the operation (empty alveola) and after suture.
Dentitio difficilis	1 J, 30 s, 2–3x/week until pain reduction.
Dolor post	2 J, 40 s, 2–3x/week in alveola, lingual, buccal and palatinal until pain reduction.
Gingivitis	75 mW, 1–2 J, 40 s, 2x/week.
Herpes labialis	75 mW, 1–2 J/cm^2, 2–3x/week. Pain reduction and the blisters dry up.
Stomatitis	75 mW, 1–2 J/cm^2, irradiation depends on the severity of the inflammation.
Aphtous and herpes	Are irradiated directly without touching the skin (infectious) and also the surroundings for 30–40s.

A significant problem for the non-expert reader when examining the literature on LLLT is obtaining a fair comparison between studies. Several well-controlled experimental studies have indicated a beneficial effect upon wounds by laser biostimulation[53]. Despite similarities of dose, and a convergence in laser choice, significant methodological differences persist regarding experimental protocols[3,26]. Potential factors that may influence the effectiveness of LLLT are shown in Table 13-3, while clinical applications of LLLT are summarized in Table 13-4.

13.6 Frontiers of Clinical Practice for LLLT

There is increasing interest in the concept of pulsing the light source to achieve greater therapeutic benefit[3,6,54–56]. Diode lasers can be pulsed at high frequencies, and continuous wave lasers can be interrupted by means of a mechanical disk that "chops" the beam.

Another novel concept is using LLLT to enhance bone regeneration after extractions or implant placement. In cell culture studies, LLLT using a He–Ne laser stimulates the proliferation, differentiation, and calcification of cultured osteoblastic cells, but only when the cells are in a phase of active growth. If the in vivo parallel holds true, LLLT of healing sites within bone would be expected to increase bone deposition and promote bone regeneration.

In a study of wound healing after tooth extraction in rats, LLLT delivered on a daily basis for 1 week using an AlGaAs laser enhanced fibroblast proliferation and accelerated the formation of bone matrix[57]. Whether LLLT exerts positive results on bone regeneration following tooth extraction in humans remains uncertain, although there are reports that the formation of granulation tissue during post-extraction healing is accelerated[35].

A stimulatory LLLT effect has been observed on fracture healing in rats using the He–Ne laser; however, studies of implant placement surgery have not found significant improvements in bone density or a positive effect of this laser on the process of osseointegration[58]. This lack of benefit may, of course, reflect a sub-optimal treatment protocol. It is important to bear in mind that the maximum benefit with LLLT occurs with repeated dosages, with the best effects being obtained when the treatment is applied daily. Less frequent treatment provides limited benefits[59]. Practically, for maximal bone stimulation, the patient may need to use a handheld LLLT device at home rather than relying on treatment administered at a dental clinic.

13.7 LLLT Technology

A key issue with bio-stimulation using LLLT is the question of whether in fact coherent (laser) light is an absolute requirement. Because of greater destructive interference effects at tissue boundaries, one would expect that bio-stimulation effects with light emitting diodes (LEDs) would be less than with a laser when used at the same parameters[1,11]. As will be discussed further below, the available evidence suggests that this is so, both in clinical and laboratory settings. Because refraction, reflection and scatter can occur at boundaries between tissue types, the physical tissue volume that is irradiated during LLLT can be difficult to estimate[13,60].

The light from an LED is neither monochromatic (singular in wavelength), nor coherent, and thus the interactions which occur as the light enters tissues and is transmitted, reflected, scattered, and absorbed can easily result in destructive interference. Nevertheless, several manufacturers of low level laser devices claim that treatment with lasers has the same effect as with LEDs[61], and they market units with LEDs for LLLT. Some so-called laser devices may be marketed with LEDs. High quality super-luminous LEDs have a spectral bandwidth of less than 15 nm, while less expensive units may have a spectral bandwidth of more than 50 nm. LEDs are much more difficult than diode lasers to focus into an optical fiber because of their wider divergence.

Several in vitro studies, with adequate blinding of the observers, have demonstrated that the effects of laser light are much greater than obtained with light from other sources, such as LEDs. Mester et al.[62] treated three groups of patients with long-standing crural ulcers with a He–Ne laser, a combination of He–Ne and GaAs lasers, and non-coherent unpolarized red light. The two laser groups demonstrated excellent healing, while only a small percentage healing response was seen in the normal red light group. In the study by Kubota and Ohshiro[55], an animal model was used in which no placebo effect is possible. In this study, LLLT with an 830-nm GaAlAs laser increased skin flap survival, with the irradiated sites showing better perfusion, and a greater number of large blood vessels. In contrast, there was no difference between non-irradiated animals, and animals treated with LEDs at $\lambda = 840$ nm.

It is unclear whether monochromaticity and coherence are of equal importance in causing photochemical responses in living tissue, which cannot be achieved by any other method. The published literature contains a number of studies which cast doubt on the specificity of treatment effects with LLLT[7,63,64]. Their main argument is that a laser could be replaced by a non-coherent light with the same optical characteristics, since some loss of coherence may occur because of scattering within the tissue. This argument was effectively disproved by Tuner and Hode[48] who reasoned that the key property of coherence is not absolute, but varies across a range. In other words, a light source can be described as more coherent or less coherent than another.

13.8 LLLT Equipment

Semiconductor diode lasers are compact and have a high conversion efficiency from electrical energy to laser energy. Unlike He–Ne lasers, semiconductor laser diodes do not require a high voltage supply, and so can be used in portable, battery-operated devices. It is also possible to pulse the light at various frequencies using simple external circuitry. Laser diodes have a typical life-expectancy of between 100,000 and 600,000 h[65].

Semiconductor diode lasers are generally variants of either aluminum:gallium:arsenide (AlGaAs) which emit in the near infrared spectrum (wavelength $\lambda = 700$ to $\lambda = 940$ nm), or indium:gallium:arsenide:phosphorus (InGaAsP) devices which emit in the red portion of the visible spectrum range (wavelength $\lambda = 600$ to $\lambda = 680$ nm). Power outputs are typically of the order of 10–50 mW, when measured at the level of the diode laser itself. It is important to note that the final usable output (from the hand piece) will be less because of losses in the internal optical path or in the delivery system.

Since increased temperature of the diode laser device during operation reduces the output power (and to a lesser extent also lengthens the wavelength), it is critical that the temperature or output of the laser diode is monitored so that control circuitry can make the necessary adjustments to maintain a constant output. This is usually accomplished using an internal photo-transistor which is fitted within the package of the laser device. With an adequate heat sink and cooling system (with Peltier cooling for higher powered devices), the potential negative effect of temperature on laser output at the level of the treatment beam can virtually be eliminated.

The beam profile from a typical diode laser is rectangular, with a high divergence on the long axis (20 degrees from the center axis), and a low divergence on the short axis (2 degrees). This gives a highly divergent oval or "sweep" profile. Diode lasers may have integrated optics which produce collimated and focused light beams. To obtain a more useful beam, a series of lenses or a self-focusing graded index fiber can be used in front of the device to either deliver the treatment beam itself or to direct the laser output into a small-diameter flexible optical fiber or a solid light guide (similar to the light tip on a curing light).

Whatever the delivery system used, it is important that the components which come into direct contact with patients are able to be protected adequately with a laser-transmissive disposable barrier, can be autoclaved, or are disposable. Similarly, it should be possible for the clinician to activate the laser into treatment mode without breaching asepsis. Some units employ footswitches or light-operated switches to allow hands-free operation.

Laser units used for LLLT are generally classified as Class III or Class IIIb in terms of the optical hazards that they pose to staff and patients. Because a low power treatment beam can be focused by the eye to give a high power density on the retina, the optical hazard is sufficiently great that laser safety standards mandate the wearing of appropriate protective glasses by patients and clinicians during treatment. Glasses are available which provide protection against common LLLT wavelengths in both the visible and near-infrared spectrum.

It is not always possible to tell by looking quickly at a device whether it is based on a laser diode or an array of LEDs, although the requirement of the manufacturer to place a laser label (e.g., Class IIIa Laser Device) because of international standards is helpful. With visible wavelengths, a simple test may help the prospective purchaser to determine the type of diode contained in the device. If the laser is visible, the beam can be pointed at a plain wall, and examined for speckle, a type of sparkling in which there are varying points of brilliance. Speckle only occurs with true laser light. The light from an LED does not speckle. For an invisible laser, the same property can be seen but with the aid of a domestic video camera, used in a darkened room to examine the impact of the beam on a wall.

The charged coupled device (CCD) used in a video camera is sensitive to light in the near-infrared region (extending to $\lambda = \sim 1100$ nm), and this feature can be used to find laser beams from near-infrared lasers, and to test the units for correct operation. An infrared phosphor board (that is capable of discriminating the wavelength of laser being tested) or a monochromator can be used in the laboratory setting to give a more detailed assessment of laser output. A monochromator will readily distinguish between a true laser diode and an LED.

13.9 Conclusions

Low level laser therapy has been found to accelerate wound healing and reduce pain, possibly by stimulating oxidative phosphorylation in mitochondria and modulating inflammatory responses. By influencing the biological function of a variety of cell types, it is able to exert a range of several beneficial effects upon inflammation and healing. LLLT exerts marked effects upon cells in all phases on wound healing, but particularly so during the proliferative phase.

There is good evidence that the enhanced cell metabolic functions seen after LLLT are the result of activation of photo-receptors within the electron transport chain of mitochondria. The effect is specific for wavelength, and cannot be gained efficiently with normal, non-coherent, non-polarized light sources, such as LEDs.

Future trials of new LLLT applications in dentistry should make use of standardized, validated outcomes, and should explore how the effectiveness of the LLLT protocol used may be influenced by wavelength, treatment duration, dosage, and the site of application.

13.10 References

1. Walsh L J: The current status of low level laser therapy in dentistry. I. Soft tissue applications. Aust Dent J 42: 247–254, 1997
2. Karu T I: Photobiology of low-power laser effects. Hlth Phys 56: 691–704, 1989
3. Laakso E L, Richardson C R, Cramond T: Factors affecting low level laser therapy. Aust J Physiol 39: 95–99, 1993
4. Walsh L J: The current status of laser applications in dentistry. Aust Dent J 48: 146–155, 2003
5. Sandford M A, Walsh L J: Thermal effects during desensitisation of teeth with gallium-aluminium-arsenide lasers. Periodontol 15: 25–30, 1994
6. Ohshiro T, Calderhead R G: Low level laser therapy: A practical introduction. John Wiley & Sons, Chichester 1988, 11–18
7. Karu T I: Photobiology of low-power laser therapy. Harwood Academic Publishers, London 1989
8. Yu W, Naim J O, Lanzafame R J: Effects of photostimulation on wound healing in diabetic mice. Lasers Surg Med 20: 56–63, 1997
9. Karu T I: Photobiological fundamentals of low-power laser therapy. IEEE J Quant Electron QE-2 3: 1703–1717, 1987
10. Karu T I: Molecular mechanism of the therapeutic effect of low-intensity laser radiation. Lasers Life Sci 2: 53–74, 1988
11. Mester E, Mester A F, Mester A: The biomedical effects of laser application. Lasers Surg Med 5: 31–39, 1985
12. Walsh L J: Ultraviolet B irradiation induces mast cell degranulation and release of tumour necrosis factor-alpha. Immunol Cell Biol 73: 226–233, 1995
13. El Sayed S O, Dyson M: A comparison of the effect of multiwavelength light produced by a cluster of semi-conductor diodes and of each individual diode on mast cell number and degranulation in intact and injured skin. Lasers Surg Med 10: 1–10, 1990
14. Walsh L J, Davis M F, Xu L J, Savage N W: Relationship between mast cell degranulation, release of TNF, and inflammation in the oral cavity. J Oral Pathol Med 26: 266–272, 1995
15. Walsh L J: Mast cells and oral inflammation. Crit Rev Oral Biol Med 14: 188–198, 2003
16. Walsh L J, Trinchieri G, Waldorf H A, Whitaker D, Murphy G F: Human dermal mast cells contain and release tumor necrosis factor-α which induces endothelial leukocyte adhesion molecule-1. Proc Natl Acad Sci USA 88: 4220–4224, 1991
17. Walsh L J, Lavker R M, Murphy G F: Determinants of immune cell trafficking in the skin. Lab Invest 63: 592–600, 1990
18. Walsh L J, Kaminer M S, Lazarus G S, Lavker R M, Murphy G F: Role of laminin in localization of human dermal mast cells. Lab Invest 65: 433–440, 1991
19. Yu W, Naim J O, Lanzafame R J: The effect of laser irradiation on the release of bFGF from 3T3 fibroblasts. Photochem Photobiol 59: 167–170, 1994
20. Bisht D, Mehrotra R, Singh P A, Atri S C, Kumar A: Effect of helium-neon laser on wound healing. Indian J Exp Biol 37: 187–189, 1999
21. Walsh L J, Murphy G F: The role of adhesion molecules in cutaneous inflammation and neoplasia. J Cutan Pathol 19: 161–171, 1992
22. Abergel R P, Lyons R F, Castel J C, Dwyer R M, Uitto J: Biostimulation of wound healing by lasers: experimental approaches in animal models and in fibroblast cultures. J Dermatol Surg Oncol 13: 127–133, 1987
23. Reddy G K, Stehno-Bittel L, Enwemeka C S: Laser photostimulation accelerates wound healing in diabetic rats. Wound Repair Regen 9: 248–255, 2001
24. Noble P B, Shields E D, Blecher P D M, Bentley K C: Locomotory characteristics of fibroblasts within a three-dimensional collagen lattice: Modulation by a Helium/Neon soft laser. Lasers Surg Med 12: 669–674, 1992
25. Pourreau-Schneider N, Ahmed A, Soudry M, Jacquemier J, Kopp F, Franquin J C, Martin P M: Helium-Neon laser treatment transforms fibroblasts into myofibroblasts. Am J Pathol 137: 171–178, 1990
26. Medrado A R, Pugliese L S, Reis S R, Andrade Z A: Influence of low level laser therapy on wound healing and its biological action upon myofibroblasts. Lasers Surg Med 32: 239–244, 2003
27. Gabbiani G, Hirschel B J, Ryan G B, Statkov P R, Majno G: Granulation tissue as a contractile organ. J Exp Med 135: 719–734, 1972
28. Gabbiani G: Modulation of fibroblastic cytoskeletal features during wound healing and fibrosis. Pathol Res Pract 190: 851–853, 1994
29. Sappino A P, Schurich W, Gabbiani G: Differentiation repertoire of fibroblastic cells; expression of cytoskeletal proteins as marker of phenotypic modulations. Lab Invest 63: 144–161, 1990
30. Schurich W, Seemayer T A, Gabbiani G: Myofibroblast. In: Sternberg S S: Histology for pathologists, 2nd ed. Lippincott/Raven, Philadelphia, 129–161
31. Kuhn C, Mcdonald J A: The roles of the myofibroblast in idiopathic pulmonary fibrosis. Am J Pathol 138: 1257–1265, 1991
32. Adler K B, Low R B, Leslie K O, Mitchell J, Evans J N: Contractile cells in normal and fibrotic lung. Lab Invest 60: 473–485, 1989
33. Lyons R F, Abergel R P, White R A, Dwyer R M, Castel J C, Uitto J: Biostimulation of wound healing in vivo by a helium-neon laser. Ann Plast Surg 18(1): 47–50, 1987
34. Marei M K, Abdel-Meguid S H, Mokhtar S A, Rizk S A: Effect of low-energy laser application in the treatment of denture-induced mucosal lesions. J Prosthet Dent 77(3): 256–264, 1997
35. Wahl G, Bastanier S: Soft laser in postoperative care in dentoalveolar treatment. ZWR 100: 512–515, 1991
36. Simunovic Z: Low level laser therapy with trigger points technique: a clinical study on 243 patients. J Clin Laser Med Surg 14: 163–167, 1996

37. Simunovic Z, Ivankovich A D, Depolo A: Wound healing of animal and human body sport and traffic accident injuries using low-level laser therapy treatment: a randomized clinical study of seventy-four patients with control group. J Clin Laser Med Surg 18: 67–73, 2000
38. Kulekcioglu S, Sivrioglu K, Ozcan O, Parlak M: Effectiveness of low-level laser therapy in temporomandibular disorder. Scand J Rheumatol 32: 114–118, 2003
39. Brosseau L, Welch V, Wells G, Tugwell P, de Bie R, Gam A, Harman K, Shea B, Morin M: Low level laser therapy for osteoarthritis and rheumatoid arthritis: a meta analysis. J Rheumatol 27: 1961–1969, 2000
40. Pinheiro A L, Cavalcanti E T, Pinheiro T I, Alves M J, Miranda E R, De Quevedo A S, Manzi C T, Vieira A L, Rolim A B: Low-level laser therapy is an important tool to treat disorders of the maxillofacial region. J Clin Laser Med Surg 16: 223–226, 1998
41. Ohshiro T, Calderhead R G: Development of low reactive-level laser therapy and its present status. J Clin Laser Med Surg 9: 267–275, 1991
42. Kitsmaniuk Z D, Demochko V B, Popovich V I: The use of low energy lasers for preventing and treating postoperative and radiation induced complications in patients with head and neck tumors. Vopr Onkol 8: 980–986, 1992
43. Mezawa S, Iwata K, Naito K, Kamogawa H: The possible analgesic effect of soft laser irradiation on heat nociceptors in the cat tongue. Arch Oral Biol 3: 693–694, 1988
44. Sato T, Kawatani M, Takeshige C, Matsumoto I: Ga Al As laser irradiation inhibits neuronal activity associated with inflammation. Acupunct Electrother Res 19: 141–215, 1994
45. Tsuchiya K, Kawatani M, Takeshige C, Matsumoto I: Laser irradiation abates neuronal responses to nociceptive stimulation of rat paw skin. Brain Res Bull 34: 369–374, 1994
46. Tsuchiya K, Kawatani M, Takeshige C, Sato T, Matsumoto I: Diode laser irradiation selectively diminishes slow component of axonal volleys to dorsal roots from the saphenous nerve in the rat. Neurosci Lett 161: 65–68, 1993
47. Baxter G D, Walsh D M, Allen J M, Lowe A S, Bell A J: Effects of low intensity infrared laser irradiation upon conduction in the human median nerve in vivo. Exp Physiol 79: 227–234, 1994
48. Tuner J, Hode L: It's all in the parameters: a critical analysis of some well-known negative studies on low-level laser therapy. J Clin Laser Med Surg 16: 245–248, 1998
49. Ghamsari S M, Taguchi K, Abe N, Acorda J A, Yamada H: Histopathological effect of low-level laser therapy on sutured wounds of the teat in dairy cattle. Vet Q 18: 17–21, 1996
50. Ghamsari S M, Taguchi K, Abe N, Acorda J A, Sato M, Yamada H: Evaluation of low level laser therapy on primary healing of experimentally induced full thickness teat wounds in dairy cattle. Vet Surg 26: 114–120, 1997
51. Neiburger E J: The effect of low-power lasers on intraoral wound healing. NY State Dent J 61: 40–43, 1995
52. Neiburger E J: Rapid healing of gingival incisions by the helium-neon diode laser. J Mass Dent Soc 48: 8–13, 40, 1999
53. Saito S, Shimizu N: Stimulatory effects of low-power laser irradiation on bone regeneration in midpalatal suture during expansion in the rat. Am J Orthod Dentofac Orthoped 111: 525–532, 1997
54. Kert J, Rose L: Clinical laser therapy: low level laser therapy. Scandinavian Medical Laser Technology, Copenhagen 1989
55. Kubota J, Ohshiro T: The effects of diode laser low reactive-level laser therapy (LLLT) on flap survival in a rat model. Laser Ther 1: 127–133, 1989
56. Bourgelais D B C, Itzkan I: The physics of lasers. In: Arndt K A, Noe J M, Rosen S (eds.): Cutaneous laser therapy: principles and methods. John Wiley & Sons, London 1983, 13–25
57. Takeda Y: Irradiation effect of low-energy laser on alveolar bone after tooth extraction. Experimental study in rats. Int J Oral Maxillofac Surg 17: 388–391, 1988
58. Kucerova H, Dostalova T, Himmlova L, Bartova J, Mazanek J: Low-level laser therapy after molar extraction. J Clin Laser Med Surg 18: 309–315, 2000
59. Walsh L J: Emerging applications for infrared lasers in implantology. Periodontol 23: 8–15, 2002
60. Anderson R R, Parrish J A: The optics of human skin. J Invest Dermatol 77: 13–19, 1981
61. Whelan H T, Smits R L Jr, Buchman E V, Whelan N T, Turner S G, Margolis D A, Cevenini V, Stinson H, Ignatius R, Martin T, Cwiklinski J, Philippi A F, Graf W R, Hodgson B, Gould L, Kane M, Chen G, Caviness J: Effect of NASA light-emitting diode irradiation on wound healing. J Clin Laser Med Surg 19: 305–314, 2001
62. Mester E, Nagylucskay S, Doklen A, Tisza S: Laser stimulation of wound healing. Acta Chir Acad Sci Hung 17: 49–55, 1976
63. Basford J R: The clinical and experimental status of low energy laser therapy. Phys Rehabil Med 1: 1–9, 1989
64. Basford J R: Low-energy laser therapy: controversies and new research findings. Lasers Surg Med 9: 1–5, 1989
65. Wheeler J, Slater N: Squaring off: The He-Ne vs red diode. Lasers Optron 16: 38–44, 1990

Index

A

ablation 90, 100
  efficiency and quality 101
  techniques 76
abscesses of the periodontium 342
absorption 7, 11, 100, 108, 197, 523
absorption
  coefficient 57, 197
  depth 206
  enhancer 387
accessory canals 242
acid
  resistance 226
  -etch preparation 96
  -etched 94
acidogenic bacteria 193
actinobacillus actinomycetemcomitans 338, 347, 348, 371, 372, 511, 512
actinomyces
  israeli 250
  viscosus 250, 511
action potential 386
acute apical parodontitis 288
adhesion 93
adhesive
  filling 141
  techniques 93, 384
a-dimethalcrylate BIS - DMA 142, 151, 155
adjacent bone 493
ad-or C-fiber nocieptors 386
ADP 511
advanced lesion 340
aggressive periodontitis 342
alexandrite laser 45
aluminium disulfonated phtalocyanine 508
amalgam 141
  alternatives 141
amelogenesis imperfecta 411
anamnesis 365
  sheet 366
anatomical root configuration 242
angel of the light source 169
anisotropic media 4
antibacterial effect 346
antibiotics 318
apex sealing 281
apical
  - coronal methods 291
  absorption 288
arc lamp 11
argon laser 39, 40, 161, 219, 423
arrangements 57
artificial caries initiation 219
atomic absorbtion spectroscopy examinations 394
ATP 523
azure B chloride 507

B

bacteraemia 454
bacteria 248, 389,505
  reduction 348
bacterial
  cells 508
  colonization 246
  flora 247
  membranes 503
bacterial
  microleakage 316
  plaque 381
  effect 82, 344
bacteroides forsythus 338
balanced force
  method 292
bandwidth 7
beam radius 19
Beer's law 15
bioactive molecules 317
biocompatible glasses 385
biofilm 511
bio-stimulative 523, 534
birefringent crystal 36
black ink 387
black staining 409
bleaching 413, 421
blebbing phenomenom 261
blood loss 457
bond strength 98, 140
bone
  regeneration 533
  resorption 242
  surgery 459
brewster's angle 29
brightness 35
brown discolorations 439
bystander injury 514

C

calcification 381
calcium 164
  fluoride 166
  hydroxide 316, 383

camphoroquinone 142, 150, 153, 154, 167
canal
debris 243
system 243
candida albicans 508, 512
capability of heat conduction 101
carbonate
content 201
loss 206
carbonated
apatite 200, 205
hydroxypatite 198
carcinoma 485
caries 77, 412
inhibitory effect 208, 211
initiation 224
prevention 99, 193
progression 224
removal 125
resistance 200
cavity
preparation 127
surfaces 96
CCD 536
cell membranes 511
cellular effects 525
ceramic inlay 130
chemical pumping 33
chemokines 530
chemo-mechanical disinfections 253
chlorhexidine 253, 408
chromogenic bacteria 409
chronic
apical parodontitis 288
periodontitis 341
classification of Periodontal Diseases 341
CO_2 Laser 1, 52, 54, 122, 198, 200, 204, 254, 390,75, 286, 315, 318, 324, 354
coagulative capacity 457
coefficient of absorption 101, 102
coherent light 2, 5, 7, 8, 9, 255, 534
collimated light 2
combined mechanical - manual preparation 295
combined periodontal - endodontic pathology 288
community index of treatment needs 367
compact-filled 142
composite resin 95, 96
compressive strength 156
concrement 338
removal 353
constructive protective arrangements 69
conventional pulp capping 316
conversion 34
rate 157
coronal- apical method 291, 292
corrective phase 343
cortico-cancelleous transplants 494
corticosteroids 318
corynebacteria 250
cracking 212
Crigler-Najjar Syndrome 411
crown down pressureless technique 293
cryosurgery 453
crytoplasmic membrane 259
cutting speed 461
cytokines 530
cytoplasm 523
cytoxic effects 503

D

decontamination 242
delivery system 76, 169, 286, 344, 346, 355, 458, 459
demineralization 161, 193, 200, 202, 219, 227
densified
composites 142, 143
composites - compact filled 145
density of the dentinal tubules 245, 377
dental cuticle 335
dentin hypersensitivity 377
dentinal
receptor mechanism 380
tubules 242, 243
diabetes 340
diffraction 5
dihematoporphyrin ester 511
dimethacrylate TEGDMA 142, 155
diode laser 11, 44, 274, 302, 306, 347, 348, 387, 389, 423, 533
direct pulp capping 315
discoloration 408
in the formative phase 409
in the post-formative phase 412
divergence 19
DNA 503
synthesis 524
doping ions 31
doppler
broadening 9
shift 9
double flared technique 293
down syndrome 340
dye 511
laser 25
dysplasia of the dentin 411

E

E. coli 261, 262, 265
E. faecalis 250, 251, 265, 276, 512
early invasive carcinoma 485
early lesion 340
edodontic problems 241
EDTA 253, 295
eikenella corrodens 338
elctrotomy 453
electric pumping 33
electron probe microanalysis 395
electronic
orbits 8
pumping 33
elektromagnetic
spectrum 4
wave 3
elliptic trajectories 8
employing birefringence 36
enamel 164, 200
resistance 196
endodontic treatment 241
endotoxins 338
energy
absorbing initiator 225
dentistry 209

enterococcus faecalis 247,249, 251, 507
epulides 472
Er,Cr:YSGG Laser 52,76, 86, 92, 94, 198, 275, 278, 363
Er: YAG Laser 76, 86, 92, 94, 197, 198, 232, 254, 265, 275, 276, 277,278, 279, 318, 355, 356, 357, 358, 359, 360, 361, 362, 372, 373, 389
erythroblastosis fetalis 411
erythroplakia 485
established lesion 340
esthetic reconstructions 134
excimer laser 1,38, 39, 76
excision 468
excite state 11
exotoxins 338
exposed pulps 315
extension for prevention 139
external source 13
extra-ordinary beams 36
extrinsic discolorations 408

F

F. nucleatum 512
facial pain 528
feed back system 362
fiber-reinforced composites 147
fibroblasts 306, 460, 525
fibromas 480
filler phase 142
fine
  compact filled composites 145
  midway - filled composites 143
finite lements 284
fissure
  sealants 195
  sealing 81, 127, 141
flash lamp 11
fluence 208
fluorescent media 9
fluoride 164, 195
  treatment 216, 222, 229,
  uptake 226
fluorosis 409
formaldehyde 382, 384
fourier limitations 5
four-level system 14
free
  radicals 417
  running laser systems 111
Frenotomy 492
frequency 4, 5, 34,
  -doubled alexandrite laser 363
front restoration 134
FTIR spectroscopy 231
fusing 388
fusobacterium nucleatum 250, 338, 510, 511,521

G

GaAIAs Laser 387, 389
GaAs 43
gamma - rays 4
gangrenous pulpitis 288
gases 29
gaussian
  beam profile 5, 19, 20, 34, 107
  bell curve 18
  pulse 7
gingiva - index 366
gingival pocket 336, 338
gingivitis- periodontitis- gingival recession 333, 341
glass ionomer cement 384
glucocorticoids 384
gold inlay 129
gram
  -negative bacteria 254,258
  -positive bacteria 260
  -positive cocci 248
granuloma interna or pink spot 412
green staining 409
grey discolorations 440
ground state 506
gutta-percha 299

H

H_2O_2 253
hard tissue treatment 77
heat 78
heat capacity 197
heisenbergs uncertainty 7
helium-neon laser 40, 510
hemangiomas 474
hemolytical anemia 411
hemophilia 457
hemorrhagic discolorations 412
HeNe laser 42,386
high energy state 503
histological specimen 468
HIV infection 340
Ho: YAG Laser 51, 75, 123, 232, 276, 286, 387, 389
holmium-thulmium laser 51
home-bleaching procedures 421
hydrodynamic mechanism 378
hydrogen peroxide 407, 417, 420
hydroxyapatite crystals 162, 193, 200, 256
hydroxyl radicals 506
hygiene index 366
hypersensitive dental necks 362

I

impact pumping 33
implant/bone interface 493
infection 242
inflammation 242, 365
inhibitors 306
initial
  lesion 340
  therapy 343
international safety standard 60
interstitial thearapy 474
intertubular dentin 96
intrinsic discolorations 408, 409
inversible pulpitis 514
ion laser 1
irradiation parameters 196
irrigation 243

K

KCP 80,81
KTP laser 234, 286, 421, 423, 429

L

L. casei 511
labeling 67

lactic acid 193
lactobacillus 193, 251
LAF Laser activated fluorides 164
laser
  Acupuncture 387
  analgesia 528
  beam 5, 23, 34, 205
  classes 60
  curing 158
  doppler flowmetry 321
  fluorescence 362
  medium 13, 29
  parameters 210
  polymerisation 153
  prepared cavities 90
  protective eyewear 67
  resonator 18
  safety officer 69, 71
  treatment 296
  wavelengths 204
laser-activated
  fluoride 162
  bleaching 407
  cavity preparation 75
  pulp capping 318
laser-supported root canal
    sterilization 254
laser-tissue interaction 196
lateral canals 242
layer requirements 171
leakage 95
LED 153, 154, 534, 535, 536
lethal photosensitization 503
leukoplakias 484
level
  schemes 15
  systems of laser 16
lichen ruber planus 340, 488
light
  conductor 368
  interactions 196
  transmission 256
linewidths of emissions 10
lipoproteins 259
liquid laser media 30
long-term failure 288
low
  level laser therapy 386, 521, 535
low
  -fluence argon laser 163
lucerin TPO 167
lymphokines 341

M

macro anatomy 242
manual preparation 291
margin 93
maryland bridge 132
mast cells 525
matrix 306
matt-finished instruments 461
maximum permissible
    exosure values 59
maxwells equations 3
measurement by X-ray 294
mechanical preparation 243
melt zone 201
metalloproteinases 306
methylene blue 507, 508, 511
micro
  anatomy 243
  -abrasion 413
  -circulation 388
  -fine composites 142
  -leakage 96
  -porosities 221
  -sive or micropore system 202
  -spaces 164
middle output power lasers 386
midway
  compact-filled composite 144
  filled 142, 144
mineral
  crystals 193
  trioxide aggregate (MTA) 317
minimal invasive 140
minimally invasive techniques 139
mirrors 13, 21
miscellaneus composites 142, 146,
    148
mitochondria 523
mobility of the teeth 365
modulation of nerve impulses 380
monochromatic 4, 5
monofluorophosphate 383
mono-infection 247
MPE-values 59
mucocele / ranula 488
murein layer 259
myofibroblasts 526

N

NADH 523
NaOCl 253, 295
Nd:YAP laser 272, 286
Nd:YAG-laser 49,50,75, 122, 196,
    197, 225, 254, 261, 265, 268, 269,
    270, 271, 272, 273, 276, 277, 281,
    286, 318, 349, 350, 351, 352, 353,
    354, 387
neck pain 528
necrotizing periodontal
    diseases 342
neisseria gonorrhea 341
neonlinear polarization 37
neural tissues 528

O

occlusal trauma 340
occlusion 388
ochronosis 411
olive oil 382
opium 382
optical
  interactions 196
  characteristics 255
  fibers 45
  materials 4
  oscillator 13
  properties 196
    pump source 11, 33
orbitals 8
osteoblast 302
osteoclasts 341
oxalate 385

P

P. acnes 250
P. gingivalis 250, 512

pain
level 378, 455
relief 528
papillary bleeding index 367
papillomas 483
papillon lefévre syndrome 340
partly sclerosed canals 288
pemphigus vulgaris 340
penetration 521
depth of chemical disinfectants 254
peptostreptococcus micros 338
perfusion indices 393
perhydroxyl radical 416
periapical
abscess 288
tissues 242
peri-implantitis 493, 513
periodontal
diseases 333
probes 365
therapy 333
periodontitis 334, 511
in combination with
endodontic lesions 342
periodontopathogenic plaque bacteria 338
peritubular dentin 96, 381
peroxide 416, 506
peventive effect 163
pH value 193, 222
phase changes 164
phenyl-propanedione 167
photo effect 4
photoactive disinfection 503
photochemical
ablation 100
interaction 39
photodynamic therapy 505
photo-inhibitors 142
photon
density 6
energy Eph 4, 6
flux 6
photopolymerization 139, 150, 151, 169
by UV light 150
stresses 158
photosensitizer 503, 507, 510
photosensitizing effect 511
placebo effect 386
plancks law of radiation 8
plancks quantum 6
plaque 193, 334, 335, 408
accumulations 365
retention 340
plaque-Index 366
plasma
arc devices 153
-mediated ablation 100, 114
pocket depth 365
polarization 5, 524
polished enamel 213
polymer chains 159
polymerisation reaction 149, 151
polymorphonuclear granulocytes 341
population inversion 17
porphyrin derivates 505
porphyromonas 507
gingivalis 338, 348, 511, 512
potassium nitrate 383
pre- eruption trauma 410
precancerous lesions 485
precipitates 166
pregnancy 472
preparation
lasers 80
techniques 241
preprosthetic surgery 491
prevention resin restoration 141
prevotella 507
intermedia 268, 348
primary hazards 64
propionibacterium endodontalis 250
prostaglandin E2 525
protective
eyewear 67
measures 67
pseudomonas 247
pulp
capping 315
necrosis 288
pulpal
analgesia 388
chamber temperature 220
defense mechanism 380
health 95
pulpal
histology 219
pressure 379
temperature 356
tolerance 388
pulpotomy 315, 323
pulse
duration 101, 205, 206, 207
energy 101
number 207
pulsed laser 204
operation 23
pulse-width 214
pumping by accelaration 33
pumping methods 33
purulent pulpitis 288

Q

Q-switched operation 23

R

radial conduction 205
radiographic findings 365
raman spectra 165
rare earths 31
reaction of the bacteria to laser light 258
reaktive oxygen species 505, 506
re-attachment 494
recall 343, 370
recession 334
reflecting surfaces 69
reflectivity 101, 102, 108
refraction 7
refractive index 197
remineralization 161
remission parameters 58
re-precipitation 202
resin
monomers 96
tags 96
resins 384
resonators 4, 13, 21,
respiratory chain 523
restorations 365

root canal
  filling 298
  preparation 290
root canal
  shaping 278
  system 242
root caries 223
rotating instruments 78
roughness 94
rubber dam 124
ruby laser 46, 75, 196

S

S. mutans 511, 512
S. sanguis 511
S. sobrinus 511
safety
  education 57
  in laser treatment 57, 284
  parameters 210, 219, 227
saliva 193
scaling 360
scalpel 452
scar
  formation 451
  tissue 316
scattering 197
  anisotropy 197
  coefficient 197
schawlow-townes formula 16
sclerosis 381
sealing 161, 390
secondary
  dentin 243, 381
  hazards 64
  odontoblasts 316
self-pase modulation 27
SEM 211, 227, 232 391
semiconductor diode laser 1, 31, 41, 535
sensitivity 393
sensitizing dye 505
shrinkage 158
silver
  iodide 382
  nitrate 382
singlet oxygen 503, 506
sintering process 201
slab laser 32
smartbleach 423
smear layer 353
sodium carbonate 382
Sodium Citrate-Pluronic-Gel 384
sodium fluoride 217, 382, 383
sodium pump mechanism 388
soft
  laser 44
  tissue surgery 360
  -laser-effects 344, 347
solid-state laser 1, 30,
sources of light 8, 9
spatial
  beam profile 101
  beam profile (TEM Modes) 105
  coherence 5
specific
  frequency 23
  heat capacity 101, 102
spectral coefficient of absorption 57
spectrum 3
spirochetes 338
spontaneous emission 9, 11, 12,
stain penetration 391
staining of pulpal ethiology 412
standing waves 21
stannous Fluoride 384, 390
step
  back technique 291
  down technique 292
sterility 450, 454
stimulated emission 1, 11
stimulating properties 306
stimulation 12, 302
streptococci sanguis 268
streptococcus 193, 251
  gordonii 252
  mutans 249, 252, 507
  sanguis 249, 250
strontium 382
structural changes 213
subgingival plaque 338
substitution 200
sulcus epithelium 494
superoxide ions 506
surface morphology 211, 221, 228
systemic diseases 342, 411, 451

T

tar 408
target cells 503, 509
tartar 338, 408
TCP 165
temperatur
  measurements 391
  rise 201, 206, 207, 284
temporal beam profile 5, 101, 104
tertacycline staining 410
tertiary dentin 316
tetracycline 440
thermal
  ablation 100
  damage 284
  damage zones 462
  decomposition 200
  diffusivity 102, 197
  injury 388, 461
  modification 210
  relaxation time 206
  side effect 389
  treatment 200
threshold condition 14
tightness 93
tin fluoride 409
TiO_2 426
titanum-sapphire laser 47
t-lymphocytes 341
TMJ disorder 528
tobacco consumption 340
tolonium
  chloride 507, 508, 514
  chloride dye 511
toluidine 505
  blue 507
tomes fibers 377
total etch technique 317
toxins 242
traditional composites 147
transition metals 31
transversal waves 3, 20
treatment scheme 369
treponema pallidum 341

trigger point 528
triplet state 503, 506

tubular
  diameters 378
tubular network 255
tubules 244, 246, 256
tumor necrosis factor-a 525
tumors 503
two photon absorbtion 4

U

ultrafine
  compact-filles composites 145
  midway-filled 144
ultra-short laser pulses 25, 114, 117,121
ultraviolet light 3
UV
  curing 139
  light 39,232

vaso-dilation 525
VCL Visible Light Curing 154, 156, 161,
veneer 128

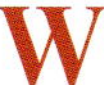

water
  induced ablation 88
  spray 86
wave
  equation 7
  vektor k 5
  -guides 4
  -length 4, 5, 6, 101, 205, 208
  -number 4, 6
  -related properties 6
worst-case hazard 60
wound
  closure 526
  healing 525, 526,

Xe-Cl excimer laser 254
x-ray
  Laser 1
  photoelectron spectroscopy 394

Yb:YAG 50
yellow discolorations 435
ytterbium laser 49

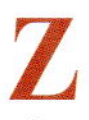

zinc
  -chloride 382
  -oxide-eugenol 325